D1226376

Encyclopedia of Medical History

Encyclopedia of Medical History

Roderick E. McGrew

with the collaboration of

Margaret P. McGrew

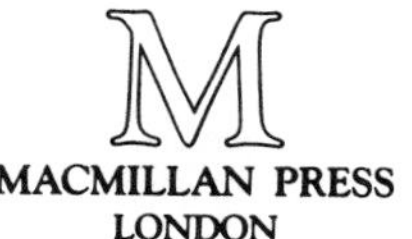

MACMILLAN PRESS
LONDON

Macmillan Reference Books

First published in the United Kingdom 1985 by
THE MACMILLAN PRESS LTD
London and Basingstoke

Associated companies in Auckland, Delhi, Dublin, Gaborone, Hamburg, Harare, Hong Kong, Johannesburg, Kuala Lumpur, Lagos, Manzini, Melbourne, Mexico City, Nairobi, New York, Singapore, Tokyo.

ISBN 0-333-28802-5

British Library Cataloguing in Publication Data

McGrew, Roderick E.
Encyclopedia of medical history.
1. Medicine – Dictionaries
I. Title
610'.3'21 R125

ISBN 0-333-28802-5

Printed in the United States of America

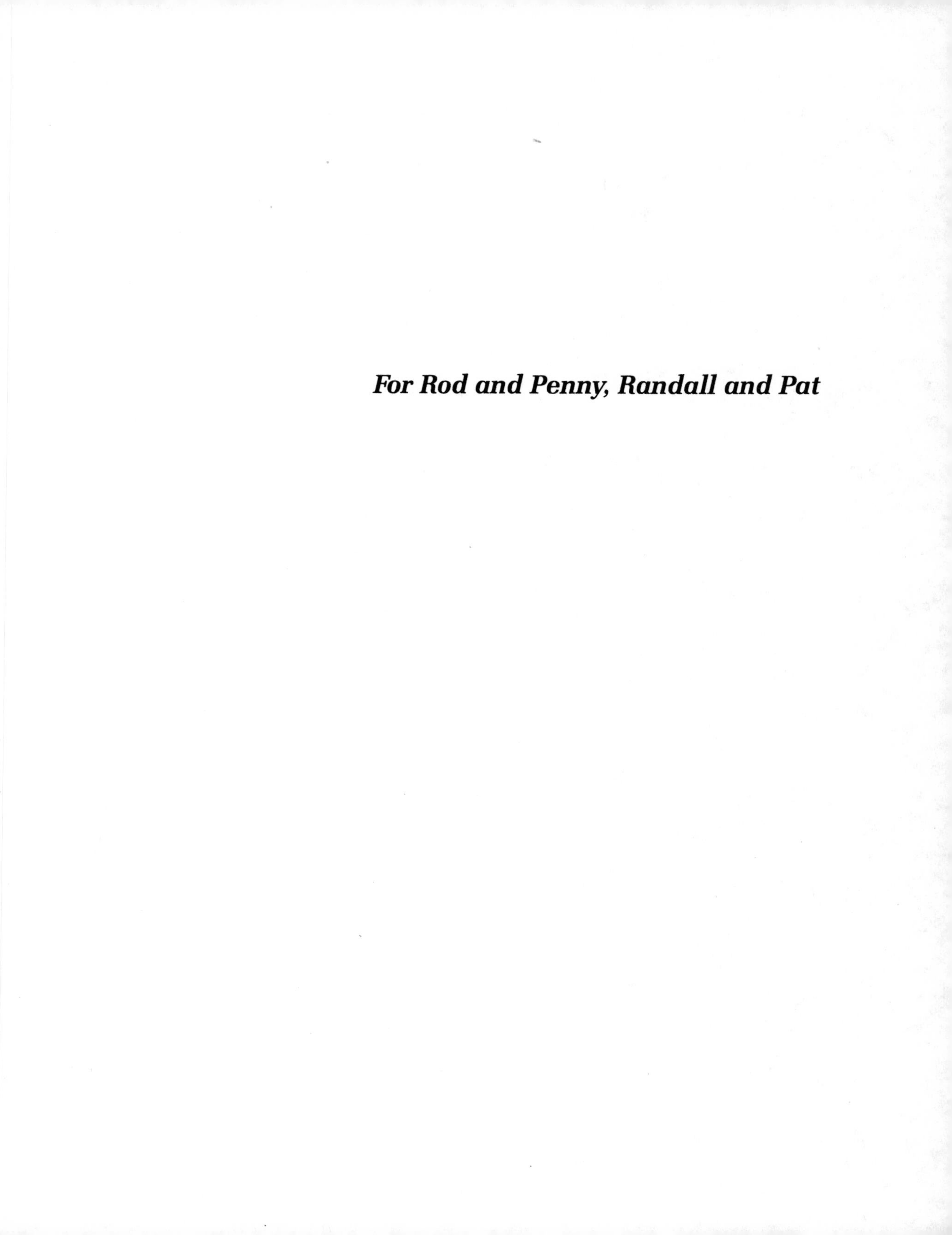

For Rod and Penny, Randall and Pat

Contents

About the Author

Roderick E. McGrew has been a Professor of History at Temple University since 1967. He has organized courses on disease and history for the graduate and undergraduate programs. Professor McGrew, the author of *Russia and the Cholera: 1823–1832*, received his Ph.D. from the University of Minnesota and lives in Princeton, N.J.

Preface

The purpose of the *Encyclopedia of Medical History* is to provide an easily accessible historical treatment of important medical topics which will engage the general reader while providing students of both history and medicine with a fund of information complementary to their specialties. Each entry has been conceived as an independent essay covering the stated topic chronologically. There are no summary or definitional entries as such, and there are no biographical articles. Individuals' contributions to medical science are discussed as part of the evolution of techniques, ideas, or institutions. The index provides a guide with page references and vital dates for the more important personages mentioned.

Each essay has a list of additional readings appended. The number of titles cited varies from subject to subject with the prime variable being the amount of historical work which has been done on the subject. At the very least the reader will find these recommendations useful for acquiring more detailed information than the entry can provide. Where there has been substantial recent historical writing or where the subject may be controversial, the reading lists are more extensive and detailed, including references to monographic literature and specialized articles. Even so, the additional readings are intended only as a supplement; they are in no sense a systematic guide to bibliography or research. Readers who require detailed current bibliographical data, including materials not available in English, may consult the U.S. Army Medical Library, *Index Catalogue*, ser. 1, 2, 3, 4, 1880–1948; the U.S. Department of Health, Education, and Welfare: National Library of Medicine, *Bibliography of the History of Medicine*, 1965–1984; and the Wellcome Institute of the History of Medicine, *Current Work in the History of Medicine: An International Bibliography,* quarterly, London, 1954–1984. In addition, reviews and review essays in the *Bulletin of the History of Medicine,* the *Journal of the History of Medicine and Allied Sciences,* and *Medical History,* to mention only three leading and easily accessible journals, provide discriminating judgments and are invaluable for following the current evolution of the field.

The author wishes to acknowledge the assistance he has received in preparing this book. Margaret P. McGrew, the author's collaborator, deserves the most particular recognition. Quite literally, without her help, the book could not have been done. Robert Rosenbaum, formerly of McGraw-Hill, proposed the idea for the book and was most helpful and supportive during the early writing phase. Thomas Quinn, senior editor at McGraw-Hill, has been enthusiastic and understanding while guiding the book through its later stages. Susan Killikelly has been an efficient, responsible, and cooperative editing supervisor. Dr. Nancy Frieden, Prof. Terry Parssinen, and Robin Price made useful suggestions and shared their work on the development of the medical profession, drugs and drug abuse, and hydropathy and irregular medicine. Especially warm recognition is owed to the administration and staff of the Wellcome Institute and Library for the History of Medicine, Euston Road, London. Unfailingly courteous, cooperative, and efficient, they gave every assistance during the 16 months the author and his collaborator worked in their collections. Temple University made it possible for the author to devote the academic year 1979–1980 to the project by granting him a leave of absence. The author accepts full responsibility for whatever errors of fact or judgment the book contains.

Princeton, New Jersey
March 1984

Encyclopedia of Medical History

Abortion

Abortion is the destruction or loss of a fetus or fertilized ovum before it is sufficiently developed to survive outside the uterus. In general, abortions are of two kinds: induced or spontaneous. Depending on the system of laws in a society, induced abortion may be legal or illegal, while in some societies even spontaneous abortion as a result of accident or neglect can result in punishment for the person held responsible, usually the mother.

There is no clear pattern in history concerning the morality or legality of induced abortions. Primitive peoples, faced with the need to limit population growth as a matter of survival, regularly practiced induced abortion. Over time, however, and as they advanced in civilization, those same peoples often would not permit abortions, and they eventually came to consider the practice immoral. The presumption is that an advancing society not only could support new lives but also needed them to continue growth. Many ancient cultures, including the Hittite, Sumerian, Assyrian, and Persian, punished any person found guilty of striking a pregnant woman and thereby causing her to abort. Self-induced abortion was punished even more severely. The Assyrian codes of about 1500 B.C., for example, decreed impaling as the punishment for such a crime.

Opinion was divided in the Greek world. Infanticide was regularly practiced by exposing newborns, particularly females, to the elements, and both Plato and Aristotle supported abortion for eugenic as well as demographic reasons. The Hippocratic oath, however, declared against aiding abortion, a position entirely consistent with the Hippocratic view that the physician's function is to assist nature and protect life.

Roman regulations appeared to be antiabortion. A law of A.D. 85 provided punishments for those who sold abortifacients rather than for the women who bought them, while the *Corpus Juris Civilis* (A.D. 533–534) of Justinian the Great prohibited abortion on the grounds that it endangered a mother's life while impinging on the father's rights and the rights of society. These laws, which held abortion socially harmful, did not, in fact, affect the majority of abortions which were carried out within the family. Jewish practice, which was derived from the Hebrew Old Testament and the Talmud, often ruled against abortion for any reason except a threat to the health or life of the mother. However, there was no specific prohibition against abortions.

Christian doctrine firmly opposed abortion, and the religious prohibitions became legal rules which were enforced throughout the Christian world. The emphasis fell on the rights of the unborn child, whose gift of life was believed to come from God rather than the biological father or mother. No attention was given to the rights of parents or society. Revulsion against abortion and the introduction of laws to prevent its practice have been characteristic of both premodern and modern western societies. Nevertheless, abortions have been regularly performed regardless of the law, though the illegal aspect vastly increased the risks of injury and death to the mother.

In the second half of the twentieth century, the conviction has grown that people should be free to decide whether they will have children or not. Family planning and the use of contraception were accepted long before abortion was, though not by the Roman Catholic church, and in the years since World War II, many legal barriers to abortion have been lowered. The reasons tend to be economic, demographic, and ethical, with the need to hold population growth stable leading the way. The claim that women should be free to control their own bodies has been vociferously put forth in advanced western societies, while the social costs of unwanted children have furnished powerful arguments in favor of abortion in poor and wealthy societies alike. Japan has permitted abortions since 1948, the Soviet Union legalized abortions in 1955, and the People's Republic of China turned to abortion as a means of population control in 1957. Great Britain relaxed its abortion laws in the 1960s, India has promoted legal abortion as well as sterilization for population control since 1971, and in 1973, the U.S. Supreme Court invalidated most state laws making abortion illegal. By the 1970s, 27 countries with 58 percent of the world's population had legalized abortion.

There have been serious second thoughts on the use of abortion as a means of population control. For example, in the Soviet Union, where abortion appears to have become more common than contraception, demographic and mortality studies indicate growing public health problems owing to the frequency of abortions. The problems are compounded by dietary deficiencies and alcoholism. An unexpectedly sharp increase in Soviet mortality rates in part correlates with the high frequency of abortions.

In western countries, most notably the United States, strong resistance on religious principles and on the basis of what is called the "right to life" has made abortion one of the most volatile issues in politics. Nor has the Catholic church abated its resistance to abortion or to contraceptives. Advocates of population control find themselves on the defensive, though their arguments gain strength as new and terrible famines are predicted for Africa as a consequence of too rapid population growth, while China's stringent birth control policies have begun to reduce the rate of population growth. Faced with dwindling resources, even the richest societies recognize the desirability of limiting population growth. But the question of legal abortion as a means to that or other social ends remains highly controversial.

Since abortion techniques are standard and reasonably safe under proper clinical control, medicine has had little to say in this debate, even though the physiological and psychological consequences of a fulfilled pregnancy or its termination may be severe. The issue has been left to politicians and legal experts, moralists, theologians, sociologists, and demographers. Abortion has been discussed in terms of moral absolutes and in an atmosphere of fevered confrontation rather than in a context of social health.

ADDITIONAL READINGS: Dan J. Callahan, *Abortion Law: Choice and Morality*, New York, 1978; Henry P. David (ed.), *Abortion Research: International Experience*, Lexington, Mass., Toronto, London, 1974; George Devereux, *A Study of Abortion in Primitive Societies*, London, 1960; David Granfield, *The Abortion Decision*, New York, 1969; Luke T. Lee, "A Brief Survey of the Abortion Laws of the Five Largest Countries," *Population Report*, ser. F, 1 (April 1973); James C. Mohr, *Abortion in America: The Origins and Evolution of National Policy, 1800–1900*, New York, 1978; John T. Noonan, *The Morality of Abortion: Legal and Historical Perspective*, Cambridge, Mass., 1970; Harold Rosen (ed.), *Abortion in America: Medical, Psychiatric, Legal, Anthropological and Religious Considerations*, Boston, 1967; Patricia Steinhoff and Milton Diamond, *Abortion Politics: The Hawaii Experience*, Honolulu, 1977.

See also: GYNECOLOGY.

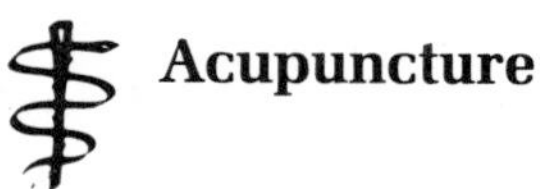

Acupuncture

Acupuncture is a medical technique that originated in China more than 2500 years ago. It is the most characteristic treatment of traditional Chinese medicine (q.v.) and has in recent years been enjoying a revival in China while attracting interest in the west. The procedure involves inserting fine metal needles one-half to several inches in length into the skin. The needles, which in some cases are driven in with great force and in others are inserted gently, are set at different depths, while the point of insertion is of particular importance. The oldest existing catalog of insertion points, the section called *"Ling shu"* in the *Huang di nei jing su wen (The Yellow Emperor's Classic of Internal Medicine)*, dates from about 100 B.C., but the points are named in an earlier collection called *He Yi's Cases* (ca. 540 B.C.). There were 360 such points in the second century. A total of 650 (some authorities say 800) loci have been identified to date. Once inserted, the needles are twirled and vibrated. A modern acupuncturist may use a battery-powered device to generate electrical stimulation.

The physiology of acupuncture rests on the Taoist doctrine that the life force (*Qi*), or energy, circulates through all the body's organs. Balance is maintained and health preserved by the interaction of two forms of energy, called yin and yang. Yin is described as feminine, dark, moist, and negative; yang, the masculine principle, is positive, dry, and bright. The acupuncture points are located on 14 lines or meridians which run the length of the body, and certain points on those meridians "control" certain physical conditions. All disease is the result of imbalance in the energy flow in the body. Pain or disease is the manifestation of imbalance, and acupuncture needles introduce a restorative and balancing *Qi*.

Though the connection between Taoism and acupuncture is clear, it is not known how acupuncture originated. It is speculated that the technique was developed in connection with studies of pain, and it may be that acupuncture is a practical application of the principle of referred pain, the tendency for a condition in one part of the body to generate pain in another. Certainly acupuncture was a specific which was supposed to relieve pain, and it was and is used for anesthetic purposes at childbirth and for some forms of surgery. Occasionally, acupuncture is used in combination with moxibustion (burning a pinch of mugwort or Chinese wormwood on the skin and rubbing the ash into the blister), and it is used more commonly with drug or herbal treatments. As an anesthetic, acupuncture has no aftereffects, and it is considered therapeutic for hay fever and headache, for certain types of blindness, and for arthritis, diarrhea, and hypertension. Some Chinese physicians believe that acupuncture can affect certain infectious diseases, sciatica, and rheumatism.

Many westerners who have had acupuncture in the People's Republic of China have been astounded by the results, while the technique has won followers in the United States as an alternative to scientific medicine. Medical researchers seeking to explain how acupuncture gives the good effect it does have noted that the insertion points correspond to places on the skin with low electrical resistance. This has led to the idea that acupuncture may influence the autonomic nervous system or stimulate the production of antibodies by the reticular endothelial system. Other suggestions include a neurosecretory effect resulting in a rise in cortisone production, and a direct influence on the pituitary gland. In China and Japan, medical researchers using advanced biochemical and physiological ideas are continuing to study what happens under acupuncture. In 1974, the National Institutes of Health agreed to a study of acupuncture as a possible management technique for chronic pain from cancer, arthritis, and neuralgia.

In the United States, though medical opinion is generally hostile, acupuncture is being used for pain relief and anesthesia. Though scientific medicine has not yet succeeded in discovering what acupuncture really does, the results are sufficiently impressive for the institutional establishment to want to have the treatment available. Acupuncture provides evidence that, while traditional explanations for the way procedures are supposed to work are often fanciful, the treatment itself may succeed at least as often as it fails. Valueless or dangerous treatments are less likely to survive than those which work, if only part of the time. Although western science cannot explain it, acupuncture has a long history of successful use.

ADDITIONAL READINGS: Robert W. Carrubba and John Z. Bowers, "The Western World's First Detailed Treatise on Acupuncture: William Ten Rhijne's *De acupunctura*," *Journal of the History of Medicine* 29 (October 1974): 371–397; Joseph Needham and Lu Gwei-Djen, "Notes on Chinese Medicine," in F. N. L. Poynter (ed.), *Medicine and Culture*, London, 1969, 255–312; Joseph R. Needham, *Science and Civilization in China*, 5 vols., Cambridge, 1974.

See also CHINESE MEDICINE.

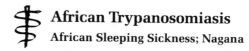

African Trypanosomiasis

African Sleeping Sickness; Nagana

Trypanosomiasis is a disease of great antiquity to which both animals and humans are susceptible. In prehistoric times, African trypanosomiasis played an important role in determining the distribution of ground-dwelling primates, including hominoids, by creating zones in which species susceptible to the disease could not exist. Later in the evolutionary process, other factors became important in determining whether susceptible species could exist with trypanosomiasis. These factors included birthrate, levels of health, and the ability to devise avoidance procedures to minimize contact with the disease. In historic times, African trypanosomiasis limited the areas open for cultural development and had a direct influence on the kinds and levels of civilization possible south of the Sahara. This influence has affected both native societies and colonizers.

Disease Characteristics The causal agents in African trypanosomiasis are flagellate protozoans called trypanosomes. There are two main types, which are morphologically indistinguishable but which produce diseases with different characteristics. Both are named for Sir David Bruce, who was instrumental in defining the trypanosome groups. The first identified trypanosome, and the one responsible for the sleeping sickness or "Negro lethargy" described in eighteenth- and nineteenth-century sources, is *Trypanosoma brucei gambiense*. This variety was isolated between 1901 and 1903 and is prevalent in central and western Africa. The second type, which was described and named in 1910, is *Trypanosoma brucei rhodesiense.* Its range is eastern Africa, including Zambia, Zimbabwe (Rhodesia), and Botswana. The vector for both trypanosomes is the tsetse fly (genus *Glossina*). The two major types of tsetse which communicate trypanosomiasis are *Glossina palpalis,* the primary vector for the Gambian trypanosome, and *Glossina morsitans,* which carries the Rhodesian variety. *G. palpalis* has a wide range, lives in brush near water, and feeds on the blood of reptiles, though humans are an acceptable substitute. *Glossina tuscipes* and *Glossina tachinoides,* which are found in eastern and central Africa and western Africa respectively, behave similarly and transmit *T. brucei gambiense. G. morsitans* is found in woodland savannahs and along watercourses in arid regions. They feed on game animals as well as humans. In addition to *G. morsitans, Glossina swynnertoni* and *Glossina pallidipes* transmit *T. brucei rhodesiense.* All are found in eastern Africa, though *G. morsitans* is in central Africa as well.

The primary reservoir for *T. brucei gambiense* is human beings, while wild animals act as reservoirs for Rhodesian trypanosomes. Wild animals are not susceptible to the Gambian trypanosome, but domestic animals are. Gambian trypanosomes are sensitive to arsenic compounds and can be treated, but the Rhodesian variety is resistant. Rhodesian trypanosomiasis is acute and often kills before the nervous system becomes involved. Gambian trypanosomiasis acts slowly, becomes chronic, and eventually involves the nervous system, producing the symptoms of sleeping sickness.

The transmission of African trypanosomiasis by the tsetse fly begins when the fly feeds on an infected host. The trypanosomes are ingested with blood and develop in the fly's lower gut. When the infected fly bites again, the trypanosomes are injected into the victim's skin with the fly's saliva. A mechanical transfer, where infective material is carried from a host to a susceptible victim without intermediate development in the fly, is possible, but it occurs very seldom. The most effective means of preventing infection is to break the infective chain by avoiding contact with flies and by excluding infected humans or animals from zones which are free of infection. Tsetse fly control by clearing undergrowth and direct attack with pesticides will give long-term protection.

Several environmental and cultural factors are important in the epidemiology of African trypanosomiasis. Drought will bring flies and people into proximity with one another around shrinking watercourses or pools. Conditions are then excellent for transmission, with a small tsetse population feeding nearly exclusively on humans. Wet conditions have an opposite effect, as tsetse spread outward from riverine centers and disperse over a wider area. Such dispersion reduces the possibility of human contact with infected flies. Apart from climatic factors, certain occupations maximize contact with flies and are dangerous. In areas where *G. palpalis* abounds and the infection threat is from the Gambian trypanosome, farmers who work rich valley soils with streams or rivers nearby are in constant danger. In woodland areas with *G. morsitans,* farmers who work on the edge of woods, or who clear brush for new fields, are in danger as are people who fish in dry river pools. Miners using canalized streams to wash dirt from ores are also exposed, as the periodic outbreaks of sleeping sickness in African mining regions show, and the same is true of road and railroad workers, especially bridge builders and timber cutters.

Clinical Symptoms The Gambian version of African trypanosomiasis develops very slowly. After initial exposure, 7 to 10 days pass before the first lesion appears in the area where the infection occurred. Swelling begins, with discoloration and a rash which finally sloughs off. This reaction is seen more often in Europeans than in Africans. Constitutional symptoms—chills and shivering or sweating—will appear within three weeks of the initial lesion, usually more swiftly in Europeans than in native Africans. The infected person suffers from headache, irritability, and insomnia, while swelling in the lymph nodes becomes generalized. Other conditions which may occur include male impotence, spontaneous abortion in females, tachycardia, and hypotension. Two months or more are required for the disease to enter the nervous system, and it is not uncommon for several years to elapse. Once the infection attacks the nerve centers, however, the prognosis becomes poor. The victim suffers from feverish attacks increasing in number, the lymph nodes shrink and harden, and the characteristic personality changes develop. Behavior becomes unfocused, insomnia is chronic, there is emotional instability, and there are periods of mania or confusion. The face takes on a vacant expression which has been called "silent grief," the tongue and hands are subject to tremors, the gait becomes uncertain, the head nods, speech is slurred, and terrible headaches develop. The headaches can drive a sufferer to suicide if he or she has energy enough. More commonly, death follows a growing somnolence and physical wasting.

Rhodesian sleeping sickness is far swifter and more violent. Most often, there are no initial symptoms, and the disease begins with a high fever and a dull headache. The fever continues, sometimes intermittently, while lassitude sets in and spreads. Rapid wasting, anemia, swelling limbs, heart involvement, tremor, and headache follow. Advanced cases show slow mental responses, slurred speech, and a flat, fishy stare. Death may come in the first few weeks from acute toxemia, and without treatment, death within nine months is virtually certain. In general there is no help for domestic animals which become infected.

Trypanosomes in Africa African trypanosomiasis appears to have existed long before there was any historical record, but since the affected African cultures produced no written tradition, evidence about the disease had to wait for non-African chroniclers. The first literary reference to sleeping sickness occurs in a passage written by the Arab world traveler, historian, and geographer of the fourteenth century, Al-Qualqueshaudî, or Ibn Khaldun. In speaking of the Malli kingdom and its rulers, he noted that the second sultan, Mârî Jâza, was "overtaken by the sleeping sickness (illat annawm) . . . a disease which frequently befalls the inhabitants of those countries, and especially their chieftains." In this case, Ibn Khaldun reported that the sultan was so overcome by sleep that he could hardly be wakened, that he was in this condition and growing progressively worse for two years, and that he died in A.H. 775 (A.D. 1373–1374).

Nagana, or animal trypanosomiasis, is suspected of playing an important role in the history of eastern Africa. The Arabs were interested in African trade and colonies, and while the Bantu people drove them out of the interior, they established a strong position on the southeast coast from which they maintained control over important trade routes. It is thought that the Arabs failed to expand their position because they were unable to rely on horses for war or transport where tsetse flies were prevalent. During the fifteenth century, the Portuguese rounded the Cape of Good Hope and challenged Arab control over trade in the Indian Ocean and the Persian Gulf. The struggle spilled onto the east coast of Africa in the early sixteenth century. The Portuguese reported heavy losses in their camel and horse herds, and they accused the Arabs of poisoning the wells. It is fairly certain, however, that the Portuguese problem was trypanosomiasis communicated by tsetse flies and not their Arab enemies. The Arabs had faced the same problem earlier, and until the second half of the nineteenth century, when steamboats and railroads revolutionized African travel, there was no choice in eastern or central Africa but to walk. Neither draft nor pack animals could survive in the tsetse regions, and this inability to keep and use large work animals may have been one important reason for the failure of central Africa to develop beyond the village stage. Human trypanosomiasis did not reach eastern and central Africa until the second half of the nineteenth century, and human bearers were used for transporting goods.

In the years after Ibn Khaldun, there is no connected account of sleeping sickness until the eighteenth century, when John Atkins, an English naval surgeon, discussed the disease in his book *The Naval Surgeon* (1734). Atkins visited the Guinea coast in 1721, where he made the acquaintance of the "sleeping distemper." He found the condition to be prevalent among the natives, to appear more frequently among the young than among the old, and to be extremely dangerous. Those few who did not die, he reported, "lose the little reason they have and turn idiots." A similar account appeared in 1794, which added the information that not only was the "Negro lethargy" widespread but slave dealers had learned to identify enlarged glands that indicated exposure to it and would refuse to take any slave showing that symptom. African slaves carried to the Americas who were captured in the interior often developed these symptoms on the voyage west or in the new slave quarters. Reports of the time which mention slaves wasting away from grief or homesickness may be describing people in the later stages of sleeping sickness. Slave masters whipped these unfortunates to arouse them or "take their minds from their troubles" and so hastened their inevitable deaths. The value of a slave dropped precipitously when sleeping sickness was suspected.

During the nineteenth century, both the European awareness of sleeping sickness and the incidence of the disease expanded. These developments were related. In 1840, Robert Clarke described what he called "narcotic dropsy" in Sierra Leone, commenting that the disease appeared to be more prevalent in the interior than it was on the coast. In 1876, a French naval surgeon named Coné produced an epidemiological survey for lower Senegal. He found sleeping sickness very widespread, leaving villages abandoned and empty or dilapidated and run-down. Reports from the Congo also described a spreading incidence of sleeping sickness. The disease was endemic as far up the river as Stanley's Pool, and increased trade on the river, especially after the introduction of steamboats in 1876, spread it more rapidly.

Henry Morton Stanley, the journalist and adventurer-explorer who "found" Dr. Livingstone, later became economic development chief for Belgium's King Leopold II. His undoubted success in developing the Congo as an avenue of commerce contributed directly to the rapid spread of sleeping sickness into central and eastern districts. Missionary reports cataloged the spread of the disease in terms of emptied villages and depleted missions. The natives brought their sick to the mission stations to be cured, thus infecting previously uninfected zones. Fatalities soared, people died by the hundreds, and the condition continued to spread. It was estimated that 500,000 people died of sleeping sickness in the Congo alone between 1895 and 1905. Even if this estimate is greatly exaggerated, which does not appear to be the case, it is apparent that the number of deaths in the area was appalling. European-sponsored commerce and industry vastly enlarged the active areas of human trypanosome infestation as infected persons traveled freely, while tsetse flies were carried on the new vehicles, especially the river boats. Sleeping sickness thereby attained a dangerously high incidence throughout sub-Saharan Africa.

Understanding African Trypanosomiasis Consciousness of the connection between nagana (that is, trypanosomiasis in animals) and the tsetse fly developed during the settlement of the Transvaal by Dutch colonists escaping British domination in the Cape colony in the early nineteenth century. These "Voortrekkers" moved into tsetse country in the 1830s and immediately suffered heavy cattle losses. they soon connected their losses with fly attacks, but they also noticed that the flies tended to remain in well-defined locations. It was possible to plan routes which avoided fly-infested zones. As their experience broadened, the Dutch colonists developed other practical measures for protection. They herded their cattle in fly-free zones; as they learned that flies were daytime feeders, they crossed infested regions at night; they found that goats seemed to be immune to nagana, so they planted goat herds in areas with fly infestations; and they recognized an association between wild game and flies, which led them to shoot out game colonies in tsetse-infested areas. Finally, they began to destroy tsetse habitats by cutting and burning brush along watercourses and by intensive agriculture. In the course of the nineteenth century, while sleeping sickness ran wild through central Africa, in South Africa and what is now Zimbabwe, Dutch and English settlers found ways to cope with fly infestation which made agriculture possible. The measures which they developed from observation and experience were ultimately confirmed to be epidemiologically sound, and some of their practices were used later in scientifically based campaigns.

The growth of scientific knowledge concerning sleeping sickness began in the early nineteenth century, but substantial progress did not come until the early twentieth. The German entomologist, zoologist, and physician Dr. Christian R. Wilhelm Wiedemann named the tsetse fly *Glossina longipalis* in 1830. At the time he did so, the fly was little known to European entomologists. R. G. Cummings, hunter, explorer, and African adventurer extraordinaire, accepted the name *tsetse* from the Tswana people and popularized it in his book *Five Years of a Hunter's Life in the Far Interior of Africa* (1850). He speculated that the name reproduced the curious buzz of the fly's approach. Another English explorer and scientific curiosity seeker, Maj. Frank Vardan, investigated the effect of the tsetse's bite on horses. He sent specimens of the fly to a London entomologist, Dr. J. O. Westwood, who identified it as *G. morsitans*, and reported his findings to the London Zoological Society in 1850.

As the craze for African exploration and colonization mounted in the second half of the nineteenth century, the information on tsetse flies, nagana, and sleeping sickness multiplied. The famous medical missionary, Dr. David Livingstone, whose accounts of his 32 years of African explorations thrilled thousands of readers, described the fly whose "bite is certain death to the ox, horse, and dog." Livingstone imported camels and water buffalo in an attempt to find work animals to substitute for the susceptible species. Dr. Livingstone firmly believed that the tsetse fly carried a sort of poison which it communicated by its bite. He was also certain that game animals and human beings were immune. In his autobiography *Travels* (1857), Dr. Livingstone recorded how he exposed himself to biting flies, and the minor inflammation which followed. Modern authority takes this as further evidence that eastern Africa, where Livingstone was exploring, was free of sleeping sickness, though infested with nagana.

In 1894, Maj. (later Sir) David Bruce was ordered to Natal and Ubombo in what was then Zululand to carry out a scientific investigation of nagana. Bruce had just completed his successful work on Malta fever. During the period 1894–1895, Major Bruce found trypanosomes in the blood of cattle and proved that the tsetse fly was responsible for transmitting them. He showed that nagana and what was called tsetse fly disease were the same thing, and that the disease resulted from the transmission of a parasitic infection from infected animal reservoirs to healthy susceptible creatures. This disposed of the poison theory, and Bruce also proved that nearly all domestic animals, with the possible exception of goats, were susceptible. Finally, Bruce answered the question of where the infection lodged by identifying *T. brucei* in wild animals such as buffalo or antelope which remained perfectly healthy. Wild animals were "reservoir hosts" where uninfected tsetse flies acquired the infection which caused nagana when injected into susceptible domestic animals.

David Bruce revealed the basic facts concerning the transmission of animal trypanosomiasis, but this achievement, though of the first importance for agriculture and African economic development, left the increasingly pressing issue of sleeping sickness open. Human trypanosomiasis was spreading, thousands were dying, and there were high economic stakes as well. Africa was rich in natural products, there were vast areas for colonization, and commercial exploitation had just begun. In response, Belgium's King Leopold II subsidized an expedition from the Liverpool School of Tropical Medicine, while the British army, the colonial office, and the recently founded London School for Tropical Medicine embarked on a series of coordinated investigations.

A severe sleeping sickness epidemic in Uganda in 1901, which claimed more than 20,000 victims, spurred the demand for action. Sir Patrick Manson's First Sleeping Sickness Commission went out from the London School of Tropical Medicine to arrive in Mombasa in June 1902. This commission, whose senior member was 39-year-old Dr. Cuthbert Christy, included Dr. Carmichael Low and Count Aldo Castellani, a brilliant 25-year-old student in bacteriology at the London School. Castellani later became embroiled in a bitter controversy over priority in discovery with Sir David Bruce. This commission looked for the cause of sleeping sickness by studying the action of *Filaria pustans*, which was thought to play a role in elephantiasis. When the investigation failed, no alternative hypothesis emerged, and the commission broke up, though Castellani remained in Africa to pursue his research.

In the meantime, Robert Mitchell Forde, a hospital surgeon in Bathhurst, Gambia, in western Africa, and Dr. J. E. Dutton, who came to Africa from the Liverpool School of Tropical Medicine, isolated a trypanosome from the blood of an English shipmaster who was suffering with an episodic fever. It was Dutton who named it *T. gambiense*. In March 1903, Alexander Maxwell-Adams published a note suggesting that human trypanosomiasis took two forms, depending on where the infection was active. When the parasite circulated freely in the blood, a chronic, irregular feverish condition resulted; but when it established itself in brain tissue, lethargy and loss of function, that is, sleeping sickness, developed. C. J. Baker, a colonial office physician in Uganda, also found trypanosomes in a fever patient and wondered if the tsetse fly was responsible. On the other hand, in 1902, the team of investigators from the Liverpool School of Tropical Medicine working in Senegambia found only 7 out of 1000 blood samples in which trypanosomes were present. They made no connection with sleeping sickness.

Castellani, working at Entebbe in Uganda, had identified a streptococcus in postmortem examination of sleeping sickness victims which he thought was the causal agent. He also found and identified trypanosomes in the cerebral fluid of 5 out of 15 moribund sleeping sickness patients. When David Bruce arrived at Entebbe at the head of the Second Sleeping Sickness Commission in 1903, Castellani reported this result. Bruce, on the basis of his work with nagana, seized on the trypanosome, and working together, the two men identified trypanosomes in the spinal fluid of 70 percent of the sleeping sickness cases. No trypanosomes appeared in healthy natives, or in natives with other diseases. Bruce gave Castellani credit for finding the trypanosomes, but it was Bruce who recognized their significance and established the research which led to the proof that trypanosomes were the causal agent in sleeping sickness.

The Bruce commission attacked the problem of controlling sleeping sickness with the hypothesis that, as in nagana, the tsetse fly was the vector. Tsetse flies were common on the shores and islands of Lake Victoria, where sleeping sickness was also common. Case-incidence maps for the Kiva region were made, and missionaries were enlisted to organize fly-trapping teams among the villagers. There was an enthusiastic response. Four hundred sixty fly collections were made and mapped; the fly- and disease-incidence maps were compared and found to coincide. Experiments were organized in which flies that had fed on sleeping sickness patients were permitted to bite monkeys. The monkeys were subsequently found to have trypanosomes in their blood. No other fly, insect, or animal was found that performed the vector function.

Sleeping sickness was eradicated from the Lake Victoria vicinity by withdrawing the people from the areas where tsetse flies prevailed. Sick humans were acting as a reservoir. Two years later, when sleeping sickness appeared on the east shore of the lake where it had not been before, the trypanosome reservoirs were found in healthy wild game. The vectoring mechanisms were the same. Subsequently, additional trypanosomes were found, beginning with *T. brucei rhodesiense*, and today there are seven different varieties associated with tsetse flies, and two more which cause American trypanosomiasis. Several insects have been found to act as vectors in the American version.

Modern Treatment and Control Early experience with sleeping sickness led to the use of arsenic compounds, which were effective if applied in the first stages of the disease. Dr. Albert Schweitzer, who went to Lambaréné and established his hospital there in 1913, and Dr. Eugene Jamot, a French army physician who was posted to Chad in 1911 and went to Brazzaville in the Congo to fight sleeping sickness in 1916, epitomize the struggle. Dr. Schweitzer operated from his hospital center, to which the victims were brought. Dr. Jamot went in search of his cases. Both men relied on chemotherapy based on arsenic. The specifics were first atoxyl and later tryparsamide, which were used to kill the trypanosomes in the bloodstream. The treatment was successful against *T. brucei gambiense.* Modern treatment has expanded the chemical base, using suramine or pentamidine where there is no nervous system involvement and such powerful and highly toxic compounds as melasoprol in advanced cases. The first principle of successful treatment is to begin as early as possible. Modern chemotherapy has materially reduced the mortality rate for sleeping sickness, but cases in their late stages are still highly dangerous and offer a poor prognosis.

Control measures against African trypanosomiasis aim at controlling tsetse flies, eliminating disease reservoirs, and preventing contact with the flies. Intensive agriculture and game destruction has been effective, while direct attacks on the flies with insecticides (most recently DDT), extensive trapping programs, and the introduction of biological enemies have all been used successfully. Before World War II, these campaigns were administered by European colonial offices. As the

African nations have gained independence, the World Health Organization has supported the efforts of the new nations at disease control. The results have been mixed. African sleeping sickness has not been eliminated, nor can it be. Constant effort is necessary to maintain control. Some ground has been lost through political unrest and economic crises, which have depopulated agricultural zones and permitted the reestablishment of tsetse fly habitats and the danger is that these conditions will lead to the reestablishment of sleeping sickness at high levels. This disease has had far-reaching consequences for the history of Africa, and its potential for damage is such that the most serious attention must be given it in the future.

ADDITIONAL READINGS: D. Brothwell and A. T. Sanderson, "Trypanosomiasis in Prehistoric and Later Human Populations," in *Diseases in Antiquity*, Springfield, Ill., 1967; J. J. McKelvey, Jr., *Man Against Tsetse*, Ithaca, N.Y., 1973; H. Harold Scott, *A History of Tropical Medicine*, 2 vols., London, 1939, 1, 454–457.

Allergy

Allergies, or allergic reactions, are part of the body's immunological defenses and involve those biochemical processes which protect the system against environmental substances. When any antigen, or substance foreign to the body, enters or makes contact with it, a process is set in motion whereby antibodies capable of resisting the invasive substances are produced. When antigens and antibodies meet, an interaction results which releases pharmacologically active substances. When there is sensitivity to these substances, they produce muscle contractions, swellings, inflammation, coughing, sneezing, and other identifiable responses. Allergic response is either immediate or delayed and may be localized or systemic. The active substances released which cause allergic reactions include histamine (the most common), serotonin, and bradykinin. Antigens may be inhaled (bacteria, molds, pollen), ingested (food, drugs), injected (serums, vaccines, drugs), or touched (plant resins, cosmetics, dyes, salves).

Allergic reaction has probably been a constant throughout human existence, but its history concerns the recognition of the reaction and the identification of its various causes. Allergies are nonepidemic, highly individual conditions. They have had no demonstrable social or cultural effect, yet their study is one of the most important fields in modern medicine, as is the study of the immunological system to which they belong. At the same time, the ability to give people relief from their reactions to pollens, house dust, dogs, cats, or whatever the allergy-causing element may be has meant a more comfortable and efficient life for the susceptible, and in some cases, it has made life possible. Also, this study has greatly increased medicine's efficiency in dealing with wounds, burns, traumatic shock, and a variety of other occurrences which trigger allergic response.

Early medical works contain numerous references to reactions which might have been allergic but were not identified as such. One fairly common reference treats reactions to foods. In the fourth century B.C., the Hippocratic writings recorded the apparent anomaly that some foods, though healthy and nourishing for most people, made a few people sick. Cheese was such a food, and to explain the phenomenon involved, it was suggested that cheese contained a poison for a few. Why this was true, or what the substance might have been, was unknown. Lucretius, the Roman philosopher and naturalist of the first century B.C., suggested in his famous scientific poem "De rerum natura" that not all foods were beneficial in the same ways for all people and what was good for some might be poison for others. Galen, in the second century A.D., noted reactions to certain plants; but detailed descriptions of what could be plant allergies did not occur until the early modern period, though Aretaeus of Cappadocia, Galen's near contemporary, gives a credible description of bronchial asthma. The "rose cold," a condition of catarrh and asthma which some people suffered near blooming roses, was described by Leonardo Botallo in 1565, and in 1607 J. B. van Helmont recorded a case of bronchial asthma, calling attention to "spasmodic attacks of difficult breathing" with periods of freedom from these symptoms between attacks. The record, however, remains very thin; historians have found only 11 such descriptions before 1700.

Allergies gained importance in the nineteenth century as systematic observation, improved research technology, the advent of bacteriological studies, and the introduction of the concept of immunity produced the main outlines for defining allergic response. In 1819, John Bostock, a London physician, described a seasonal catarrhal nose infection which came to be known as "Bostock's summer catarrh." This was one of the first efforts systematically to classify one group of cases within the larger stock of catarrhal infections. Bostock's summer catarrh corresponds closely with the concept of hay fever, or pollenosis. John Elliotson gave a detailed account of this condition in 1831, including a patient's prescient suggestion that the condition was brought on by pollen. By 1851, Charles Blackley, another English scientist, and Morrill Wyman at Harvard University were working separately on research which proved Elliotson's surmise that grass and weed pollens were the irritants in hay fever. Their results were published in 1872 and 1873. Henry Salter, who was studying the causes of asthma in this same period, reached the conclusion that the causal mechanism in asthma and that in hay fever might well be identical, as he was able to ascribe asthma attacks to contact with hay, dogs, cats, horses, and cattle.

The nature of the allergic reaction was still unknown, though it was coming to be suspected. Dr. Wilhelm P. Dunbar, of Hamburg, who was familiar with Blackley's work, believed that a toxin was at work, and in 1903 he proved that the pollen reaction was not a mechanical irritation by inducing it by use of a saline or alcoholic extract of the pollen grains. Dunbar attempted to produce an antitoxin for hay fever allergy, which he called "pollatin." Put into a nasal spray, pollatin had no discernible curative effect, but it did bring on negative reactions in some patients. Dunbar ascribed the reactions to sensitivity to the spray's horse serum base. In 1902, Charles Richet, professor of physiology at Paris, published the results of his research on an antitoxin for the poisons produced by the jellyfish and the sea anemone. It was he who noted that, in laboratory tests, a substance which produced no discernible reaction when first administered would in subsequent applications bring on an increasing sensitivity to it in the organism. This idea began to be applied to human reactions, and in 1906 Dr. Clemens Pirquet of Vienna suggested the word "allergy" to denote hypersensitivity, or a capacity for reaction.

In 1910, Sir Henry Dale, who was then studying ergot of rye poisoning, identified a specific substance in the ergot which was to be called histamine. This substance caused "smooth" muscles to contract, produced a decline in blood pressure, and brought on most of the characteristics of the shock response which the substances known as Witte's peptone and Popielski's vasodilatin also generated. It was also noticed that a histamine injection produced reactions similar to the anaphylaxis which resulted when a protein was injected into a previously sensitized animal. The discovery remained at this point for nearly 16 years, until it was determined that there was histamine in vital organs in sufficient quantity to be of effect, and that, in fact, something comparable to histamine was released during the destruction of invading protein or would appear when cells were damaged. This substance appeared to produce the changes responsible for the symptoms of allergic reaction. Britain's Sir Thomas Lewis carried this assessment forward when he showed that injured cells do, in fact, manufacture histamine, thus accounting for sun, heat, or cold allergies; while an American, Dr. Charles F. Cole, discovered how to test for histamines. By 1924, William Duke, another American, was using the phrase "physical allergy" to describe skin reactions to heat and cold. The final demonstration that, in the anaphylactic reaction, histamine was released by the injured cells was made in 1932 by Wilhelm S. Feldberg in Berlin and by Carl Draystedt of Northwestern University. Once histamines were identified as active agents in the allergic reaction, attention turned to controlling their production, an achievement which was accomplished after World War II. The discovery of histamine and the way it worked completed an intellectual model for the mechanisms of allergic reaction, thus providing medicine with a new and important analytic tool, as well as a method for dealing with the myriad discomforts and occasional mortal danger of allergies.

ADDITIONAL READINGS: J. H. Parish, *The History of Immunization*, London, 1965; Sidney Raffal, *Immunity*, New York, 1961; M. Samter and H. I. Alexander (eds.), *Immunology Diseases*, New York, 1965; Warren T. Vaughn, *The Story of Allergy*, New York, 1941.

See also IMMUNOLOGY.

Anatomy

Anatomy is an ancient discipline concerned with the identification, description, and classification of body structures. Comparative anatomy treats similar structures in different species; gross anatomy explores major segments of bodies through dissection, observation, and comparison; the anatomy of fine structures requires advanced microscopal systems. Gross anatomy developed between 1500 and 1850. Since then, anatomical research has concentrated on fine structures, becoming an integral part of such specialized fields as histology, neurology, and embryology. In this respect, the history of anatomy has followed and joined with the history of physiology. General anatomy is also part of the history of pathology, surgery, and, in the early modern period, art.

Most cultures prior to the modern era gained anatomical knowledge by accident. In many cultures, religious views which mandated reverence for the body prevented systematic dissection and analysis of human remains. As a result, much of what was thought or known about human anatomy came from hunters, butchers, and priests, who dismembered animals and birds in the course of their work. Efforts to heal wounds, to repair broken limbs, and to assist women in childbirth provided some opportunities to learn directly about human body structure. Some practices which should have yielded anatomical information did not. The Egyptian custom of embalming the dead gave very little useful anatomical information because the evisceration was carried out through slits in the body rather than a substantial opening. Where the information seems better, as in Greek Hippocratic medicine, it would appear to have been acquired through clinical observation and some animal dissections.

Post-Hippocratic medicine in the Hellenistic and Roman worlds was different. There is clear evidence of anatomical studies, though prevailing humoral physiology blinded anatomists to what they saw. The Alexandrian medical school, which achieved its greatest eminence between 250 B.C. and 48 B.C., was particularly significant. It was the only center in the ancient world where human dissections were regularly performed for scientific reasons. The Alexandrian anatomists are also said to have practiced human vivisection on condemned criminals. The most important among the Alexandrians were Herophilus, a medical scholar trained in the Hippocratic tradition, who carried out dissections of the human skull, eye, brain, and liver, and Erasistratus of Chios, a contemporary of Herophilus in the early third century, who did similar work, though his interests were physiological rather than anatomical. Unfortunately, the Alexandrians' voluminous writings have been entirely lost. What is known about them comes from later medical writers who quote them or dispute them. The most comprehensive references are in the writings of Galen of Pergamum in the second century A.D.

Alexandrian medicine developed at a late stage in Greek culture, when, as it has been suggested, traditional religious ideas lost their vitality, skepticism abounded, and a marked dualism between body and soul could rationalize the former into meaningless matter. Alexandria was also far from Greece proper. Subsequently, the rise of Christianity and its acceptance in the fourth century as the official faith in the Roman empire reinforced the accepted prohibitions on human dissection. In this case, it was belief in the resurrection of the body which made the church a firm opponent of postmortem examination. Judaism and Islam took a similar stance. Jewish rabbis, Christian priests, and, after the seventh century, Moslem mullahs stood against the desecration of the human body. Thus the anatomical tradition transmitted in Galen's writings formed the foundation for physiology and medicine in Christian Europe and the Moslem world until the sixteenth century.

Modern anatomical studies using human subjects became possible only when the church relaxed its stand against autopsying the dead. Even before that came, however, practical needs, including wound care and forensic medicine, opened up possibilities for certain kinds of observation and allowed some anatomical probing. Some secular authorities were prepared to go much farther. Early in the thirteenth century, Emperor Frederick II, who founded the universities at Padua and Naples and fought bitterly with the papacy over the boundaries of monarchical authority, ruled that all physicians in his domain were to learn anatomy by studying the human body, and all physicians were required to produce documents showing they had had such training.

In fact, the rule was applied only in Frederick's holdings in Italy and Sicily. In the fourteenth century the papacy further relaxed its prohibitions on dissection, and the first documented necropsy took place at Padua in 1341. When the black death arrived in 1348, the papacy approved postmortems to find the cause of the plague, but it was not until 1537 that Pope Clement VII finally endorsed teaching anatomy by dissection.

The early anatomy demonstrations followed Galen and his Moslem synthesizers. They were public events at which a professor read out the Galenic text while a demonstrator pointed to the parts mentioned and a dissector did the cutting. So powerful was the force of tradition that contradictions between the texts and what the dissections revealed were commonly ignored. Even the greatest of the sixteenth-century anatomists, Andreas Vesalius, a professor at the University of Padua, at first hesitated to challenge what the authorities said on the basis of what he saw, or seemed to see. Consequently, his early work repeated the Galenic tradition. The tide was turning, however, with the aid of artists who had no commitment to or foundation in the works of established anatomical authorities. Leonardo da Vinci's anatomical drawings are remarkable for their perception and accuracy. They are also remarkable for the absence of any debt to the past. In this area, art served and supported science.

In 1543, Vesalius published his masterwork, *De fabrica corporis humani (Concerning the Composition of the Human Body)*. The richly illustrated text confronted the Galenic tradition squarely, giving precedence to observation over authority. The realization that many of Galen's proofs rested on observation of animals rather than humans helped to explain anomalies in Galen's treatment. In the end, Vesalius's greatest contribution was to establish anatomical study on a strong foundation of observed fact and demonstration. His work contains no startling revelations or great discoveries. Yet it marked a revolutionary change in method. Appeals to traditional authority lost validity, and the controversies which followed concerned accuracy and the techniques of observation rather than philosophy or literary scholarship.

Vesalius's work presented exact descriptions of the skeleton and muscles, the nervous system, blood vessels, and viscera. His followers worked out the details. The Vesalian anatomy spread rapidly. His student and successor as professor at Padua, Gabriel Fallopius, published a volume of anatomical observations in 1561 which clarified and corrected aspects of Vesalius's own work, while Ambroise Paré, the leading surgeon of the sixteenth century, used Vesalius as a reference for the anatomical section of his classic work on surgery, published in 1564. Paré translated large parts of Vesalius into French, thereby putting the Vesalian anatomy into the hands of practicing barber-surgeons.

By the end of the century, Vesalian anatomy had entered into the daily practice of surgery and medicine and had become the standard for anatomical studies throughout Europe. A new generation of anatomists, who began with an understanding of the skeleton and muscles, the viscera, and the central nervous system was firmly in control of the field, and detailed work on the components of the gross anatomy was beginning. Hieronymus Fabricius published a study on the veins in 1603 which contained the first accurate descriptions and representations of the venous valves. William Harvey was studying at Padua while this book was in preparation; it was he who provided the explanation of the purpose and function of the valves when he published his classic work on circulation of the blood (q.v.) in 1628. This was the first modern work in physiology; the anatomy came directly from the Vesalian school.

Anatomical discoveries which opened new fields for study multiplied in the seventeenth century. Gaspare Aselli of Padua described the lacteal vessels of the mesentery and correctly identified their function with carrying chyle from food. His work, which introduced color plates for the first time in anatomical studies, led to subsequent studies of the lymphatic system and the thoracic duct. The pancreatic duct was identified in 1644 at Padua, the submaxillary duct in 1656, and the parotid duct in 1659. By the late seventeenth century, anatomists had gained a substantial grasp of the accessory glandular structures of the digestive system, and it was possible by the end of the century for Franciscus Sylvius of Leyden to outline a chemical theory of digestion. There was also work on the general structure of the kidney, while Regnier de Graaf provided a detailed and accurate description of the reproductive system. The development of microscopy (q.v.) in the course of the seventeenth century also contributed to anatomical advance. Marcello Malpighi took the lead in using microscopic techniques systematically for anatomical purposes.

During the seventeenth and eighteenth centuries, surgery (q.v.) advanced in training and technique, and as it did so, anatomy became increasingly important to it. In the absence of anesthesias, surgeons did their work at high speed. A specialized knowledge of anatomy was essential. Under the influence of such men as John and William Hunter, Edinburgh's three Alexander Monros, Pierre Dionis, William Cheselden, and Antonio Scarpa, a practical anatomy for surgeons took shape which stressed a topographical approach to the body. Anatomical atlases were produced with special aids to memory which included triangles or quadrangles used to identify surgically significant areas.

In the late eighteenth and early nineteenth centuries, demonstration of human body structures by the dissection of cadavers had become accepted practice, and as medical study expanded and the formal demonstration was complemented by student dissection, the demand for subjects increased. The demand was hard to meet, especially where laws restricted the disposition of bodies, and was the case in England and Scotland. The illegal acquisition of cadavers led to scandals which involved anatomists and surgeons in body snatching and finally murder.

The most famous incident was the case of William Burke and William Hare, who murdered at least 16 persons in 1823 to supply Dr. Robert Knox's Edinburgh dissecting theater. Eventually apprehended, Burke was hanged, his skin was tanned and sold in strips, and his body was made the subject of a two-hour dissection demonstration by the well-known Edinburgh lecturer Dr. Alexander Monro. A riot in the street forced the authorities to let the public into the lecture, and 20,000 people filed through the theater. William Hare turned king's evidence and escaped prosecution. Dr. Robert Knox, who was not implicated in the murders, was sharply attacked for buying bodies. He was supported by other anatomists, who stressed the difficulties in finding subjects for dissection. Knox publicly defended what he had done and declared he would do it again. An angry mob burned his house, and he left Edinburgh with his career ruined.

In 1832, it became legal for custodians of a body to turn it over to a medical school. However, acquiring an adequate supply of cadavers remained a serious problem in the United Kingdom into the twentieth century.

By the middle of the nineteenth century, the subject matter of gross anatomy was firmly established, and it changed comparatively little over the ensuing 130 years. Research scientists working in anatomy turned to fine structures and issues which involved functions and growth. These problems were increasingly physiological and required dynamic conceptions to frame hypotheses rather than the static descriptive portrayals of traditional dissecting room anatomy. This was particularly true of work on the structure of cells and mammalian reproduction. Studies of the nervous system (see Neurology) remained closer to traditional anatomy than either histology or embryology, however, due to the relatively large structures involved. There was also more traditional material with which to work. But the traditional analytical approach also confronted the need to explain nerve function, and this essentially physiological requirement lived uncomfortably with a static and descriptive method.

Modern anatomy has become progressively more specialized and complex. It is also entirely interdisciplinary and, in a classic sense, physiological (i.e., concerned with function). The indissoluble union of structure and function, together with the emphasis on dynamics and development, has left traditional descriptive anatomy to surgery, while the specialized disciplines which have developed as knowledge and research techniques advance suggest a holistic view of the human organism in its total environment. Traditional anatomy reached its fulfillment as a field of study at the middle of the nineteenth century. A structural-functional approach has superseded it.

ADDITIONAL READINGS: Jacques Barzun (ed.), *Burke and Hare: The Resurrection Men*, New York, 1979; Herbert Cole, *Things for the Surgeon: A History of the Body Snatchers*, London, 1964; J. H. Cole, *A History of Comparative Anatomy*, London, 1944; George W. Corner, *Anatomy: Clio Medica* III, New York, 1930; J. Kevorkian, *The Story of Dissection*, New York, 1959; Bernard Knight, *Discovering the Human Body: How Pioneers of Medicine Solved the Mysteries of the Body's Structure and Function*, New York, 1980; Charles Singer, *The Evolution of Anatomy*, London, 1925.

See also CIRCULATION OF THE BLOOD; MICROSCOPY; NEUROLOGY; PHYSIOLOGY; SURGERY.

Anesthesia

"Anesthesia" was the word suggested by Oliver Wendell Holmes in 1846 to designate the effects of ether, the volatile gas whose introduction into surgery began a revolution in medical practice. Anesthesia, as Holmes pointed out, "signifies insensibility—more particularly (as used by Linnaeus and Cullen) to objects of touch," and he thought a correct adjectival use would be to speak of an "anti-aesthetic agent." To speak of an "anaesthetic agent" was, to Holmes' mind, less certain. Today, "anesthetic" is a general noun referring to the many agents which produce cessation of feeling. Anesthesiology is a major medical discipline whose boundaries extend far beyond the act of administering an anesthetic, and the anesthesiologist is a highly trained medical specialist. The foundations for the anesthesiologist's specialty were laid in the nineteenth century; the systematization of the art was accomplished in the twentieth century.

Early Anesthetics Both pain and the effort to alleviate it have been constants in human history. There is a vast array of natural products which produce altered states of consciousness and which have been important for rituals as well as relaxation at different times and in different cultures. In some cases, as in ancient China and India and pre-Columbian America, it appears that natural anesthetics or soporifics were used to ease the pain of certain medical treatments, surgery included. Knowledge about such practices, however, is uncertain, and there is no established connection between them and the traditions which fostered rational or scientific medicine.

Most early traditions are far clearer in identifying substances known to affect consciousness than in connecting those substances with interdicting pain. Even so, in the first century A.D., the Greek physician and naturalist Dioscorides suggested that the root of the mandragora plant steeped in wine be given to patients before surgery, and it appears that mandragora was used in Asia both to induce confessions from criminals and to effect some relief from the agonies of torture. The Roman naturalist Pliny reported that mandragora, the "potion of the condemned," was used to reduce the pain of crucifixion, though the concoction reportedly offered to and refused by Christ was variously described as vinegar or wine, combined with gall, myrrh, or hyssop. There is evidence that cannabis was used by the Scythians of the Pontic steppe, by the Egyptians, and by the Arabs, though not to combat pain; records from the third century A.D. in China mention its use to render a physician's patients unconscious.

Alcohol was also widely used. In the form of wine or brandy, alcohol could numb responses, though its effects were superficial and often produced violent behavior. In the early Middle Ages, European physicians used a "soporific sponge," recipes for which have been found in materials as early as the ninth century. A fresh sponge was soaked with a concoction of opium, hyoscyamine, unripened blackberries, lettuce seed, juice of hemlock, mandragora, and ivy. The sponge was then sun-dried, and when it was needed, it was dipped in lukewarm water and applied to the patient's nose.

Opium was the most important single agent against pain before the discovery of ether. Opium poppy seeds have been found in Swiss lake dwellings of the fourth millennium B.C., and opium was in use in Egypt in the second millennium. Avicenna referred to it in the eleventh century as "the most powerful of stupefacients," and it was freely used in western medicine from the sixteenth to the twentieth century. Thomas Sydenham recommended it for treatment of strangulated bowel in the seventeenth century, and in the nineteenth century it was still recommended for that purpose and for amputations. When used for such surgical purposes, massive doses were given. In the nineteenth century, for a lithotomy (removal of bladder stone), a male adult would receive 8 to 10 grains.

Some mechanical measures reduced pain in some cases. Compression to cut off the blood supply produced numbness and, when applied to the carotid artery, unconsciousness. Such techniques were reported as part of various surgical practices. Efforts to develop a clamp or screw whose effect would be sufficient to ease the pain of amputation ran up against the problem that such an instrument was itself extremely painful and could do severe damage to the limb. Bleeding to excess began to be used for some anesthetic purposes in the eighteenth century. The second Alexander Monro of Edinburgh proposed the idea in 1777, and Philip Syng Physick of Philadelphia bled a patient into a state of collapse before manipulating a dislocated joint. The patient was entirely relaxed and seemed insensitive to pain. This method was also used to ease births in the early nineteenth century.

The techniques of induced somnambulism developed by the followers of Franz Anton Mesmer found some favor with surgeons. John Elliotson of Edinburgh and London experimented with the mesmeric trance as a surgical anesthesia, as did James Esdaile in India. Mesmerism, termed "hypnotism" by James Braid of Manchester, proved successful in operations. It was held useless for emergencies, however, and not all persons were equally susceptible. The chemical agents which came into use just after the mesmeric trance were considered more effective, more efficient, and far less exotic. The potential for hypnotism as an anesthetic has never been fully realized.

Chemistry and Anesthetic Gases Eighteenth-century chemistry provided the immediate antecedents for anesthesia, especially the work on combustion and gases which was crowned by the virtually simultaneous discovery of oxygen in 1771 by Joseph Priestley and Karl Wilhelm Scheele of Sweden. Priestley also identified carbonic acid gas and, in 1772, nitrous oxide. Valerius Cordus had synthesized ether from sulfuric acid and alcohol in the sixteenth century. He called his compound "sweet vitriol," and though he considered it to be medically useful, he did not identify its anesthetic properties. Paracelsus, who was Valerius Cordus's contemporary, mistakenly considered the compound to be stable, but he also recognized its sleep-inducing properties, and he remarked that it "quiets all suffering without any harm, and relieves all pain, and quenches all fevers, and prevents complications in all disease." For all its healing powers, however, sweet vitriol came into the eighteenth century known as ether or sulfuric ether, without recognition as an effective anesthetic.

The first gas recognized to have anesthetic powers was nitrous oxide, which was commonly supposed to be deadly. The young Humphry Davy inhaled nitrous oxide in 1795 with distinctly pleasant results. There was a certain giddiness, his muscles relaxed, and his hearing seemed more acute. It also made him want to laugh, and he dubbed the compound "laughing gas." In 1800 Davy published a monograph on nitrous oxide in which he reported that inhaling the gas gave him temporary relief from an inflamed gum, and he noted later on: "As nitrous oxide . . . appears capable of destroying physical pain, it may probably be used with advantage during surgical operations in which no great effusion of blood takes place."

Eighteen years later, Davy's student, Michael Faraday, who had pressed ahead with the study of gases, noted anesthetic effects from sulfuric ether and compared the results from inhaling it with those of inhaling nitrous oxide. Henry Hill Hickman, a contemporary of Faraday and Davy, went farther. Hickman was a member of both the Edinburgh and London royal colleges of surgeons, and in 1824 he carried out painless operations on animals using carbon dioxide as an anesthetic. He called the condition he induced "suspended animation," but he failed to arouse any interest in it in England or in France, though his memorandum to the French Academy of Sciences won the approval of Baron Dominique-Jean Larrey, the most famous surgeon of Napoleon's day, who was still greatly admired.

Although surgeons and the medical historians writing about them have deplored the sheer terror which surgery without anesthetics bred and have described at length the ghastly scenes accompanying any operation, there was no systematic search for effective anesthesia, and when one was finally discovered, its discovery was fortuitous. Both ether and nitrous oxide were familiar substances in the first half of the nineteenth century. Physicians in the United States used ether to treat pulmonary tuberculosis, while ordinary citizens attended public lectures by itinerant professors expounding on the new chemistry and the properties of gases. The demonstrations often included giving volunteers from the audience doses of ether or nitrous oxide, which brought on a kind of drunkenness and hilarity.

Laughing gas parties and ether frolics were popular entertainments, especially for medical students, and such familiarity with the gases inevitably led some medical students to consider them for more serious uses. It was just such entertainments which probably inspired William E. Clarke, a student of chemistry and medicine who lived in Rochester, New York, to promote a tooth extraction under ether in January 1842. The patient was a certain Miss Hobbie, the dentist was Dr. Elijah Pope, and the operation, the first of its kind on record, was entirely successful. Clarke made no effort to record the event; he seems to have considered it unimportant. Two months later, a young Georgia doctor, Crawford W. Long, who was trained at the University of Pennsylvania, suggested to a friend that he could remove a tumor from the friend's neck painlessly. Long appears to have been inspired by reports of a nitrous oxide demonstration, though he knew about ether from his partying days in medical school. His friend agreed, and the operation was performed painlessly and successfully on March 30, 1842. Ether was the anesthetic. Long made no attempt to publicize what he had done until 1849, three years after a public demonstration of ether's anesthetic properties had been made in Boston.

The First Anesthetic Ether as a surgical anesthetic was discovered in the United States. Several men, Long included, worked with the substance and could claim priority of discovery (or at least conception), but the man commonly regarded as the discoverer of anesthesia was a Boston dentist, William T. G. Morton. Another dentist, Horace Wells, thought of using nitrous oxide for extractions, and he had one of his own teeth pulled on December 11, 1844, without pain. Granted permission to show the procedure in Dr. John C. Warren's surgery class at Harvard, Wells botched the demonstration. Though the patient, a young boy, later said he had felt nothing, he cried out as if in pain, and Wells was hooted out of the auditorium. This failure started a long decline of fortunes, and Wells was arrested for throwing acid on pedestrians in New York. He killed himself on January 24, 1848.

T. G. Morton gained a resounding success using ether in the same forum where Wells failed. Morton first used ether as a local anesthetic when preparing a tooth for filling, but he came to consider its possibilities as a general anesthetic when he noted its numbing effect on adjacent tissues. Animal tests showed that inhaling sufficient ether to produce anesthesia was not fatal, so Morton tried the substance on himself and his assistants. The first trial failed as the assistants only became excited, but Morton then switched to sulfuric ether on the advice of Dr. Charles A. Jackson. This substance worked. On September 30, 1846, Morton extracted a tooth from a patient, Eben H. Frost, using the ether anesthetic. He arranged for his operation to be reported in the Boston *Journal* the following day, and he requested the opportunity to demonstrate his anesthetic in Dr. Warren's operating theater. An invitation was extended for October 16, 1846. Morton administered ether to the patient, Gilbert Abbot, from whom Warren removed a tumor located at the angle of the jaw. There was no outcry; the operation was painless and a success.

The use of ether as an anesthetic quickly spread to Europe. It was used in Paris on December 15, in London four days later, and on December 21, 1846, Robert Liston, one of the most famous London surgeons of his day, amputated a diseased thigh while the patient was insensible from ether. Anesthesia became accepted and acceptable. Childbirth excepted, medical opposition to its use was virtually nonexistent, though François Magendie, the great French physiologist, spoke out fiercely, if ineffectually, against it. Unlike antisepsis, which took nearly 50 years to gain acceptance, anesthesia carried all resistance before it.

No fatalities were reported in anesthesia's initial stages. This was fortuitous. The procedures used were crude, and anesthetics which produced insensibility were dangerous. Chloroform claimed its first recorded victim in 1848, and within 10 years, John Snow listed 50 chloroform fatalities. This was only the tip of the iceberg. The systematic development of anesthesiology into a specialized and highly professional field in the twentieth century was in large part a response to the dangers any person faced when anesthetized. Those dangers were neither understood nor appreciated in the early days of anesthetic practice, and even had they been, liberation from pain was so welcome an achievement that the attendant dangers could be disregarded.

The Expansion of Anesthesia Though ether was the first successful anesthetic, the long-term importance of nitrous oxide was greater. In the 1970s, though ether virtually had disappeared from the scene, nitrous oxide in some form or combination was used in well over half of all surgical interventions. In the nineteenth century, however, the first challenge to ether came from chloroform.

Discovered virtually simultaneously in 1831 by Samuel Guthrie in the United States, Eugene Soubeiran in France, and Justus von Liebig in Germany, chloroform waited until 1847 to be put to use. Dr. James Young Simpson, who held the chair of surgery in Edinburgh, experimented with ether in childbirth, but he wanted something better. A Liverpool chemist, David Waldie, recommended chloroform to him, and after trying it on himself and guests at a dinner party, Simpson introduced it into his obstetrical practice. Objections were raised immediately, though not on medical grounds. Preachers argued that God intended birth to be painful, while the laity found something immoral in reducing women to a state of unconsciousness at such a critical point in their lives. When it began to be said that the anesthetic brought on erotic fantasies, transforming birth into an imagined orgasm, new fears for the fate of the child, if not for the mother, were voiced.

The public reaction against chloroform anesthesia for childbirth died down when Queen Victoria chose to have chloroform administered to aid in the birth of her son, Prince Leopold, on April 7, 1853. Four years later she chose chloroform again for the birth of Princess Beatrice. In both cases, the anesthetic was administered by John Snow, the first physician to make a systematic study of anesthesiology. By the time of his death in 1858, Snow was England's leading specialist on anesthetics, and probably history's first anesthesiologist.

Once anesthetics had been identified and their value appreciated, there was a rush to find additional substances, to refine techniques for administration, and to develop more specialized applications. Charles Gabriel Pravaz invented the hypodermic syringe in 1853, and two years later Alexander Wood of Edinburgh used it for injecting narcotics. In 1847, Nikolai Ivanovich Pirigov, the man who became Russia's most famous medical figure and leading surgeon, described the rectal application of ether anesthetic, and he subsequently developed the technique. Marc Duprès published on the subject in the same year.

Sir Benjamin Richardson, a popular Victorian physician, devoted the early years of his career to identifying various anesthetic substances. He resurrected mandragora, acquired a root, prepared and tested it. There was an undoubted if unpredictable narcotic effect. In all, Richardson identified 14 anesthetic substances, but his most important contribution was to identify and promote extreme cold through rapid evaporation of volatile substances as a local anesthetic. In 1867, he introduced a successful ether spray which continued in use for many years.

Cocaine, a white powder refined from the leaves of the Peruvian coca plant, was found in 1860 by Albert Niemann, working in the Wöhler laboratory at Göttingen University. The Peruvian coca and its narcotic powers had been known in the west since the sixteenth century, but its characteristics had never been systematically explored before. Sigmund Freud, who thought cocaine would be useful in combating morphine addiction, brought the substance to the attention of his Vienna colleague, Carl Koller, an ophthalmologist interested in local anesthetics for eye surgery. Koller tested cocaine, found it effective, and had his findings presented in 1884 to the Congress of Ophthalmology, which met in Heidelberg. The substance was greeted with enthusiasm as the most important discovery for the field since Helmholtz invented the ophthalmoscope.

New materials and growing experience with the physiology of anesthesia brought further achievements. One of the most important was William Stewart Halsted's work on conduction anesthesia at Johns Hopkins. Halsted showed that by injecting local anesthetic drugs into the nerve areas controlling the area to be operated, almost any part of the body could be anesthetized. He used cocaine for the purpose, and, just a year after Koller's demonstration, he had established neuroregional anesthesia. He reported success with more than 1000 surgical cases. Halsted also became addicted to cocaine, and though he broke his habit, his experience pointed to the dangers inherent in this most effective anesthetic substance. Attempts to synthesize the anesthetic agent in cocaine were successful in the early twentieth century. Ernst Fourneau's stovaine was quickly followed in 1904 by Alfred Einhorn's procaine. This substance, best known under its trade name, Novocain, was introduced into medical and dental practice in 1905, and it remains a favorite local anesthetic.

In the modern era, intravenous administration of anesthetics began with the work of Pierre-Cyprien Oré, who published a monograph on the subject in 1875. Sir Christopher Wren, the great seventeenth-century English architect and scientist, is credited with administering the first successful intravenous anesthetic in 1659 when he injected a dog with opium in warm sack (sherry). The dog reportedly was stupefied. This venture, however, had no consequences for anesthesia until the nineteenth century. Oré's work developed very slowly, possibly owing to the material (chloral hydrate) he attempted to use. Following the discovery of the barbiturates early in the twentieth century, intravenous anesthetics gained ground to become firmly established with patients, surgeons, and anesthesiologists.

Conclusion During the twentieth century, the techniques of anesthesiology have become increasingly sophisticated, the instrumentation for administering anesthetics and monitoring patients' responses has been infinitely refined, and the substances used to achieve anesthetic effects have been multiplied again and again. These developments have come through the combined work of physiologists and chemists, pharmacologists, anesthetists, and physicians. Together with antiseptics, anesthetics have revolutionized surgery (q.v.). The conquest of pain during operations made the surgeon's work more certain—it was no longer necessary to control a struggling patient by force while attempting to manipulate the scalpel—and thousands of people came to accept surgery as routine treatment for conditions which in other times they would have endured rather than have repaired. The major achievement in this process was the discovery and implementation of the anesthetic principle itself at the midpoint of the nineteenth century. That discovery, once made, has been infinitely elaborated upon to provide safer and more effective ways of blocking pain and thereby vastly to enlarge the scope of modern medical treatment.

ADDITIONAL READINGS: T. E. Keys, *The History of Surgical Anesthesia*, rev. ed., New York, 1963; T. E. Keys and Albert Falconer (eds.), *Foundations of Anesthesiology*, 2 vols., Springfield, Ill., 1965; Victor Robinson, *Victory over Pain: A History of Anesthesia*, New York, 1946; W. Stanley Sykes, *Essays on the First Hundred Years of Anesthesia*, 3 vols. [vols. 1 and 2 are reprints of 1960 edition], Edinburgh, 1982; Owen Wangensteen and S. D. Wangensteen, *The Rise of Surgery: From Empiric Craft to Scientific Discipline*, Minneapolis, Minn., and Folkestone, Kent, 1978.

See also SURGERY.

Antibiotics

Antibiotics are chemical substances produced by microorganisms which destroy or prevent the growth of bacteria or other microorganisms. When such inhibiting or destructive action is taken against microorganisms pathogenic for man, the antibiotic can become important for therapeutic purposes, provided it is not harmful to the human system. Penicillin (q.v.), which was identified in 1928, was demonstrated to have systemic therapeutic powers in 1940, and by 1944 it had become important in treating gram-positive bacterial infections and wounds. Streptomycin, which was isolated in 1943, was the second antibiotic with demonstrated therapeutic effect, and it was increasingly employed after World War II against gram-negative bacteria and gram-positive bacteria which were resistant to penicillin and in the treatment of tuberculosis. Other antibiotics with therapeutic effect have subsequently been identified, including bacitracin, chloramphenicol, chlortetracycline, oxytetracycline, tetracycline, erythromycin, and aureomycin. Since 1940, the development of antibiotics has revolutionized disease therapy and vastly increased the expectation of successful treatment when diseases strike.

Though antibiotics are the product of the present medical scientific world, the tradition that nature (or God) provides certain natural products which will cure diseases is as old as humankind. One of the most persistently recommended substances is mold, which was commonly used in treating wounds or cuts, presumably to inhibit infection. In the Mayan Indian culture, for example, green corn was roasted and then left to produce a mold which was gathered and used as a specific for ulcer and intestinal infections. In Brazil, people gathered a dry, free-growing fungus called *puf* to apply to cuts or minor abrasions, while throughout the Ukraine and in central and southern Europe, mold was highly regarded for its wound-cleansing powers. A loaf of bread purposely left on a rafter in the peasant's house would become moldy, and when anyone was injured, it would be available to be sliced, made into a paste with water, and applied to the wound. Similar prescriptions appeared in formal medical treatises, with one seventeenth-century English work praising mold grown on a human skull. How the therapeutic effect of molds was discovered is entirely obscure, but the fact that such prescriptions are nearly universal is significant.

In 1852, a communication to Britain's leading medical journal, the *Lancet*, recorded an early systemic use of microorganisms for healing a specific condition, and there were numerous hints in papers published in the 1870s and 1880s that fungi were antibacterial. The first clear observation of antibacterial action, however, was made by Louis Pasteur, the French founder of bacteriology, and his associate, Joubert. In 1877, they described how rapidly anthrax bacilli multiplied in sterile urine, while the addition of "common bacteria" halted the development of anthrax. Pasteur was primarily interested in immunity reactions, but he came very near to stating the principle of bacterial antagonism. In 1885, an Italian scientist, Arnaldo Cantani, not only stated that principle but proposed a specific therapy based on it. Using a mixture of bacterial strains, he painted the throat of a tubercular child and reported that the bacteria in his mixture displaced tubercle bacilli while bringing about a decline in fever. This idea, though without any understanding of the biochemical elements involved, appeared again and again in the 1880s and 1890s. It was also paralleled by the idea that one infective pathogen would drive out another. An attack of erysipelas, for example, was reported to have desirable effects on patients with lupus or chronic syphilis, and in 1887, Rudolf Emmerich inoculated rabbits with streptococci from erysipelas as a counter to anthrax infection. The results were favorable. Well over half the rabbits survived the anthrax infection, which in untreated animals was commonly fatal.

Interest in the "natural antagonism" of one bacterial species for another fitted with the Darwinism prevalent in late-nineteenth-century thought which made the "struggle for existence" and "natural selection" household phrases. A French bacteriologist, Paul Vuillemin, coined the word "antibiosis" in 1889 to describe that condition in nature when "one creature destroys the life of another to preserve his own." Vuillemin compared the lion attacking its prey with the behavior of antagonistic bacteria, and he called the killer or active agent the "antibiote," while the victim was, logically enough, the "support." In 1889, Marshall Ward accepted the term "antibiosis" as the opposite of "symbiosis," and as a word descriptive of natural antagonism.

This rather crude pseudo-Darwinian idea remained to describe bacterial antagonism and to serve as the context for hundreds of research projects until 1928, when G. Papacostas and J. Gaté refined the idea. In a monograph published that year, which reviewed microbial associations and their applications in nature, the concept of antibiosis was accepted, but qualifiers were added. Antibiosis was "reciprocal" (i.e., both participants might be affected); "unilateral" (i.e., one affected the other while remaining unaffected itself); and "organic." The organic qualification was the most interesting, for that suggested an interference through metabolism with the rate of growth and reproduction of the affected bacteria.

The early work on bacterial antagonism had suggested finding parallel actions with the bactericidal actions of metals such as mercury or the arsenicals or of acids used as antiseptics. The bacteriostatic idea, which was contained in "organic" antibiosis, is the one which describes the action of most modern antibiotics against bacteria. Selman Waksman turned the words "antibiosis" and "antibiote" into "antibiotic" in 1945. He suggested that the term be applied to describe "a chemical substance of microbial origin, that possesses antibiotic powers." The practice, however, is to use it to include antimicrobial substances from any living source, including plant and animal tissues.

Between 1889 and 1945, literally hundreds of individual studies concerning antibiosis or bacterial antagonism were published, but relatively little was known about the biochemistry of the processes described. Chemotherapy (q.v.) concentrated on metals and synthetic products, a position which proponents of antibiosis tended to deplore. There was evidence that, at least in wound treatment, bacteria useful to the healing process were actually destroyed by strong antiseptics, and this without eliminating infective bacteria. Almroth Wright, one of the most interesting medical figures of the early twentieth century, proposed an approach to disease therapy based on a generalized immunization principle. His Inoculation Division at St. Mary's Hospital at Paddington, in London, attracted brilliant young scientists, among them Alexander Fleming, and during World War I, Wright's research team, transplanted to France, did important work on wounds. Fleming was particularly effective in demonstrating the frequently destructive effects of antiseptics on tissues and cells and the absence of effect on pathogens. This negative achievement did not greatly advance understanding of natural defenses against bacteria, though Fleming's discovery in 1922 of the enzyme lysozyme did. In 1936, a deliberate search for the antibiotic produced by *Trichoderma lignorum* led to the isolation of gliotoxin. In 1939, René Dubos began studying tyrothricin systematically, and in 1940 Ernst Boris Chain demonstrated that penicillin acted as a systemic therapeutic agent.

Though medical science has achieved a more sophisticated view on bacterial antagonisms, no theoretical structure has evolved to guide the search for antibiotic substances. Literally hundreds of antibiotic products have been discovered in the years since World War II, but only a few have been found to be both safe and effective. Techniques have become highly developed, and the necessity for using an interedisciplinary approach with bacteriology, biochemistry, and biology at its core has been generally accepted. However, the methodology still requires the product of microbial action to be isolated, identified, purified into crystalline form, assayed, and tested for effect, side effect, and toxicity. These processes are admirably suited to pharmaceutical companies' laboratories, and work on producing new antibiotics has moved away from research institutes and universities.

But the study of antibiotics is relatively young. In 1940, when René Dubos asked Selman Waksman to organize a panel on antibiotics for the annual convention of the Society of American Bacteriologists, the two men failed to find enough people to constitute a panel. By 1946, however, it was possible to organize a special conference on antibiotic substances. The problem on this occasion, Waksman told the opening session, was one of selecting the best prepared among the many available to speak on the subject.

Today, antibiotics occupy an established place in our medical system, providing sound and acceptable therapeutic agents for the successful treatment of a wide range of bacterial infections, and a major defense against secondary infections which accompany virally caused diseases. They have also expanded the scope of surgical work. But the antibiotics, whether taken individually or as a class of drugs, are by no means a panacea, or entirely trouble-free. Physicians have learned that toxic effect and allergic reaction are constant dangers to be weighed, while the tendency for resistant bacterial strains to appear argues the necessity for controlled use. Ironically, the nearly miraculous effect of antibiotic treatment on both syphilis and gonorrhea undoubtedly strengthened the tendency to drop cautionary attitudes toward sex, a change in view which has contributed to the new epidemic of venereal infections which has startled public health officials during the past decade. Clearly, prevention is always better than cure, but with the antibiotic arsenal, cures have come to be the expected outcome of treatment.

ADDITIONAL READINGS: Herbert M. Boettcher, *Miracle Drugs: A History of Antibiotics*, Einhart Krawer (trans.), London, 1963; H. F. Dowling, *Fighting Infection: Conquests of the Twentieth Century*, Cambridge, Mass., 1977; H. W. Florey, E. B. Chain, et al., *Antibiotics: A Survey of Penicillin, Streptomycin, and Other Antimicrobial Substances from Fungi, Actinomycetes, Bacteria, and Plants*, 2 vols. London, New York, and Toronto, 1949; Hubert A. LeChevalier and Morris Salotorovsky, *Three Centuries of Microbiology*, New York, 1965; John Parascandola (ed.), *The History of Antibiotics: A Symposium*, Madison, Wisc., 1980; Selman A. Waksman, "Antibiotics," *Encyclopedia Americana*, New York, 1977, 54–56; Selman A. Waksman, *The Conquest of Tuberculosis*, Berkeley, 1964.

See also CHEMOTHERAPY; PENICILLIN; SULFONAMIDES.

Antiseptic

Antiseptics are substances which prevent the spread of bacteria when applied to living tissues. Highly concentrated antiseptic agents may kill microorganisms; low-concentration antiseptics generally inhibit growth. Unlike sulfonamides or antibiotics, which work within the organism, antiseptics are applied to the surface of bodies, or to cavities which can be reached from the outside. Antiseptics generally are toxic when ingested and can result in dangerous, even fatal poisoning. The current understanding of antiseptic action rests on the discovery of bacteria and their role in putrefaction, fermentation, and infection. Those principles were defined by Louis Pasteur and Robert Koch in the second half of the nineteenth century. Efforts to prevent spoilage or infection are much older.

The word "antiseptic" was first used in an English pamphlet entitled *An Hypothetical Notion of the Plague and Some Out of the Way Thoughts About It* (1721). The author, a Mr. Place, wrote of "antiseptick" as a counter to spoilage or corruption. The well-known physician John Pringle used the word in the same way in 1752. In 1767, the Dijon Academy sponsored an essay competition dealing with antiseptics. The prize essay was a historical survey which discussed cautery, gangrenous ulcer, and putrefaction, especially in wounds; second prize went to a paper which reviewed the action of such antiseptic agents as alcohol, turpentine, pitch, aloes, styrax, benzoin, and Peru balsam.

The history of wound care and surgery shows that a variety of substances was used to control infection and spoilage. Among the earliest and most successful were resins and balsams, which are mentioned in the Hippocratic writings of the fifth and fourth centuries B.C. The Egyptians used ethereal oils, gums, and various spices to arrest the decomposition of dead bodies. Turpentine was widely recommended in the Middle Ages and early modern period and was still in favor at the time of the Civil War (1861–1865). Frankincense and myrrh were native gum resins of the Middle East whose use continued into the eighteenth century, while styrax and benzoin were among the oldest and most popular balsams in popular use. Mentioned in Pliny's writings, styrax originated in southeast Asia, was valued in the medieval world for treating scrofula, and was still used for wounds in the Napoleonic era. Peru balsam, an Indian medication from the new world, was recommended by Spanish authorities in the sixteenth century and was still in use in 1876.

Ancient Greek medicine employed wine and vinegar in wound dressings. Alcohol gained favor during the nineteenth century when Auguste Nélaton used alcohol soaks to disinfect wounds in elective surgery, achieving a mortality rate below 5 percent in the period 1863–1864. Fifty years earlier, Napoleon Bonaparte had commissioned Bernard Courtois to make nitrate, and he discovered iodine (1811). Humphry Davy and Joseph Louis Gay-Lussac showed iodine's elementary nature, and by 1820 it was recommended for internal use against goiter and externally for scrofula. Iodine became popular in France for treating wounds, and some surgeons used it as a finger dip. Other materials which gained popularity as antiseptics included bromine, creosote, ferric chloride, zinc chloride, and nitric acid. In 1847, Ignaz Semmelweis built his prophylaxis against puerperal fever on carbolic acid, the same substance Joseph Lister later used in his antiseptic treatment.

During the eighteenth century, a strong hygienic movement developed which stressed fresh air and cleanliness. It came in response to mounting fatalities from childbed fever, hospital fever, and repeated outbreaks of yellow fever, typhus, and other epidemic diseases. Foul smells and infection were thought to be causally linked, and hygienists joined with social reformers to create a front against noxious odors, corruption, and disease. When Semmelweis argued that it was actually the physicians' hands which carried cadaveric fever from the dissecting room to the maternity wards, he was running counter to conventional beliefs, and he could not explain what was carried. Joseph Lister's attack on wound sepsis, which came just 18 years later, benefited from Pasteur's early work on fermentation and made prevention of bacterial infection a primary goal.

Joseph Lister did not invent antisepsis, but he did develop a systematic and successful method for achieving it. His technique is now obsolete, but in the second half of the nineteenth century it was one of the most important innovations in the history of medicine. Joseph Lister (later Baron Lister) was born in 1827, the son of J. J. Lister, the amateur physicist and microscopist who discovered the achromatic lens. He received early training from his father in microscopy, which helped him to an early appreciation of Pasteur's work. Lister was trained in medicine at University College, London, which he entered in 1848, emerging four years later with a bachelor of medicine degree with honors. After appointment as a fellow of the Royal College of Surgeons, and a year spent as house surgeon at University College Hospital, he went to Edinburgh as assistant to James Syme, an eminent surgeon and noted teacher. In 1859 he was appointed regius professor of surgery at Glasgow. In 1861, he was given charge of the new surgical block in Glasgow's Royal Infirmary, and it was there that he developed his antiseptic method.

The Glasgow Royal Infirmary was built according to the latest principles of hygienic hospital construction to prevent the ravages of hospital disease, but the mortality rate there was no better than that in other institutions. In the Male Accident Ward, which was under Lister's direction, the death rate from infection in amputation cases ran between 45 and 50 percent during the period 1861–1865. Lister had studied and published on aspects of wound healing, particularly coagulation and inflammation, and he employed microscopic analysis in his work. He rejected the theory which connected infection with bad air, and he postulated a kind of infectious agent similar to dust or pollen carried by the air. There is no evidence that he considered the dust to be, or to contain, a living organism.

In 1865, Lister learned about Pasteur's work on fermentation and putrefaction. He also concluded that carbolic acid affected bacteria, a conclusion reached after considering its reported effects in reducing entozoic infection among cattle pastured on a sewage farm near Carlisle and its successful use against typhoid in Carlisle. Lister had tried various methods for washing infection away. He became convinced, however, that not only was it necessary to cleanse the wound, but that a barrier against further infection had to be created, and that the scab should become part of that defense.

Lister made his first trial on August 12, 1865, dressing a compound fracture of the tibia with lint soaked in carbolic acid. The dressing remained in place four days. The wound did not become infected and remained free of infection through the subsequent healing period, when it was dressed first with water and carbolic acid and then with carbolic acid and olive oil. All compound fractures were extremely dangerous, but since the wound in this case was considered to be less serious than some, Lister admitted that it might have healed successfully without his treatment. The success, however, was an important pointer. On May 19, 1866, Lister took up a far more serious case, a compound fracture of the leg which showed extensive bruising and bleeding. The carbolic treatment was again applied, the wound healed without infection, and Lister wrote to his father that "a most dangerous accident seems to have been entirely deprived of its most dangerous element."

The technique Lister evolved varied in details when it was practiced but included six basic steps. As much as possible of the clotted blood was squeezed from the wound; the wound was swabbed out with crude carbolic; carbolic-soaked lint was applied directly to it; a cover of malleable tin was put over the dressing and was taped on; absorbent wool was packed around the wound and splinted into place; and the tin was lifted and fresh carbolic painted on the lint when redressing was necessary. The Listerian principle involved both antisepsis (killing infective agents already present in the wound) and asepsis (preventing the entrance of infective bacteria into the wound). Both were essential to the success of the procedure.

Lister published his first results in the *Lancet* for March 16, 1867. In 11 cases of compound fracture, none of the patients died of sepsis. One was lost to a hemorrhage, and two others contracted infections, one of which resulted in an amputation. The other 8 recovered uneventfully. Lister was also expanding his field. In 1866, he began to use his method on abscesses, and in April 1867, he first used antisepsis during a surgical operation. Operating under an "antiseptic curtain" and irrigating the wound with carbolic lotion, Lister removed a tumor from an old man's upper arm. The patient recovered without complications.

In reporting his successes to the British Medical Association, Lister wrote in August 1867 that "since the antiseptic system has been brought into full operation and wounds and abscesses no longer poison the atmosphere with putrid exhalations, my wards, although in other respects under precisely the same circumstances as before, have completely changed their character, so that during the last nine months not a single instance of pyaemia, hospital gangrene, or erysypelas has occurred in them." Despite the miasmal vocabulary, Lister was reporting a major victory in the control of bacterially caused disease. Between 1865 and 1869, surgical mortality in the Male Accident Ward dropped from 45 to 15 percent. In the course of his career, Lister's overall surgical mortality was only 4.2 percent as against the pre-Lister surgeons' records of about 9 percent. Lister's operative mortality was even lower, amounting to no more than 1.5 percent, but this very low figure also reflected the fact that his practice, like that of most surgeons of his day, was quite an ordinary one, and most of his operations were minor.

The reception to Lister's work was mixed.

While his techniques improved and his reputation spread, resistance gathered as well. Despite Rudolf Virchow's skepticism, Lister gained a substantial German following, but he met with strong opposition in France, Britain, and the United States. Apart from English prejudice against Glasgow and Edinburgh, where Lister returned in 1869, the basic problem was that his technique assumed that Pasteur's germ theory of disease was correct, and that point was hotly disputed. Moreover, in many places, what was thought to be Lister's method failed to work. The Lister technique involved a series of steps, all of which were important. Some surgeons used one part or another with mixed and unpredictable results. The conclusion was that Lister was wrong. Lister himself contributed to the controversy by refusing to publish further results. He had been harshly criticized for the implication in his earlier reports that surgery was mismanaged in Glasgow before his work there, and he had no interest in creating further problems for himself.

The *Lancet* remained firmly pro-Lister but was never able to arrange a formal test comparison between surgical outcome under Lister and that under others. Nevertheless, Lister's fame spread. Between 1869 and 1876, his Edinburgh wards were crowded with students and foreign visitors. The Prussian military medical staff introduced some of his ideas during the Franco-Prussian War (1870–1871), achieving somewhat better results with battle wounds than did the French, who ignored Lister completely. In 1875, Lister made a triumphal tour of German medical research centers, where he was warmly and enthusiastically received, but an American tour the following year was less successful. His reception in Boston and New York was warm, but American resistance to antiseptic surgery remained firm, and in 1882 the American Surgical Association formally rejected the Lister doctrine.

In 1877, Lister was offered and accepted the chair of clinical surgery at King's College Hospital, London. This put him at the epicenter of resistance to his ideas, and he accepted the challenge by undertaking almost at once what was considered to be a very dangerous operation. On October 26, 1877, he undertook to repair and wire a fractured kneecap, a procedure which required him to convert a simple fracture into a compound one. It was the danger of infection which made this a daring feat, but Lister performed it successfully, and then he repeated the operation six more times. This achievement proved convincing, and with the definitive proofs which Koch was offering that germs cause disease, the antiseptic method was soon established.

Lister became one of medicine's most famous figures during his own lifetime, yet the rapid movement of scientific development in the last quarter of the nineteenth century outpaced him even before his retirement from active practice in 1892. The carbolic spray, or curtain, which saturated surgeon, assistants, and patient was the symbol of the Lister method, but it came under early criticism from Lister's followers, and he himself abandoned it in 1880. Carbolic-soaked bandages proved their worth in the Franco-Prussian War, but Koch's researches proved that chemical measures were less effective for sterilizing instruments than heat. The wearing of face masks, rubber gloves, and surgical gowns and the abandonment of the large operating theater with its crowds of students and spectators further reduced the potential for infection.

Lister's lasting contribution concerned preventing contact between contaminated surfaces and open wounds. Theodor Billroth used Lister's techniques to achieve a remarkable degree of operative success in abdominal procedures. Billroth was unconvinced by the germ theory of disease, but he followed Lister's methods faithfully. Lister, as a recent biographer put it, "made surgery safe," while Billroth showed how Lister's work expanded the field.

While the antiseptic principle remains firmly in place, methods for combating bacterial infection have changed radically. No general antiseptic which can safely be used against all infective microorganisms has ever been found, but better methods for dealing with infection have been identified. Chemotherapy, which began with Paul Ehrlich's pioneering work, opened an entire field for dealing with infection; penicillin, sulfonamides, and antibiotics have proved far more effective than external antiseptics. Nevertheless, scores of products have become available to resist different sorts of microorganisms in different situations. These are the children and grandchildren of Joseph Lister's antiseptic principle, and they attest to the importance of his achievement.

ADDITIONAL READINGS: Frederick F. Cartwright, *The Development of Modern Surgery,* London, 1967; Frederick F. Cartwright, *Joseph Lister,* London, 1963; Sir Rickman J.

Godless, *Lord Lister*, London, 1917; C. A. Lawrence and S. S. Block (eds.), *Disinfection, Sterilization, and Preservation*, Philadelphia, 1968, 1971; Owen Wangensteen and S. D. Wangensteen, *The Rise of Surgery from European Craft to Scientific Discipline*, Minneapolis, Minn., and Folkestone, Kent, 1978.

See also BACTERIOLOGY; GYNECOLOGY; PUERPERAL FEVER; SURGERY.

Arthritis

"Arthritis" is a generic term for any disease which produces swelling in the joints and pain in the limbs. The most common forms are osteoarthritis, gout, and rheumatoid arthritis. Osteoarthritis is any chronic, multiple, degenerative joint disease. Gout and rheumatoid arthritis are particular arthritic forms resulting from excessive concentrations of uric acid and rheumatic infection, respectively. Other more specialized conditions include ankylosing spondylitis, a degenerative syndrome in which the entire spinal column becomes enclosed in a bony casing from ossification of the spinal ligament, and osteophyles, a joint condition which may result from improper diet.

Arthritic conditions have been identified in dinosaur and Neanderthal man skeleton remains as well as in bones from Egyptian burial sites which cover over 3000 years of history (ca. 2900 B.C. to A.D. 200). There is also evidence from early Anglo-Saxon remains. Literary evidence begins with the Egyptian medical papyri of the second millennium B.C., and there is at least one Assyrian letter of the eighth century B.C. which describes arthritic pains, ascribing them to bad teeth. Although paleopathology has been unable to identify rhomboid arthritis, there are passages in the Hippocratic writings of the fifth century B.C. and in the works of Soranus of Ephesus, a Byzantine Greek physician of the second century A.D., which seem to refer to that disease. Soranus described a chronic arthritic condition which spread rapidly and which affected people above the age of 35, especially women. He also referred to morning stiffness and identified a hot and cold chronic arthritis which may have been an attempt to distinguish between an infective arthritis and the rheumatoid type.

Later European authorities were inclined to link arthritis with prevalent infective diseases. In the seventeenth and eighteenth centuries, it was suggested that arthritis was a consequence of gonorrhea, and in the nineteenth century, both tuberculosis and syphilis were thought to cause arthritic conditions. In the first decade of the twentieth century, scarlet fever, pneumonia, dysentery, and brucellosis were all implicated as causes for arthritis.

Rheumatoid arthritis was recognized as a specific condition in the early nineteenth century. The first complete clinical description appeared in 1800 in an M.D. thesis by Augustin Landré-Beauvais, who also distinguished it from gout. In 1859, Sir Alfred Garrod not only separated gout from all other forms of arthritis by discovering an excess of uric acid in the blood of all gout sufferers but also argued that "rheumatoid arthritis" was a phrase which should "imply an inflammatory condition of the joints not unlike rheumatism . . . but differing materially from it." Discovering what caused rheumatoid arthritis, or polyarthritis, was more difficult. Though it had been noted that arthritis seemed to occur in the wake of other conditions, that observation left the largest part of arthritis syndrome unexplained. It was theorized that a poison-generating focus of infection might produce toxic elements which in turn would cause arthritis, and this hypothesis led physicians to recommend tooth extractions, tonsillectomies, appendectomies, and even gall bladder removals in an effort to halt the development of arthritic conditions. In 1940, however, research scientists identified a substance similar to an antibody which circulated in the blood of arthritis sufferers and which they named the "rheumatoid factor." The nature of that factor remained obscure until it was shown that a group A hemolytic streptococcus caused rheumatic infections. It then became clear that the elusive rheumatoid factor in at least 75 percent of those afflicted with rheumatoid arthritis was immunological reaction to group A streptococcus.

The historical incidence of arthritis sufferers is difficult to estimate. The association between arthritis and such common conditions as gonorrhea, syphilis, and tuberculosis suggests a broad incidence, but there are no firm data until the early nineteenth century, and even those are suggestive rather than definitive. It was estimated in 1805 that 1 out of every 310 persons in the general population was rheumatic, while in 1818 the *London Directory* claimed that out of every 25 hospitalized patients, 1 suffered from "chronic rheumatism." In recent years, the Empire Rheumatism Council found that rheumatoid arthritis accounted for between 2 and 4 percent of all diseases for which treatment was applied in England and Wales, while in 1956 the United States was estimated to have between 4 and 6 million rheumatoid arthritis sufferers, though a more recent authority prefers a far lower figure of 1 percent of the population.

Arthritis is a disease which can cripple but does not kill. Palliatives apart, there is relatively little that can be done for its victims, and this, of course, has been true historically as well. Bleeding, purging, and violent counterirritants were all prescribed in the past to little effect. Rest and attention to diet proved more useful, while splints and bandages to relieve pain and forestall deformities had some successes in the late nineteenth and early twentieth centuries. The most effective medicines have been the salicylate family, especially aspirin (acetylsalicylate); injections with gold salts; and treatment with steroid hormones. The latter were developed by Philip Hench and E. C. Kendall of the Mayo Clinic, Rochester, Minnesota. In 1949 Hench and Kendall demonstrated the dramatic if temporary effect of cortisone treatments, for which they received a Nobel prize in 1950. Since cortisone, synthetic anti-inflammation drugs of the phenylbutazone group have appeared which offer further relief, but the search continues for some method to cure or, even better, to prevent arthritis.

ADDITIONAL READINGS: W. S. C. Copeman, *A Short History of the Gout and Rheumatic Diseases*, Berkeley and Los Angeles, 1964; Joseph Lee Hollander, *Arthritis and Allied Conditions*, Philadelphia, 1966.

See also GOUT; RHEUMATISM.

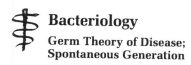

Bacteriology

Germ Theory of Disease; Spontaneous Generation

Bacteriology, the systematic study of microorganisms, is a branch of microbiology and has a close affinity with several medical disciplines, most notably immunology, epidemiology, and public health. As a discipline in its own right, bacteriology came of age in the third quarter of the nineteenth century when it established proofs for the germ theory of disease, probably the most important single concept for the history of modern medicine, and then contributed to the understanding of immune reactions and the discovery of sulfonamides and antibiotics. One important offshoot of bacteriology is virology, the study of submicroscopic organisms in plants and animals. Together, bacteriology and virology have given modern medicine the means to understand the causes for most of humankind's major infectious diseases and, through that understanding, to develop techniques for their identification, treatment, and control.

Early Beginnings The idea that entities too small to be seen exist and play a role in human illness occurs in various forms before the early modern period, though it seems to have been more a folk tradition than a part of scientific thought. The Roman author Varro, in the first century B.C., speculated on the possibility that disease was caused by "tiny animals," invisible to the naked eye, which were carried on the air to enter the body through the mouth or nose. Pliny the Elder shared Varro's speculations, but the first developed theory which ascribed disease causation to tiny, autonomous living entities was Girolamo Fracastoro's *On Contagion* (1546). This author spoke of disease seeds (*seminaria contagiosa*) which could be carried by the wind or communicated by touch or by contact with infected objects.

Popular opinion blamed visible parasites for human diseases, and the parasites that could be seen inspired speculation about minuscule or invisible creatures which also affected human health. There was a German folk myth, for example, that the bodies of sick people produced minute wormlike creatures which exited from the nostrils, eyes, and ears to enter the bodies of the healthy. Parasitic guinea worms were thought to cause dracontiasis, possibly the "plague of fiery serpents" which the Israelites suffered. In medieval times it was not unusual to find references to heart worms in cases of sudden death, while tooth decay was laid to tooth worms.

Spontaneous Generation While parasites seen and unseen were considered part of disease and were often cited as the cause for disease, they were not necessarily believed to enter the body from outside as autonomous entities. And those parasites that acted as a cause for disease in a particular body were often thought to have been generated spontaneously within the body by mysterious processes. The doctrine of spontaneous generation accounted for the presence of parasites, which by their actions created disease symptoms. The later and more sophisticated version, which was conventional wisdom until the second half of the nineteenth century, held that parasites, and the bacteria associated with diseases, were themselves symptoms, that is, products of the disease. The same argument was used to explain the bacteria present in fermentations.

Fracastoro could only assume the existence of disease-bearing seeds. The discovery of the microscope (see Microscopy) at the beginning of the seventeenth century produced proof that microorganisms did exist. By the middle of the century, Athanasius Kircher claimed to have seen tiny creatures in the blood of plague victims, which he asserted to be the plague's cause. The century's most notable reports on microorganisms came in Antonj van Leeuwenhoek's letters to the Royal Society in London after 1676. But microscopes were too primitive for refined observations, and the study of microorganisms remained at an elementary level. Nevertheless, interest in parasites as disease-causing (or symptom-causing) agents continued. Dr. G. Bonomo made the first identification of a disease-causing parasite when he ascribed the skin condition called scabies to a "minute living creature" shaped like a tortoise which was "whitish in color, a little dark upon the back, with some thin and long hairs." Dr. Bonomo used a low-power microscope to collect these and other details, and in his paper (1687) he described how the animal was propagated, how it produced the characteristic scabies symptoms, and why internal medication did no good. Since the animal moved freely, the condition was obviously contagious, and anything a patient used, especially linens, bedclothes, gloves, towels, and handkerchiefs, was liable to transfer it.

Bonomo's achievement was virtually unique. There was no sequel to it for a century and a half, and the doctrine of parasitic infection itself reached its summit around 1700 and then declined in favor. The standard work which summarized the position was Nicholas Andry's *On the Generation of Worms in the Human Body* (1699), an exhaustive study of parasites on humans, the diseases associated with them, and their treatment. The book was expanded and improved in 1718 and 1741. Andry rejected the spontaneous generation theory, asserting that the parasites' "seeds entered the body from without," and he held that some foods were particularly liable to convey them. He had no experimental data to support his positions. Even when proofs were available, however, belief in spontaneous generation remained dominant.

In 1668, Francesco Redi at Florence showed experimentally that maggots did not appear on meat that was protected against flies. His conclusions were ignored, as were the even more definitive proofs presented by the Abbé Lazaro Spallanzani, professor of physiology at the University of Pavia. In 1748, Father John Needham, a Welsh Catholic priest in exile in Europe, claimed to have proved spontaneous generation. He boiled a meat infusion, corked it, and then heated it again. After it cooled, he was able to identify "animalcules" in the broth which, he said, could only have appeared spontaneously. Buffon, the great French naturalist, accepted his proofs, but Spallanzani pointed out that Needham had not protected his infusion from the air. He also showed that broth heated above boiling point for 45 minutes and hermetically sealed would keep indefinitely without generating life. These conclusions, published in 1767 and 1776, failed to convince, and belief in spontaneous generation persisted for yet another century.

Background to Discovery: 1830 to 1860 After 1830, improvement in microscopy and better laboratory techniques brought more of the world of "little animals" into view. At the same time, medicine had moved toward the position that each disease was a particular entity with recognizable symptoms and pathology. The process of differentiation had begun with Thomas Sydenham's classification of fevers in the seventeenth century, and it had been nourished by developments in pathology and morbid anatomy during the eighteenth century. The man commonly identified as the founder of the modern doctrine of specificity was Pierre Bretonneau (1778–1862), a provincial French doctor who did his most important work at Tours. Bretonneau published very little, but he had devoted students who spread his ideas. Working with diphtheria (q.v.), which he named, Bretonneau contended that diphtheric conditions, whether in the throat, the nose, or the lower respiratory tract, were pathologically the same, and at the same time they were different from all other inflammatory and ulcerative conditions of the throat. He also separated typhoid from all other fevers by identifying characteristic lesions in the small intestine. Bretonneau concluded that a unique cause was responsible for each condition. He thought in terms of a "morbid seed" for each specific disease, "as every seed in natural history gives rise to a determined species."

Specificity of disease might lead logically to specificity of cause, but apart from Bonomo's scabies parasite, there was no evidence that particular seeds or animals caused particular diseases. There was, of course, a great deal of evidence that parasites and bacteria existed, but it was commonly believed that they were all alike. That conviction, however, began to be challenged in 1835, when a lawyer and estate manager, Agostino Bassi, published a book on muscarine in silkworms which showed that the fungus found on dead silkworms contained the cause of the disease. The point was proved by inoculating healthy silkworms with the fungus and so inducing the sickness. Bassi never went farther with this interest because his eyes failed, but his conclusions inspired Johann Schoenlein of Zurich to investigate ringworm. He found a fungus in ringworm pustules and concluded in 1839 that the fungus accompanied ringworm. He did not show that the fungus caused the condition, though he inferred that conclusion.

In 1840, Jacob Henle, also of Zurich, published an essay on miasmas and contagia in which he argued that infectious diseases formed a specific group with subheadings of miasmal, miasmal-contagious, and contagious. The differences he saw argued for different causes, and Henle believed that infectious diseases were caused by a living agent. The eminent biochemist Justus von Liebig expressed the general skepticism when he wrote, with some justice, that pathologists were too apt to consider "two things which occur frequently in conjunction, as standing in the mutual relation of cause and effect." And in 1850, when John Simon delivered a series of lectures on pathology at St. Thomas' Hospital in London, he characterized Henle's conclusions as unproved and probably unprovable.

Fermentation and putrescence were also closely studied in the 1830s and 1840s, though the results were inconclusive. Theodor Schwann, working between 1834 and 1837 in Johannes Mueller's Berlin laboratory, showed that heat would destroy the "infusoria" responsible for putrefaction, and in common with several other men, he reported in 1837 that yeast cells were responsible for fermentations. Schwann was a meticulous researcher who did surprising things with the microscopes available. He was one of the early proponents of cell theory, and some authorities regard him as the founder of the germ theory of disease. The last laurel is probably not deserved, but his work before 1850 was well to the fore of the bacteriological vanguard.

Pasteur, Fermentation, and Germ Theory Between 1857 and 1863, the French chemist Louis Pasteur undertook a series of studies which showed that the "fermentations" which occurred in different substances were different, and he set out to identify the causal agents. He concluded that fermenting agents were living forms and that fermentation was the result of their life cycles. Without such organisms, there was no fermentation. Pasteur also held that fermenting agents were not generated spontaneously but were carried by the air. Like Spallanzani a century earlier, Pasteur set up an experiment which proved conclusively that fermentation only occurred when air could reach a previously sterilized substance. The fermenting agent entered the substance from outside it. It was this work that caught the attention of Joseph Lister, who applied Pasteur's ideas to create an antiseptic wound dressing in 1866 and to lay the basis for aseptic surgery.

Pasteur's work on fermentation continued for another decade. He was able to show the wine industry that *Mycoderma aceti* was responsible for souring wine and that heating to 55°C eliminated the problem. Later, he applied the same principle to beer and to milk. Pasteurization, as the process came to be known, marked a major step toward purifying foods, and it was particularly important for controlling tuberculosis.

Pasteur's solution to a devastating silkworm infection became a demonstration in how disease spread. He proved that the silkworm disease was caused by a living organism which could be communicated, and he revealed the life cycle of the organism from moth through egg, worm, and chrysalis. His work in 1877 on anthrax, a disease deadly to cattle and sheep which humans sometimes contracted, was his first effort to understand a bacterially caused condition which could affect man. In this case, his most important contribution was to develop an attenuated vaccine which gave protection against infection. The anthrax bacillus had been identified by Casimir Davaine in 1863 and cultured by Robert Koch in 1876. It was Pasteur, however, who gave the most complete demonstration of the environments in which anthrax thrived and showed that the disease was caused by the anthrax bacillus and nothing else.

Pasteur was an outspoken proponent of the germ theory of infection, which he argued before the French Academy of Medicine on February 19, 1878. Later that same year, in a joint paper with Jules Joubert and Charles E. Chamberland, Pasteur summarized his conviction that microorganisms were responsible for disease, infection, putrefaction, and fermentation; that only particular organisms could produce specific conditions; and that once those organisms were known, it would be possible to prevent or at least resist infection. He considered surgical procedures particularly dangerous, since "germs and microbes" could be expected to be found "on the surfaces of all objects, particularly in hospitals," and he recommended heat treatments to purify surgical instruments, sponges, and bandages. Here Pasteur's work again intersected with that of Joseph Lister, though Lister was inclined to rely on chemical agents rather than heat.

Robert Koch and Scientific Bacteriology Proving the germ theory of disease established bacteriology as a scientific discipline. Pasteur, though a firm believer in germ theory, was much less successful in defending or proving it than was Robert Koch (1843–1910). Pasteur was an excellent microscopist, recognizing and discriminating among the still unnamed and unclassified streptococcus, staphylococcus, and pneumococcus. But it was Koch's meticulous, step-by-step demonstrations which established the bacterial concept of disease causation once and for all. His portrayal of the life cycle of the anthrax bacillus, presented to Friedrich Cohn's seminar at Breslau in the spring of 1876, led Julius Cohnheim to remark: "It leaves nothing more to be proved. I regard it as the greatest discovery ever made with bacteria."

Robert Koch's paper "The Etiology of Traumatic Infective Diseases," first published in 1879 and translated into English in 1880, was a monument to his method, and it proved the germ theory of disease beyond the shadow of a doubt. This paper dealt with wound infections of all sorts, but the basic problems it set were to discriminate among bacteria, to connect specific bacteria with specific effects, and so to settle whether bacteria were a consequence of infection or its cause. To answer these questions, Koch laid down a series of principles which were later expanded and refined into what came to be known as Koch's Postulates. In their final form these held that to prove a particular bacterium produced a specific condition, four requirements must be met: (1) The organism must be shown to be present in every case of the disease; (2) the organism can be cultivated in pure culture; (3) inoculating an animal with the culture will reproduce the disease; and (4) the organism can be recovered from the inoculated animal and grown again in a pure culture. Some disease-causing entities, most notably viruses, have to be accepted without fulfilling all these conditions, but in general, these rules have provided the criteria for accepting the demonstration of particular bacterial causes for specific diseases. This has refined the germ theory of disease into a bacterial explanation of disease causation.

Among Koch's technical innovations, the use of solid cultures for growing bacteria was probably the most important. Pasteur had shown that it was essential to isolate specific bacterial strains. Artificial cultivation in liquid media served his purposes. Koch's more advanced microscopic and micrographic techniques showed up the distortions and inconveniences which liquid media produced. Indeed, with characteristic certainty and arrogance Koch criticized Pasteur's liquid media as an example of his careless and unconvincing methods "which describe incredible facts with regard to pure cultivations of the organisms of hydrophobia, sheep pox, pleuropneumonia, etc." Convinced that liquid cultures were unsatisfactory, Koch began his search for solid media by growing bacteria colonies on the surface of a cut potato. He was not the first to do so, but he was the first to realize the value of solid media and to demonstrate how, with this aid, "pure cultures of bacteria could be grown regularly with the greatest ease." Potato cultures could be used for some pathogenic bacteria, but not all, and Koch eventually chose to solidify the standard "nutrient broth" by adding gelatin to develop a universal medium. Unfortunately, the nutrient gelatin liquified at body temperature, and some bacteria digested it. This problem was solved when a colleague suggested using agar-agar, an extract of Japanese seaweed, to solidify the culture medium.

Robert Koch's insistence on demonstrating each step of his proofs, his technical skill, and his ability to devise the means to find the information he needed established the basis for laboratory techniques and a regular methodology. Koch's own research declined in significance and quality as his administrative and teaching responsibilities mounted, but his reputation as the world's foremost bacteriologist gave his opinions a Jovian authority. This was not entirely fortunate, for it meant that his word carried great weight even when he was wrong. His premature announcement of an immunizing agent (tuberculin) effective against tuberculosis produced a scandal, while his erroneous belief that cows did not transmit diseases to human beings temporarily closed off an important area of research in preventive medicine. Nevertheless, his achievements were enormous, and while he spent the last years of his life in Africa and Asia studying the causes of tropical diseases, his students, followers, and competitors used his methods to discover the causal agents for diphtheria, typhoid, lobar pneumonia, gonorrhea, undulant fever, cerebrospinal meningitis, leprosy, tetanus, plague, syphilis, whooping cough, and streptococcal and staphylococcal infections. This age of discovery had ended by the time World War I began, and new generations of scientists began working on the implications of bacteriology's golden age.

Twentieth-Century Development In the twentieth century, bacteriology has vastly expanded its area of work while refining its techniques. New discoveries have been few, but the refinement of information has produced new levels of understanding that are comparable in significance to the original discoveries. In the early part of the century, the most important achievements were actually by-products of the failure to develop effective serum therapies. In the case of pneumococci, for example, the attempt to develop a serum showed that there were different strains of pneumococci which could be identified by serological reactions. Lobar pneumonia attracted attention because it had a high (25 percent) case mortality, and in 1912 the Rockefeller Institute and Hospital put a team to work on it. The result was a classification system for pneumococci based on serological characteristics.

Classifying pneumococci was an important achievement, but it set the stage for an even more significant development. F. Griffith, an English bacteriologist, wanted to improve epidemiological practices through more precise knowledge of the nature and action of specific bacterial strains. In 1928 he wrote a paper entitled "The Significance of Pneumococcal Types" in which he used the Rockefeller typologies to classify sputum samples collected between 1920 and 1928. His figures showed an actual transformation of pneumococci and, on closer examination, a regular sequence of changes in type of pneumococcus before the development of pneumonia and during recovery from it. Griffith was not much interested in these facts and did not investigate the mechanism behind them. Nobody considered the matter particularly significant until 1944, when the transforming agent was identified as deoxyribonucleic acid (DNA), thus opening the way to understanding the chemical bases of heredity. Griffith's 1928 paper, as one recent commentator put it, was "the fuse of a time-bomb" which exploded to extraordinary scientific effect 16 years later.

The attempt to find a serum therapy for streptococcal infection had similarly broad significance. Never successful, it nonetheless established the basis for a highly effective system, or combination of systems, for typing streptococci, which led to important clinical and epidemiological results. The first system was developed in 1897, while the basis for the modern system was established by J. H. Brown in 1919. Brown set up three categories: (1) alpha, in which there was a green stain which resulted from contact with blood; (2)

beta, in which there was a complete hemolysis; and (3) gamma, in which neither change occurred. Beginning in 1918, the Rockefeller Institute was also working on streptococcal infection. Rebecca Lancefield, a member of the research team, has given her name to the grouping system which resulted. Griffith, whose paper on pneumococci was of such broad significance, had worked out a serological typing system for streptococci, but Lancefield rejected both the Brown and Griffith systems to build one based on precipitation tests which classified groups according to the source of the streptococcal strain used. Group A included most strains from human disease, including scarlet fever. In 1934, Griffith showed that group A included 27 different serotypes. In the end, the Lancefield grouping was combined with the Griffith typing to permit a clear distinction between pathogenic and nonpathogenic strains and, for epidemiological purposes, discrimination among the strains of pathogenic group A.

Conclusion Bacteriology has been both the cause and the product of the modern revolution in medicine. Its contributions to antiseptic surgery, its proofs for the germ theory of disease, its role in modern epidemiology, and its contributions to the more effective diagnosis and treatment of bacterial and viral diseases helped to change the practice of medicine from an art (or craft) to a disciplined, systematic application of scientific knowledge. In its broadest applications, bacteriology has done much to transform the essential character of life into its modern form. Like so much else connected with medicine, however, bacteriology's period of greatest achievements correlates exactly with the industrialization of the modern world, and its most significant accomplishments have been produced in the world's most rapidly developing societies. Those societies which fostered the development of bacteriology have become the best placed to gain from its achievements.

Knowledge can be exported; the social and economic prerequisites for implementing that knowledge for social good have to be developed. In this respect, scientific advances have widened the differences between the lives which people live in developed and undeveloped societies. The ability to identify specific disease causes has often outpaced broader social perceptions of disease. The establishment of a firm scientific basis for medical work demanded that medical training become scientific; as a result, the cost of medical care has risen and accessibility to medical care has been restricted. Nevertheless, bacteriology is a branch of science whose history is a fascinating and inspiring record of achievement and whose contribution to the improved quality and longevity of life in modern affluent societies is unquestionable, yet its role in modern life has yet to be systematically understood.

ADDITIONAL READINGS: Peter Baldry, *The Battle Against Bacteria: A Fresh Look*, Cambridge, Melbourne, New York, and London, 1976; William Bulloch, *A History of Bacteriology*, Oxford, 1938, 1960; Patrick Collard, *The Development of Microbiology*, Cambridge, New York, London, and Melbourne, 1976; Harry W. Dowling, *The Battle Against Infectious Diseases*, Cambridge, Mass., 1977; J. Farley, *The Spontaneous Generation Controversy from Descartes to Oparin*, Baltimore, 1977; William Ford, *Bacteriology*, New York, 1939; W. D. Foster, *A History of Medical Bacteriology and Immunology*, London, 1970.

See also CONTAGION; IMMUNOLOGY.

Barber-Surgeons

Barbers, beard trimmers, bath attendants, and similar functionaries were ubiquitous in medieval society, where they performed a variety of services, some of which were medical. Attendants at German public baths clipped, trimmed, and shaved their clients, but they also bled, cupped, leeched, gave enemas, pulled teeth, and sold ointments. Monastic regulations requiring the tonsure and regular bleeding made the barber, who also performed minor surgery, a necessity, and the first recognized barber-surgeons appeared in monasteries around the year A.D. 1000.

These barber-surgeons were part of a motley crowd selling medical services, which included stonecutters (lithotomists), bonesetters, cataract couchers, herniotomists, pig gelders, midwives, and, on a somewhat more exalted level, surgeons. University-trained physicians formed a learned professional elite, whose members occupied academic chairs, served as the trustees of an established medical tradition, and ostentatiously held themselves aloof from the common herd. Especially in northern Europe, physicians considered themselves to be observers and consultants, not active participants in the healing process. They thought surgery in any form to be a menial task beneath their dignity, and the Paris medical faculty went so far as to require their students to swear an oath that they would perform no surgery, including bleeding. This meant an enlarged opportunity for barbers, and as early as 1254, one of the thirteenth century's great surgical writers, Bruno di Longoburgo, complained that barbers were performing surgical operations, including scarifications and phlebotomies.

Barber-surgeons began to gain recognition and status in the thirteenth century. In 1210, the College of St. Cosme (Côme) was established in Paris. The members of the college were divided into those who wore a long robe and those who wore a short robe. The distinction was that long-robed surgeons were entitled to operate, while the wearers of the short robe could only operate after passing a special examination. The college granted three degrees: a bachelor's, a licentiate, and a master's. The main part of the training was practical, but there was some theoretical instruction as well.

Members of the Paris medical faculty disliked the pretensions of the long-robed surgeons and so formed an alliance with the barber-surgeons, supporting their claims against the surgeons' monopolies on most operations. The physicians began secretly to lecture on anatomy in French to the barber-surgeons, who in their turn swore to be the perpetual dependents and supporters of the physicians. Lecture activities included cadaver dissections and demonstrations. In the fourteenth century, the barber-surgeons organized a guild, and as they became more numerous and powerful, they demanded more of the physicians than the physicians were willing to grant. In 1499, the barber-surgeons asked for their own cadaver for anatomical demonstration, but this was carrying independence too far, and the physicians withdrew their support.

The struggle between the surgeons and the medical faculty continued until 1660, when the surgeons capitulated, recognizing the physicians' dominance. The barber-surgeons then declined in quality and influence, though their numbers actually increased. In 1301, it is estimated, there were 29 barber-surgeons in Paris; in 1634 the number was 40; in 1743, there were more than 300.

In England, the pattern was somewhat different. English physicians in the Middle Ages were at least as inclined as the French to avoid surgical tasks. A master surgeons' guild was organized in 1368, and it joined the physicians in 1421. The Mystery or Guild of the Barbers of London received its charter from Edward IV in 1462, and a special charter for surgeons was created 13 years later. In 1540 the Guild of Surgeons joined the Company of Barbers to form the United Barber-Surgeon Company. Its first master was Thomas Vicary. This organization lasted until 1745, when the surgeons and the barbers again parted company. As surgeons became university-trained and won social approval, the barber-surgeons lost their medical functions, though some continued to pull teeth. In the nineteenth century their medical importance faded away entirely. Only the barber's pole remained as a reminder of what the barber had once been.

In the German states, where surgery did not develop until the nineteenth century, the barber-surgeon held the field, but in Italy, Spain, and southern France, the barber-surgeon never acquired the medical importance enjoyed in the north. Salerno, the first important medieval medical school, did not divide surgery from medicine, so there was little conflict between physicians and surgeons; the medical schools at Padua and Bologna were particularly strong in anatomical studies, and they honored surgery. And where physicians and surgeons were separated, as in the Florentine Statute concerning the Art of Physicians and Pharmacists (1349), physicians and surgeons were held to be equals, while the barbers were given an inferior status. Barbers never gained the standing that conflict between surgeons and physicians opened to them farther north, and their medical functions remained under the surgeons' control.

ADDITIONAL READINGS: Arturo Castiglioni, *History of Medicine*, E. Krumbhaar, (trans.), New York, 1947; Jesse Dobson and R. Milnes Walker, *Barbers and Barber-Surgeons of London: A History of the Barbers' and Barber-Surgeons' Companies*, Oxford, 1980; Benjamin Lee Gordon, *Mediaeval and Renaissance Medicine*, New York, 1959; John Malbon Mynors, *The Barber's Progress*, Salisbury, Zimbabwe, 1969; David Riesman, *The Story of Medicine in the Middle Ages*, New York, 1935.

See also MEDICAL PROFESSION; MEDIEVAL MEDICINE; SURGERY.

Beriberi

Beriberi is a complex of conditions arising from vitamin B_1 (thiamine) deficiency. There are three generally recognized forms; wet, dry, and infantile beriberi. The wet form is an acute condition with edema present, and it frequently results in death from heart failure. Dry beriberi is a chronic condition with peripheral nerve lesions affecting different muscular systems. As the disease progresses, it often brings on paralysis or paresis of the lower limbs. Infantile beriberi shows different aspects of the adult forms, and it is an acute condition considered dangerous. Beriberi is not a tropical disease, though it appears most often in tropical zones.

Beriberi is said to be described in a Chinese medical text of the second millennium B.C., and there are references to the disease scattered through the medical literature. The most serious wave of beriberi, however, occurred in south and southeast Asia between 1870 and 1910. Fishing villages in Newfoundland and Labrador had outbreaks of beriberi in the twentieth century, and it also appeared among Brazilian naval personnel, Panama Canal laborers, and African military police teams. All these groups are "closed" or isolated societies living on diets of milled rice or wheat which were notably deficient in thiamine. Whole grains are the most common source of vitamin B_1, and even isolated peoples who eat whole grains escape beriberi.

The late-nineteenth-century beriberi epidemic was a by-product of advancing technology and colonial economic developments. Steam-driven rice mills were introduced, which produced a cheap and more attractive food product than did traditional hand milling, but the process destroyed the thiamine-bearing outer husk. People who lived mainly on this food fell ill with beriberi. Chinese plantation and tin mine workers in Malaya, for example, consumed from 2500 to 3200 calories in milled rice daily, and they sickened at a rate of 120 per 1000. Mortality was high. In one two-year period, 800 out of 2400 Chinese laborers died of beriberi. South Indian Tamils working on nearby rubber estates and native Malays living in coastal villages were generally unaffected by beriberi. The Malays pounded their own rice by hand in the traditional way, while the Tamils parboiled their rice before pounding or milling it. Parboiling shifted the thiamine location from the husk to the inner kernel, rendering it impervious to modern milling processes or to loss through washing.

Beriberi had severe effects in the Japanese navy, where milled rice was also issued, and where by 1878 incidence had reached 300 cases per 1000. When the Japanese changed from a ration that was predominantly milled rice to one of wheat, barley, beans, milk, meat, and some milled rice, beriberi disappeared within two years. This experience dramatically demonstrated a connection between diet and beriberi, but its nature was not understood until Christiaan Eijkman, working in Java, observed that pigeons and chickens fed on milled rice developed conditions similar to beriberi. Eijkman then focused his attention on the rice components in beriberi-producing diets and isolated the milling process as the proximate cause. His conclusions meant that controlled populations whose diet could be regulated would seldom suffer beriberi in the future. But the disease remained a serious threat to life among the urban populations of southeast Asia who were forced to depend on milled rice.

During World War II, beriberi became a major problem in Japanese prison camps, where limited rice diets were the rule. But since 1945, epidemiologists have reported a gradual decline of beriberi in its areas of greatest incidence. In Asia this decline owed less to the synthesis and commercial production of vitamin B_1 in 1926 than it did to more general social and economic factors. Among these, the most significant appear to be a general rise in living standards resulting in a more varied and better diet; an increase in the consumption of fats (which do not require thiamine to be metabolized) as well as other foods; the rising cost of rice; and an improved public understanding of nutrition. Whichever cause applies, beriberi appears to be receding, and the means are available to eradicate it completely. It is improbable, however, even if eradication fails, that a wave of beriberi comparable to that of the late nineteenth century will occur again.

ADDITIONAL READINGS: W. R. Aykroyd, *Conquest of Deficiency Diseases: Achievements and Prospects*, Geneva, 1970; R. R. Williams, *Towards the Conquest of Beriberi*, Cambridge, Mass., 1961.

See also DEFICIENCY DISEASES.

Bloodletting

Bleeding; Cupping; Venesection

Bloodletting, or bleeding, was a long-established medical practice. The Hippocratic writings accepted bleeding as a recognized therapy for specific conditions. Erasistratus of the Alexandrian school was skeptical, and some of his followers avoided bleeding entirely, but Galen firmly supported the procedure, and after Galen, bleeding tended to be done regularly, and in some periods enthusiastically, for many conditions and diseases. There were occasional critics, and there were differences of opinion concerning when bleeding should occur, where the blood should be drawn, the amount that should be taken, the method that should be used, how often it should be done, and whether it should be followed by a purge. On the whole, however, the efficacy of bleeding was considered an established fact until the middle of the nineteenth century. Then bleeding faded away, a victim of cellular pathology, the germ theory of disease, and a profoundly altered view of how illness should be treated.

The most common technique for bleeding was to tie a bandage around the arm so the veins of the forearm would swell up and then open the exposed vein with a sharp knife. The blood would be collected in a bowl or basin. By the Middle Ages, this operation was commonly performed by barber-surgeons. Cupping was another method for drawing blood which was also used to "draw" boils or other surface eruptions. A cup was heated by dropping burning material into it, its lip was greased, and the cup was then inverted over a scarified point on the skin. The cup developed suction as the burning material consumed the oxygen, and blood or pus was drawn through the skin opening. Leeches also were placed on the skin to draw blood. The number and distribution would depend on the physician's view of the disease. The practice was common enough to make leeches a sought-after commodity. Early in the nineteenth century, normal annual demand for the bloodsuckers in France for example, ran to 2 to 3 million; during the bleeding craze which crested in the 1830s that demand increased eightfold.

Bleeding followed humoral doctrines and finally departed with them. Because the humors (q.v.) were believed to control the body's functioning, and blood to contain all the humors, bleeding was thought to provide a method for directly manipulating or correcting the conditions which could be traced to any humor. In particular, it was believed to be effective against conditions arising from plethora, the accumulation of too much of the vital humor from overeating, too little exercise, dissipation, and just living. Purging was thought to be effective as well, and bloodletting with purging was considered a sovereign remedy against plethora. Inflammations and fevers, which were believed to result from humoral concentrations were thought to be aided by bleeding, which could draw off the inflammatory humor.

There was some doubt that a fever caused by an outside substance or contagium could be effectively treated by bleeding, and that doubt, expressed in the sixteenth century, became an issue in nineteenth-century arguments over fever treatments. A further problem was posed by those who believed fevers resulted from a weakened constitution which was unable to resist unhealthy miasmas. In such cases, debility rather than plethora obtained, and there seemed to be no basis for bleeding. This argument was important during the partial retreat from bleeding in the eighteenth century, and it reappeared in the nineteenth. It was countered by exponents of bleeding who claimed that the appearance of debility was really plethora in another guise, and that only a dramatic bloodletting could restore blood vessels which had collapsed under the weight of too much blood.

Resistance to bloodletting took the form of limiting its application by employing the Hippocratic idea of acting only to aid nature, by specifying diseases which could not be cured by bleeding, or by identifying persons for whom bleeding was dangerous. The major debate was not over whether or not to bleed but over how to employ the treatment. The heroic school, which included Guy Patin, dean of the faculty of medicine in Paris in the seventeenth century, Benjamin Rush of Philadelphia in the eighteenth century, and François Broussais, the radical Parisian bloodletter of the nineteenth century, all held with copious bleeding on all occasions. This was often combined with heavy purgatives and gargantuan dosing with drugs, including opium. In the early nineteenth century, the radical bleeders dominated. Broussais's influence was such in France that bloodletting was never so popular nor so widely practiced as it was between 1825 and 1835. Bloodletting declined in England in the eighteenth century, but it became popular once more in the early nineteenth century. Its resurgence reflected the return of hundreds of medical men from the wars, where heroic methods were standard. Henry Clutterbuck led the heroic bloodletting movement in England, supported by Benjamin Walsh.

Statistical proofs were employed on both sides of the argument to demonstrate the efficacy or uselessness of bleeding. In 1840, Pierre Louis, who has been called the founder of medical statistics, argued persuasively that in pneumonia cases bleeding had no positive effect, a conclusion which fitted both a mounting skepticism concerning the effectiveness of established therapies in general and new conceptions of disease. In the end, venesection and the heroic therapies gave way in the face of bacterial theories of disease causation, a better understanding of what fever was, cellular pathology, and a growing sophistication about human physiology and the blood's role. Included in this last was the realization that debility was a serious problem.

Nevertheless, bloodletting continues to be practiced, though on a greatly reduced scale. Ironically, in the light of Pierre Louis's work, it continued to be used in France until the 1920s for pneumonia therapy. In some areas of the world, leeches are still applied to remove blood from bruises and black eyes. Moreover, venesection is a recognized treatment for overproduction of red blood cells (erythremia) and for blood congestion in cases of acute heart failure. However, the conviction that bleeding was a generally effective therapy faded in the course of the nineteenth century with the advent of modern scientific medicine.

ADDITIONAL READINGS: Erwin H. Ackerknecht, "Broussais: Or a Forgotten Medical Revolution," *Bulletin of the History of Medicine* 27 (July–August 1953): 320–343; Leon S. Bryan, Jr., "Blood-Letting in American Medicine, 1830–1892," *Bulletin of the History of Medicine* 38 (September–December 1964): 516–529; Fielding H. Garrison, *Introduction to the History of Medicine*, 4th rev. ed., Philadelphia and London, 1929; Earle Hackett, *Blood: The Paramount Humour*, London, 1973; Peter H. Niebyl, "The English Blood-Letting Revolution: Modern Medicine Before 1850," *Bulletin of the History of Medicine* 51 (Fall 1977): 464–483; Guenter B. Risse, "A Renaissance of Bloodletting: A Chapter in Modern Therapeutics," *Journal of the History of Medicine and Allied Sciences* 35 (January 1979): 3–22.

See also HEMATOLOGY.

Blood Transfusion

Folklore and ancient medical practice both reflect the conviction that blood introduced into the body from an outside source could cure illness, preserve health, and save life. The Egyptians believed that the pelican fed her young with blood from her own breast; the blood of ducks, geese, pigeons, goats, sheep, and cattle was prescribed for a variety of internal and external conditions. In Rome, epileptics were supposed to be cured by swallowing fresh human blood, and those afflicted went to the gladiatorial games hoping to catch a drop from a fallen fighter. In the fifteenth century, physicians proposed to preserve the life of aged Pope Innocent VIII with blood from three young boys. There was no theoretical or anatomical basis for injecting blood into a vein until William Harvey established the principle of blood circulation in 1628.

The first attempts to pass blood from one creature to another by injecting it into a vein were made in the middle of the seventeenth century. The earliest experiments appear to have been the work of a reclusive English cleric, Francis Potter, between 1650 and 1653. He had conceived the idea of transfusion as early as 1639. It is unclear whether Potter's work affected what came after it, though there is a case to be made that it did. Robert Boyle described Sir Christopher Wren's use of a quill and bladder to give an intravenous injection to Boyle's dog in 1659, and during 1665 several attempts were made by members of the Royal Society to effect a transfusion. One attempt, by John Wilkins, in which blood was drawn from a dog and then injected into the vein of a bitch, was the first successful indirect transfer. In 1666, Richard Lower, also of the Royal Society, made the first successful direct transfusion from the artery of one animal into the vein of another. He used quills for the connection, but later he abandoned them for silver tubes.

A French physician, Jean Denis, is credited with

the first successful medical transfusion. On June 15, 1667, he gave a lamb's blood to a 15-year-old boy. Richard Lower did a similar transfusion from a sheep to a man five months later. The British experimenters were interested in a biological phenomenon; Jean Denis was developing a medical procedure which he introduced into his practice. In 1668, one of his transfused patients died, and an action was brought against him. Though Denis was cleared—the patient was poisoned by his wife—transfusion was considered too dangerous to be continued in France. In England, apart from speculation on the transfer of personal or cultural characteristics through blood transfusion, the process lost its scientific interest and failed to develop as part of medical practice. The predominance of humoral therapies undoubtedly contributed to the general lack of interest; the very real dangers of antigenic reaction and bacterial infection were also significant.

Interest in blood transfusions languished until the early nineteenth century when John Henry Leacock took up the subject as a treatment in hemorrhage. It was his conclusion, set out in a dissertation published in 1817, that it was safer to transfuse blood from like to like (dog to dog; human to human) than across species lines. James Blundell accepted Leacock's thesis and expanded it. A successful physician, lecturer, and obstetrician at Guy's Hospital, London, he began using blood from his assistants to inject into patients with hopeless prognoses. He used a syringe to inject the blood, and in 1827 he began to publish his lectures on the results. In 1829, he successfully transfused blood from his assistant to a woman suffering postpartum hemorrhage. She recovered. Blundell's work was followed by that of James N. Aveling, who was also able to make a successful medical transfusion and who invented a rubber bulb syringe to pump blood more quickly from donor to recipient. During the Franco-Prussian War (1870–1871), J. Roussel is credited with the first battlefield blood transfusion, and the apparatus which he had invented in 1865 was subsequently adopted in the French, Austrian, Belgian, and Russian armies.

Though hardly a common practice in the second half of the nineteenth century, blood transfusions were done with sufficient frequency for observers to see problems. The first was the tendency for the donor's blood to coagulate before it could be absorbed into the recipient's system. Anticoagulants began to be used in 1869—sodium phosphate was the earliest. There were also attempts to remove the fibrin from blood before administering it. Though useful against coagulation, this method also destroyed many valuable blood components. A purely mechanical measure to prevent triggering the clotting process was to coat tubes and containers with moisture-resistant grease or wax. At the time of the outbreak of World War I, it was found that sodium citrate was an innocuous and effective anticoagulant. This vastly eased and enlarged the use of blood transfusions. With an effective anticoagulant, blood could be stored in bottles to be used as needed, and the physical presence of the donor was no longer necessary.

The discovery and antiseptic control of bacteria reduced the danger of infection from transfusions, while the discovery and exploration of antigenic reactions led to blood classification. In 1900, Karl Landsteiner began to develop a classification system based on the presence of two agglutinating substances. The resulting ABO system permitted typing of all blood and made it possible to match the types of donor and recipient. This work drastically reduced the possibility of antigen reaction and made blood transfusions practicable. Transfusions could be used routinely in surgery, for accident victims of all kinds, and as a major element for treating the wounded in World War II. Better transfusion techniques, including the use of plasma, were responsible for steadily improving results from battlefield first aid through World War II, the Korean war, and the Vietnamese war.

Substantial supplies of blood maintained in blood banks provide a ready source in case of need. The blood transfusion, which has become a staple of medical practice since World War I, is one of the most important practical developments in modern medical treatment.

ADDITIONAL READINGS: Earle Hackett, *Blood: The Paramount Humour,* London, 1973; G. L. Keynes (ed.), *Blood Transfusion,* Bristol, 1949; Richard M. Titmuss, *The Gift Relationship: From Human Blood to Social Policy,* New York, 1971; Charles Webster, "The Origins of Blood Transfusion: A Reassessment," *Medical History* 4 (Fall 1971): 387–392.

See also HEMATOLOGY; SURGERY.

Brownian System

Brunonianism

The Brownian system was a unitary philosophy of medicine which explained disease and recommended treatment according to fluctuations in the quality of "excitability," defined as the ability inherent in every living thing to perceive or receive impressions from outside itself and respond to them. The system was created by John Brown (1735–1788), a Scottish physician who studied under William Cullen. Cullen was interested in the irritability-sensibility thesis which Albrecht von Haller systematized in 1752. Like Théophile de Bordeu, his contemporary at Montpellier, Cullen believed that sensibility and irritability were balanced in all organs and not simply characteristics of different tissues. He also considered muscles to be extensions of nerves, and he therefore defined life as a function of nervous energy.

Brown took parts of William Cullen's thesis, transformed "irritability" into "excitability," and went on to build a comprehensive medical theory which attracted widespread attention for nearly 50 years. Brown's system was favorably received in northern Italy and Germany; it had fewer supporters in England and Scotland, while French empirical medicine flatly rejected it. In the first decade of the nineteenth century, Friedrich von Schelling, the youthful inventor of Nature Philosophy, accepted and promoted Brownianism, bringing it into the mainstream of what now is called romantic science. Dr. Benjamin Rush of Philadelphia, who was himself an enthusiastic systematizer, brought Brownianism to America.

John Brown outlined his basic ideas in a book entitled *Elementa medicinae* (1780), which he then translated into English as *The Elements of Medicine* and published with added commentaries in 1787 and 1788. Brown's system postulated that, while the main concentration of excitability was in the neuromuscular system, life and all the vital functions which compose it were the sum of the constant responses by the living thing to its environment. Hence Brown compared himself to Newton, for the principle of excitability, like the law of gravitation, was irreducible and represented the long-sought first principle for biology.

There was no hint of a life force, or any determination to live. On the contrary, Brown was a radical mechanist whose views were similar to those of Julien Offroy de la Mettrie, the atheistic physician whose *L'homme machine* (1747) scandalized even relatively enlightened readers. Health in Brown's system meant achieving a balance between stimuli and excitability. A disposition to ill health followed when the stimuli were either excessive or inadequate, and the excitability factor fluctuated in inverse proportion to the stimulus. The alert physician worked to balance these influences before his charge became sick. Brown emphasized preventive care rather than a cure as such.

The conditions which led to illness were sthenia (excessive stimulation) and asthenia, its reverse. All diseases were the result of these conditions. Disease symptoms—fever, rash, nausea, or headache—were not significant; they were simply manifestations of the underlying disorder. Treating them was only palliative, and traditional medicines, without Brownian principles, were at best innocuous and could be harmful. The only effective treatment for any illness was to manage the level of stimulation. For the sthenic condition, debilitating measures were required to lower the level of excitement. In the most serious cases, moderate bloodletting could be done, though Brown regarded bleeding with disfavor. In general, occasional sweats and vomiting, gentle purges, and a strictly vegetarian diet with watery drinks were prescribed. For an asthenic condition, the physician prescribed highly seasoned foods, rich soups, and undiluted wines. Musk, camphor, ether, and opium were the drugs of choice, and Brown gave special emphasis to alcohol, primarily in the form of brandy, with opium to counteract any surplus stimulus. Brown dosed himself with four or five glasses of brandy at a time, and he is reported to have died of opium and alcohol abuse.

Brownian medicine enjoyed a wide reputation. Its partisans were fully persuaded of its value; its opponents were equally convinced of its dangers. In 1802, feelings became so inflamed among Göttingen students that a riot broke out which lasted until cavalry was sent into the city to end it. Leading physicians endorsed the system only to be refuted by their colleagues, and while the judgment that Brown's treatment "was responsible for more deaths than Napoleon and the French Revolution combined" is exaggerated, there was much in the system that was dangerous.

Modern historians are inclined to give John Brown some credit. His concept of disease has been compared to the concept of stress, which can be responsible for numerous physical symptoms. His idea of the organism's constant adjustment to its many environments and his belief that the physician must actively promote health by stimulating the organism's natural functions have resonance for modern medicine. On the other hand, the Brownian system contributed little to a scientific understanding of disease. Given the state of medical knowledge at the end of the eighteenth century, the harm it did can be vastly overrated, as undoubtedly the contemporary claims for its success were exaggerated. The Brownian system is most important for what it reveals concerning methods of thinking about disease and treatment at the end of the eighteenth century, when it seemed to offer an acceptable and even popular alternative to established medical strategies.

ADDITIONAL READINGS: "John Brown," *Dictionary of National Biography*, vol. 3, London, 1908, 14–17; G. B. Risse, "The Brownian System of Medicine; Its Theoretical and Practical Implications," *Clio Medicinae* 5 (1970): 45–51; G. B. Risse, "The Quest for Certainty in Medicine, John Brown's System of Medicine in France," *Bulletin of The History of Medicine* 45 (January 1971): 1–12; G. B. Risse, "Schelling's 'Naturephilosophie' and John Brown's System of Medicine," *Bulletin of the History of Medicine* 50 (Fall 1976): 321–334.

See also PHYSIOLOGY.

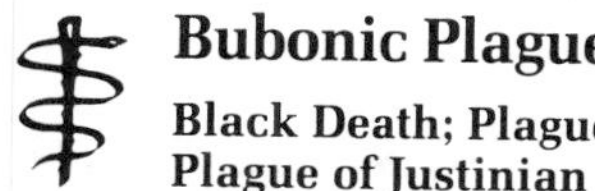

Bubonic Plague

Black Death; Plague; Plague of Justinian

Introduction Bubonic plague is an epidemic disease of extraordinary ferocity which has claimed untold millions of lives. There have been three great waves of plague infection in recorded world history. The first began in the sixth century A.D., the second began in the fourteenth century, and the third erupted in the second half of the nineteenth century and continued through World War II. The fourteenth-century plague, which is more commonly known as the black death, initiated 500 years of bubonic infections, closed the Middle Ages in Europe, and made "plague" a household word. The nineteenth-century pandemics were devastating for China, India, and southeast Asia, but they were also responsible for introducing plague into the western United States, where the disease has become endemic. In the years since 1945, there have been sporadic outbreaks of plague which have occasionally reached epidemic proportions, the most recent coming during the Vietnamese war. No other epidemic disease compares with plague in longevity and mortality. For at least 1500 years bubonic plague has returned again and again to devastate human settlements, and while it is currently controlled, especially in advanced societies, it remains a continuing and present danger.

The Disease Plague is primarily a disease of densely populated zones, households above all else, and its perpetuation and reinforcement involve a complex relationship among commensal and wild rodents, bacteria, insect vectors, and humans. Occasional plague outbreaks can occur almost anywhere, but for the disease to become rooted and recur, an environment must exist which can support a high density of rodent hosts living in proximity with human beings. Endemic plague among rodents remote from human habitation poses a danger only to humans who invade those zones.

The bacterium responsible for bubonic plague is *Yersinia* (formerly *Pasteurella*) *pestis*, one of the most pervasive, persistent, and dangerous life forms in the world. It lives in the bloodstream of dozens of varieties of rodents (rats, ground squirrels, marmots, etc.), but it is most commonly found among rats. The simple presence of *Y. pestis* in the rodent population has not always meant an immediate threat to humankind. Once the disease becomes epizootic among rodents in proximity to people, however, epidemic outbreaks have followed with consequences equally disastrous to humans and to the rodent hosts.

Why an epizootic starts is not clear. The bacterium begins to multiply. As it does so, it poisons its host's blood, and the rodent dies. This is why a "rat-fall," the sudden appearance of dead or dying rats, has come to be regarded as the precursor of a human epidemic. The most common vector for transferring *Y. pestis* from one body to another is the rat flea, *Xenopsylla cheopis,* though other flea types are almost as efficient. Among the some 200 known fleas which transfer plague, one of the least efficient is the human body flea (*Pulex irritans*), and it therefore seldom happens that flea-borne plague will travel from one person to another.

Feeding fleas transfer *Y. pestis* from rat to rat or from rat to human. The flea lives in the rat's fur and feeds on blood through the skin. When the flea is on an infected rat, it draws *Y. pestis* into its own stomach with the blood it ingests. In turn, the plague bacterium multiplies in the flea's stomach, eventually plugging it with live bacteria. The flea, which can no longer swallow fresh blood, regurgitates live bacteria when next it tries to feed, and those bacteria pass through the break in the skin's surface. The flea defecates as it attempts to feed, and this provides another source for infective material.

When the host rat dies and its body cools, the blocked or engorged flea moves on to the next living creature available. If that creature is human, the flea will bite in an effort to feed, thereby introducing *Y. pestis* into the human bloodstream. A bubonic infection follows. Rats are the essential plague incubators. Even humans dying of plague have too little of the bacterial agent in their bloodstreams to continue the infective chain, and modern physicians believe that plague victims can be nursed in an open ward without danger. The exceptions are patients with pneumonic plague, where the bacteria have entered the lungs (rather than remaining in the bloodstream) to be expelled in droplets with every breath or cough. Pneumonic plague is highly contagious, and it is almost always fatal.

Plague Rats With few exceptions, the history of plague epidemics has been a function of rodent populations, particularly rats. Two types of rat are involved. Both are susceptible to plague infection, but the common house rat, *Rattus rattus*, which is also known as the black rat, ship rat, or plague rat, has been the more dangerous of the two to humans. *R. rattus* is a gregarious creature which probably originated in India or Burma. It is not known when *R. rattus* was transferred from Asia to the eastern Mediterranean, but it may have occurred in the fourth century B.C., when Alexander the Great's empire bridged Asia and Europe. *R. rattus* is not an independent traveler. Its natural range is relatively narrow, and when it does move, it is by some conveyance, most commonly by ship. The evidence of its presence in west Asia and the Nile delta is indirect, but it appears to have been firmly established there by the sixth century A.D. It is thought likely that merchants or returning Crusaders were responsible for bringing *R. rattus* into central and western Europe between the eleventh and thirteenth centuries, as there is incontrovertible evidence of its presence there by the fourteenth century. *R. rattus* remained in Europe until the eighteenth century, when it disappeared for reasons which are still obscure.

The brown field rat, or sewer rat (*Rattus norvegicus*) is larger, stronger, and fiercer than *R. rattus*, but its role as a plague bearer has been less significant. The brown rat avoids people, though it will use human facilities for its burrows, is adventuresome, loves water, and is an excellent swimmer. *R. norvegicus* originated in temperate Asia east of the Caspian. It began moving westward in the eighteenth century, was identified in England in 1728, and was found throughout the Continent two decades later. Whether the brown rat displaced the black rat, whether changes in construction practices made European dwellings less habitable for rats, or whether a combination of environmental and genetic factors was responsible, the rat population in Europe changed. This change coincided with the disappearance of plague as a major European disease, though it must be added that there was a worldwide decline in plague incidence as well.

Plague Symptoms Bubonic plague has shown a stable diagnostic image since its first recorded descriptions. The premonitory symptoms include general discomfort, headache, giddiness, apathy or restlessness, nausea, and pains in the limbs and lower back. Often there are chills and fever with temperatures rising to 103 or 104°F. The pulse is very rapid. Patients tend to deteriorate quickly. In some cases, the disease develops fully in a few hours. At most, it requires a day. Notable external symptoms include a flushed, often bloated face with staring or wandering eyes, dilated nostrils, hot, dry skin, and dry lips. Patients suffer from insomnia, delirium, stupor, and loss of coordination. A staggering gait and jerky, uncontrolled hand movements are classic symptoms and go with vertigo, a hesitant, thick, lisping speech, and memory failure.

The characteristic buboes which give plague its name are most commonly swellings in the lymph nodes in the groin, armpit, and neck. These buboes vary in size from a walnut to a hen's egg—some sources reported swellings the size of a small apple—and are excruciatingly painful. Even a comatose patient may react when they are lightly touched, and historical sources record that pain drove some victims into such a frenzy that they tore off their clothes and rushed into the streets or hurled themselves from rooftops or out of windows. Without treatment, from 60 to 90 percent of those infected die, and death comes in one to five days.

Pneumonic plague is faster and more deadly. Though the premonitory symptoms are similar, the victim soon coughs blood and in a matter of hours, certainly no more than three days, will be dead. Some modern plague specialists identify a third variant, septicemic plague, in which the infection either overwhelms the body's lymphatic defenses or enters the bloodstream directly. This version, like pneumonic plague, is always fatal when untreated.

The History of Plague Western historians know the first pandemic as Justinian's plague because it arrived from lower Egypt or Ethiopia during the reign of Justinian the Great (527–565). Infection became general in the eastern Mediterranean, with the most notable outbreak in 542 in Constantinople, where, according to Procopius of Caesarea, the death rate reached 10,000 per day. It recurred repeatedly during the next five years, though it probably went no farther west than southern France. Contemporary sources recorded as many as 100 million deaths. Edward Gibbon, the great Enlightenment historian of Rome's decline, found these figures "not impossible," and a contemporary chronicle spoke of a terrible depopulation which "turned the country into a desert, and made the habitations of men to become the haunts of wild beasts." Modern historians are rightly skeptical of such reports. Even so, the sixth-century plague probably claimed 20 to 25 percent of the existing population, while the combined effects of social disorder, war, and diseases over the entire period from the sixth to the eighth centuries may have reduced populations by as much as one-half.

Plague in Islam Arab sources also record a series of major plague outbreaks in the seventh century. The newly established Moslem religious leadership declared that the plague was sent by God as a mercy and a martyrdom for the faithful, an invitation to Paradise. For the infidel, the plague was simply a horrible death with no hope for the world beyond. The faithful should therefore face the plague with equanimity, especially as the disease could not be contagious—it had been sent by God to take only those whom God intended to claim. The religious explanations stopped short of prohibiting treatment of plague victims, and Arab medical literature, like that in the medieval west, developed a vocabulary for describing plague, an etiology for the disease, some preventive measures, and recommended treatments for the stricken.

Plague in Asia The picture of the plague's first appearance in east Asia is fragmentary and unsatisfactory. The best information concerns China, where two compilations on epidemic diseases exist, one made under the Song dynasty (960–1279) by a certain Sima Guang, and the other a section in an encyclopedia compiled in 1726. Bubonic plague was common in Guangdong province, a region served by the port city of Guangzhou, but it was seldom met in the interior. Thus it appears that bubonic plague came to China by sea, possibly arriving as much as two generations after it attacked the Mediterranean. In 762 the Chinese coastal provinces sustained a severe bubonic outbreak with characteristically high mortality. One contemporary estimated that it carried off over half the population of Shandong province, and there were recurrent epidemics into the first decade of the ninth century. It is also possible, though by no means certain, that there was plague in Japan between 800 and 810.

The plague's effects in China paralleled those in the west. There was a significant drop in population, with particularly heavy losses in the southern maritime provinces, though diseases other than plague were active as well. Moreover, Buddhism, imported from India, became well-established during the plague era, offering a comforting influence not unlike that of Christianity and Islam.

The Black Death The black death, which initiated the second wave of plague infection, is historically the best known plague and the one that has been the most thoroughly studied. Though contemporary soures located the origin of the black death on China's inner frontiers, modern historians have begun to consider the Caspian region as the active center from which the disease may have sprung. Passage through the grasslands was very slow, moving from one rodent colony to the next contiguous one. Occasional contacts with human settlements resulted in sporadic outbreaks, but the disease did not appear with epidemic force until 1346, when it broke out among the Tatars engaged in expelling Italian merchants from the Crimea. Gabriel de Mussis, a contemporary chronicler, though not an eye witness, told how the Christians took refuge in the citadel at Kaffa (Feodosia), where the Tatars beseiged them. Plague forced the Tatars to raise the siege, but before withdrawing, they used catapults to lob the corpses of plague victims over the citadel walls. Plague then broke out among the Christians, and when they fled by ship, the plague traveled with them into the Mediterranean.

It would be incorrect to take this story as a literal explanation for the introduction of bubonic plague to the west, but it does dramatize the importance of trade and war in spreading plague infestation. Shipborne rats and fleas carried plague along commercial routes to establish it in Sicily and southern Italy and then in Genoa and Venice. Sicily was the transfer point for diffusing plague to north Africa, Sardinia, Corsica, and the Spanish coast. Venice, Genoa, and later Pisa were the portals through which it passed into central and northern Italy, France, Germany, the Scandinavian countries, and England. Eventually the plague reached Moscow by way of western Europe and the Hansa ports.

Bubonic plague arrived in Europe at a time when natural and human problems had reached a crisis. By the fourteenth century, population growth had outstripped the productive capacity of the late medieval economy, bringing underemployment, social and political instability, poverty, disease, and famine. These conditions created an environment which maximized the plague's impact, and most historians now accept the plague's role in destroying traditional political authority, thinning out existing oligarchies, leveling feudal barriers to economic growth, and creating an instant demand for labor which had to be satisfied from a drastically reduced work force. In effect, the fourteenth-century plague intensified the action of powerful structural forces which were turning Europe toward modernity.

The black death was particularly severe. Contemporary accounts spoke of a stunning mortality. Boccaccio believed that more than 100,000 persons died in Florence between March and June 1348, while the pope was told that exactly 42,836,486 Europeans perished. Such figures convey the contemporary belief in massive losses and are symbolically rather than statistically significant. Cities were especially hard-hit. Venice, whose figures are more reliable than most, lost 600 persons a day at the peak of the epidemic; modern historians estimate that such towns as Florence, Siena, Orvieto, and San Gimignano probably lost from 50 to 60 percent of their pre-epidemic populations. Plague incidence, however, was very uneven. Where some communities were devastated, others were untouched. Moreover, general population figures are difficult to establish with any certainty. It is, therefore, extremely hard to arrive at any credible mortality figures for Europe as a whole. Estimates that half Europe's population perished are probably as exaggerated as the pope's 42 million, but there is good reason to believe that at least 25 percent of Europe's population died, and 30 percent is not improbable.

Plague in Early Modern Europe During the next 300 years, the plague returned again and again. Centers of infection capable of generating epidemics were established, and the rhythms of plague outbreaks reflected the changing seasons of the year as well as the cycles of bacterial, rodent, and insect life. Although an extraordinary number of mortalities continued to occur, the mortality reinforcement from repeated attacks in the same areas, which characterized the black death, was uncommon. Hence long-term or structural changes in population and social institutions were exceptional, and where they are suspected of occurring, they almost always correspond with changes developing from more deeply rooted trends in the society.

England suffered a succession of plague outbreaks in the fifteenth, sixteenth, and seventeenth centuries, ending with the great plague of London in 1665, whose total death toll reached 68,596. There were, however, no further epidemic outbreaks, and after 1679 plague entirely disappeared from the English bills of mortality. On the European continent, fifteenth-century outbreaks were especially severe in Spain and Italy. Germany, Holland, Italy, and Spain all had heavy plague infections in the first half of the sixteenth century, while Moscow had a particularly severe outbreak in 1572 in which 200,000 deaths were reported for the city and the region. That same year, Mediterranean Europe underwent a new general outbreak which moved northward into the Hapsburg lands and finally Germany.

Plague incidence dropped in the course of the seventeenth century, though in 1656 Naples suffered one of the worst of all recorded epidemics, in which 300,000 people died in just five months. In the first quarter of the eighteenth century, plague was active in Istanbul, the Danubian basin, Poland, Galicia, and the Ukraine. It appeared for the last time in Germany, Scandinavia, and Austria in 1713, with Vienna suffering a major outbreak. After 1714, the year of the great February hurricane, plague was seen no more in central and northern Europe. The last severe western outbreak occurred in the south of France between 1720 and 1722. This was a particularly virulent epidemic which took an estimated 50,000 lives in Marseilles and two-thirds of the population of Toulon. For the rest of the eighteenth century, however, the Mediterranean and eastern Europe were the main areas of suffering. There was a serious epidemic in Kiev in 1770, and in 1771 Moscow underwent the last of the great European plague outbreaks.

The Middle East, Africa, and Asia The Middle East suffered equally with Europe from plague. It attacked north Africa, Egypt, Iraq, Iran, and the Asian as well as European holdings of the Ottoman empire. Istanbul had repeated outbreaks, and through the middle of the nineteenth century, Turkish territories remained the center of plague infection which was closest to Europe. There was also, however, a gradual decline in the frequency and severity of the attacks. Istanbul had its last outbreak in 1841, and by 1843 the plague had disappeared from the Turkish borderlands and Armenia. The last attack in Egypt came in 1845, and north Africa was free of plague by 1873. There were scattered outbreaks, however, in western Arabia, Mesopotamia, and Kurdistan.

Although the sources on it are scant, the plague appears to have been epidemic during the seventeenth and eighteenth centuries in China, India, and southeast Asia, but with a declining incidence. India, after heavy outbreaks in the fifteenth and sixteenth centuries, appears to have become plague-free by the end of the seventeenth century. One hundred years later, new outbreaks occurred at Cutch, Gujarat, and Kathyawar, and from 1836 to 1838 in Rajputava. These were isolated incidents, however, and by the middle of the nineteenth century the second great wave of plague outbreaks was finished.

Plague in Modern Times The third wave of plague infection started out from endemic centers in China between 1856 and 1866 and had its most serious effects in east Asia, though outbreaks also occurred in western Asia, Egypt, and north Africa. This wave had no effects in Europe, but it established plague among wild rodents in the western United States. Precisely when this happened is not certain, though it was no earlier than 1866 and may well have been as late as 1894. In that year, the third wave of plague infection reached the Chinese coast in Guangdong province, appearing in the ports of Guangzhou, Hong Kong, and Beihai. Once into the arteries of coastal trade, it spread northward, breaking out in southern Manchuria in 1899 and appearing in Fujian in 1901. The Fujian epidemic was extremely serious. The disease moved along inland waterways until every country in the province was infected. It remained active over the next three decades. Intensive campaigns with rat-killing pesticides and DDT were finally successful in controlling human plague in this area, and by 1950, Wenzhou was the only major port where it was still reported.

Away from the coastal regions, there were severe outbreaks of pneumonic plague in 1910 and 1911 and 1920 and 1921 in northern Manchuria. Inexperienced hunters became infected when they harvested plague-infected wild rodents. These outbreaks, though destroying whole communities, did not become endemic, and the plague soon disappeared. Both Inner and Outer Mongolia suffered periodic plague outbreaks, as did the northwest provinces of China proper. In 1931, for example, some 20,000 people died in Shanxi and Shaanxi provinces, though the disease then faded away. Other outbreaks during the period occurred in Yunnan province, with a particularly bad epidemic beginning in 1939. In 1941 it was charged that Japan deliberately introduced plague at Changde, Hunan province. If the charge is true, the effort proved unsuccessful. There was an epizootic in 1942, and perhaps 100 human cases were reported. By 1943, however, the plague had entirely disappeared.

Burma, Indochina, Thailand, Java, and India had varying experiences. Plague was very serious in Indochina but much less so in Thailand and Burma. Java, however, suffered heavy losses in 1910 and 1911, while the annual plague mortalities from 1920 to 1927 ran between 8000 and 10,000. The year 1934, when 23,239 deaths were reported, was Java's worst plague year. By 1942, only 339 cases were reported, although there was an increase after World War II. India was especially hard hit. Between 1898 and 1948, India suffered over 12.5 million plague deaths, an annual mortality of nearly 0.25 million. The early losses were most severe, with over 6 million deaths recorded between 1898 and 1908, and 4.25 million between 1909 and 1918. Plague has steadily declined in India since 1918, and with improving control devices in cities, bubonic plague in India has become essentially a rural disease with hut-dwelling commensal rats the main carriers and *Xenopsylla cheopis* the primary vector. This differs notably from western Asia, where plague is endemic in the mountains of Kurdistan among wild rodents. *X. cheopis* is again the primary vector, but there appear to be no rats. It is from this center that plague moved through Persian and Turkish Kurdistan, Mesopotamia, and Iran to Syria.

In Africa, Egypt was relatively plague-free through the second half of the nineteenth century, but the disease was reimported from Asia in 1900. The plague was less serious here than in China or India. Between 1899 and 1930, there were 19,386 cases reported, with 10,272 deaths. Plague was most active in upper Egypt rather than the lower region and the port cities, and it largely disappeared between 1930 and 1941. There was some plague in Suez during World War II, but Egypt has been comparatively plague-free since then. Finally, though Uganda was probably the oldest endemic plague center in Africa, the disease has been in decline there as well. Conditions in South America are similar to those in the western United States. Infection of wild rodents came relatively late, and so far there have been no major outbreaks in the human population, though cases are on record of sporadic infection.

Western Society and the Plague The horrors which attended plague have left us graphic evidences, from pictures and cartoons to the hundreds of plague monuments which dot central European landscapes. Early modern plague literature, from Boccaccio to Defoe, portrayed societies confronting a total moral breakdown; Boccaccio is particularly affecting as he describes how parents abandoned children, or servants fled their masters. The workers who remained were too few to do what had to be done; hence, funeral customs collapsed. Corpses were tumbled into the streets to be hauled away and buried in huge pits. Brigandage was common, and no one was safe from the so-called body gatherers, the scavengers employed to collect and dispose of corpses. Armed with special powers, they demanded bribes in exchange for protection, and, when they were dissatisfied or rejected, they broke into houses to rob, murder, and rape. Some preventive measures were as terrible as the disease they were intended to prevent. In Milan, for example, plague victims were walled up in their houses or abandoned in open fields to die.

With the passage of time, however, the horrors dissipated, and reactions became routinized. Nonetheless, a city in the grip of plague was a fearsome sight, with palls of smoke hanging over it from fumigations and the fires which burned up victims' belongings, while death carts creaked and rumbled through the streets. Physicians and plague inspectors stalked through the gloom wearing masks which gave them the look of predatory birds. Flight was always the individual's most effective preventive measure, and infected zones became entirely depopulated. Problems of robbery and murder remained serious, but in later epidemics the panic which attended the black death became less common.

Anti-Semitism When plague first appeared, people blamed their enemies for propagating it. These convictions began with belief in the Devil as the source of evil, but they ended by finding human scapegoats who were thought to do the

Devil's work. Even before plague reached Europe, lepers had been denounced for poisoning wells, and the lepers in their turn denounced the Jews. When the epidemics began, this was remembered. Jews were accused of responsibility for plague outbreaks, and the result was a wave of anti-Semitic violence which was not surpassed until the twentieth century.

The persecutions began in May 1348, in southern France, when the Jews of Narbonne and Carcasson were literally exterminated. As the plague spread, anti-Jewish feeling mounted. Jews were tried at Chillon for poisoning wells. Confessions were extracted under torture, and these confessions were then widely circulated and raised the intensity of violence. In Basel, Jews were herded into a wooden building and burned alive; at Strasbourg, 16,000 Jews were reported killed, with 2,000 murdered on St. Valentine's Day alone; while in Mainz, where the Jews resisted, 12,000 were said to have been slaughtered. The religious order of Flagellants, who did public penance in the hope of appeasing God's wrath, identified the Jews as instruments of the Antichrist and incited the total destruction of Frankfurt's Jewish quarter. By the end of 1351, 60 large and 150 smaller Jewish settlements had been obliterated, and some 350 individual massacres have been identified in which tens of thousands died.

Prevention and Control Whether God or Allah was said to have willed the plague, its spread was believed to be miasmal or atmospheric, and through direct human contact. In the early days, it was not unusual to find these explanations linked together. The theory of contagion (q.v.) may well have gained early adherents as a result of experience with pneumonic plague, and contagionist theories were strengthened by the way plague concentrated its attack. When whole groups of people sickened, it was natural to believe that the first to fall had infected the rest. One fourteenth-century observer noted, "The contagious nature of the disease is indeed the most terrible of all the terrors, for when anyone who is infected by it dies, all who see him in his sickness, or visit him, or do any business with him, or even carry him to the grave, quickly follow him thither."

The miasmists laid the appearance of plague to "a corruption of the air . . . visible in the form of mist or smoke . . . spreading over the land." If one followed Galen, such a miasma generated an energizing spirit, or *pneuma*, which was carried through the atmosphere and entered the body, where it spread to all the vital organs. The cause for miasma was said to be the putrefaction of unburied corpses or, more generally, "putrid" fumes arising from any decaying matter. Other causes included natural disturbances, irregularity in the progression of the seasons, sharp temperature fluctuations, strong winds from a dangerous quarter, and astrological events.

The techniques advised for avoiding plague reflected contemporary interpretations of its dynamics. The miasmal theorist identified dark, crowded areas as dangerous and recommended sheltered, dry, light, and airy resorts. Burial was mandatory. Venice stipulated that all graves for plague victims had to be at least five feet deep, and beggars were prohibited from exhibiting plague corpses in their quest for alms. Streets were cleared of refuse, personal cleanliness was stressed, and people were encouraged to move slowly to avoid exhaustion and to restrain those passions which led to overeating, drunkenness, and sexual indulgence. As preventives, they were advised to suck pomegranates or sour plums, to eat lentils, Indian peas, or pumpkin seeds, and to drink lemon, pomegranate, and onion juices. Pickled onions were considered healthful at breakfast, as were eggs with vinegar, though not hard-boiled. The safest houses were believed to be those facing north, away from the dangerous south wind, and windows were to be glazed or covered. Burning dry, highly scented woods such as juniper, ash, vine and rosemary was considered healthful, as were such aromatics as wood of aloes, amber, musk, cypress, laurel, and mastic. In fact, none of the recommended substances had any practical effect, with the possible exception of a disinfectant containing sulfur, arsenic, and antimony, but the rest at least combated odors and gave their users a sense of doing something in their own behalf.

Some specifics against plague were complex, and others were expensive. A mixture of 10-year-old treacle with chopped-up snakes, wine, and 50-odd additional ingredients was one of the more complicated, while a mixture of powdered emeralds and gold dust was one of the more expensive (and dangerous) prescriptions. Bleeding was in favor, as was the curious conviction that the stench of human waste was protective. Some people sat for hours with their heads hanging over the latrine to inhale the richly fetid smells. Soothing potions helped to reduce the pain of the buboes and other sores or eruptions on the body, and some physicians believed in opening and cauterizing the buboes when they became "ripe" in four to seven days. Since nothing was really effective, the best physicians could offer was some comfort. Unfortunately, their ministrations more commonly increased debilitation and pain.

Quarantines Local authorities treated the plague as if contagion had been proved, and those responses remained an established pattern into the nineteenth century. Early in 1348, vessels suspected of carrying plague were turned away from some Italian ports, but it was Venice which codified the first systematic quarantine policy, on March 20, 1348. The Venetians closed their port to all suspected vehicles, travelers, and ships for a period of 40 days. Other cities used similar procedures. In 1374, Visconti Duke Bernabo ordered Milan cleared of all plague victims, while new arrivals in the city, together with attendants for the sick, were held for 14 days in isolation. Three years later, Ragusa invoked a regulation ordering travelers from plague zones to be isolated and observed for 30 days; this period later was extended to 40. In 1383, Marseilles established a 40-day quarantine, and in subsequent years, most communities experimented with various exclusions and measures of isolation.

By the seventeenth century, the techniques and policies for fighting plague had become routine over much of Europe, with emphasis on isolating those already sick while trying to exclude further infection with more or less rigorous quarantine regulations. Observance of the rules tended to be perfunctory, as experience taught what seemed to be dangerous. Thus, while physicians and plague officials covered themselves to avoid contamination on their rounds, most people showed no fear of returning to where the plague had been, using the possessions of the deceased, and even sleeping in their unchanged beds. There was a distinct class bias to plague infection. The well-to-do, who were better housed and less commonly exposed to rat fleas, were also much more mobile and free to leave plague areas. They were further benefited by plague regulations which paid little heed to egress but concentrated on preventing entrance.

The Modern Era In the nineteenth century, the medical tide turned, beginning with the pioneering work of Louis Pasteur and Robert Koch, who established the bacterial causes for many diseases. When plague reached the Chinese coast in 1893 and 1894, teams of investigators, trained in their methods were sent to study it, and the search turned immediately toward finding a bacteriological cause. The discovery was made simultaneously and independently by Alexandre Yersin, a French-Swiss bacteriologist who trained under Pasteur and who had worked on anthrax with P. P. E. Roux, and by a Japanese physician, Shibasaburo Kitasato, who had studied with Koch and Emil Behring. Yersin noted in his diary for June 23, 1894, that he looked for and found the plague organism in the corpses of dead rats, and in his formal report he concluded that plague was contagious, that it could be controlled by inoculation, and that rats were the principal vector. Yersin's drawings and descriptions make it clear that he had, indeed, discovered the bacterium causing plague. Kitasato first disagreed with and then later accepted Yersin's descriptions, and his reports show that he too had discovered what Yersin named *Pasteurella pestis*.

Yersin's identification of the rat's role was less easily accepted, and his recommendations for a campaign to control rats were only gradually developed. By 1905, however, the supporting evidence was in, and a joint advisory committee of the Royal Society and the Lister Institute was working on plague rats and bacteria. They also began studying rat fleas. The idea that the flea was the plague vector was offered in 1897 by both P. L. Simond and M. Ogatia, and it was accepted as a basis for research by 1905. Still not understood were the mechanics of passing the infectious agent from one host to another. The critical mechanisms of blocking and regurgitation were finally established by A. W. Bacot and C. J. Martin in 1914. With this epochal discovery, the central mystery of bubonic plague stood revealed.

No effective measures for controlling or curing plague appeared until the causal agent was known. Then, for nearly 30 years, vaccination was the primary method. Eighteenth-century attempts to immunize against plague had been unsuccessful, and the idea had faded away. In 1894 and 1895, Alexandre Yersin and his associates successfully immunized rabbits against plague, and a year later, the famed Russian physician and medical scientist Waldemar M. W. Haffkine established the standard method for plague immunization until the appearance of live vaccines. The Haffkine vaccine often produced a violent reaction which occasionally incapacitated the recipient, but it also reduced plague mortality by 20 to 30 percent.

Live vaccines, which seemed effective and which avoided reactions, were developed in Java and Madagascar in the early 1930s, but killed vaccines remained important. When World War II broke out, the U.S. government vaccinated all its armed forces with killed vaccines, but the other Allies, Russia included, used live vaccines. The war experiences validated both. By the end of the war, no American bubonic plague deaths had been reported despite service in plague-infested areas while the British lost just five men to plague in their Middle East force. Since World War II, aerosols and oral administration have provided a speedy alternative for immunizing large numbers of people in a short period of time. Vaccination, to be effective, requires a series of injections over a nine-month period.

Modern rodenticides and pesticides have greatly enlarged the potential for stopping a plague attack. At the time Yersin identified rats as plague bearers, the means for killing the animals were limited. Hunting them was never effective, and while such poisons as arsenic, cyanide, and strychnine do kill rats, they kill people and domestic animals as well. Three highly effective rodenticides were developed during World War II: 1080 (sodium monofluoroacetate), ANTU (alphanaphthylthiourea), and warfarin. 1080, though effective, is dangerous; ANTU, though not very toxic to humans, is deadly for dogs, cats, and pigs; but warfarin, which was synthesized in 1948, is both effective and safe, though it has the disadvantage of being very slow-acting. DDT (dichlorodiphenyltrichloroethane), which was developed in 1938, has proved as deadly for plague fleas as for lice and mosquitoes, and in Peru in 1945, it was effective in halting a plague outbreak by destroying rat fleas. DDT, which infiltrates the food chain and affects plant and animal life in adverse ways, is not immediately dangerous and can be called nontoxic. When freely used as an agricultural insecticide, however, it has produced significant environmental side effects, and this has led to restrictions on its general use.

Rodenticides, insecticides, and vaccines have greatly increased humankind's capacity for fighting plague, and there have been developments in treatment as well. In 1896 Alexandre Yersin created a therapeutic serum by immunizing horses. This and similar serums remained the sole means for effecting plague cures until the discovery of sulfonamides (q.v.). Sulfanilamide was developed in 1908 as a dye, but it was not until 1932 that sulfonamide compounds were used medically, and they were not used against plague until 1938. Once introduced, they were very effective, reducing mortality among those treated from 40 or 50 percent to 10 percent. Even septicemic plague responded, and the death rate dropped from over 90 percent to between 20 and 50 percent. In 1928, penicillin appeared to promise a weapon against plague, but though it destroyed plague bacilli in the laboratory, penicillin was ineffectual when the bacillus was in the body. However, streptomycin, discovered in 1941, proved deadly to *Y. pestis*, and while there were problems to be resolved in dosage and timing, this substance was the first to be effective against pneumonic as well as septicemic and bubonic plague. By 1950, two more antimicrobials, the tetracyclines and chloramphenicals, supplemented streptomycin.

Conclusion In the last quarter of the twentieth century, sporadic plague outbreaks have continued to occur, and plague remains endemic through the western United States, on the China-India border, in southeast Asia, and in central Africa. Moreover, recent evidence strongly suggests that *Y. pestis* can develop strains resistant to the currently available antimicrobials, while the very breadth of infection among commensal and wild rodents makes any thought of eradication impractical. Nevertheless, it is unlikely that modern man will be forced to relive the experiences which accompanied Justinian's plague or the black death. On the other hand, in a world as uncertain and as interconnected as the modern world, nobody can rule out the possibility that either a cataclysmic war or a succession of natural disasters will break down the public health systems which form society's primary defenses against disease. Nor is it impossible that the still-obscure mechanisms which generate virulent plague will again be activated. Either situation could produce a significant increase in plague incidence. Together, they could have catastrophic results.

ADDITIONAL READINGS: John T. Alexander, *Bubonic Plague in Early Modern Russia*, Baltimore and London, 1980; D. H. S. Davis, A. F. Hallet, and M. Isaacson, "Plague," in W. T. Hubbert, W. F. McCulloch, and P. R. Schnurrenberger (eds.), *Disease Transmitted from Animals to Man*, Springfield, Ill., 1975; Michael W. Dols, *The Black Death in the Middle East*, Princeton, 1977; Alan D. Dyer, "The Influence of the Bubonic Plague in England," *Journal of the History of Medicine and Allied Sciences* (July 1978): 308–326; Robert S. Gottfried, *The Black Death: Natural and Human Disaster in Medieval Europe*, New York and London, 1983; Charles T. Gregg, *Plague!*, New York, 1978; L. F. Hirst, *The Conquest of Plague: A Study of the Evolution of Epidemiology*, Oxford, 1953; Charles F. Mullett, *The Bubonic Plague and England: An Essay in the History of Preventive Medicine*, Lexington, Ky., 1956; John Norris, "East or West? The Geographic Origin of the Black Death," *Bulletin of the History of Medicine* 51, 1 (1977): 1–24; R. Pollitzer, *Plague*, Geneva, 1954; J. F. D. Shrewsbury, *A History of Bubonic Plague in the British Isles*, Cambridge, 1971; Philip Ziegler, *The Black Death*, New York, 1969.

Cancer

Although cancer is a disease of great antiquity, it is also preeminently a modern disease. Its rising incidence and mortality in industrialized societies of the twentieth century owe a debt both to those societies' success in controlling other diseases, with a consequent increase in the average age of the population, and to the environmental dangers which are inherent in technologically sophisticated civilizations. Since World War II, cancer has been a primary target for intensive research which has enlarged understanding of cancer's epidemiology and has produced improved diagnostic and therapeutic techniques. Nevertheless, the essential question of why cancer occurs when and where it does remains unanswered. Most authorities believe that cancer's secrets will eventually be revealed, but until that time, the best that medicine can do is to give cancer sufferers the longest possible period of survival under acceptable conditions of life.

The Disease "Cancer" is the term used to define any condition arising from the uncontrolled division and multiplication of cells. It is a condition which occurs in all living forms. The uncontrolled division and multiplication of cells result in two basic types of tumor, or neoplasm, called benign and malignant. A benign tumor remains localized where it originally occurred; a malignant tumor has the power to metastasize, that is, to communicate itself beyond its point of occurrence and thus produce malignancies elsewhere in the body. Malignancies are responsible for the high mortality in cancer cases.

The classification of neoplasms begins with the location of the condition. Carcinomas are neoplasms which occur on the skin, in lining tissues, and in organs. Sarcomas are tumors of bone, muscle, or connective tissue, while leukemias involve bone marrow and the white corpuscles of the blood. Lymphomas are associated with lymph nodes. Depending on the system of classification used, there are 100 or more types of cancer, and they may appear in nearly any part of the body.

Nothing comparable to the bacteriological explanation for infective diseases is in sight for cancer, but it is possible to identify certain conditions which are favorable to cancer growth. Many substances have been shown to be cancer-causing. Soot was one of the earliest carcinogenic agents to be identified. It was found to be responsible for a high incidence of cancer of the scrotum among eighteenth-century chimney sweeps. Other related carcinogens are tars, pitch, and industrial oils. Aniline dyes have cancer-causing properties, while radiation exposure is a certain and highly dangerous cancer cause. Soon after x-rays came into use, it was noticed that ionizing radiation produced severe irritation on skin surfaces, and later it was proved that people working with x-rays, radium, or radioactive material had a high cancer rate. Diagnostic and therapeutic uses for x-rays have also been implicated, and it is not uncommon for cancer treatment with radioisotopes to generate additional cancerous conditions.

The development of atomic power has significantly enlarged the problem of cancer from radiation exposure. Studies of the victims of the American atomic attacks on Hiroshima and Nagasaki in Japan provide overwhelming evidence of the correlation between radiation exposure and cancer. Persons located 1¼ miles from the blast center had 3 times the normal incidence of leukemia, while those who were only ¾ mile from the blast center had a leukemia incidence 20 times the normal rate.

Other materials or activities known to cause cancer include cigarette smoking, nutritional deficiencies, alcohol abuse (which has been linked with cancer of the larynx), and overexposure to the direct rays of the sun. Some cancer causes are as commonplace as ill-fitting false teeth. Mouth cancer has also been traced to the Indian practice of smoking a cigar or cigarette with the burning end in the mouth. A high incidence of abdominal skin cancer has been found in Kashmir, where people will hold a pot of coals against their stomachs to ward off the cold.

Before the twentieth century, cancer was diagnosed most readily in females, leading to the conclusion that women were more susceptible than men. In 1969, however, in a study of cancer mortality in 24 countries, the rate for men per 100,000 of population was 181.8; the rate for women was 150.8. The most common cause of cancer death among men was lung cancer (41.7 per 100,000), followed by stomach cancer at 31.9. Breast cancer was responsible for the highest rate among women (23.9 per 100,000), followed by stomach cancer at 21.6. In 1969, women died of lung cancer at the low 7.6 rate, though that figure is rising now. In all living things, cancer tends to appear later rather than earlier, though leukemias and lymphomas are most serious for ages 5 to 15. It is now thought that advancing age reduces the effectiveness of the immunological system and contributes to a rise in cancer incidence. It is clear that where life expectancy has increased, more cancer has appeared. The highest cancer incidence and mortality fall in the age group 40–65, while 80 percent of deaths from the five major types of cancer occur in people 55 years of age or older.

With greater life expectancy and increased environmental hazards, there has been a dramatic overall increase in cancer mortalities in advanced societies. In 1930, in the United States, the death rate from cancer stood at 112 per 100,000 of population. In 1968 it had reached 130. On the other hand, the survival rate also has improved. In 1930, less than one person in five lived five years after cancer was diagnosed. By the end of the 1950s that figure had reached one person in three. Early diagnosis and treatment have a significant effect on certain types of cancer. The five-year survival rate with skin cancer, the easiest to diagnose early and the most accessible for treatment, is 90 percent. But even in lung cancer, the five-year survival rate is 29 percent when the cancer is found and treated while still localized. That rate drops to 9 percent when regional involvement has occurred. Breast cancer has a five-year survival rate of 85 percent when treated while localized, but that figure drops to 53 percent when regional involvement has taken place.

There are now three basic treatments for cancer: surgery, radiation treatment, and chemotherapy. Surgery is the oldest and most common, though by itself it almost never cures a cancer. This is because surgery usually is performed when the tumor is apparent and therefore has probably metastasized. The exception is cervical cancers, which, given early identification, are considered 90 percent curable by surgery. Surgery also appears to strengthen immunological defenses.

Radiation treatment is often used with surgery. It is effective in slowing tumor growth so that surgery can be performed, and in the case of Hodgkin's disease it has been used to effect cures. Radiation treatment is also valuable for treating cancer of the cervix, prostate and testicles, small breast tumors, and some nasopharyngeal tumors.

The third form of treatment, chemotherapy, has developed since World War II. It uses chemical agents to inhibit cell development, and while it is, with radiation treatment, largely palliative once dispersion has occurred, it is effective against leukemias and lymphoses. The best hope for the immediate future is improved chemotherapy supported by radiation treatment. The more distant hope appears to lie with immunotherapy, which even now can offer some assistance to natural resistance in a cancer-attacked organism.

Early History Living creatures have suffered cancer from the earliest times. Traces of tumors have been found in dinosaurs from the Cretaceous Age as well as in a Pleistocene cave bear. Egyptian mummies from the third to fifth dynasties (ca. 3000–2500 B.C.) display evidence of neoplasms. There are similar indications in Inca remains from about 500 B.C. The Edwin Smith papyrus of Egypt (dating from ca. 1660 B.C.) deals with surgery and summarizes earlier treatises. It speaks of a "bulging tumor of the breast" for which there is no cure. The Ebers papyrus (ca. 1550 B.C.) describes a "large," "loathsome tumor" which generates pustules and which may rise "as though the wind were in it." Such tumors are said to be better left alone. Some modern authorities suggest that the papyrus describes a tropical ulcer or gas gangrene. However, the description also fits Kaposi's sarcoma, a neoplastic entity known to be endemic to the region. Other Egyptian medical fragments show familiarity with accessible tumors which can be removed surgically or cauterized and suggest palliatives to ease the suffering from stomach or uterine cancers.

After the sixth century B.C., cancer is mentioned regularly in European medical literature. The treatment recommended varies with the dominant system of medical thought. The actual incidence of cancer before the nineteenth century remains a mystery. But physicians had enough experience with the condition to classify it, to propose procedures for treating it, to describe its varied clinical characteristics, and to be skeptical about prognosis. This suggests that cancer with visible manifestations was met often.

The most commonly diagnosed cancers appeared in women. Breast cancer was the archetypal form whose massy profile, spreading filaments, and swollen veins, like legs and feelers, suggest the appearance of a crab. Hence the Greek *karcinos* (cancer, or the crab). Cancers were crablike in other ways. The exterior surface was thought comparable to the texture of the crab's shell; the condition was persistent, literally refusing to let go; while the pain was like sharp claws seizing hold in the depths of the body.

Cancer and the Humors Cancer's history as a concept began in Greece, and it found its first significant expression in the writings ascribed to Hippocrates of Cos. A variety of terms—"phyma," "oidema," "karkinos," and "karkinoma"—is used to identify different kinds of growths or swellings. There is no sure way of telling which ones were cancerous by modern definition. The conditions described were thought to result from an accumulation of black bile, the melancholic humor. Superficial growths or swellings which were easily accessible could be cut out or cauterized. But conditions deep within the system, the so-called occult growths, were to be left alone, since the patient would live longer with the disease untouched. Various palliatives to reduce pain were recommended, but the occult growths were considered to be infallibly fatal.

Although Hippocratic medicine introduced a humoral physiology, it was the Roman physician Galen of Pergamum who codified it in the second century A.D. He held that inflammation occurred when there was a flow of humors (q.v.) to any part of the body. The type of inflammation which resulted showed which humor was responsible. Most commonly, the humors were carried in the flow of blood called to a particular site by wounds, contusions, fractures, or any other event which caused swelling and inflammation. A tumor could also develop because there was too much blood in the veins. A flux of black bile mixed with the blood produced a scirrhus, a type of tumor which could cause or be converted into a cancer. A flux of black bile unmixed with blood produced cancers directly. Galen believed that cancers could occur in any part of the body but that they were most common in the female breast. He considered surgery effective so long as all the tumor was removed, but he repeated Hippocrates's warnings against attempting to treat deep, occult, or hidden cancers.

After Galen synthesized humoral doctrine, subsequent writers repeated his agruments and fitted their information into his system for nearly 1500 years. In the fourteenth century, for example, John of Arderne, who has been called the father of English surgery, described a rectal carcinoma, or bubo, which he considered "nothing more than a hidden cancer." He also reported that he never "saw nor heard of any man that was cured" of this condition, but he did know many that had died of it. At the end of the fifteenth century, Antonio Benivieni, who did his work in Florence and contributed to the foundations of morbid anatomy, gave a detailed description of a stomach cancer; and in 1553, Giovanni Filippo Ingrassi published a list of tumors, though without any basis for classifying them. In the late sixteenth century, professor of medicine at Basel Felix Plater (Platter) did an autopsy on a knight whose behavior for two years prior to his death had become increasingly irrational. Plater found a brain tumor which, he argued, caused the knight's mental problems. As the tumor enlarged, so Plater theorized, it compressed the brain, interfering with the venous system and thus producing irrational actions. In the early seventeenth century, Gaspare Aselli of Padua identified lacteal fluid in lymph channels. This contributed a physiological basis for the long-postulated lymphatic involvement in breast cancers, directed attention to lymph nodes, and made lymphatic drainage a consideration in proposing more extensive surgical resections. Hieronymus Fabricius recommended the removal of lymph nodes in mastectomies and developed a specialized surgical tool for the operation. Finally, a small book published in 1700 by Deshaies Gendron argued against the prevalent humoral doctrine on cancer causes. Cancers, in his view, were not inflammatory masses composed of "fluted humors" but were solid structures which were created out of nervous, glandular, and lymphatic vascular parts to form a compact, uniform, and cancerous substance capable of destructive growth. Gendron built his argument on clinical studies and observation of cancerous materials. His break with nearly 2000 years of medical tradition had no influence at all, however, and his work remained (and remains) largely unknown.

Cell Theory and Cancer In the eighteenth century, cancer was still considered the most unfavorable outcome of inflammation. Inflammation generally was believed to occur when a mixture of "liquid lymph" or "salty serum and gelatinous lymph" with true blood was trapped in solid parts of the body. If the fluid contained a "cancerous element," the inflammation would become cancerous. In the later eighteenth century, John Hunter, a Scot who practiced in London, reformulated the traditional view by adding the idea that "coagulating lymph," that is, that part of the blood which clots spontaneously, was the basic formative substance for both healthy and diseased animal tissues. Hunter's coagulable lymph emerged as "blastema" in the first half of the nineteenth century. Blastema, or plastic lymph, was thought to be the fluid, formative substance carried in the blood and circulated to the tissues to provide the material for maintenance, growth, and repair. Blastema was also considered to be the original formative material from which the solid parts of the body were made.

In 1800 and 1801, Marie François Xavier Bichat, a brilliant young French anatomist (who died suddenly in 1802, possibly by accidental infection from an autopsy knife), laid down the principles that all tissue was similar in structure, that each type of tissue was a unit of life capable of reproducing itself, and that tumors, cicatrices, and cysts were not inflammations but an overgrowth of cellular tissue. All tumors were composed of cellular tissue, and they differed only in the character of the "morbid matter" deposited in the cellular base. The ideas of blastema and cellular tissue then were joined to form a physiological concept in which blastema was considered the nutritive, generative substance out of which the cellular structures emerged. Tumors or cancers were thought to result from the introduction of a perverting or exaggerating "principle" which generated destructive growth.

Neither blastema theory nor the concept of cellular tissue was of long duration. Blood's nutritive function was established fact, but the idea that the solid parts of the body developed from a plastic lymph was abandoned by the end of the 1860s. Microscopic lenses with sufficient magnification and resolution to identify cells in normal animal tissues began to be used after 1830, and they provided evidence that the cell actually contained its own generative nucleus. Similarly, cells were identified as the fundamental unit in tumor tissue. Moreover, botanists were finding evidence to reject the fibrous theory of plant structures. Mathias Schleiden concluded that plants were aggregates of cells, and early in 1838 Theodor Schwann carried this idea over to animal tissues, arguing that the cell was the structural unit and the nucleus was the reproductive organ. The latter point was not accepted, but the idea that animals, like plants, were structural aggregates of autonomous cells was gradually accepted.

Johannes Mueller, who was the most influential physiologist of his day in Germany, accepted Schwann's cellular ideas. Ultimately, Schwann and Mueller together framed the cellular concepts which were current at mid-century: Both normal and pathological tissues were aggregates of transformed cells which developed from an amorphous cytoblastema derived from circulating blood. Karl von Rokitansky, head of the department of pathological anatomy at the University of Vienna, attempted a final synthesis of cell theory (see Cells) with humoral doctrines to define the laws of histogenesis. His arguments, however, went beyond what he could demonstrate, leading Rudolf Virchow to refute him in 1846. Mueller supported Virchow's criticisms, and Virchow began to expound the doctrine which became the basis for the modern cellular approach to cancer.

In 1867, Wilhelm Waldeyer published two papers which outlined an approach to cancer pathology which is still current. Blastema theory had disappeared, as had the idea of an outside infective or "corrupting" principle. Cancer cells developed from normal cells, growing and multiplying by cell division. Local spread of cancer cells could occur only by their movement into adjacent tissues. Long-distance spread (metastasis) resulted from the transportation of cancer cells by blood, lymph, or other fluid to another site. The transformation of normal epithelium into cancerous epithelium did not involve cell dissolution, nor could there be any distant transformation of connective tissue cells into epithelial cancer cells. The multiplication of cancer cells would generate or would be accompanied by connective tissue proliferation, while the stroma of some carcinomas could appear as fibrous, fatty, or cartilaginous. All the stated propositions applied with equal force to sarcomas, which are the true connective tissue cancers. Finally, benign growths, whether in epithelial or connective tissue, will arise in their normal respective cell types. Waldeyer's account of the genesis and spread of carcinomas, as one recent authority has said, "is essentially the account that is found in all textbooks of oncology and pathology in use today [1978]."

Science, Society, and Cancer: The Twentieth Century The disappearance of humoralism and the establishment of cell theory provided a solid conceptual foundation for twentieth-century cancer research. The most important work dealt with the acquisition and transfer of neoplasms in plants and laboratory animals, the creation of laboratory techniques for pursuing that work, statistical studies which contributed to the epidemiology of cancer, and research on environmental causes for cancer. Speculative investigations into heredity, sexual behavior, viruses as causal agents, and the applicability of immunological reactions as a control and cure for cancer have opened new horizons.

Germany, closely followed by France and England, was the main center for biological research in the late nineteenth century, but German preeminence failed to outlive World War I. Both France and England retained active research organizations through the years between the World Wars, but neither generated the massive quantities of particularized research which came to be the hallmark of the American scientific community and which had been a feature of German science between 1850 and the Hitler regime. America's domination of oncological research, although prefigured in the 1920s and 1930s, emerged after World War II. This development reflected American economic power, the rapid maturation of the American scientific and academic establishments during the first half of the twentieth century, the dislocations in European culture between 1914 and 1945, including the flight of Jewish scientists and intellectuals from Nazism, and the mounting preoccupation of the American public with health and the eradication of diseases.

Awareness of cancer as a significant social problem in the United States began in the early twentieth century. Statistical studies demonstrated that cancer mortalities were increasing and that early treatment was the only hope. In 1913, prompted by the American Medical Association and the American College of Surgeons, the American Society for the Control of Cancer was formed to educate the American public to the danger signs of cancer and to convince people that "the risk is not in surgery, but in delayed surgery." In May 1913, the *Ladies' Home Journal* carried an article by Samuel Hopkins Adams which was the first of what became millions of words on cancer aimed at the general public. In 1935, the Women's Field Army for the War Against Cancer was established to educate women to cancer's danger signals, and in 1937 this organization played a prominent role in lobbying for government support for cancer research. Congress passed the National Cancer Act in that year. In 1944, the American Society for the Control of Cancer became the American Cancer Society.

There were very few institutions created specifically to treat or study cancer before the twentieth century. The earliest cancer facility was built at Rheims in France in 1740 with funds bequeathed by the canon of the cathedral. In 1791, Samuel Whitbread, the London brewer, endowed a cancer ward at Middlesex Hospital, and in 1828 William Marsden founded the Royal Free and Cancer Hospital in London. With the new century, the situation changed radically as public concern mounted and societies to support cancer studies proliferated. The German Central Committee for Cancer Research was organized in 1900. Two years later the Royal College of Physicians and the Royal College of Surgeons of England founded the Imperial Cancer Research Fund, and the French Association for Cancer Research was organized in 1906. The American Association for Cancer Research was organized in 1907, the same year the Japanese established their Society for Cancer Research. The Memorial Sloan-Kettering Cancer Center in New York City grew up over the first half of the twentieth century, with the Sloan-Kettering endowment made in 1939. The Leningrad Institute for Oncology was founded in 1926, but the largest center for cancer research in the Soviet Union, the Institute of Experimental and Clinical Oncology of the Academy of Medical Sciences of the U.S.S.R., was not established until 1951.

Japan had to reconstruct its program of cancer research after World War II, but in 1953, the Japanese Foundation for Cancer Research began a new program concentrating on cancer from radiation. West Germany was unable to reconstitute a cancer research program until 1964, when the German Cancer Research Center opened at Heidelberg, where the Institute for Experimental Cancer Research had been active since 1906. The Drahji Tata Fund established a cancer research center in 1941 in Bombay. It began to receive public funds in 1947, following India's independence. In 1957 it was brought under the control of the Ministry of Health; in 1962, it was moved again to the Department of Atomic Energy. The Tata Cancer Center accepts some 12,000 cases annually and provides information on cancer in an agrarian, nonindustrial society. Critics consider the center a luxury which the Indian government can ill afford in a country where millions die annually from cholera, malaria, and bubonic plague.

Although private giving was at the base of American cancer studies, public funding has become the main support for cancer research. Individual states such as Texas, Wisconsin, and New York have subsidized cancer research at university-based institutes, while strong federal support has subsidized a national program. In 1937, Congress voted funds to establish a National Cancer Institute of the United States. In October 1939, a research facility was opened. Federal support for cancer research steadily increased from 1937 to 1970, aggregating $2 billion, with the average appropriation level reaching $200 million in 1970. When reductions in cancer funds were threatened by planned reductions in government spending, a powerful health lobby led by Mary Woodard Lasker and supported by the Lasker Foundation not only successfully resisted cuts but also promoted and helped steer through Congress a National Cancer Act, which President Nixon signed on December 23, 1971. The new act guaranteed a rising budget for the next five years, with the initial appropriation at $500 million. Annual increases would then carry the cancer budget to above $1 billion by 1976. Other elements in the act included a programmed research plan, the creation of a new cancer institute independent of the National Institutes of Health, a provision for clinical application of research findings, an international cancer data bank, and a three-person President's Cancer Panel to report directly to the President. The plan was a blueprint for what was called a "Crusade Against Cancer," and its proponents based their arguments on "the very natural and intense desire of the American people to be free of the threat of cancer." Opnion sampling showed that cancer was the disease the public most feared, and recent figures on rapidly rising cancer incidence were used to drive home the need for immediate action. The National Cancer Act of 1971, like its predecessor in 1937, passed by large majorities in both houses of Congress.

All cancer-related issues gained in importance throughout the 1960s and 1970s. The discovery that many items routinely consumed in everyday life had the power to start cancers led to federal actions banning, limiting, or warning against carcinogenic products. Major controversies have resulted. The multi-million-dollar tobacco industry was hit hard by reports published under the auspices of the surgeon general of the United States in 1964 showing the connection between smoking and lung cancer. The industry organized to resist, and criticisms of the surgeon general's report have continuously emanated from the National Tobacco Institute's research organization. The government's warnings against cigarette smoking remain, and a major shift in smoking habits has taken place. Nonsmoking areas in public places and on public conveyances have been requested and accepted, though efforts to convince people that they should not smoke at all have been less successful. In health-sensitive sectors of society, however, the individual's freedom to smoke is being inhibited by nonsmokers' insistence on their right to breathe air free of tobacco smoke pollution. There have also been controversies over sweeteners, hair dyes, food preservatives, and a host of other products which been declared carcinogenic.

Such controversies have kept the cancer issue alive and before the public. There have been controversies as well within the medical-scientific community about the allocation of funds for cancer work, the organization of research priorities, the emphasis on the crusade mentality, and above all the effectiveness of the cancer program. But if there are questions about the efficacy of what is being done, there seems to be no serious conflict over whether it should be done. And there seems to be a growing certainty that, in time, medical science will dissolve the mysteries surrounding cancer's cause and ultimate control. Until that happens, cancer will remain a significant medical problem with major ramifications for society and politics. In that sense, it is very much the disease of twentieth-century advanced societies.

ADDITIONAL READINGS: Ernst Baumler, *Cancer: A Review of International Research*, Geoffrey Lapage (trans.), London, 1968; Edward J. Beattie, Jr., *Toward the Conquest of Cancer*, New York, 1980; John Cairns, *Cancer, Science, and Society*, San Francisco, 1978; Thelma Burnfield Dunn, *The Unseen Fight Against Cancer*, Charlottesville, Va., 1977; Sigismund Peller, *Cancer Research Since 1900: An Evaluation*, New York, 1979; L. D. Rather, *The Genesis of Cancer*, Baltimore, 1976; Richard A. Rettig, *Cancer Crusade: The Story of the National Cancer Act of 1971*, Princeton, 1977; Victor Richards, *Cancer: The Wayward Cell*, Berkeley, 1978; Michael B. Shimkin, *Contrary to Nature*, Washington, D.C., 1977.

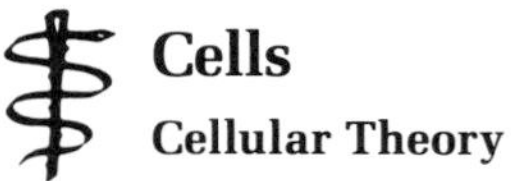

Cells

Cellular Theory

The emergence of modern medicine came about with a series of major discoveries in the nineteenth century which revolutionized methods for defining, studying, and managing disease. Probably the two most important were cellular theory and the germ theory of disease (see Bacteriology). Only William Harvey's explanation of the circulation of the blood (q.v.), which was published in 1628, can compare in significance with these concepts, and if we add modern biochemistry to circulation, germ theory, and cells, we have the intellectual underpinnings for twentieth-century medicine.

The English microscopist Robert Hooke first used "cell" as a descriptive word for biological structures in 1664. He was describing the "pores" in petrified wood, which he saw were identical with the "microscopical pores" in normal wood. When he observed similar openings in charcoal and cork, he also referred to them as cells. The term meant an enclosed space, and it retained that meaning into the first half of the nineteenth century. When anatomy began to use the idea of a cell in the eighteenth century, it was still with the implication of an enclosed space. "Cellular tissue," for example, referred to loosely constructed connective tissue which could be blown up with air or fluid to fill the spaces or compartments (cells) between the membranes. The idea of the cell as a living unit capable of reproducing itself did not appear until the early nineteenth century.

The problems of microscopy were particularly difficult when the subject was soft tissues. Staining, freezing, and slicing techniques were all in the future, and the preparation of specimens was rudimentary. Problems in studying plants were less serious because the material was more rigid and easier to handle. Here, the interspatial cellular concept gave way rather early to the concept of the cell as both a structural unit and a growing entity. Cell theories developed in connection with plant studies during the first third of the nineteenth century, and in the 1830s, the idea was carried over from plant studies to research on animals, including humans. Theodor Schwann, a student of Johannes Mueller, published a series of papers in 1838 under the general title of "On the Analogy in the Structure and Growth of Animals and Plants." Schwann took the idea for the comparison from his friend and colleague Matthias Schleiden, a botanist at Jena, who had worked on the concept of the cell in his plant studies.

Matthias Schleiden claimed that plants were aggregates of living units (cells), which both contributed to the plant as a whole and lived an existence of their own. The cells he described were living structural and functional entities which reproduced themselves. The nucleus, which was located in the cell wall and which Robert Brown had identified in 1831, was the reproductive unit. New cells were believed to be generated from nuclei within mature cells. Schwann was certain that, as he wrote in 1838, "all these phenomena can be demonstrated in animal structures," and that, in fact, the living cell was the basic component in all living things. Schwann claimed that he had observed the process he described in cartilage tissue, and that it appeared in the thin-walled cells of the frog notochord Mueller reported. None of this amounted to a demonstration, and while Schwann asserted a cellular theory, he lacked evidence at critical points to sustain it.

An even more serious question concerned the cells' specificity of function and raised the difficult problem of cellular genesis. Schleiden and Schwann both tried to find the answer by combining the reproduction of cells from cells with the concept of a nurturing fluid out of which cell forms arose in a kind of spontaneous generation. The fluid, which was called blastema, can be traced back to John Hunter's "coagulable lymph" in the preceding century and even older humoral ideas which explained the formation of the solid portions of the body. Schwann referred to blastema as a "structureless substance, which lies either within or between already present cells." New cells formed within this substance "in accordance with prescribed laws" to develop into "the elementary parts of organisms." The different kinds of cells which resulted produced the basis for a fivefold classification of tissues: blood and lymph; tissues such as the crystalline lens of the eye, the chordal dorsalis, and all epithelial tissues; "fused wall" tissues such as cartilage, bones, and tooth enamel; fibrous cells, including loose connective tissues and tendons; and cells with fused walls but with intercommunicating cell cavities, that is, nerve, muscle, capillary, and vascular tissues.

Though evidence for defining and even classifying cells existed, there was no evidence on which to establish Schwann's theories of cytogenesis. Even so, for nearly two decades, the genesis of cells was referred to as "blastema," and when the brilliant and prolific Karl von Rokitansky published his *Handbook of Pathology* between 1842 and 1846, he tried to use blastema theory as the basis for a comprehensive explanation of disease process. Rudolf Virchow, who attacked Rokitansky in 1846 for asserting what he could not prove, himself accepted much of Schwann's explanation, and Virchow did not make a final break with the blastema concept for 12 more years.

Embryologists should have been better placed to comment on the problem of cell genesis, but as it happened, only two men took up Schwann's view of the cell as the basic unit of life; and only one of them, Karl Reichert, entirely denied the blastema theory (1854). The other, Rudolf Koelliker, followed Schwann's cellular ideas, but at least until 1851 he supported the concept of "free formation" of cells in adults and under pathological conditions. Robert Remak was actually the first to dispense entirely with blastema, "free formation," and spontaneous generation to assert that all cells without exception, both normal and pathological, came from preexisting cells. Remak published his conclusions in 1852, two years before Reichert, and six years before Virchow's great handbook on pathology. Even so, it is Virchow's formulation of the principle, *omnis cellula a cellula* "every cell from a preceding cell", that is remembered. This is owed in part to Virchow's extraordinary charisma (his detractors speak of flamboyance and self-dramatization) and in part to the fact that Virchow was an outstanding controversationalist whose strong opinions were heard on most of the leading issues debated in the second half of the nineteenth century. These included social and political questions as well as arguments over disease, medicine, and natural science.

In 1855, August Förster published his handbook for pathology in which he set out the new viewpoint based on Remak and Reichert. Blastema was no longer the generative substance. Cells arise from the division of cells with the process beginning in the egg, with cleavage of the yolk forming embryonal cells which separate into three germ layers which become the substance for future tissues. There are no new cells, either pathological or normal, in the sense of cells created or generated from noncellular material. All cells come from preexisting cells. Förster was close to Virchow, and his book and Virchow's present exactly the same view. The publication of Virchow's study in 1858 completed the establishment of the cell as the basic unit in understanding the human body.

During the next half century, cell theory was central to arguments over disease, particularly cancer (q.v.). A revised and increasingly precise physiology developed based on the analysis and description of cellular characteristics, while the empirical evidence to correct and complete the ideas offered at mid-century accumulated. The successful solution to the problem of cell genesis, however, left the concept of specificity in function open, as well as the related question of the reason for cell transformation and pathological growth. The latter question remains unanswered after a century and a quarter of research on cancer. The former has led to analysis of the molecular structure of cells, and work on genetic coding.

In common with bacteriology, cell theory introduced a specific, verifiable unit into medical studies and seemed to promise a factual foundation for future generalizations concerning structure and function. Undoubtedly, acceptance of the cell did much to dispel vague and arbitrary theories, but it also raised new questions, many of which remain unsolved. Though cells are central to modern physiological and pathological work, they are important as units of definition. Studies seeking explanation for cell behavior, whether normal or pathological, turn to the complex biochemistry of the body, including immune response and genetic codes. Having become the unit to be studied, the cell is now the target for an arsenal of new techniques, each aiming at more precise information concerning it, while the basic principles laid down in the middle of the last century either have been dispersed or have become so well established that they can serve as untested postulates while research progresses on other levels. The cell, once discovered, has proved to be the beginning of new possibilities for understanding the body and its problems.

ADDITIONAL READINGS: Erwin Ackerknecht, *Rudolf Virchow: Doctor, Statesman, Anthropologist*, Madison, Wisc., 1953; John R. Baker, "The Cell Theory: A Restatement, History, and Critique," *Quarterly Journal of Microscopal Science 59* (1948), 90 (1949), 93 (1952), 94 (1953), 96 (1955); Arthur Hughes, *A History of Cytology*, London and New York, 1959; Lester S. King, *The Growth of Medical Thought*, Chicago, 1963; L. J. Rather, *The Genesis of Cancer: A Study in the History of Ideas*, Baltimore and London, 1978; Rudolf Virchow, *Disease, Life, and Man: Selected Essays*, trans. and with intro. by L. J. Rather, Stanford and London, 1959.

See also CANCER; PATHOLOGY; PHYSIOLOGY.

Chemotherapy

Chemotherapy treats disease by administering drugs which inhibit or destroy disease-producing agents without attacking the system in which they are found. Chemotherapy is best known as the current leading treatment in cancer cases, but the so-called combined therapy which has made it possible to cure pulmonary tuberculosis is also a chemotherapy; the uses of sulfonamides, penicillin, and other antibiotics to limit the multiplication of bacteria or to destroy them are additional examples.

Treatment with agents which attacked the disease-bearing microorganism was employed long before the germ theory of disease was proved. Ancient Greek medicine used the male fern as a specific agent against intestinal worms, while Hindu medicine treated leprosy with chaulmoogra oil, a substance extracted from a species of *Hyanocarpus*. Mercury was found effective for treating syphilis at the beginning of the sixteenth century, and in the seventeenth century, cinchona bark began to be used to control malaria. There was no basis other than experience for selecting these materials from thousands of other items in nature, and even after the discovery that microorganisms were responsible for certain diseases, there was no established theory to guide the search for elements which would attack the causes of disease. Robert Koch, who, with Louis Pasteur, led the bacteriological revolution, submitted a report in 1881 which called attention to the variations in bactericidal effect of different disinfectants, and he raised the further problem of why an antiseptic known to kill bacteria under laboratory conditions (in vitro) failed to do so in the living organism (in vivo). Emil Behring, another of the pioneers in bacteriological work, interested himself in Koch's problem, but it was Paul Ehrlich in Frankfurt who had the necessary background in chemistry to contribute a solution. Ehrlich stayed with the problem, and while he cannot be said to have solved it, he is generally credited with laying the foundations for chemotherapy.

While studying aspects of diphtheria, Ehrlich was surprised by the body's ability to generate antibodies which were specific to particular infective organisms. This phenomenon was similar to the one which Emil Heubel noted in lead poisoning, where there appeared to be a "preferential disposition" for lead in certain tissues but not in others. "Chemical affinity" and "side-chain effect" were phrases Ehrlich used to define this phenomenon, and he made it his goal to apply the principle to controlling disease-causing microorganisms. He set out to find agents which were specifically bound to and toxic for particular bacteria but which would have no effect on the bacteria's host. In 1891, Ehrlich and an associate successfully treated malaria with methylene blue, and then they turned their attention to the treponemes responsible for syphilis (q.v.). Arsenical compounds were known to be effective against trypanosomes which were protozoans, that is, single-celled animals, but the preparation used, an organic arsenical called atoxyl, was liable to damage the optic nerve. Ehrlich applied arsenical compounds to treponemes, which, as bacteria, are single-celled members of the vegetable kingdom, and in 1907 he took patents on the 606th preparation which he tried, which proved strikingly successful against syphilis. The compound was marketed as Salvarsan in 1910. Ehrlich called the process at work against disease-bearing bacteria "chemotherapy," and he defined the process in 1911 as destroying parasites chemically, but only with such substances as the parasites themselves would attract.

Subsequent progress in chemotherapy was very slow. Close cooperation between chemists and biologists was difficult to arrange. Pharmaceutical companies were still immature, and drug development occurred either as a by-product of scientific investigations or as part of the development of industrial chemistry (see Pharmacy). Germany's acknowledged superiority in the dye industry also conferred leadership in the early development of chemotherapeutic agents. The critical problem was the lack of any systematic method for pairing disease-causing organisms and chemical compounds. This meant that developing any specific drug was a long, drawn-out, time-consuming process that could only be shortened by unexpected insights, a kind of scientific serendipity. There were, in fact, only a few compounds available until 1935 for chemotherapeutic use. These included quinine and quinicrine for malaria, emetine for amebiasis, the arsenicals which affected trypanosomiasis and amebiasis, and antimony preparations for schistosomiasis. In most other cases, potentially bactericidal compounds damaged other tissue as well. Ehrlich's "silver bullet," the remedy which would go straight to its target and nowhere else, appeared to have been a myth.

The situation changed in the middle 1930s when Gerhard Domagk announced the first sulfa drug. Domagk was research director for the German Bayer Company. Following a program of empirical research comparable to Ehrlich's and aimed at the similar goal of discovering compounds with bactericidal properties, Domagk had tested a variety of metal-based compounds—gold, tin, antimony, and arsenics—only to discover that either their antibacterial actions were too weak or their toxic side effects were too dangerous. Early in the 1930s, however, Domagk became interested in the azo dyes that his company produced, and, in the course of working with a new dye compound which would penetrate fabric more deeply and be colorfast, he identified antibacterial effects as well. The dye compound was called Prontosil, and it proved effective against hemolytic streptococci in laboratory mice. Curiously, Prontosil had no effect on bacteria in a test tube. The element in Prontosil which affected streptococci was sulfanilamide; it was, as Domagk called it, a true chemotherapeutic agent. Dr. and Mme. Jacques Tréfouël confirmed Domagk's findings at the Pasteur Institute in Paris, and they showed that chemical action in the body released the active antibacterial agent from the dye compound. Domagk's announcement was delayed to permit additional testing to confirm the apparent anomaly of an agent which was ineffective in vitro but which proved effective in vivo. Fifteen hundred human tests preceded the final announcement. It also seems that Domagk's company delayed announcement in the hope that a patentable substance would be found. Sulfanilamide had been discovered, and the discovery had been published, in 1908. There had also been a research project in the United States in 1919 which used a substance analogous to Prontosil and reached similar though much less positive conclusions. Without patents, sulfanilamide went directly into competitive production.

The discovery of sulfanilamide led to further work which soon produced several important members of the sulfonamide family, including sulfathiazole, sulfadiazine, and M and B 693.

These compounds, like sulfanilamide, are bacteriostatic; that is, they affect the bacterial metabolism and prevent its multiplying in the host. This permits natural body defenses to function effectively against the invader. The new drugs affected the causal agents in erysipelas, puerperal fever, streptococcus infection, pneumococcus, gonorrhea, meningitis, and some infective bowel and urinary diseases. Their discovery and introduction vastly enlarged the therapeutic options for treating bacterial infections and gave chemotherapy a critical role in medical practice.

The discovery of penicillin (q.v.) and subsequent families of antibiotics further enlarged the scope of chemotherapeutic attack. Penicillin was first identified by Sir Alexander Fleming in 1928 and proved to be one of the most effective chemotherapeutic agents of all, with demonstrated effectiveness against most pus-forming cocci as well as pneumococcus, gonococcus, meningococcus, anthrax, diphtheria bacterium b, tetanus, and syphilis. A further weapon was added in the mid-1940s when Selman A. Waksman, a soil microbiologist at Rutgers University who was working with various fungi, isolated actinomycin. This antibiotic proved to have dangerous toxic effects and was useless for therapy. In 1944, however, Waksman found another species of fungus, *Streptomyces griseus*, from which he isolated streptomycin. This substance proved effective against the tubercle bacillus, and, with other compounds, it opened the way to an ultimately successful chemotherapy for tuberculosis (q.v.).

Since World War II, with chemotherapy a demonstrably sound principle of treatment, and with pharmaceutical houses fully developed enterprises, an intensive search for effective chemical agents for particular diseases has produced a steadily lengthening list of compounds. Furthermore, the experience with sulfonamides and antibiotics led to a more rational attack on the problem of discovering effective agents, and the emphasis shifted from finding effective elements in nature which could be matched to diseases to developing synthetic compounds which are made with prior knowledge of the biological character and chemical composition of the target. This development began as early as 1938, when two British scientists, D. D. Woods and (Sir) Paul Fildes, showed that sulfonamides worked their effects by preventing bacteria from using para-aminobenzoic acid (PABA), an element necessary for growth. Sulfonamides became attached to bacteria in place of PABA, but since they could not be metabolized, bacterial growth stopped. Fildes suggested that an effective chemotherapeutic agent was one which interfered with essential metabolic processes in the pathogenic microorganism, and he argued that such a substance would have a close chemical affinity with the element required. Though the successful application came much later, the Fildes-Woods theory was basic to chemotherapy for cancer.

At present, chemotherapy is one of the most active fields in medicine. Research aims not only at developing new drugs and discovering new therapeutic substances but also at learning more about the action of established drugs. Apart from toxic effect, the sulfonamides, the antibiotics, and penicillin have all been reduced in effectiveness by the development of bacterial strains which are immune to the drugs' actions. Combinations of drugs can counter some immunity problems while the search for acceptable alternatives continues. In the case of penicillin, the appearance of severe allergic reactions led to the development of cephalothin, a compound which can be given safely to persons allergic to penicillin to achieve a similar effect, and the number of such compounds continues to expand with need.

ADDITIONAL READINGS: H. F. Dowling, *Fighting Infection: Conquests of the Twentieth Century,* Cambridge, Mass., 1977; Iago Galdston, "Some Notes on the Early History of Chemotherapy," *Bulletin of the History of Medicine* 8 (June 1940): 806–818; Sir Charles Harrington, "Modern Trends in Chemotherapy," *Nature* 176 (September 3, 1955): 1–7; Lucien Israël, *Conquering Cancer,* Joan Pinkham (trans.), New York, 1978; R. Y. Keers, *Pulmonary Tuberculosis,* London, 1978; David Wilson, *Penicillin in Perspective,* London 1976.

See also ANTIBIOTICS; CANCER; PENICILLIN; SULFONAMIDES; SYPHILIS; TUBERCULOSIS.

Chinese Medicine

Traditional Chinese medicine originated in folk and religious practices which had become infinitely elaborated by the first millennium B.C. Organized medicine developed between the middle of the first millennium B.C. and the end of the first millennium A.D. and was contemporary with ayurvedic medicine in India and the Hippocratic tradition in Greece. The period of greatest institutional growth paralleled the later Roman (Byzantine) and Moslem eras and the early stages of the western high Middle Ages.

The most important source for early Chinese medicine is the *Huang di nei jing su wen (The Yellow Emperor's Classic of Internal Medicine)*, which was given its present form in the first century B.C. This work summarized some 600 years of actual medical practice. *Nei jing* covers all aspects of body function, with the information organized for medical purposes under the categories of diagnosis, prognosis, therapy, and regimens. Some nonmedical sources also included medical information. The first in the series of Chinese dynastic histories, for example, the *Shi ji* (*Historical Memoirs*) of Sima Qian, describes the work of one Bian Que, a physician consulted on behalf of the prince of Qin, around 500 B.C. Bian Que's method was to judge "the history and condition of the patient as a whole," and his diagnostic techniques included observations on color and tongue conditions, an early version of auscultation, anamnesis and medical history, sphygmology, and palpation. This text also refers to many of the therapeutic practices noted in the later *Nei jing*, including acupuncture (q.v.), radiant heat, counterirritants, aqueous and alcoholic decoctions of drugs, massage, gymnastics, and medicated plasters.

Beliefs and Practices A complex physiology comparable to Greek theories was used to explain the onset of illness, though the earliest explanations for disease were demonological and called for ritual exorcisms. In the historic period, demonology remained as an explanation for disease, especially in the folk tradition, and persisted to modern times. The physiological basis for explaining body function was the interaction of yin and yang, the two dynamic principles which were believed to control all existence. Yin was the moist, dark, female aspect of the universe. Yang was masculine, joyful, bright, and dry. Yin or yang produced illness when there was too much of the one or the other, and they joined four meteorological influences—wind, rain, twilight, and brightness of day—to form the causes for the six basic classes of disease.

The classification by sixes persisted despite the introduction of a parallel system for classifying all natural phenomena into five groups based on earth, fire, water, wood, and metal. *Qi* was a vital spirit comparable to *pneuma*, or air (breath), in the Greek system. It suffused the body, and its balance was disturbed by one of the six active disease-producing influences. Therapies concentrated on affecting or adjusting the flow of *Qi*. This was the principle behind acupuncture as well as various drug and dietetic treatments. Traditional Chinese medicine stressed preventing sickness rather than curing it, and the treatises abounded in recommendations for maintaining proper balance within the system. Surgery played only a small part in traditional Chinese medicine. Surgeons were relegated to an inferior status, and the only major surgical procedure that was common was creating a eunuch by removing the genitalia.

The medical philosophy built on yin–yang and the five- or six-part classification of diseases formed a system of medical correspondences which emphasized mutuality, interdependence, balance, and harmony. These concepts paralleled the ideals defined in the same period by Kong Fuzi (Confucius) as the bases for right governance. Before Kong Fuzi time, combinations of warring states struggled for control of China. Contemporary medicine, which portrayed a hostile world filled with enemies to health, paralleled the political and social situations. The therapies involved—rituals to engage stronger spirits to protect the body and campaigns to expel conditions from the body—reflected the essentially amoral politics of power practiced by the warring states. Confucian doctrine, a product of the period of conflict, proposed to maintain order by rigid adherence to stated ethical norms, seeking health for the body politic by emphasizing moral responsibility, a hierarchy of obligations, and the achievement of harmony. The major medical philosophies of the same period built on similar principles of harmony, order, and balance, thus following the pattern of political thought.

Taoism made a third approach to the question of health through medicinal drugs. The harmony Taoism pursued was between the organism and the natural laws which controlled its function. Drugs were considered a means to bring a malfunctioning system back into accord with the demands of nature. Since this method was pragmatic rather than systematic and moral, Confucians avoided it.

The end of the period of warring states in the third century B.C. also introduced a period of institutional organization in medicine. Physicians began to be recognized as a group separate from shamans, alchemists, invocators, liturgiologists, pharmacists, veterinarians, leeches, and priests. The physician rose in social status from a kind of artisan or technical specialist (*mu*) to a learned Confucian scholar (*shi*) with a recognized specialty. The transformation was not total. A large number of practitioners still were called *Fang shi*, a category which included many with skills which did not qualify for advanced status. Among these were magicians and technologists of all kinds, including pharmacists. All performed medical functions. The state took control over physicians' qualifications, and in 165 B.C. government examinations were introduced to qualify practitioners. An imperial university was founded in 124 B.C. which taught medicine as one of a group of scientific disciplines which included astronomy and hydraulic engineering. Subsequently, professorships and lectureships in medicine were set up, and in the seventh century A.D., the Imperial Medical College was established together with medical colleges in the chief provincial cities. In licensing and education, the Chinese system led both the Arabs and the west, as the first qualifying examinations in Islam were not introduced until the tenth century, while Roger of Sicily's twelfth-century decree on licensing doctors was probably the first in Europe.

During this same period (ca. 200 B.C.–A.D. 200), the Chinese laid the basis for a statewide medical service which was later divided into a service for the imperial palace and a public service. These state institutions took responsibility for medical administration in the provinces and in the military. The state medical service also took over hostels, hospices, and hospitals built by Taoist and Buddhist communities. The first permanent hospice with dispensary was founded by the Buddhist prince of southern Qi, Xiao Ziliang, in A.D. 491, while the first state-sponsored hospital was built in A.D. 510 by Taibo Yü, prince of northern Wei. The office called the Court of Imperial Sacrifices administered the Imperial Medical Service and was given responsibility for the hospital's physical plant. Ultimately the state assumed full control over all medical functions, hospitals included. Buddhist and Taoist monks and nuns were forbidden to practice medicine (A.D. 653), orphanages and infirmaries for the destitute were established by the state in the capital (A.D. 734), and in the year 845 temple lands and properties were appropriated by the emperor to be used for hospitals. In the period from 1050 to 1250, a number of state-sponsored health institutions were established throughout the empire. These included infirmaries for the aged and sick poor, hospitals for special groups including foreigners, officials, war prisoners, and the Jin Tatars, orphanages, outpatient clinics, and in 1076, subsidized apothecaries. The state also took responsibility for pharmacopeias, and in the eighth century it produced *Guang Ji Fang (A General Formulary of Prescriptions)*, from which certain common prescriptions were taken to be written on notice boards and displayed at crossroads where the common people could take advantage of them.

The institutional structures for Chinese medicine declined with the weakening of the empire, especially after the seventeenth century, and by the nineteenth century only vestiges remained. There were, however, historic achievements. Technically advanced and conceptually sophisticated, Chinese medicine had many characteristics consistent with the development of scientific medicine, but continuity, tradition, and authority created a cultural atmosphere which was not conducive to innovation. The adequacy of existing practice and its congruity with the contemporary value system militated against radical changes. Thus traditional Chinese medicine has remained firmly rooted in modern Chinese culture, and, in the form of acupuncture, it has made a bid for acceptance outside China. Given the heavy economic burden which modernization represents, traditional medicine offers today's China an alternative to the prohibitively costly development of a scientific medical system. Traditional medicine is in place, is widely accepted, and represents a legitimate solution for certain aspects of medical care in the People's Republic of China.

ADDITIONAL READINGS: Chi-Min Wang and Lien-Tê Wu, *History of Chinese Medicine: Being a Chronicle of Medical Happenings in China from Ancient Times to the Present Period*, Tien-Tsin, 1932; E. H. Hume, *The Chinese Way in Medicine*, Baltimore, 1940; Frederick F. Kao and John J. Kao (eds.), *Chinese Medicine-New Medicine*, New York, 1977; Lu Gwei-Djen and Joseph Needham, "Records of Diseases in Ancient China," in D. Brothwell and A. T. Sanderson (eds.), *Diseases in Antiquity,* Springfield, Ill., 1967, 222–237; Guido Majno, *The Healing Hand: Man and Wound in the Ancient World,* Cambridge, Mass., 1975, chap. 6; Joseph Needham, *Science in Traditional China: A Comparative Perspective,* Cambridge, Mass., 1981; Joseph R. Needham, *Science and Civilization in China,* 5 vols., Cambridge, 1974; Joseph R. Needham and Lu Gwei-Djen, "Chinese Medicine," in F. N. L. Poynter (ed.), *Medicine and Culture,* London, 1969, 255–312; S. Pálos, *The Chinese Art of Healing,* New York, 1971; M. Porkert, *The Theoretical Foundations of Chinese Medicine; Systems of Correspondence,* Cambridge, Mass., and London, 1973; Sung Tz'u, *The Washing Away of Wrongs,* Brian E. McKnight (trans.), *Science, Medicine, and Technology in East Asia,* I, Ann Arbor, 1981; René Taton, *History of Science: Ancient and Medieval Science from the Beginnings to 1450,* A. J. Pomerans (trans.), New York, 1963, pt. I, chap. 5, pt. III, chap. 4; Paul U. Unschuld, *Medical Ethics in Imperial China: A Study in Historical Anthropology,* Berkeley and London, 1979; I. Veith, *Huang ti Nei Ching Su Wên: The Yellow Emperor's Classic of Internal Medicine,* Berkeley, 1966.

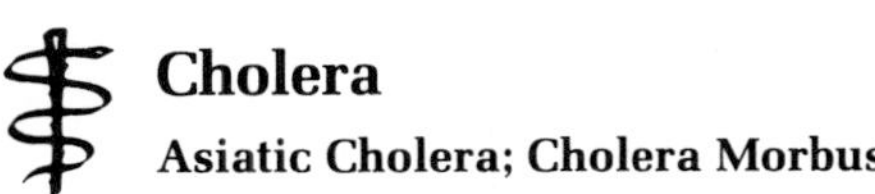

Cholera

Asiatic Cholera; Cholera Morbus

Asiatic cholera is an epidemic disease which became pandemic in the nineteenth century, attacking nearly every major country in the world. By the third decade of the twentieth century, cholera had retreated to its traditional endemic centers in south Asia, but it has showed no signs of disappearing there, remaining extremely dangerous to India, Pakistan, and far northwest Burma. Sporadic outbreaks since World War II in Egypt, southeast Asia, the Philippines, China, and Africa underline the continuing need for vigilance against a disease which now surpasses bubonic plague as a threat.

The Disease The bacterial cause for cholera is the *Vibrio cholerae,* or *Vibrio comma,* bacillus, which was isolated by Robert Koch in 1883. The vibrio lives in the human intestine. It is exposed in fecal matter and is most commonly communicated by polluted water. Even before the bacterial cause was known, therefore, it was possible to reduce cholera incidence by control of public water supplies. Effective sanitary policies have proved to be the best means for controlling cholera, and in modern times the disease remains a serious threat primarily in those societies where sanitation is primitive and there are large concentrations of population.

While only laboratory tests to prove the presence of the vibrio can confirm a cholera diagnosis, the disease has distinctive clinical characteristics. At the onset, a patient will fell anxious or oppressed, and there are internal disturbances, nausea, and dizziness. These conditions quickly give way to a violent vomiting and diarrhea, with stools turning to a grayish liquid often described as "rice water." The liquid is expelled from the body with no visible strain or trauma. Intense muscular cramps or seizures follow, and there is a burning sensation in the stomach, with an insatiable craving for water. This violent period is generally followed by a "sinking stage" during which the pulse fades, body temperature drops, and lethargy sets in. At this point the patient is near death and shows the classic cholera physiognomy: a sunken and cadaverous face with a marked liverish color around the eyes, and lips tight-drawn, puckered, and blue. A bluish tinge appears around the fingernails, the tongue seems cold and is often coated, and the voice sinks to a husky whisper. In most cases, death follows soon after.

Throughout most of the nineteenth century, cholera's mortality averaged approximately half of its incidence, and there was relatively little that physicians could do for those who contracted it. Contemporary reports noted that at the beginning of an outbreak no treatment was successful, while during the period when the disease was declining, all treatments worked equally well. Modern therapies are more successful and have reduced mortality to under 10 percent of incidence, though when treatment is not given, mortalities return to their nineteenth-century levels.

The cholera's action probably results from the multiplication of the *V. cholerae* in the middle and lower small intestine, where it produces a toxic substance which interferes with the normal functioning of the intestinal membrane. The result is that water and salts are not absorbed but are expelled in the watery diarrhea. Water which may be drunk only contributes to the diarrhea, so the most effective way to counter the effects of radical dehydration is to replace fluids and salts intravenously. Once begun, this treatment is maintained by replacing the quantity of the last stool with an equal quantity of water and salt solution. Though effective in halting the symptoms resulting from dehydration, the maintenance therapy has to be continued until the vibrio either evolves out of its toxic phase or is destroyed. It has been found that such oral antibiotics as tetracycline, chloramphenicol, and streptomycin can reduce bacterial action and hence the diarrhea by half, while tetracycline in sufficient quantity can actually eradicate the bacteria. Vaccination is of marginal utility for prevention and of no use for cures. Effective cholera treatment requires trained personnel more than technology, though in underdeveloped countries this is hardly an advantage, because paramedics and nurses capable of dealing in a disciplined way with massive numbers of cholera cases are virtually always in short supply. The recent development of prepackaged replacement fluids offers a solution to this problem.

History The history of cholera began on the subcontinent of India. Both literary records and religious practices suggest that cholera was endemic to that region for at least 2000 years, but it was not until the sixteenth century that European travelers, explorers, traders, and officials gave detailed descriptions of a terrible plague whose symptoms were those of cholera and which was reported to reach epidemic proportions. One authority has identified 64 separate and authoritative accounts of cholera in India between 1503 and 1817, and no less than 10 of those refer specifically to epidemics. It is equally certain that cholera did not reach Europe before the nineteenth century. Hence the diseases described in European medical classics from the Hippocratic writings to Thomas Sydenham, though designated as cholera or a "bilious flux," were not true Asiatic cholera. The evidence concerning European border zones is not so clear. There is a tradition, for example, that cholera attacked the Crimean Tatar capital of Bakhchiserai in the seventeenth century, but even if the disease were cholera, there is no evidence that it proceeded any farther inland. It is also questionable whether cholera reached China before the modern era. There may have been an outbreak in the seventh century A.D., but there is no further evidence of cholera in China for the next 1200 years. Cholera may well have been present in Ceylon and Burma before the later eighteenth century, but only as sporadic outbreaks connected with the centers in India. The areas of cholera's historic endemicity were in south Asia, and specifically the delta regions of east and west Bengal.

After Britain expelled the French from India and began to develop a regular colonial administration, information concerning the diseases of the region multiplied. Europe's best and earliest data on cholera were from British Indian reports which dominated both medical and political decisions until experience supplanted them in 1830. The British reports showed increased cholera activity in the later eighteenth century and accurately reported the beginnings of the first pandemic in 1816 and 1817. The reasons that the disease broke out of its endemic centers at that time are still obscure, though climatic factors probably played a role. World weather patterns were violently disturbed in the second decade of the nineteenth century, possibly as a result of massive volcanic activity, and there was a dramatic increase in the quantity of volcanic dust present in the atmosphere. This appears to have resulted in heavy rainfalls which were followed in India by an unusually dry, hot summer in 1816. In the midst of flooding and harvest failures, the cholera reached epidemic proportions in Bengal during 1817, and by 1820 it had spread throughout the subcontinent. It subsided into local outbreaks in 1821, but the damage had been done. Moving with the masses of religious pilgrims who came to take the holy waters of the Ganges or transported by traders and soldiers along the main commercial routes, cholera spread east and west into the regions contiguous with India. By 1824, it had passed through southeast Asia all the way to the Philippines; it had gone by sea and by land to China; and from China it may have gone west toward the Russian borders; it certainly went east into Japan. To the south, the disease spilled out of India into Ceylon; to the west, it followed well-traveled routes through the Persian Gulf into Mesopotamia; and northward, it moved through Persia to the boundaries of the Turkish and Russian empires. When it reached the Russian port of Astrakhan at the head of the Caspian and the mouth of the Volga, the cholera stood at the gateway to Europe. It then receded, however, and the first pandemic period ended in 1826.

The first pandemic remained geographically in Asia, though it approached Europe, and it may have touched Africa at Zanzibar. The second, third, and fourth pandemics affected the entire world, though with considerable regional variation, while in the fifth and sixth pandemics the areas of incidence receded significantly. The second pandemic began in 1829 and lasted through 1852. In that period, cholera returned repeatedly to the Asiatic countries, broke into Egypt and north Africa, and in 1829 and 1830 entered Russia via Astrakhan and Orenburg. Russia was the staging area for cholera's movement across Europe from 1830 to 1832. The cholera reached North America from Europe in 1832, attacking New York and the eastern seaboard, then moving through the interior of the country across the Rocky Mountains to the Pacific coast by 1834. The disease also moved south to Mexico and Central America, Cuba, and possibly Peru and Chile. It reentered the southern United States from Cuba, passed north through New Orleans and Charleston, and eventually reached Canada. Cholera remained a major threat in the western hemisphere until the last decades of the nineteenth century.

The third pandemic began in 1852 and 1853 and met a residue of local infections still active from the second to achieve an extraordinary intensity as well as extent. The year 1854 proved to be one of the worst cholera years on record. The fourth and fifth pandemics continued the patterns begun in the second. The fourth pandemic started in 1863 and lasted until 1875. It was notable for opening a new route into Europe. Moslem pilgrims to Mecca in the jubilee year of 1865 carried cholera throughout Arabia and Mesopotamia, but they brought it as well to Alexandria, which became a transfer point for the disease to other Mediterranean ports including Istanbul, Ancona, and Marseilles. This seaborne route supplemented the traditional northerly routes from Persia through the Caspian region and across Russia. The fourth pandemic also saw dangerous outbreaks in central Europe in the wake of the Austro-Prussian War (1866) and a very broad extension in Africa, where it moved from the seacoasts into Ethiopia, the Kilimanjaro region, Tanganyika, and the upper Congo.

By the end of the nineteenth century, most European countries had recognized that cholera could be controlled through active public health measures, and this work was made more effective by the isolation of cholera's bacterial cause in 1883. As a consequence, the sixth pandemic, which lasted from 1899 to 1926, had only slight effects in western Europe and failed to reach the Americas at all. The disease was very severe in Russia early in the period, however, and it returned to ravage that country during World War I and the revolution which followed. 1921 and 1922 were particularly bad years, but the disease was then brought under control, and cholera has not been a problem in the Soviet Union since 1926.

The sixth pandemic had significant effects outside the western world, but in the years since 1926 one after another of its areas of incidence has been reduced. By 1945, cholera was stabilized in its zone of endemicity. Since 1945, the disease's influence outside that zone has been sporadic, though often violent, and there have been some new developments. In 1961, a variant of *V. cholerae* called El Tor (named after the quarantine camp on the Red Sea where it was isolated in 1905) spread cholera in the western Pacific and southeast Asia. It had long been believed that the El Tor variant did not produce true cholera. Outbreaks in the 1960s and 1970s have been locally violent, especially in Asia, where it appears that the People's Republic of China has had some serious experiences. Precise information, however, is lacking. Though nothing comparable to the nineteenth-century pandemics has appeared, cholera remains a significant disease today, especially in Asia.

Cholera's Effects There are no reliable general statistics on cholera's mortality, but in localities where accurate figures are available, it is difficult to discern any significant demographic consequences. Cholera death tolls in Europe do not compare to those ascribed to bubonic plague, and cholera incidence represented only fractions of whole populations. Here the Russian case is instructive. Between 1823 and 1926, Russia had an aggregate total of 5,537,358 reported cholera cases. Of that total, approximately 40 percent, or 2,140,558, died. The largest part of both cases and deaths was recorded between 1847 and 1861. In those 14 years, 2,589,843 Russians were reported to have contracted cholera and 1,032,864 to have died. The most intense epidemic experience Russia had was between 1892 and 1896, when there were 822,648 cases with 385,985 deaths. Over the entire period, Russia's aggregate figures show 55,000 cases annually and 21,000 deaths. Russia's population in 1823 approached 30 million. It grew steadily throughout the nineteenth century to reach 150 million in 1906. In even the worst cholera years, therefore, incidence was only a small fraction of the population, and the death tolls were a smaller fraction still.

Cholera's most important historical effects were functions of how and whom it attacked rather than how many it killed. Cholera was hardest on the poor and destitute. This made it a powerful influence for social reform, urban development, and public health programs. But the disease also underlined the dangers of poverty and intensified class bitterness. The well-to-do had their fears of the unwashed mob reinforced, while the poor believed that cholera was a new instrument of oppression or even a conspiracy aimed at their destruction. Cholera epidemics often were scenes of social violence. Mobs repeatedly broke loose to destroy hospitals, attack physicians, and vent their fury on innocent strangers who appeared as sinister enemies of the people. Violence was a particular feature of the first cholera epidemics, creating scenes of riot and destruction from St. Petersburg to Paris, London, and New York. Efforts by the authorities to enforce sanitary regulations regularly triggered the violence. The relaxation of controls and the greater intensity of later cholera attacks appear to have had the effect of defusing the most explosive situations. Even so, Russian peasants rioted in 1893 and 1894 just as they had done in 1830 and 1831. Some local health boards won the peasants' confidence, but these were exceptions, and most peasants remained suspicious of governmental agents, terrified of hospitals, and horrified by cholera.

In the nonwestern world, so long as authorities did not interfere, the populace seemed to suffer passively. Partial exceptions were the Moslem societies of north Africa and the Middle East. There, the inability of established authority to control the disease and the helplessness of the religious leadership weakened the credibility of the governing establishment and contributed to a growing interest among the elite in scientific medicine and cultural westernization. Here cholera became an element in an important process of cultural transformation.

In the west, the social dimension was of prime importance. Because both cholera and violence were worst where the urban poor huddled, plans for renovating their dark and filthy warrens were a recognized necessity. Cholera forced governments to acknowledge the inadequacy of existing housing, water and sanitary systems, cemeteries, clinics, and hospitals. The cholera influenced the emperor Napoleon III's decision to rebuild the city of Paris, and it contributed to a host of urban improvements in London, where Sir Edwin Chadwick agitated for the installation of sewer pipe and a regular disposal system. All around Europe, the establishment of cholera councils to deal with local outbreaks marked a significant beginning of modern public health institutions. The cholera created needs which required government responses, and by the second half of the nineteenth century, most European governments actively accepted broader responsibilities for living conditions and were creating the administrative systems to fulfill their obligations. So important was cholera in their development that, as one authority put it, from the point of view of the social sciences, the cholera era was one of revolutionary change.

Cholera Control Neither effective treatment nor rational control policies were possible until the active cause for cholera had been identified. The crucial work on this problem was done in the second half of the nineteenth century and forms an integral part of the history of bacteriology (q.v.) When cholera first reached Europe in 1830, scientists had already developed the elements of a germ theory, but they lacked the means to prove it. With microscopy and its supporting laboratory techniques still in their infancy, the arguments for and against such theories tended to be historical, epidemical, and clinical. The issue was drawn around the concept of contagion (q.v.), and this brought up the problem of quarantines. Those who believed that disease was communicated directly from person to person or indirectly by objects or material carrying the disease-bearing agent argued for severe quarantine policies and supported sequestration of the ill, fumigation of goods, and interdiction of crowds and processions. It was this approach which shaped European policies when cholera first appeared, and it was the attempt to enforce stringent regulations which generated much of the social violence experienced in the early cholera outbreaks. Severe control measures proved unsuccessful, and thus scientists who believed that disease was the product of spontaneous generation, an "epidemic constitution," or a miasma pointed to the quarantine failures to demonstrate how wrong the contagionists were. Since quarantines also affected economic interests adversely, there were powerful reasons for governments to deny the contagionist position or at least to modify restrictive policies.

Though "localists" contributed to social reform movements, it was the contagionists arguing for an infective "principle" or microorganism who advanced a scientific understanding of cholera. Various hypotheses were advanced in 1830 and 1831 which postulated "tiny animals" as the agent of infection and suggested that water supplies were possible carriers of cholera. But the first major breakthrough came in 1854, when John Snow, a young physician from the north of England, was able to establish a direct connection between 500 fatal cholera cases in a London neighborhood and the pump which supplied their water. His pointed suggestion that the best thing the authorities could do to control cholera in the neighborhood would be to shut off the Broad Street pump echoes in today's literature on cholera control. Snow did more, however. He studied cholera incidence among subscribers to the Southwark, Vauxhall, and Lambeth water companies. The Lambeth company drew its water upstream from London at Thames Ditton; the others drew directly from the river in the city. Cholera mortality was eight to nine times greater among the Southwark and Vauxhall subscribers than it was among Lambeth's customers. The controlling factor was the source of water supplies.

Though Snow's arguments carried great force, they were not accepted as final. The causal agent had to be identified, and that result could only be obtained in the laboratory. By 1862, Louis Pasteur had disproved spontaneous generation, had established the existence of bacteria, and had laid the empirical foundations for the germ theory of disease. In Germany, Jacob Henle, an anatomist and histologist who anticipated Pasteur's conclusions on microorganisms as the cause of disease, had Robert Koch as one of his students at Göttingen. Koch's work on anthrax, presented in 1876, and an 1879 paper on infection in wounds established the bacterial theory of disease on firm scientific footing. In 1883, Koch and a student of Pasteur, Pierre Paul Emile Roux, headed separate expeditions to study the cholera in Egypt. Roux used the Pasteur method, which was to reproduce the disease in animals and then look for the organism. Since cholera only affects man, the method failed. Koch, who worked directly on cholera victims, successfully isolated and identified *V. cholerae* in Alexandria in 1883. He then went to Calcutta, where he confirmed his findings, and in February 1884, he reported his success to the German government.

Though Koch's findings were not universally accepted, they were basically correct and established an empirical foundation for rational policy decisions. The results came quickly. Laboratory analysis was used successfully for the first time in New York in 1887 to identify cholera on an infected ship, and the subsequent foundation of a city laboratory paid dividends in 1892 by identifying cholera on newly arrived vessels, thus permitting measures to be taken which may well have forestalled a major outbreak. From this point on, control over cholera became steadily more effective.

Current recommendations include the following points: (1) an adequate intelligence service with laboratories for rapid diagnosis; (2) adequate facilities for isolating patients; (3) a sanitary engineering service to deal with—and, if necessary, replace—contaminated water supplies; (4) control measures against the sale of potentially dangerous cold foods and drinks; and (5) large-scale publicity campaigns to ensure that people take all necessary personal precautions—including personal cleanliness, especially washing hands after toilet use, avoiding excesses in eating or drinking, and avoiding overexertion. The most important preventive measure is to guarantee clean water.

Conclusion Though the last pandemic ended by 1926, cholera remains a public health problem. Outside the endemic centers, it is necessary to guard against unexpected sporadic outbreaks; in the endemic areas, constant vigilance is necessary to keep down the incidence and mortality rates. Despite repeated efforts, no progress has been made toward eliminating endemic cholera. The chance appears to be slight that cholera could again become a worldwide threat. But the danger of serious sporadic cholera outbreaks will remain as long as the disease is active. Since the final eradication of endemic cholera does not appear to be a reasonable expectation, it is all the more important for modern societies to make every effort to maintain intact the various control systems, public and private, local and regional, national and international, which have built effective barriers against cholera and which have kept substantial segments of the world's population free from its effects for over half a century.

ADDITIONAL READINGS: P. B. Beeson and W. McDermott, "Cholera," *Cecil Loeb Textbook of Medicine*, 13th ed., 1971; Geoffrey Bilson, *A Darkened House: Cholera in Nineteenth Century Canada*, Toronto, 1980; D. Burria and W. Burrows (eds.), *Cholera*, Philadelphia, 1974; C. C. J. Carpenter, "Cholera," in George W. Hunter et al. (eds.), *A Manual of Tropical Medicines*, Philadelphia, 1966; J. S. Chambers, *The Conquest of Cholera, America's Greatest Scourge*, New York, 1938; Norman Longmate, *King Cholera: The Biography of a Disease*, London, 1966; Roderick E. McGrew, *Russia and the Cholera, 1823–1832* Madison, Wis., 1965; R. J. Morris, *Cholera: 1832*, London, 1976; M. Pelling, *Cholera, Fever, and English Medicine*, Oxford, 1978; R. Pollitzer, *Cholera*, Geneva, 1959; Charles Rosenberg, *The Cholera Years: The United States in 1832, 1849, and 1866*, Chicago, 1962.

Circulation of the Blood

From the earliest times, blood has held a place of honor among the body's constituents as the life-giving fluid, the primary humor, and a medium for nutrition and tissue building as well as a cause for fevers and inflammations.

There was, however, little understanding of the mechanisms by which the blood served the body. Galen, whose influence on medical questions was paramount until the early modern period, failed to comprehend how the circulatory system worked, believing that the veins which carried blood originated in the liver, while the arteries originated in the heart. He thought that blood was prepared in the liver and then moved to the body's periphery through veins into organs, where it was consumed. The portion of this blood which went from the liver to the right ventricle of the heart divided into two streams. The first passed to the lungs via the pulmonary artery. The second crossed the heart through "interseptal pores" into the left ventricle, where it mixed with *pneuma* (air), became heated, and passed from the left ventricle to the aorta, to the lungs, and to the periphery. The connection of arteries with veins allowed some *pneuma* to enter the veins, while the arteries received some blood.

Galen's description of the blood system, involving regeneration rather than circulation, went largely though not entirely unchallenged for 14 centuries. Modern scholarship has unearthed a thirteenth-century commentary on Avicenna's Galenic anatomy. The author, a certain Ibn an-Nafis, could see no way for blood to pass from the right side of the heart to the left, and he suggested that "the attenuated blood reaches the lung through the *vena interiosa* (pulmonary artery) where it spreads across the pulmonary substance and mixes with the air. Subsequently, the finer parts of the blood, mixed with air, flow into the *arteria venosa* (pulmonary vein) in order to reach the left cardiac chamber." Others who may have noticed the weakness in Galen's descriptions remained silent, or their commentaries have been lost, and Ibn an-Nafis has the distinction of being the only critic known to have proposed a circulation through the lungs.

By the sixteenth century there were several hints that the Galenic doctrine on blood distribution would be overthrown. Leonardo da Vinci produced accurate drawings of cardiac valves, but he was not engaged with the larger problem and remained a traditionalist where circulation was concerned. Michael Servetus, the Spanish theologian and physician, theorized about a "smaller circulation" through the lungs and suggested that blood could not flow through the septum but must find its way across the lungs to the left side of the heart. Servetus had only an idea; there was as yet no evidence, and he died a martyr's death at the stake in Geneva without developing his idea farther. John Calvin had denounced him to the authorities for holding heretical opinions. Servetus' ideas were repeated by the Italian anatomist Mattheo Colombo in 1559. Colombo's theory was widely known, but it failed to move him or his contemporaries to anything more than a modification of Galen's doctrines. In 1603, Hieronymus Fabricius published a treatise on venous valves, but he drew no conclusions from it. Andrea Cesalpino, one of Fabricius's contemporaries, came closer to the issue. A botanist as well as a physician, Cesalpino described the heart's valve action correctly in 1571, and he began to use the term "circulatio." His analogue appears to have been the stages of the distillation process. In 1593, Cesalpino was talking about a return of venous blood to the heart and an outflow of blood to the arteries. This was a beginning point, but it fell short of defining the circulatory system.

William Harvey, who studied with Fabricius at Padua from 1600 to 1602, was also familiar with the earlier Italians' thinking. He showed no evidence of developing the circulation concept, however, until much later, formulating his ideas over more than two decades while building a successful medical practice in London. He finally published his conclusions on the subject in 1628 under the title *Exercitatio anatomica de motu cordis et sanguinis (An Anatomical Disquisition Concerning the Motion of the Heart and the Blood).*

Harvey developed his theory of blood circulation by meticulous observation and careful reasoning. He made no use of microscopes, which had just reached their first stage of development, and he followed a traditional Aristotelian approach to the philosophy of science. In practical terms, this translated into the conviction that because the body's formation was purposive, its structures should be appropriate to the functions they performed. Yet when he compared the contemporary understanding of the arterial, venous, and cardiac systems with the actual structures through which the supposed functions were carried out, he found only anomaly and contradiction. "Why," he queried, "when the structure of both ventricles is identical . . . should their uses be imagined to be different, when the action, motion, and pulse of both are the same?" Put in this way, absurdity followed absurdity until the investigator had to believe either that nature was irrational or that the explanation was wrong. "Why," Harvey persisted, "was nature reduced to the necessity of adding another ventricle for the sole purpose of nourishing the lungs? . . . How comes it that spirits and fulginous vapours can pass hither and thither without admixture or confusion." And in exasperation, "Good God! how should the mitral valves prevent regurgitation of air and not of blood? Why should the pulmonary vein be presumed to be made for many—three or four different usages?" And then there was the puzzle that the pulmonary veins, "though destined for the conveyance of air," had a blood vessels' structure. In this case, "Nature had rather need of annular tubes such as those of the bronchiae, in order that they might always remain open."

Such questions framed the work. Harvey studied and retested each element in the system, beginning from the assumption that available explanations and physical reality did not match. Nor was he simply attacking tradition. Vesalius, for example, had held that the heart extended itself physically during contraction, giving it the effect of a cupping glass absorbing or drawing up blood. But Harvey showed that what actually happened was that the heart chamber became hard during systole and ejected blood.

Though Harvey may have taken the concept of circulation from the Aristotelian idea of a circle as the perfect form and circularity as perfect movement, his explanation for circulation was built on demonstrable functions carried out through appropriate structures. The missing link in his chain, where hypothesis rather than demonstration had to serve, was his inability to show the structure by which the blood passed over from the arterial to the venous system. Marcello Malpighi supplied this deficiency in 1661 with microscopic analysis of the frog's lung, showing the capillary system. The rest of Harvey's conception was built on firm factual foundations and is now entirely familiar. The heart functions as a pump which drives the flow of blood through the arterial system to the various organs of the body, reaching to the extremities and then returning through the veins. The volume of blood moved in a day, with the left cardiac ventricle pushing about 15 grams (½ ounce) with each stroke, meant a flow of such magnitude through the aorta that there was no possible way the liver could manufacture it from the materials which could be ingested. Consumption and regeneration were physically impossible; the blood circulated and was constantly reused and refurbished by the intake of foods. Harvey stated his basic position in Chapter 14 of his book, recording that "it is absolutely necessary to conclude that the blood in the animal body is impelled in a circle, and is in a state of ceaseless motion." The heart is the organ responsible for this action, which it "performs by means of its pulse," and Harvey concluded that the maintenance of the blood's circulation is "the sole and only end of the motion and contraction of the heart."

William Harvey's work was quickly recognized, but there was also criticism, especially from his countryman, James Primrose, and from the French physician Jean Riolan. He won support from the Dutch physician Jan de Waal, who added new empirical data to strengthen the argument on the passage of blood from the arteries to the veins as well as on the unidirectional flow of blood in arteries and veins. Malpighi's discovery of the capillary system was the final and most valuable evidence confirming Harvey's thesis. From that point forward, there was an accepted factual explanation for circulation which could then become a foundation for work on related body functions.

William Harvey's explanation of circulation compares in significance with the discovery and demonstration of cell theory, or the establishment of the bacterial causes for disease. These achievements belonged to the nineteenth century, however, and nothing comparable to Harvey's theory appeared for 200 years. There were historical reasons both for what Harvey was able to accomplish and for the long gap between his work and comparably significant work in the nineteenth century. William Harvey lived at a time when there was great activity in the field of gross anatomy (q.v.) and when empiricism was making headway against established doctrines of philosophical necessity based on revealed authority. Harvey was also fortunate that his mentors and older contemporaries were working on issues which could illumine the problems which interested him and that he himself held to a world view which assumed a necessary connection between form and function. Harvey's Aristotelian leanings were exactly suited to the issues posed by physiological study, and his philosophy and the search for empirical truth precisely complemented one another. Finally, the subject was one which did not require an advanced technology for effective investigation. Perhaps it was the only one in physiology. The intellectual model for the system, a pump, was entirely familiar, while the one point which required a measure of technology to confirm could be done within the limits of seventeenth-century microscopy, though Harvey did not do it.

William Harvey stayed entirely within the limits of what he was able to control. He avoided building speculations into his conclusions, and he was fortunate that his subject matter was such that he could demonstrate his conclusions with the methods available to him. Literally thousands of researchers over the next 200 years would be able to make similar controlled discoveries of particular phenomena, but an infinitely advanced technology would be required before similarly controlled, empirical results on a physiological system would be possible. Moreover, Harvey's discovery had virtually no effect on actual medical practice until the nineteenth century. The discovery of blood circulation opened the doors to a modern physiology, but at least two centuries elapsed before western science had developed sufficiently to pass through them.

ADDITIONAL READINGS: Jerome Joseph Bylebyl (ed.), *William Harvey and His Age: The Professional and Social Context of the Discovery of the Circulation of the Blood*, Baltimore, 1979; William Harvey, *Movement of the Heart and Blood in Animals: An Anatomical Essay*, Kenneth J. Franklin (trans.), Oxford, 1957; Sir Geoffrey Keynes, *The Life of William Harvey*, Oxford, 1966; Lester S. King, *The Growth of Medical Thought*, Chicago, 1963; Walter Pagel, *New Light on William Harvey*, Basel, 1976; Karl E. Rothschuh, *History of Physiology*, G. B. Risse, (trans. and ed.) Huntington, N.Y., 1973.

See also ANATOMY; HEMATOLOGY; PHYSIOLOGY.

Clinical Medicine

Introduction The clinical concept is at the root of all modern medical practice. It involves identifying, recording, and analyzing symptoms presented in individual cases as a basis for diagnosis and treatment. Relentlessly inductive, clinical medicine requires accuracy in observation and testing to determine deviations from established norms. Both techniques and instruments for observation, therefore, have played a critical part in its historical development, as has physiological research to demonstrate what normal conditions or functions may be.

Therapeutically, the clinical approach emphasizes aiding the organism to resist disease and to repair damage. Until the end of the nineteenth century, therapeutic techniques combined traditional medical philosophies with an ad hoc empirical approach, and it could be said that disease was managed rather than cured. In the course of the twentieth century, this emphasis has shifted dramatically. Scientific research isolated the causes for diseases in such areas as bacterial or viral infection, nutritional deficiencies, physiological or psychological dysfunction, and environmental influences, and it became possible to choose treatments on the basis of what was known to be effective against specific causes. Not all disease conditions succumbed, and there are substantial gray areas in both the understanding of disease causation and the development of successful treatments. Even so, what has been termed the therapeutic revolution has given the modern clinician a degree of effectiveness which is unique in recorded history.

Origins of the Clinical Concept The patron of clinical medicine is Hippocrates. Whatever he may have been historically, Hippocrates has been endowed with the attributes of the ideal physician: compassion, knowledge, and dedication to the patient's welfare. Three ideas drawn from the Hippocratic heritage have been particularly influential: detailed observation and reporting, nature's healing power, and the physician's personal responsibility for the patient. The morality embodied in these principles is epitomized in the Hippocratic oath. In the seventeenth century, the men who originated modern clinical medicine chose Hippocrates as their guide and called themselves Hippocratics. Today, though the technology of medicine has vastly changed, the Hippocratic tradition as interpreted in the early modern period remains a powerful influence in shaping the ideals which clinical medicine pursues.

The clinical approach to medicine can be differentiated from traditional—that is, classical or medieval—medical philosophies by the way it conceptualizes disease. Traditional medical systems considered disease to be a unitary phenomenon which arose from malfunctions in the fluid (humoral) or tissue (solidist) composition of the body. Such thinking, as Henry Sigerist argued, could only conceive of *disease* and not *diseases.* For the plural to become possible, illness had to be thought of as a condition alien to the body's normal state, which was caused by influences located outside the body, which invaded the body, and whose effects could be identified with particular organs or groups of organs. Not all these prerequisites appeared at once, but by the seventeenth century the specificity of diseases was established, if not universally accepted.

One of the earliest modern medical thinkers to move toward the clinical concept was Theophrastus von Hohenheim, better known as Paracelsus, who, in the sixteenth century, openly challenged the unitary theory of disease. Paracelsus believed that diseases were entities separate from man and antagonistic to life, that they were the product of external causes, that they affected particular organs, and that they produced anatomical changes in those organs. Organ change, in fact, determined the nature of disease, as Paracelsus saw it, and as the way an organ worked was gradually transformed, the effects were felt throughout the whole system. Paracelsus was particularly interested in chemical reactions, and he claimed to find both diagnostic clues and effective treatment in the body's chemistry. His "chemistry" was, however, as philosophical as Galen's physiology, owing relatively little to observation and the accumulation of data, and a great deal to a priori reasoning. Even so, Paracelsus appears as a forerunner of ideas central to the clinical concept, while his detailed descriptions of the diseases miners suffered can be considered a positive clinical contribution. It might also be noted that Paracelsus identified himself with Hippocrates (as against Galen), and in the medical world of the sixteenth century he was as knowledgeable about the methods and skills of irregular practitioners as he was familiar with the esoterica of academic medicine.

Paracelsus was at least a century ahead of his time. The unitary philosophies which he attacked remained firmly in place, and Paracelsus himself, when all was said, retained much in common with them. But 100 years later, the picture was very different. The most important influences pointing toward a reorientation in medical thought and the development of a clinical approach appeared in England and Holland. The man who epitomized the new outlook was Thomas Sydenham (1624–1689), the leading exponent of clinical medicine in England and a major personality in the history of modern medicine.

Sydenham's medical philosophy was eclectic and showed the continuing influence of traditional ideas as well as the shape of a new approach. In his pathology, for example, Sydenham was a humoralist. He also accepted the idea of "constitutions" or predispositions to disease in nature, and he followed a therapy built on diet, purgatives, and bleeding. On the other hand, he came to accept cinchona bark as a specific against fevers, and he believed firmly in opium (Sydenham's drops), especially for the heart. But Sydenham's most important contribution was his emphasis on clinical observation. He thought in terms of different diseases with different characteristics which should be described "with the same minuteness and accuracy observed by a painter in painting a portrait." Diseases also should be classified by species as botanists classify plants, while the most careful distinctions needed to be made between those phenomena which were "particular and constant" in a disease and those which owed to accidental causes such as age, physical constitution, or the treatments applied. He left excellent clinical descriptions of a variety of diseases, including smallpox, malaria, consumption, rheumatic polyarthritis, scarlatina (which he differentiated from measles), the acute febrile form of St. Vitus' dance (Sydenham's chorea), and hysteria, which he identified in both men and women. Called the English Hippocrates by his contemporaries, Thomas Sydenham marked the emergence of the clinical approach to medicine, and his example proved influential in England and on the Continent.

Hermann Boerhaave was the acknowledged master of clinical medicine in the eighteenth century and the man responsible for its spread in Europe. Boerhaave was trained at Leyden, where bedside clinical teaching began in Europe in 1626. Boerhaave was appointed to Leyden's chair of theoretical medicine in 1701, and his inaugural lecture was an argument for returning to the study of the Hippocratic texts. Boerhaave knew and admired Sydenham's work (he is supposed to have raised his hat when the English Hippocrates's name was mentioned), and in one sense he improved upon it. What Sydenham did as an individual physician, Boerhaave systematized and taught as a basic approach to medicine. Students from all over Europe flocked to attend his classes, carrying his ideas away with them as the basis for their own practice and teaching. Boerhaave's influence was particularly important at the universities of Vienna and Edinburgh, two of the leading centers for medical training in the eighteenth century, but it was felt strongly throughout Germany and England as well.

Boerhaave was not an original thinker. He made no great discoveries and apart from teaching was best known for treatises which summarized current knowledge. He compiled what has been called the first textbook in physiology, but he also published on chemistry, nervous diseases, eye diseases, syphilis, and medical pedagogy. He considered himself a true disciple of Hippocrates whose first interest was to assist the patient. He was fond of pointing out that theoretical discussion ended at the patient's bedside, and, following the Hippocratic style, he tried in lecture and writing to reduce his conclusions to pithy aphorisms. Boerhaave taught his students to place the examination of the patient first. Careful observation was the key. Once the observation had been made, Boerhaave became eclectic, using iatrochemical and iatrophysical explanations as well as elements of the humoralism and solidism from which they were descended. The treatments recommended followed conventional wisdom at its widest stretch. Neither therapeutics nor causal explanations were especially significant, however. The essence of what Boerhaave taught lay in observing the patient and his or her symptoms. It was this clinical orientation which Boerhaave's pupils carried across Europe.

Rise of the Qualitative Approach In the seventeenth and eighteenth centuries, the techniques for identifying symptoms and formulating diagnoses were entirely a matter of external observation. Some store was set in urine samples, though chemical analysis had barely begun, and the urine gazers who claimed to make judgments about an individual's health by looking at a sample while muttering incantations crossed the line between irregular medicine and quackery. Blood, apart from its color, its copiousness, and its flow, was hardly more revealing, and while pulse taking had a history at least as old as Galen, its adepts had to be extraordinarily skilled to identify the nuances of beat which were considered diagnostically significant. There was, in fact, no clear idea of what constituted normal function, and so any attempt to identify abnormalities quantitatively was bound to fail. Qualitative judgments, therefore, were the norm, and this was true of all those physical signs which could be taken to indicate disease.

Successful quantification awaited the establishment of standards for normal function and the discovery of instruments which could accurately record the body's workings, or methods of analysis which could reveal significant changes in chemical composition. Neither existed before the nineteenth century. But the problem went further. Even those physicians who followed Sydenham or Boerhaave dealt basically in what they were able to observe and what the patient told them. Far from exploring the surface and orifaces of the body, the early clinicians remained quite literally at arm's length, nor did that circumstance change in any marked way until the early nineteenth century. Postmortem investigations, on the other hand, were frequent and detailed as pathology (q.v.) advanced, providing evidence concerning the effects of disease conditions which could be correlated with the observations physicians were accumulating. The outstanding compilation for this purpose was Giovanni Battista Morgagni's classic *The Seats and Causes of Diseases Investigated by Anatomy* (1761), which demonstrated that diseases are located in specific organs, that disease symptoms correlate with anatomical lesions, and that pathological organ changes are responsible for most disease symptoms. Two years later, François de Boissier de Sauvages published a *Methodical Nosology* attempting to use symptoms as the basis for disease classification. Too little was known concerning the relationships between organic pathology and clinical symptoms, however, for the Sauvages classification to be anything but confusing and misleading. It remained to the next century effectively to correlate clinical descriptions with morbid anatomy and pathology.

The correlation between symptoms and conditions revealed postmortem became the basis for classifying diseases by the early nineteenth century and provided the essential elements in clinical diagnosis. In 1826, René Laënnec, a leading figure in the important French school of clinical medicine, summarized the goals of the observational-anatomical approach under three headings: (1) to characterize a pathological condition in the cadaver according to the physical consequences of organ changes, (2) to recognize certain signs in the living patient which indicated the existence of such pathological conditions and which were physical and independent of the superficial disturbances in vital action which often accompanied them, and (3) to treat the condition with those remedies experience had shown to be most effective. Laënnec himself contributed to more accurate identification of disease conditions in the chest cavity when he developed his method of "mediate auscultation" and the instrument he called the stethoscope. Earlier, in the eighteenth century, Leopold Auenbrugger proposed the method called "percussion" to identify thoracic conditions. Both were indications that clinicians were beginning to study the body in life to gain more accurate and comprehensive indications to compare against the postmortem results.

The Paris clinicians led the development of clinical medicine in the early nineteenth century. In addition to Laënnec the group included Marie François Xavier Bichat, Jean-Nicolas Corvisart, Gabriel Andral, and Pierre-Charles-Alexandre Louis. And their efforts in turn were supported by the work of two major physiologists, François Magendie early in the century and Claude Bernard in the middle years. British medicine was strongly disposed to the clinical approach, and the French school found ready acceptance in London, where Guy's Hospital was an early center. Its staff included Richard Bright, whose *Reports on Medical Cases* (1827) published among other original observations his association of a fatal dropsy with kidney disease; Thomas Addison, whose book *On the Constitutional and Local Effects of Disease of the Supra-renal Capsules* (1855) has been called one of the most important works in clinical medicine; and Thomas Hodgkin, who first described lymphadenoma in 1832 and whose name later was attached to that disease. The clinical approach also gained support in Dublin, where its leading practitioners included Robert James Graves, known for his work on exophthalmic goiter; William Stokes, a follower of Laënnec who published major studies on chest diseases (1837) and diseases of the heart and the aorta (1854); and Sir Dominic John Corrigan, known for his work on water-hammer pulse and fibroid phthisis.

Close observation produced new instruments designed for specialist analysis. In the eighteenth century, Anton de Haen in Vienna promoted the use of a thermometer to measure body temperature for diagnostic purposes, and the sphygmomanometer (q.v.) developed in the nineteenth century from various experiments in recording blood pressure. Laënnec's stethoscope was followed by a variety of instruments to permit physicians to investigate hidden or hard-to-approach regions of the body. The laryngoscope, for example, was conceived by a Dr. Bozzini of Frankfurt-am-Main in 1804. Bozzini thought that it would be possible to see into various body cavities by using a mirror to reflect light onto the surfaces to be examined. The larynx was the subject for a series of attempts to apply Bozzini's principle, but the first successful instrument was invented in 1855 by a singing teacher, Manuel Garcia, who was apparently unaware of previous efforts to illumine the throat. Garcia's instrument was taken over by two Austrian clinicians, Türck and Czermak, who put it on spectacle frames, and Voltolini, who added an oxyhydrogen incandescent lamp to give steady and high-intensity light for larynx and ear examinations. The new instrument gave instant results, producing new pathological data from the larynx, and in 1859, Czermak began to use it in examinations of the nasopharyngeal cavity. The following year the first photographs were attempted, but it was not until 1882 that Thomas R. French, of Brooklyn, New York, devised consistently effective methods for photographing the larynx and nasopharynx. Between 1868 and 1897, the laryngeal mirror was used to investigate the upper air and food passages (bronchoscopy and esophagoscopy), and by 1904 bronchoscopy had become a common practice, while experiments in investigating the esophagus and the stomach were in train. Wilhelm Conrad Roentgen's discovery of x-rays (see Radiology) a decade earlier opened the way to more effective investigation of the chest and gastrointestinal system than either the stethoscope or variations on the laryngoscope could offer, though both earlier instruments remained staples in clinical diagnosis.

Hermann Ludwig Ferdinand von Helmholtz's invention of the ophthalmoscope in 1851 was one of the most significant advances in instrumentation. Critically important to the development of modern ophthalmology (q.v.), the ophthalmoscope opened hitherto unknown worlds of observation. Eye diseases generally had been diagnosed by visual examination with, at most, a magnifying glass to assist the diagnostician, but the ophthalmoscope permitted investigation of the ocular fundus, the interior of the eye itself, and revealed connections between fundal pathologies and primary systemic or organic disease. In particular, the ophthalmoscope established a direct connection between internal medicine, especially neurology, and ophthalmology. Its success also generated a family of similar instruments designed for more specialized purposes, including the ophthalmometer, tonometer, instruments for transillumination, visual test types, the phorometer, and the perimeter and split-lamp corneal microscopes.

Development of Quantitative Methods The original clinical concept of disease involved alterations in body structures and assumed an invasive causal mechanism. In the nineteenth century, however, as physiology advanced, functions appeared to be more significant than static structures, and physicians turned toward changes in such fundamental indices as temperature, blood pressure, and breathing rates to find the basic indications of illness. Moreover, the physiological approach to disease appeared to be more objective, more susceptible to quantification, and ultimately more accurate than the original clinical method. The more extreme among the physiologically oriented claimed that clinical descriptions of disease represented an artificial or composite reality, that the disease categories were themselves no more than definitions contrived on the basis of a greater or lesser number of particular phenomena, which were then "averaged" to arrive at a classification. Such a process, according to the Johannes Mueller school of German physiologists, was purely "ontological" and did not deserve the designation of scientific. Only "experimentation combined with observation can make pathology what it should be, an exact science," was the German school's position, and Rudolf Virchow, one of its most outspoken exponents, pushed the matter farther. In his view, "practical medicine shall become applied theoretical medicine, and theoretical medicine shall become pathological physiology." Ultimately, as Virchow saw it, "The subjects of therapy are not diseases but conditions; we are everywhere only concerned with changes in the conditions of life. Disease is nothing but life under altered conditions."

The physiologists' challenge to the methods of French and English clinical medicine promoted an ideological division whose influence reverberated through the medical controversies of the nineteenth century. But ideological conflict, in this instance, proved less significant than practical results. What the German school actually accomplished was to broaden clinical medicine's base by introducing the idea that the goal of medical science was to arrive at an "understanding of morbid processes" and of the relationships which existed among pathological phenomena. In the pursuit of these goals, German experimental physiology added new dimensions to the clinical field, and in particular to the development of techniques for measuring and recording organ functions, while establishing norms which would determine what results suggested deviation and hence a pathological condition. In effect, by the end of the nineteenth century, clinical medicine had absorbed the physiological or functional approach, though the stress on science and its technology left a lasting mark.

While nineteenth-century German physiologists accused clinicians of "ontology" and insufficient scientific rigor, clinical specialists had serious reservations about disease classifications and hence diagnoses built on the appraisal of organ function. Organ dysfunction, unless it was a long-standing problem, generally did not correlate with structural defects, yet physicians had developed a basic confidence in indications of disease which were reflected in altered or defective structures. In sum, they were skeptical of symptoms which could not be "proved" in anatomical pathology. And this skepticism was reinforced when autopsies seemed to show that many so-called functional indices were unreliable indicators for specific diseases. What helped to change these attitudes was the invention of instruments which could measure and record vital actions. This sort of record could become a "factual transcription of pathology" and came to be considered the equivalent of finding an abnormal lesion. Advanced instrumentation filled the clinicians' need for reliable data on function and was responsible for drawing physiology into the service of clinical work.

Analytical Tools: Monitoring Vital Signs The beginning point for measuring vital functions and establishing a quantitative method dated from a monograph by John Hutchinson, published in 1846, which was titled *On the Capacity of the Lungs, and on the Respiratory Functions, with a View of Establishing a Precise and Easy Method of Detecting Disease by the Spirometer.* Hutchinson defined five variables which required measuring and which related the quantity of air breathed to motions in the chest wall. They included "residual air," the amount of air remaining after the deepest breathing; "breathing air," the quantity necessary for normal inspiration and expiration; "complemental air," the amount beyond normal inspiration by deep breathing; "reserve air," the amount of air left after gentle expiration; and "vital capacity," the quantity expelled in the greatest possible voluntary expiration following the deepest possible inspiration. The spirometer mentioned in the title of Hutchinson's monograph applied only to vital capacity, but it was of particular importance. Hutchinson recorded the vital capacity of more than 2,000 healthy persons in the process of checking them for various public jobs. On the basis of that experience, he claimed that the spirometer could detect the presence of lung disease earlier than either percussion or auscultation. One dramatic test seemed to support the claim. The British public became fascinated with an American named Freeman, a giant for the time who stood more than 7 feet tall. Hutchinson took spirometric readings on him when he first visited England and then was able to do a comparative reading two years later. The second reading revealed that there had been a 20 percent reduction in vital capacity over the two-year period. A year later, Freeman developed tuberculosis, from which he never recovered. Hutchinson and the spirometer had recognized a problem which neither of two auscultators noticed, and this led some physicians to the conclusion that the spirometer might well displace the stethoscope for investigating lung diseases.

Unlike the stethoscope, the spirometer needed no skilled interpreter to read the results. Since the Hutchinson method was quantitative, its use involved no special feeling, no intuition for disease. Any doctor could read the numerical valuations given and arrive at a judgment. The problems appeared later. It was noted that so-called deficiencies of vital capacity occurred in healthy people, and there was some difficulty in determining what might be a pathological reading in any given case. But while arguments over the spirometer continued through the century, it was clear that the Hutchinson method provided a new and noteworthy way of approaching certain diagnoses.

Other vital signs which the nineteenth century learned to measure and to use for diagnostic purposes were the pulse, blood pressure, and body temperature. Interpreting the pulse's beat had been an important factor in Galenic medicine, but it involved a series of judgments, none of which could be considered objective or subject to quantification. Nicholas of Cusa was interested in pulse counting in the mid-fifteenth century, as was Galileo 130 years later. Early in the seventeenth century, Santorio Santorio of Padua, that most persistent of the weighers and measurers, devised an instrument for counting the pulse called a pulsilogium. In 1707, England's Sir John Floyer published *The Physician's Pulse Watch*, in which he recognized the Galenists' skill in identifying various beats but deplored the absence of any objective standard for determining abnormality. He recommended counting the pulse against a watch or clock, and he had a special 60-second pulse watch made.

None of these early developments had any significant influence on practicing physicians, though by the nineteenth century the Galenist method was generally considered to be too subjective and complicated to be useful. On the other hand, even the most advanced clinicians saw little to recommend in pulse counting. Théophile de Bordeu thought the pulse was significant, but he concentrated on the equality or inequality of pulsations together with the intervals between and discounted pulse counting as such, while Laënnec concluded that the pulse was not a reliable indicator for the state of the heart or blood circulation, and he warned against its use. In 1835, Julius Hérisson invented a sphygmomanometer, which showed the beat of the pulse in a column of mercury, and his instrument was the first for reading pulse or blood pressure which did not require opening an artery to insert it. The instrument was, nevertheless, clumsy, difficult to use, and inconsistent. Twelve years later, Carl Ludwig, one of Germany's leading experimental physiologists, modified the advanced instrument (which was required to be inserted in an artery) by adding a pen-and-drum arrangement to record the pulse beat automatically. This so-called kymographion was only used for animal experiments. In 1854, Karl Vierordt combined Ludwig's recording apparatus with a modification of Hérisson's machine to create what was called a sphygmograph, a pulse recorder which could be used for routine monitoring on humans. Étienne-Jules Marey refined and improved the design in 1860, and a body of evidence began to accumulate which was clinically significant, particularly for early warning against the onset of some heart conditions as well as defects in the blood vessels. A beginning had been made on objective study of the pulse for diagnostic purposes.

Pulse and blood pressure were related, and the development of the sphygmomanometer made possible the more accurate monitoring for diagnostic work that the pulse counters and recorders were seeking. Samuel von Basch invented a workable instrument for measuring blood pressure accurately in 1876, but the basic design for the instrument was established 25 years later by Scipione Riva-Rocci. Riva-Rocci's instrument was the prototype for today's sphygmomanometers. Nikolai Korotkoff suggested in 1905 that the instrument could be used more effectively if the physician, instead of feeling for the pulse to determine the pressure end points, listened in the pit of the elbow as the blood flow stopped and then, as pressure was released, was allowed to return. The reading on the manometer when the first sound appeared was the maximum; fading to disappearance gave the minimum. Korotkoff's method proved accurate for both and continues in use.

Blood pressure measurement quickly became an accepted clinical technique. The American brain surgeon Harvey Cushing promoted blood pressure readings during surgery to provide an accurate and continuing record of cardiac strength. More generally, as machine design improved and the number of available readings expanded, physicians were able to establish a standard for normal blood pressure range and thus to identify abnormalities which pointed toward specific pathological conditions in the venous and arterial system, in the heart, and in the kidneys. These data were of major diagnostic importance, and in 1912, Massachusetts General

Hospital mandated measuring the blood pressure of all entering patients. For diagnostic and monitoring purposes, measuring blood pressure, checking pulse rates, and recording body temperature have become routine processes fundamental to clinical practice.

Although the realization that temperature change is important in following the course of illness dates from very early times, as with the other vital indications, the ability to measure temperatures and determine what is abnormal belongs to the modern period. At the end of the sixteenth century, Galileo devised an instrument to indicate changes in temperature, but he made no medical application. Santorio Santorio in the seventeenth century made several attempts to estimate body heat. His efforts failed, and many scientists even questioned whether creating a thermometer was worthwhile. In 1683 Robert Boyle referred to the thermometer as "a work of needless curiosity, or superfluous diligence" and went on to argue that one could tell all that it was necessary to know by feel. Since no instrument had yet been devised which gave consistent readings, and since until the eighteenth century there was no standard measure for temperature, Boyle's view is understandable. Even the resolution of those problems, however, did not mean that thermometry would be accepted into medicine. A standard for normal body temperatures had to be established, while correlations between abnormalities in temperature and diseases needed to be defined.

Most of the basic problems in dealing with temperature were resolved in the eighteenth century. Gabriel David Fahrenheit developed a workable mercury thermometer with a temperature scale pegged to three points: 0°, a point determined by a mixture of ice, water, and sal ammoniac or sea salt; 32°, which was the freezing point of water; and 96° which was the external human body temperature. Hermann Boerhaave used Fahrenheit's thermometer in fever cases. Anton de Haen, who was one of Boerhaave's students, began to use temperature change as a guide to treatment, regarding movement toward a normal temperature as a positive sign. On the whole, however, physicians made little use of temperature, and Gerard van Swieten, another of Boerhaave's students, claimed that the pulse gave more important information concerning fever than temperature could. Nor were the early-nineteenth-century clinicians much interested in body temperatures. Their attention was concentrated on physical diagnoses and autopsies. Thermometers for measuring temperature were available, but there seemed to be no strong reason for using them.

A shift toward interest in temperature studies took place toward the middle of the nineteenth century. In 1841, Gabriel Andral published a series of recordings of temperature variations in certain diseases, and three years later, Henri Roger presented his findings on temperature levels in the newborn together with further correlations of temperature and illness. George Zimmerman, an army surgeon, provided evidence on temperature patterns in local inflammations. In 1850 and 1851, F. W. F. von Bärensprung and Ludwig Traube gathered these and additional observations together to argue that body temperature was a key indicator for diagnosis and prognosis and an important guide for therapy. With more and better information available, interest in thermometry waxed strong over the next two decades, with the definitive work on the subject for clinical medicine appearing in 1868. Carl Wunderlich's classic *The Temperature in Diseases* presented data collected on nearly 25,000 patients, with the total number of readings in the millions. Temperature variations in 32 diseases were analyzed, and the components for using temperature effectively became generally available.

Wunderlich's book was both an explanation of clinical use and a much-needed guide for everyday practice. Several myths were dispelled. For clinical purposes, absolute accuracy was unnecessary; frequency of reading was more important, and a minimum of two readings a day was essential. Doctors were unnecessary for taking temperatures. Nurses, clinical assistants, even relatives (provided they were intelligent and well instructed) could do what was necessary. Wunderlich laid down the position that normal temperature was a sign of health while mobility of temperature indicated disease, and he showed that certain types of temperature fluctuation were characteristic of certain diseases. Some of this was controversial, and arguments over the accuracy of measurement and the meaning of the readings when they were available continued through the century. Nevertheless, thermometry was established and reinforced the idea of specific, graphic, and objective data as fundamental to clinical practice.

The instrumentation necessary for pulse, blood pressure, and temperature readings was easily accommodated to bedside practice and, together with the various pre-x-ray visual aids, could be maintained in a normal office. Clinical medicine tended to be individual medicine and to involve a personal relationship between the physician and the patient. This was particularly true in the growing middle-class practices of the nineteenth century, and the relations between the physician and the person who could pay for his services became a kind of paradigm for doctor-patient relationships in general. Clinical medicine belonged to the affluent classes, which could afford privacy and personal attention. People too poor to afford personal attention obtained what health care they could at dispensaries and in hospitals, or from irregular and folk practitioners. But there were tendencies in the development of medical science itself that militated against treating each individual as an individual by promoting specialization, centralization of facilities, and a significant dilution of the prized personal attention for purposes of diagnosis and treatment which had developed in the nineteenth century. Instrumentation played an important role in this process. Monitoring some vital functions was possible with portable instruments appropriate to the bedside or the office, but others required extensive facilities and a degree of technical expertise which general practitioners were not likely to possess. Microscopy and radiology (qq.v.) are examples of the latter; biochemistry for diagnostic purposes is an example of the former.

Biochemistry Chemistry as a diagnostic tool appeared in the sixteenth century, but its period of greatest significance came much later. Analyses of blood and urine began to be applied to specific disease conditions in the second half of the eighteenth century. William Hewson held in 1772 that it was possible to draw diagnostic conclusions and recommend therapies on the basis of chemical investigations of blood serum and solids, while Matthew Dobson set out to find the origin of the sweetness of diabetic urine. In 1776 he reported experiments in which he evaporated urine and found a residue which smelled and tasted like sugar. Further studies on diabetic urine by John Rollo, a physician, and William Cruikshank, a chemist as well as a surgeon, noted that the sugar-like residue varied in quantity and intensity during the course of the disease. Some clinical applications followed. The tests provided diagnostic evidence for the presence of diabetes mellitus (q.v.), offered data useful for evaluating a patient's response to therapy, and appeared to give some insight into the causes of the disease. The last, however, was more apparent than real. Cruikshank continued to study body fluids, looking for chemical keys to dropsy, rheumatism, gout, jaundice, and scurvy. However, his example was not widely followed. Physicians were not prepared to do chemical analysis, and such scientists as were interested in chemistry were not interested in studying medical problems. Nevertheless, a tradition was begun.

Chemistry took on new importance in 1827 when Richard Bright published his *Reports of Medical Cases*. Bright was able to show that the accumulation of fluid in the tissues known as dropsy was accompanied by a shriveling of the kidneys, while heating the urine of a dropsy victim precipitated a large quantity of albumin in the form of an opaque white material. Bright's demonstration of albumin in dropsy patients forged a link between an alteration in a living patient and a lesion which appeared on autopsy. The form of kidney disease subsequently called Bright's disease could be diagnosed in the living patient by a single, simple chemical test. Later work showed that albumin in the urine could arise from other causes, and that Bright's test was not an infallible or definitive sign that dropsy was developing. Even so, Bright's work was of major importance in connecting chemistry with clinical observation and anatomical dissection.

Bright's work was only the beginning of a mounting assault on body fluids with chemical analysis to arrive at firm diagnoses of illness. Gabriel Andral, who called on medicine in 1841 to initiate studies of pathological conditions in body fluids, published his *Pathological Hematology* in 1843. Andral considered both the appearance of the blood and its chemical properties, but it was the latter which received the most attention. He noted that the four constituents of blood—globules, fibrin, solids, and water—were present both in sickness and in health but that the proportions among them changed. He established normal ratios for each part and then connected changes in the ratios with different diseases. An excess of red globules, for example, was the condition known as plethora and was accompanied by dizziness, fever, singing in the ears, and rapid heartbeat. Anemia was the reverse condition. The red globules were in short supply, and this condition meant low vitality and sluggish body functions.

In all of his chemical work, Andral followed a quantitative method. He separated and weighed the blood's constituents to arrive at a picture in numbers of the blood's condition. His work aroused widespread interest and argument; it also fostered blood studies for diabetes and research on the role of uric acid in gout. Alfred Becquerel did similar studies in 1841 on the composition of urine, establishing the average amounts of water, urea, uric acid, lactic acid, albumin, and inorganic salts secreted in a 24-hour period and correlating these data with various disease conditions. His methods were also entirely quantitative.

By the middle of the nineteenth century, it had become clear that counting red blood cells would provide additional diagnostic evidence, but the first efforts to accomplish this task were failures. In 1877, however, William R. Gowers, an English doctor, published his *On the Numeration of the Red Corpuscles,* in which he argued that an accurate count of red blood cells provided the best index for diagnosing anemia. Gowers invented a device called the "haemocytometer," which could be attached to any microscope and which gave a more accurate accounting of the red blood cells than any other method. He was able to demonstrate that iron therapy worked by increasing the number of red blood cells and that skin color did not accurately reflect red cell counts and was a poor indicator for anemia. Gower's methods and his instruments were not infallible. The haemocytometer was difficult to use, and different investigators found different results. The error margin amounted to a variation of 15 to 25 percent. Other techniques were found to substitute for counting. The best alternative was to use centrifugal force to pack the blood cells together and then measure their volume. This method and the instrumentation to carry it out pointed the way toward the centrifuge.

Laboratories As chemistry and microscopy became increasingly important, access to a diagnostic laboratory became essential to the practicing physician, and this institution began to appear in the later nineteenth century. The clinical laboratories were offshoots of research laboratories and initially were intended to channel knowledge about biological processes into new methods for diagnosing and treating illness. Providing diagnostic services to physicians was at best a secondary goal, and while they served it, it was also clear that there was a larger need to be met. One means for meeting that need was the ward laboratory. This laboratory was usually established in space adjacent to the main hospital wards, and its sole purpose was to support patient care. Ward laboratories became ubiquitous and increasingly complex as they acquired more sophisticated instrumentation and employed more and better-trained technicians while absorbing more and more of the house physicians' assigned work time. These laboratories, as Sir William Osler pointed out, had become "as essential to the proper equipment of the hospital as the internes. They are to the physician just as the knife and scalpel are to the surgeon." And this dependency increased rapidly. Laboratory techniques soon passed out of the competence of individual physicians to become highly developed specialties. Bacterial studies were as complicated as they were necessary. There were, for example, 689 different methods for distinguishing the germ which caused typhoid from other microorganisms which resembled it. The everyday tools of the bacteriologist—chemical staining, magnifying instruments, culture media—required special training and a great deal of time, nor were other specialties notably easier. The laboratory and the laboratory specialist had become an integral part of clinical medicine by the early twentieth century, and as their importance rose, the physician found himself or herself making judgments on the basis of data someone else had compiled. This was the shape of the diagnostic world to come.

Hospitals and research institutions established

laboratories, but the demand for services grew so rapidly that it could not be met institutionally. As a result, commercial laboratories for chemical and microscopic work appeared in major cities, and the demand for their services simply exploded in the course of World War I. It is estimated that nearly 300 laboratories were supplying analyses to physicians with the American expeditionary forces, and as more and more physicians learned to use and trust the commercial laboratories, their number expanded further. This meant a continually deepening dependency of physicians on data which were essential to their work whose acquisition and primary analysis they could not control. In general, this was not considered to be unhealthy. On the contrary, it appeared to be making science and technology serve the real interests of both physicians and patients, and the result was a revolution in clinical practice. The price has only begun to become apparent.

The great shift in clinical medicine from the individual toward the institutional and mechanical grew out of the need to monitor physiological functions and the need for instrumentation for that purpose, together with the bacteriological revolution, which multiplied already existing demands for specialized laboratory work. Chemical analyses of body fluids, organ scans, electrocardiograms, and x-rays were only the beginning of the techniques used to diagnose disease and monitor treatments. Testing in all its forms became a routine element in diagnosis, so routine, in fact, that testing was done regardless of whether any special value was attached to the tests for any individual patient. This pattern has been most apparent in the United States, and there are abundant data which demonstrate it. In five Michigan hospitals, for example, which were studied for the period 1938–1958, there was a 100 percent increase in the number of tests given to patients in six diagnostic categories. At Yale-New Haven, the number of laboratory procedures increased from 48,000 in 1954 to 200,000 10 years later, with only a slight increase in the number of patients involved. And the rate of expansion accelerated in the 1970s. United States statistics showed a total of 2 billion recorded laboratory tests in 1971. By 1976, the number had more than doubled to 4.5 billion, and comparative studies have shown a comparable expansion in Canada and Great Britain.

The problems associated with an excessive dependency on instrumentation cut deeper than a dehumanized medical culture and go to the root of modern clinical practice. Sound diagnosis and treatment rest on intelligent interpretation of accurate information, and there are troubling indications that at the very time physicians have been moving away from patients to deal more objectively with cases, the technology on which they must rely has been shown to be inherently prone to a relatively high level of error. This, of course, was true in the early days of instrumentation's development, and there was a healthy skepticism about the results which the magical machines could produce. But the extraordinary successes won by a scientifically based medicine have reinforced faith in all its routine procedures, though the evidence has been accumulating for a long time that this faith needed to be qualified.

Studies concerning the accuracy achieved by diagnostic laboratories and the medical value of tests and screenings routinely administered have been carried on regularly in the United States since the end of World War I. An initial survey which the government sponsored in 1919 showed such an incidence of error and disparity of result in laboratory work that the American Medical Association created an oversight committee to review the situation. Apart from confirming the existence of a continuing problem, this adventure into regulation had little practical effect. A Public Health Service investigation of city and state laboratories testing for syphilis in the late 1930s concluded that many of these centers could not meet "minimum standards of efficiency," while a commission which studied 18 laboratories in 1949 calculated that test results were unacceptable on more than one-third of the specimens submitted. A Pennsylvania commission undertaking a similar study found comparable results. Part of the problem was the absence of either a federal regulatory code or effective state licensing requirements for laboratories. As late as 1964, only 16 states had established performance standards, and where standards did exist, enforcement was uneven.

A Clinical Laboratory Act was passed by Congress in 1967 which established federal overseer powers, and by 1977 just over half of the states had established scientific standards for laboratory performance or required licensing for technicians. But regulatory legislation hardly touched the problem, and the testing explosion which occurred in the 1960s and 1970s multiplied its effects. The state of New Jersey investigated 257 laboratories over the period 1967–1973 for one of the basic, most common, and least complicated analyses: the level of hemoglobin in blood. They found that nearly one in five laboratories failed to give an acceptable result over 70 percent of the time. Other aspects of blood analysis carried an error rate of from 20 to 25 percent. The conclusion is that as clinical medicine has moved toward an ever greater dependence on laboratories, the level of error has become an increasingly important factor, reaching the stage of a significant problem for accuracy of diagnosis.

The issue scarcely ends with laboratories. Clinicians have become dependent on various medical specialties for assistance in their work, and there, too, problems have emerged. X-rays were, until recently, used extensively for all manner of diagnostic work, but apart from the potential danger of repeated exposures, investigations have showed that interpreting the results, even for skilled specialists, was at best an uncertain art. During World War II, x-ray was used to screen recruits for military service, but when the films were reviewed in 1942 for diagnostic accuracy, a confusing picture emerged. Doctors reading the films found that they were in disagreement with their colleagues about one-third of the time and, on rereading, that they disagreed with their own previous interpretation 20 percent of the time. A Danish study carried out in the early 1950s produced similar results. Three experienced radiologists studied 2500 x-ray films. They found that when any one of them declared a particular film to depict a pathological condition, agreement among the three was achieved in only 12 percent of the cases. Tests dealing with electrocardiograms showed a comparable lack of agreement in reading what the machine recorded.

Conclusion The instruments available to the modern clinician are extraordinary, but they are by no means infallible, nor are the specialists who read them. Data gathering for modern clinical purposes requires at some point to be brought back and focused on the particular patient. To the extent that this part of the process has been lost, and that instrumentation and specialist analysis have become a substitute for more personalized clinical skills, the physician faces a potential for error and a reduction in effectiveness. Clinical medicine began with physicians working with patients. It has evolved, in its most advanced forms, toward a position where diseases rather than patients have become the focus. There appears to be a growing conviction, however, that a return to the patient is necessary if the miracles that medical science offers are to be fully realized.

ADDITIONAL READINGS: Arturo Castiglioni, *History of Medicine*, E. B. Krumbhaar (trans. and ed.), New York, 1941, 545–550, 615–624, 698–712, 818–835; Audrey B. Davis, *Medicine and Its Technology: An Introduction to the History of Medical Instrumentation*, Westport, Conn., 1981; Kenneth Dewhurst, *Dr. Thomas Sydenham, 1624–1689: His Life and Original Writings*, Berkeley, 1966; Knud Helge Faber, *Nosography: The Evolution of Clinical Medicine in Modern Times*, 2d rev. ed., New York, 1930, 1978; David Kenneth Keele, *The Evolution of Clinical Methods in Medicine*, London, 1963; Garret Arie Lindbom, *Hermann Boerhaave: The Man and His Work*, London, 1968; S. J. Reiser, *Medicine and the Reign of Technology*, Cambridge, Mass., 1978; S. E. D. Shortt, "Clinical Practice and the Social History of Medicine: A Theoretical Accord," *Bulletin of the History of Medicine* 55 (Winter 1981): 533–542; E. Ashworth Underwood, *Boerhaave's Men at Leyden and After*, Edinburgh, 1977; David M. Vess, *Medical Revolution in France, 1789–1796*, Gainesville, Fla., 1975; Morris J. Vogel and Charles E. Rosenberg (eds.), *The Therapeutic Revolution: Essays in the Social History of American Medicine*, Philadelphia, 1979.

See also MEDICAL PROFESSION; MICROSCOPY; PATHOLOGY; RADIOLOGY; SPHYGMOMANOMETER.

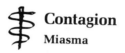

Contagion

Miasma

Contagion, the idea that a disease is communicated directly or indirectly from one individual to another, is an ancient doctrine which became an important issue in the eighteenth and nineteenth centuries. Until the bacteriological discoveries of Louis Pasteur and Robert Koch ended speculation over the causes of most epidemic disease, there was no scientific basis for proving contagion or its opposite, yet to protect the community decisions had to be made. The basic issue was whether or not to impose quarantines to control the spread of disease, but with no clear scientific evidence, social, economic, and political factors determined the stance which governments took.

The idea of contagion was foreign to the classic medical tradition and found no place in the voluminous Hippocratic writings. The Old Testament, however, is a rich source for contagionist sentiment, especially in regard to leprosy and venereal disease. Varro, a Roman writer of the first century B.C., and Cicero both speculated on the possibility that fevers were communicated by "tiny animals" which might be carried on the wind, but the doctrine received its classic statement in 1546, when Girolamo Fracastoro published his treatise *On Contagion*. Fracastoro held that contagious diseases were probably caused by living disease seeds which could be communicated, and he strongly recommended quarantine, sequestration, and fumigation.

In the seventeenth century, contagionist sentiment was reinforced by sightings of microscopic "animalcules" by Athanasius Kircher (1659) and Antonj van Leeuwenhoek (1676). Parasites, bacteria, and worms all went together, or as Nicholas Hartsoeker wrote, "I believe that the worms cause most of the diseases which attack mankind." In 1699, Nicholas Andry published his treatise *On the Generation of Worms in the Human Body*, in which he rejected spontaneous generation and asserted that parasites were active in causing disease and that "their seeds entered the body from without." His views, of course, were firmly contagionist.

Anticontagionist thinking ascribed epidemics to atmospheric factors, diet, the conjunction of planets, miasma generated by decaying matter, and other environmental causes. But in the sixteenth and seventeenth centuries, anticontagionism did not fit the political climate. This was an age which valued stability and accepted unlimited political power as a necessity. Contagions could be resisted in the same way an invading enemy was fought, while the rules enforced for sanitary reasons had the further effect of demonstrating the ruler's determination to maintain order. Such regulatory authority was accepted by merchants and householders who looked to the prince as their protector, and even in the commercial republics of Italy and Germany, where merchants made the decisions, this authoritarian approach prevailed.

Attitudes toward quarantine changed in the eighteenth century, and by the second decade of the nineteenth, the balance had swung sharply against contagion. This swing corresponded with what might be called the revolutionary century (1760–1860). Political values shifted as European societies grew more populous, more affluent, and more open. Strong monarchists still believed in the government's protective role, but public sentiment opposed such paternalistic interference. Merchants complained bitterly about the interruption of trade, the politically minded saw quarantines as an effort to reimpose royal rule by force or to destroy a liberal opposition, while physicians argued that there was no medical justification for quarantines.

Anticontagionist sentiment developed in the midst of a succession of new and devastating epidemics which ushered in the nineteenth century. Plague was a fading problem in all but eastern Europe, but outbreaks in the Levant set off a campaign by convinced contagionists to protect English ports in the early 1820s. The other diseases at issue were yellow fever (q.v.), which had its most important effects in the new world, typhus (q.v.), which could not be distinguished with any degree of certainty from typhoid, and cholera (q.v.). There was no question in most minds about the contagiousness of leprosy, syphilis, and smallpox (qq.v.).

The first wave of aggressive anticontagion sentiment came from America in the wake of the yellow fever epidemic of 1793. An observation of the outbreak in Philadelphia, the contentious (though always influential) Benjamin Rush abandoned his view that yellow fever was contagious, implicating rotting vegetable matter—a cargo of coffee dumped and spoiling on the Philadelphia docks—as the source of an infectious miasma, and he declared firmly against quarantine measures. His opinions won a large following among Philadelphia physicians, though local authorities in Pennsylvania, New Jersey, and Delaware vacillated between quarantines and free movement.

In post-Napoleonic Europe, yellow fever outbreaks at Gibraltar resulted in quarantines along the Spanish-French frontier. Anticontagionists, led by J. A. Rochoux from France and Charles Maclean, an English physician who devoted much of his brief career to fighting contagionist policies, published a manifesto in 1822 and lobbied successfully against quarantine legislation in the Spanish Cortes (parliament). Nicholas Chervin, a French physician who had spent nearly a decade in America, visited Spain and then campaigned aggressively in the French Chamber of Deputies against the yellow fever quarantine. The Academy of Medicine was called in, an investigative commission was appointed, and, following another year of study, the commission reported in favor of the anticontagionists. The academy, despite heavy pressure from the government, accepted the report, and the chamber withdrew financing for the quarantine. It was a stunning victory for anticontagion, and it brought Chervin the Grand Prix de Médecine for 1828.

The arguments which carried the day against yellow fever quarantines were scarcely definitive, but they were effectively presented. They held that the outbreaks of yellow fever and the arrival of ships from infected regions were coincidental; that nursing mothers did not communicate the disease to their babies; that people attending the sick did not become sick; that the disease was prevalent in defined localities; and that there was no discernible pattern of infection connected with the movement of goods and refugees or other traffic. Ignorant of the epidemiology of yellow fever, the anticontagionist looked for evidence that would prove communication by contact. Of course, such evidence did not exist.

The cholera pandemics which crossed Europe and the Americas during the nineteenth century reinforced anticontagionism between 1826 and 1866 and left a residue of resistance even after the bacterial cause for cholera was demonstrated in 1883. During the first pandemic (1816–1826), most governments established quarantines and invoked coercive sanitary regulations. These efforts proved entirely fruitless, while violence on the quarantine lines in Russia in 1830 and 1831, upheavals in Paris and London in 1832, and riots in New York underlined the social dangers of restrictive policies. Medical opinion became strongly anticontagionist, and by the time the second pandemic arrived in the period 1848–1849, the cholera's devastating effects among the poor were taken for proof that this epidemic disease and possibly epidemic diseases in general were essentially the product of unhealthy living conditions. In 1849, Britain's General Board of Health issued a report on the 1848 cholera outbreak in which it attributed its severity to an increase in those social conditions which generated the miasmas which caused epidemics. Those conditions included overcrowded housing, bad drains, damp, filth, inadequate and unwholesome food, and unsanitary water. No blame was attached to the relaxation of quarantines. On the contrary, the failure of quarantines to stop the cholera in earlier outbreaks was considered significant, and governments were also impressed with the violence which enforced sanitary regulations produced.

Anticontagion sentiment reached its peak around 1850 and then began to decline. There were several reasons. In the wake of the revolutions of 1848, and with the onset of the Crimean War, attitudes toward political authority again changed. Revolutionary upheavals brought a new taste for order and a greater willingness to consider coercion as a necessary evil, though interruptions in international trade were only accepted reluctantly. There was also some persuasive evidence that diseases were, in fact, communicable. Here the work done by William Budd and John Snow on typhoid and cholera became important. Third, the quantity of information concerning microorganisms was increasing, though the effective application of that knowledge to disease causation was still in the future. Finally, the anticontagionists had been so strong that a correction was almost inevitable. Their positions were no more scientifically secure than the contagionists', and there was always room for revision. It is more than likely that this factor, when combined with the changed attitude toward authority, produced the swing. Governments in the 1850s and 1860s reintroduced quarantine policies, and by 1869, even Rudolf Virchow, the most outpoken of anticontagionists an political liberals, had moved toward contagionism.

These events took placed before the germ theory of disease had been established. Once that was done, the argument over contagion shifted to studies of disease agents and modes of transmission. In modern terms, the anticontagionists were justified in resisting quarantines as doing more social harm than medical good. Because the question of contagion was scientifically moot, its resolution in the era before germ theory reflected the dominant political culture and serves historians as an index of important social attitudes.

ADDITIONAL READINGS: Erwin H. Ackerknecht, "Anti-contagionism Between 1821 and 1867," *Bulletin of the History of Medicine* 22 (September–October 1948): 562–593; Geoffrey Marks and William K. Beatty, *Epidemics*, New York, 1976; *Wesley W. Spink, *Infectious Diseases: Prevention and Treatment in the Nineteenth and Twentieth Centuries*, Minneapolis, 1979; C. E. A. Winslow, *The Conquest of Epidemic Disease*, Princeton, 1943.

See also BACTERIOLOGY; EPIDEMIOLOGY.

Coronary Heart Disease

The cardiovascular system, which is responsible for blood circulation, includes both the heart and the blood vessels. The heart acts to circulate the blood throughout the entire system. When the heart stops functioning, the system dies, and the cessation of heart function is a definition of death. In modern society, malfunction in the heart itself, arising from pathological conditions in the cardiovascular system, has become a significant cause of death. Malformed hearts produce a variety of congenital heart diseases. Bacterial infections, which cause inflammation of the lining of the heart muscle called rheumatic heart disease, generate severe pathological effects. But the most common and hence the most dangerous condition is the deterioration of the vascular system which results in coronary heart disease. Disease processes such as arteriosclerosis reduce blood flow, producing a condition of inadequacy called ischemia and resulting in the death of a portion of the heart muscle (infarction), which can produce a fatal heart attack.

The term for such an attack is "myocardial infarction," which refers to a complex of symptoms including prolonged chest pain. Originally described in 1912 by James Herrick as a coronary thrombosis, or coronary attack brought on by blockage of the coronary arteries, the disease has been given a broader etiology as a result of a more complete understanding of the effects of arterial disease. An older term, still in use to describe the violent, stabbing pains which come with underlying coronary artery disease, is "angina pectoris." This condition was first described clinically and connected with arterial degeneration in the second half of the eighteenth century. Its application to a specific clinical condition came after Herrick's work in the twentieth century.

Heart disease has been present from ancient times. Studies of Egyptian mummies from the third millennium B.C. show degenerative heart, arterial, and vascular conditions, and there is similar evidence in Peruvian remains from the first millennium B.C. Written sources including the Ebers papyrus, the Bible, the Talmud, and the Hippocratic writings contain references to anginal and myocardial diseases, and the Hippocratic writings of the fourth century B.C mention vascular obstruction and sudden death in connection with an anginal attack. There is no way of determining, however, how widespread these conditions were.

Galen of Pergamum, who wrote in the second century A.D., attached great importance to the blood and blood vessels, noted that without respiration the heart dies at once, and identified three different heart lesions, which he called "dyscrasias." The first was a slight version, which produced palpitations. The second was more severe and affected parts of the heart. The third, or "organic dyscrasia," affected the whole heart and resulted in instantaneous death. Though offering no explanation for these variations, Galen quoted Hippocrates to the effect that the terminal attacks were often preceded by "frequent and serious faintings." Modern authority suggests that Galen's organic dyscrasia resembles myocarditis rather than a coronary thrombosis. Myocarditis would have involved a severe chronic condition resulting in death, while a thrombosis would have been a sudden, unannounced attack resulting from some foreign object's blocking the blood flow. Other writers after Galen touched on subjects relevant to heart disease but did not refer to it directly. Caelius Aurelianus, for example, who wrote in the fifth century A.D., included a chapter on "the cardiac passion" which included a description of what appears to be the type of shock which accompanies a coronary attack.

Though scattered references to heart conditions continued to appear through the next 1000 years, neither Latin, Islamic, nor Hebrew medical sources went much farther than the classic writers. In the sixteenth century, however, as postmortem examination became more common and anatomical dissection was practiced more regularly, new evidence on heart failures began to accumulate. In 1507, for example, Antonio Benivieni described a case of heart pain followed by death in which the postmortem revealed a small piece of dark flesh in the left ventricle. The idea that this was the cause for death is hardly credible, but the search for pathological evidence in the heart was significant. In 1560, Amatus Lusitanus gave a precisely detailed report describing a sudden death owing to "an obstruction in the heart." In this case, however, there was no autopsy. Five years earlier, Andreas Vesalius had reported on the death of a man whose heart was found to be distended in the left ventricle. In 1586 Petrus Salius Diversus presented his suggested hypothesis that cardiac syncope and sudden death were owed to obstruction of the blood vessels. Nearly 200 years passed before this insight gained factual support.

The anatomical studies of the sixteenth century built the foundations for William Harvey's explanation of blood circulation published in 1628. Yet that momentous achievement had little immediate effect on understanding heart disease. Nevertheless, evidence was accumulating. In 1649, Harvey himself described two cases of what appears to have been myocardial infarction in a letter to Jean Riolan. In one case, that of Sir Robert Davy, there were repeated seizures with pain in the chest and a feeling of suffocation. The patient finally died in the midst of one of those seizures, and an autopsy showed a large tear in the left ventricle. In the other case, a greatly enlarged heart was found. There was no suggestion of blockage or any other cause, though in the second case Harvey noted that the patient kept his emotions hidden, with the clear implication that this had some significance for his condition. Though Harvey reported on the so-called third circulation through the coronary arteries and veins, he did not recognize its importance for heart conditions, nor were he and his contemporaries prepared to see the possible relationship between conditions in the veins and arteries and the onset of heart disease. This did not mean, of course, that arterial occlusion was not noticed. In the previous century Leonardo da Vinci had drawn veins and arteries which clearly showed degeneration, and in 1683 Luigi Bellini reported his observations on calcification of coronary vessels, their subsequent cloture, and the clinical signs which might follow. Even so, it was not until the eighteenth century that the importance of such developments for heart disease was generally appreciated.

In the eighteenth century the study of heart disease moved substantially forward. Progress began with general texts on the heart, its function and diseases. J. B. Sénac published the best and most comprehensive of these in 1749. Such books included clinical data, postmortem findings, and theoretical discussions which involved both modern and classical authors. The strictly cardiological literature was supported by pathology collections, especially the work of Giovanni Morgagni, whose masterwork on morbid anatomy published in 1761 contained much evidence of heart damage. There was no correlation, however, with the pathology of the coronary vessels, though Morgagni did note that the heart lost force as its parts became "tendinous" instead of fleshy.

The first clinical description of the condition known as angina pectoris was read by William Heberden before the College of Physicians in London in July 1768. It was published in 1772. Entitled *"Some Account of a Disorder of the Breast,"* this classic paper was just nine pages long. It marks the beginning, however, of modern observation on heart disease and provides a convincing diagnostic image. Heberden dealt only with clinical description and employed neither ancient authority nor postmortem evidence. Indeed, Heberden was apparently unaware that others had mentioned what he described, for the condition which he identified he considered to be unnoticed and virtually unknown. Heberden's stress on precardial pain as a diagnostic concept and his conviction that the prognosis for such conditions was very serious led a number of his contemporaries to consider blockage or shrinkage in the circulatory system as a cause. Dr. Edward Jenner was apparently the first to correlate angina pectoris with impaired circulation which would produce a morbid change in the heart's structure. Jenner also identified a thrombus in the coronary artery of a person who died of an angina attack. In 1799, C. H. Parry published his *Inquiry into the Symptoms and Causes of the Syncope Anginosa, Commonly Called Angina Pectoris*, in which he summarized the clinical findings and discussed a number of cases with their postmortem results. These cases demonstrated "ossification" and obstruction of the coronary arteries together with gross pathology of the aorta. There was no evidence of myocardial damage, however. Allen Burns, writing in 1809, extended the ideas of Heberden, Jenner, and Parry, particularly with experimental data on ischemia and further evidence of change in the structure of the heart's substance. He did not, however, articulate the idea of infarction.

Though the work on angina of eighteenth-century English physicians gained wide acceptance, there was a great deal concerning ischemic heart disease that was still not clear, and there was a feeling that the Heberden-Jenner-Parry view oversimplified the processes involved. In 1804, however, Antonio Scarpa had presented the description of arteriosclerosis, an entity which Jean G. C. F. M. Lobstein refined in 1833. Using evidence from dissections, Scarpa explained what is now called atherosclerosis. He noted that "the interal coat (of the vessel) is subject from slow internal cause, to an ulcerated and steatomatous disorganization," and he referred as well to a "squamous and earthy rigidity and brittleness." He also described cases in which there were "ulcerated corrosions" of the heart, a phenomenon which, while recognized still, is not fully understood. Arteriosclerosis, a term invented later by Lobstein, became the focal point in the study of coronary artery disease. In 1846, the greatest of the nineteenth-century pathologists, Rudolf Virchow, introduced the idea of thrombosis when he described a clot in the pulmonary artery.

Other studies on coronary problems looked more specifically at the heart. It had been known since the end of the seventeenth century that interruption of blood flow by ligation could produce cardiac arrest, and this lead was followed again in the nineteenth century by John Ericksen, P. I. Panum, Albert von Bezold, and especially Julius Cohnheim. Cohnheim was a pathologist who identified "fibrous myocarditio" and "heart aneurysm" with obstructions in the coronary, and he believed that failure of oxygen supply was responsible for myocardial damage. Even so, it was Carl Weigert in 1880 who provided a classic description of myocardial infarction, which was then refined over the next two decades. Clinicians added to what the pathologists reported. The most notable effort was by E. von Leyden, in a work entitled *On Sclerosis of the Coronary Arteries and the Morbid Conditions Dependent on It* (1884). Though he did not identify myocardial infarction as such, Leyden did establish various types of lesions and their clinical consequences.

By the end of the nineteenth century, a substantial quantity of information on coronary heart diseases was available. Moreover, the processes of arterial degeneration and morbid consequences to the heart itself had been recognized, with emphasis falling on the latter. This material was rationalized in a series of important papers, books, and lectures in the first decade of the twentieth century by Sir William Osler, W. P. Obrastzow, N. D. Straschesko, and finally James D. Herrick. It was Herrick's paper in particular, published in 1912, which provided the definitive synthesis on coronary heart disease, or coronary thrombosis as he called it. But neither Herrick nor his colleagues discovered anything new. Rather, they put together with studied care and great precision what was known concerning coronary occlusion and its effect on the heart. As a recent authority wrote, "they deserve the credit given to them for having initiated the definitive understanding of cardiac infarction as a clinically recognizable morbid entity."

Herrick's paper appeared in 1912, but the ideas he had to offer caused no stir at all. More than two decades passed before his conclusions had filtered through the journals and medical schools to become accepted in the profession at large. Certain individuals grasped and used them before that, but Herrick himself, writing in 1942, noted that for at least six years his message seemed to go unheard. Subsequent developments refined the initial understanding of coronary heart disease, greatly improved diagnostic techniques, introduced measures for providing first aid and treatment for heart victims, and opened the area of cardiac surgery, the use of pacemakers, and finally heart transplants. These developments have greatly expanded the recognized varieties of heart disease, while markedly improving the chances an individual has of surviving a heart attack.

Despite the achievements which have followed Herrick's work, the degenerative conditions in the circulatory system responsible for damage to the heart are not well understood. They appear to be associated with aging, though it is also believed that metabolic abnormalities in the vascular tissue begin the processes which eventually create occlusion and ischemia. Epidemiological studies suggest that coronary heart disease, like cancer, is particularly prevalent in affluent and advanced societies. More specialized investigations have identified rich, high-fat diet, low exercise levels, psychic stress, and cigarette consumption as contributing causes. These ideas have won broad acceptance, bringing about revolutionary changes in modern styles of living. These include a powerful reaction against obesity and smoking, a new interest in exercise programs, particularly jogging, a turn away from high-cholesterol foods, and a general stress on the importance of good health. These preoccupations are most marked among urban citizens of middle-class status. Even so, the question of whether heart diseases have increased with the advance of modernized, industrial societies or whether a long-existing condition has finally been identified and quantified remains unanswered. However this question may finally be answered, the greater attention to health and personal fitness which the study of heart disease has provoked appears to be a clear social gain.

ADDITIONAL READINGS: P. E. Baldry, *The Battle Against Heart Disease*, Cambridge, 1971; James B. Herrick, *A Short History of Cardiology*, Springfield, Ill., 1942; J. O. Leibowitz, *The History of Coronary Heart Disease*, London, 1970; Rex N. MacAlapin, "Coronary Arterial Spasm: A Historical Perspective," *Journal of the History of Medicine and Allied Sciences* 35 (July 1980): 288–300.

See also HEART.

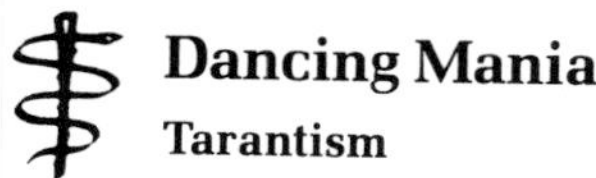

Dancing Mania

Tarantism

Dancing mania was a well-defined, ritualistic behavior pattern which appeared in late medieval times. It represented popular reactions to stress, danger, or disorder expressed in forms appropriate to medieval culture. Modern analogies for the dancing mania include the controlled leaping of the Shaker communities, the speaking in tongues of charismatic Christians, and the rhythmic chanting of revival meetings. Chorea, or St. Vitus' dance, is sometimes confused with the dancing mania but actually is a different phenomenon. First described by Sir Thomas Sydenham in 1686, chorea is a severe nerve disorder caused by the streptococcus responsible for rheumatic fever. There is no such bacterial etiology involved in the dancing mania.

Dancing manias appeared in central Europe, southern Italy, and Spain. All versions had a religious foundation. St. John the Baptist and St. Vitus were the patron saints in central Europe, while tarantism in southern Italy reflected the tension between pre-Christian and Christian cultural patterns. The dancing manias took on epidemic characteristics, and modern medical historians, recognizing their psychocultural genesis, have treated them as pathological manifestations which had a specific causal mechanism. Recent studies have concentrated on the causal aspect in a European context. Additional work on comparable phenomena in non-European cultures is needed.

Medieval Dancing During the later years of the fourteenth century, and in the wake of the black death, there was an outbreak of hysteria which took the form of compulsive dancing by men and women alike. Beginning in 1374 near Aachen (Aix-la-Chapelle), the phenomenon spread rapidly across the low countries to France and throughout Germany. There was a distinct pattern or ritual to the dancing. Men and women spontaneously and without preliminaries jumped up wherever they were and began to dance. They went out into the streets, joined hands, formed circles, and, "appearing to have lost all control over their senses, continued dancing, regardless of the by-standers, for hours together in wild delirium." Only total exhaustion halted the cavorting, but when the dancers stopped, they fell down and groaned, complaining of a terrible oppression. Cloths bound around their waists gave some relief, and this "tight binding" became an integral part of the dancing phenomenon.

While in the dance, the dancers were oblivious to anything around them. Some seemed possessed and screamed out the names of the devils tormenting them. Others claimed they were in danger of immersion in a river of blood, which was why they leaped so high. Still others claimed visions of Heaven's open gates with Jesus and Mary on their thrones. In advanced cases, dancers would fall to the ground, writhe, foam at the mouth, and show signs of being in the grip of epileptic fits, but such interludes were usually short, and they soon were dancing again. At any given time, hundreds of people might be dancing, but apparently no community ever gave itself up entirely to the mania.

In those areas where the dancers appeared, normal life came to a halt. Crowds gathered to watch, and religious ceremonies, including special masses, were invoked to aid the afflicted. The participants were primarily peasants, artisans, and the indigent, with only a few well-to-do townspeople and nobles. There was also an anticlerical side. When the dancers danced in Liège, they taunted and cursed the priests. Priests preached against dancing, asserting that the dancers were possessed of devils, and carried out formal ceremonies of exorcism.

The dancing mania had points of similarity with the flagellant movement (see Bubonic Plague), which it followed. Born in the emotional upheavals generated by famine, pestilence, and war, it reflected the torments of the time and contributed to them. Unlike the flagellants, who claimed to do penance before an angry God, the dancers were considered victims who needed to be helped. The saints were called upon to intercede for them and end their torment, while the dancing itself became a response to need and a form of therapy. The dancers became victims in another sense. Rogues pretended ecstasies to prey sexually on the women, while thieves and cutthroats used the dances as cover for their crimes.

There were scattered incidents of dancing in the fifteenth century, but another epidemic began in the sixteenth century, and by the eighteenth century the dance mania had largely disappeared. Dancing was not an unusual form for this kind of reaction to take in European society. Before the fourteenth century, there were instances of dancing for punishment (Kölbrück, 1071), or because of possession by devils (Erfurt, 1273; Maastrick, 1278). Moreover, dancing was an accepted form of religious expression as well as a mode of behavior appropriate for stressful situations. Hungarian pilgrims who followed a route to holy places in western Germany and the Rhineland performed their acts of adoration by dancing. By the seventeenth century, however, values had changed, dancing was no longer an appropriate reaction, and the phenomenon disappeared. Finally, the mania affected only a small part of the population, suggesting that the usual or accepted methods for living with tension or stress were successful for most but not all the people.

Tarantism Conclusions concerning the medieval dancing mania have been supported by analogy with tarantism, a specialized form of dancing localized in Apulia in southern Italy. Developing in the fifteenth century and reaching its height in the seventeenth century, tarantism appeared as a ritual in which the individual, usually a woman, was supposedly bitten by a tarantula spider. This spider, though nonpoisonous elsewhere in Europe, "poisoned" the victim, who then became dull and lethargic. When chords of a version of the dance known from the ritual as the tarantella were struck, the victim, if the tune were keyed to his or her response, would get up and begin to dance. The dance became a furious, erotic, and finally orgiastic performance which lasted until the victim was exhausted. Tarantism usually occurred in July or August, and people, once "bitten," would show the signs of their "disease" approaching as the anniversary of the dance came around. Then, after exhausting themselves in a new tarantella, they would be free for another year. Observers point out that Apulia was very poor, and that the women of Apulia were depressed, exploited, and profoundly repressed. Their anxieties and repressions, shaped in the culture of their land, formed the causal nexus for tarantism.

Apulia had been part of Magna Graecia, and as it was backward, traditional behavior patterns lasted longer than in more developed regions. The explosion of repressed sexual energy in the dance correlated closely with both classical Greek psychic practices particularly the stress on catharsis and the Dionysian revels, ancient rituals of a violent and orgiastic nature which were of fundamental importance to Greek religion. The church repressed the Dionysian orgies and tried to stamp out the dancing. To circumvent the church, and to validate the dancing, the idea emerged that a person poisoned by spider bite had to dance to be "cured." The disappearance of tarantism in the eighteenth century indicated that the maniacal dancing had ceased to be an acceptable or appropriate cultural response to problems. The tarantella remains as a particularly vigorous dance with formalized movements which are vestiges of the former dancing mania and preserves the tunes by which earlier generations freed themselves of psychic burdens.

ADDITIONAL READINGS: J. F. C. Hecker, *The Epidemics of the Middle Ages*, B. G. Babbington (trans.), 3d ed., London, 1859; George Mora, "An Historical Sociopsychiatric Appraisal of Tarantism and Its Importance in the Tradition of Psychotherapy of Mental Disorders," *Bulletin of the History of Medicine* 37 (September–October 1963): 417–439; George Rosen, "Psychopathology in the Social Process: Dance Frenzies, Demonic Possession, Revival Movements, and Similar So-Called Psychic Epidemics: An Interpretation," *Bulletin of the History of Medicine* 36 (January–February 1962): 13–14; Henry E. Sigerist, *Civilization and Disease*, Ithaca, N.Y., 1943, chap. 11.

Deficiency Diseases

Deficiency diseases are pathological conditions arising from the absence of necessary elements in the diet. The discovery and synthesis of vitamins (q.v.) and the development of scientific nutrition in the early years of the twentieth century led to successful campaigns against such vitamin deficiency diseases as scurvy, rickets, pellagra, and beriberi (qq.v.). The deficiency diseases which continue to be widespread are those for which acceptable solutions may be available but which are difficult to control for cultural, economic, or technical reasons.

Since World War II, the most serious problems with deficiency diseases have appeared in underdeveloped and developing nations. Developed nations are less prone to deficiency disease, though they have not always been so. In 1900, Great Britain, for example, suffered the effects of dietary deficiency at a rate comparable to that of developing societies today. Food technology, especially the creation of synthetic supplements, makes radical changes in the incidence of deficiency disease practical. Gross insufficiency of food supplies clearly will affect the incidence and intensity of deficiency diseases, but famine is not the central problem, because the deficiency diseases also occur where there is a sufficient quantity of food. Quality is the basic problem, and this involves methods of preparation as well as the types of food eaten. Since most deficiency diseases develop in infancy or early childhood, prenatal care, customs governing nursing and weaning, early solid food offerings, and the prevalence of intestinal disorders which affect the degree to which food constituents are used are all significant factors. Finally, the deficiency diseases have broad social consequences which are only beginning to be studied systematically but which appear to be influential in retarding social, cultural, and economic growth in much the same way that they adversely affect growth and maturation in individuals. Poverty is a major causal factor in deficiency diseases, and overcoming poverty would obviously affect deficiency diseases drastically. Recent work in this field does not, however, view long-term structural changes in society and economics as prerequisite to solving the problem. The emphasis is on the possibilities inherent in the world as it is.

The deficiency diseases currently at the center of health studies include protein-energy malnutrition (PEM), nutritional anemias, goiter, and xerophthalmia. Although it is probable that these diseases have affected human life over long periods of time, systematic study of their etiology and epidemiology belongs to the very recent past. The foundations for this work were created by the League of Nations, and it has been carried forward by the World Health Organization, the United Nations International Children's Emergency Fund (UNICEF), the Food and Agricultural Organization, and such nongovernmental agencies as the Cooperative of American Relief Everywhere (CARE), Catholic Relief, and the Oxford Committee for Famine Relief.

Protein-energy malnutrition (once called protein-calorie malnutrition) is the most serious and widespread of the deficiency diseases. It is actually a variety of pathological conditions arising from simultaneous deficiencies in proteins and calories, and it is commonly associated with various infections. It is found most frequently among infants and small children. There are two recognized manifestations of this disease which form the extremes of a spectrum from calorie to protein deficiency. The symptoms for both will often be found in the same population. Calorie deficiency is called nutritional marasmus and is characterized by muscle wasting, loss of subcutaneous fat, and low body weight. Apart from gross deficiency of calories, protein shortages and infection are involved in the causal system. Protein deficiency results in a disease called kwashiorkor, a severe clinical syndrome often resulting from a shortage of amino acids necessary for protein synthesis, with calorie deficiency as well. Kwashiorkor results in some (and sometimes all) of the following symptoms: edema and muscle wasting, dermatosis, hair changes, enlarged liver, diarrhea, mental apathy, and general misery. Laboratory tests will show low levels of serum albumin. This syndrome occurs most frequently during and after weaning, and it is often precipitated by infection. Between these identifiable extremes is a host of protein deficiency and calorie deficiency conditions.

Though kwashiorkor and marasmus are common phenomena throughout the developing world, there appear to be changes in incidence which are significant. Kwashiorkor dominates in tropical Africa and tends to occur after weaning. It has been called a village disease, and it appears to be declining. Marasmus, on the other hand, tends to occur before the age of 15 months, is widespread throughout the developing world, and appears to be increasing. It has been called an urban disease, and it is common in the shantytowns which ring nearly every urban center in the developing world. As the tendency in modern world development is toward urbanization, it seems that marasmus should become the most common deficiency disease in the developing world.

After age three or four, children with protein-energy deficiencies seldom require medical attention, but the effects persist in slow and often incomplete rehabilitation, retardation of both physical and mental development, and often permanent injury to mental capacities from brain damage and injury to the central nervous system and the skull from deficiency-induced metabolic disturbances. It is thought that the physiological consequences to mental health and stability are reinforced by withdrawal of the child from normal contacts due to illness in a vital stage of development. In sum, there seems to be a strong likelihood that preschool malnutrition produces irreversible mental and emotional damage.

Since the complex of conditions associated with protein-energy malnutrition is extremely widespread, it must be accounted one of the most important problems confronting the world today. A general rise in living standards, improved information on infant care, the importance of mothers' diet, breastfeeding, correct weaning procedures, and balanced food intake will begin to make some headway on the problem possible. The imbalances in human diet between developed and developing countries and the relatively low per-capita resources of the latter promise continued significant problems in this area.

Apart from protein-energy deficiency, there are some 30 deficiency diseases which affect the world's population. Xerophthalmia, a syndrome of vitamin A deficiency diseases in which eye lesions predominate, is one of the most widespread. Night blindness is an early sign of A deficiency, but as the deficiency continues to affect the cornea and conjunctiva, lesions, scarring, and ultimately blindness may follow. Keratomalacia is an extreme form in which the cornea is destroyed. This complex of conditions appears early in medical literature. There is a reference in an Egyptian medical treatise of about 1500 B.C. to the use of liver against night blindness, a recommendation which appears in the Hippocratic writings and in Hebrew medical practice as well. Xerophthalmia was widely discussed in the nineteenth century, and it appeared with a notably high incidence during the Irish potato famine (1846–1847). Another outbreak of special interest occurred in Denmark during World War I when the Danes sold their butter to Germany, turned to margarine, yet continued to use separated (skimmed) milk in feeding infants.

Historically, xerophthalmia was associated with poor diets, but it was only in 1912, when a food factor called fat-soluble A was identified, that the causal mechanisms became clear. Today, xerophthalmia appears most commonly among children aged one to three. It is a disease prevalent among the poor, and it is most common in developing countries. It is especially widespread in urban areas of south and southeast Asia, with notable incidence in Indonesia. It is less common in urban areas of the eastern Mediterranean, north Africa, sub-Saharan Africa, and Latin America. It is very rare in west Africa, where red palm oil, the most common cooking oil, is carotene-rich, and it is relatively rare in rural communities. Xerophthalmia is almost never seen in developed countries. Epidemiologists find it difficult to evaluate xerophthalmia's contribution to blindness, but it is considerable. In Vietnam, xerophthalmia is considered to be a principal cause of blindness; its effects are severe in south India, with estimates going as high as 50 percent of all blindness; in the Philippines it is thought to be of the first importance.

One deficiency disease whose incidence has been significantly reduced is the swelling of the thyroid gland called endemic goiter. A disease which results from a reduced availability of iodine, goiter was widespread in history, appearing in both well-to-do and poor communities. It was known in England as "Derbyshire neck," and there are references to its presence in North and South America, throughout Europe, and in Asia. Marco Polo commented on it while traversing Chinese Turkestan, and the disease was known from early times in China proper. It was a long-standing problem in Italy, and it apparently was common among the Incas. Goiter has been especially notable in the Alpine valleys of Switzerland, in the high Pyrenees, in the Himalayas, and in the Cordillera of the Andes. But it was prevalent as well in North America's Great Lakes region, in Lombardy, in glaciated southern Finland, and in the Netherlands. What linked the Alpine valleys and the lowland plains was glaciation and flooding, which together removed iodine from the soils and water, and the deficiency of natural iodine brought on goiter among long-term residents.

Apart from unsightliness, goiter produced serious consequences, including deaf-mutism, cretinism, and idiocy. It has been estimated that a goiter incidence of 50 percent in a given population would result in 4 percent of the population's suffering mental deficiencies or deaf-mutism. Iodizing salt has proved to be the most effective solution. Switzerland introduced the first iodization program in 1923 and in 25 years had reduced the incidence of goiter by 90 percent while recording a substantial drop in cretinism and deaf-mutism. The second program was introduced in Michigan in 1924. Unfortunately, on a world basis, only 32 political units out of some 120 have introduced iodization programs, and goiter remains an active deficiency disease, though the means for ending it are known and readily available.

Nutritional anemias, a condition in which the hemoglobin content of the blood is lower than normal, also pose significant problems, particularly in developing countries. The discovery of vitamin B_{12} provides an effective weapon against the often-fatal pernicious anemia, but blood deficiencies remain a widespread problem, particularly for infants and children to the age of two, adolescent girls, and pregnant women. Blood deficiencies affect energy levels, alertness, disease resistance, and general health. A survey in Kenya found 80 percent of the population with iron deficiencies; in Sierra Leone and Nigeria, some 40 percent of adult females showed iron deficiency anemia; and India throughout the twentieth century has been troubled with widespread anemia. One survey of 4000 men and women found 14 percent of the sample suffering severe anemia, and 85 percent of the pregnant women were deficient. Such incidences suggest a very large disease potential. Anemia in its critical forms is often fatal, and here again the distinction between the developing and developed societies appears. The United States has a death rate from anemia of 2 per 100,000; in Latin America, the rate varies from 12 to 32 per 100,000. Education, iron supplements, and a generally improved diet from a better standard of living appear to offer the best opportunities for reducing this problem.

The deficiency diseases are of particular interest for what they reveal concerning the intersection among medical science, social awareness, and cultural development. The classic deficiency diseases—scurvy, beriberi, rickets, and pellagra—could be ascribed to a particular cause. Observation and increasingly sophisticated biochemical research identified the controlling factors responsible for each condition. Generally rising living standards in the urban-industrial world helped to create an environmental improvement which included diet. And in vitamins, science gave enlightened governments a weapon for these nutritional wars which could be used precisely and effectively. The nonspecific deficiency diseases, and particularly the protein-energy malnutrition syndrome, are infinitely more complex etiologically and epidemiologically. Scientific advances have vastly enlarged understanding of the processes involved, but the recognition of these conditions as diseases and any plan to eradicate them demand social and cultural insight, political organization, and economic power. The nutritional sciences have advanced significantly, but the resolution for deficiency diseases requires a type of knowledge only the social sciences provide. In addition, this problem must be seen in a global context rather than in terms of disease incidences in particular localities. Today's deficiency diseases highlight issues which are fundamental to the stability and welfare of the late-twentieth-century world.

ADDITIONAL READINGS: W. R. Aykroyd, *Conquest of Deficiency Diseases: Achievements and Prospects*, Geneva, 1970; G. H. Beaton and J. M. Bengoa, *Nutrition in Preventive Medicine: The Major Deficiency Syndromes, Epidemiology, and Approaches to Control*, Geneva, 1976.

See also BERIBERI; NUTRITION; PELLAGRA; SCURVY; VITAMINS.

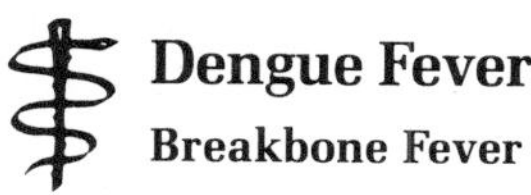

Dengue Fever

Breakbone Fever

Dengue fever is a mosquito-borne, virus-caused disease which has been prevalent in the Caribbean and the southern United States in the western hemisphere and throughout the tropical and subtropical zones of the eastern hemisphere. It is especially notable for the rapidity of its attack, the extreme discomfort which it produces, and its large incidences. Most dengue fevers have low mortalities, though a variant called dengue hemorrhagic fever is very severe and highly dangerous. No vaccine is effective against the dengue fevers, and there is no specific treatment. Preventing or managing shock is the most important feature of treating dengue hemorrhagic fever. Prevention, as in yellow fever or malaria, is largely a matter of mosquito control.

There are four distinct antigenic types of virus which cause dengue and at least three other anthropod-borne viruses which produce denguelike diseases. Moreover, there appears to be an antigenic overlap between dengue viruses and the viruses which cause yellow fever, Japanese encephalitis, and West Nile fever. There are no mutual immunities, but dengue and yellow fever tend not to occupy the same areas, though both use the same vector, the mosquito *Aëdes aegypti*. In those few cases where both dengue and yellow fever have appeared, they have generally done so at different times of the year.

Unless a positive serological identification can be made, modern clinicians are warned that they should refer to denguelike infections, and there is the further problem that dengue fevers have many symptoms similar to those of influenzalike disease and to those of the early stages of malaria, typhus, hepatitis, and leptospirosis. There are also close similarities between the course run by dengue fevers and that run by sand fly fever, Colorado tick fever, and Rift Valley fever, though, unlike dengue, these generally show no rash.

Classic dengue fever comes on suddenly from two days to a week after the initial inoculation by a mosquito bite. The temperature rises swiftly to 104°F or more, a severe frontal headache develops, and there are excruciating pains in the joints. These pains are so intense that patients can hardly bear to be touched; lying in bed can be agonizing, and even to lift an affected finger will be intensely painful. There is severe vomiting and a foul taste in the mouth. A rash appears which may disappear in one to five days. Convalescence is long and difficult, often lasting for weeks or even months. The pain retreats slowly, and dengue patients develop a tightly restrained or mincing gait to avoid the pain of moving the affected joints. Symptoms vary greatly in intensity from place to place, but the popular names which the disease bears indicate the common characteristics. "Breakbone fever" is one of the most common in English, though the extraordinary depression which attends some convalescences led two young women who were recovering from the disease to suggest that "break heart fever" would be more appropriate. The word "dengue" itself is Spanish and means "affectation," an idea translated directly into English as "dandy fever." The French *bouquet* as applied to this disease carried the connotation of an affected, mincing gait.

History Though it is probable that denguelike diseases occurred before the eighteenth century, there is no record of them. The first description of a denguelike attack was written in 1779 by David Bylon, a medical officer for Batavia in the Dutch East Indies who suffered the disease himself. He called it "knuckle fever," or "joint fever," (*knokel koorts*) and he noted the swiftness of the illness' attack. At 5 P.M. he was perfectly well; four hours later he was in bed, feverish, restless, sleepless, and suffering severe pain, especially in the legs, arms, and joints. Bylon referred to this as "a very well known disease" but one which had never before been epidemic in Batavia. The following year, Dr. Benjamin Rush of Philadelphia reported on "a bilious remitting fever" which people called "breakbone fever" and which prevailed from July to October. What he described was clearly dengue. He wrote of "exquisitely severe pains" which were so acute that some of his patients could not lie in bed. He also described the vomiting, rash, and depression during recovery. During this same period there was a report from Cairo of a prevalent "knee sickness," while reports from the Coromandel Coast in India described a disease which attacked everyone, though its victims all recovered. They commented as well on the pain in the joints and limbs. No explanation has been offered for these four widely separated epidemic outbreaks in 1779 and 1780.

Throughout the nineteenth and twentieth centuries there have been repeated dengue pandemics in the Caribbean and along the southern coasts of the United States, as well as in Mediterranean Europe, South Africa, throughout Asia, and in Australia.The places commonly attacked include the Virgin Islands, Cuba, Jamaica, Venezuela, Mexico, Panama, and Puerto Rico. In the United States, dengue was a regular visitor to Charleston, South Carolina; Savannah, Georgia; Mobile, Alabama; and New Orleans, Louisiana. Texas had a dengue epidemic in 1885 and 1886 both in the coastal cities and along the railroads leading into the interior.

In the eastern hemisphere, dengue was active in India in 1824 and 1825 and again in 1853 and 1854. A severe outbreak swept from east Africa through Arabia, India, and China in the period 1870–1873, and at the end of the century, Brisbane, Australia, had its first attack. The epidemic there was particularly bad, with hemorrhagic symptoms appearing, and at least 60 deaths. It was estimated that 75 percent of the population fell ill. In 1927, Durban, South Africa, recorded over 40,000 cases, while that same year and the year following, a dengue outbreak in Athens and Piraeus affected an estimated 90 percent of the population. There were 239,000 cases in Athens alone, hemorrhagic symptoms were common, and there were numerous fatalities. A similar epidemic occurred on Formosa in 1931. Dengue was reported from the Caribbean in epidemic force in 1969, and there is a strong presumption that the disease will remain active for the foreseeable future.

Until the twentieth century, nothing was known of dengue's epidemiology, though an insect vector was strongly suspected. In Beirut in 1905, volunteers were successfully infected using a mosquito, but the experiment was inconclusive because there was suspicion that the recipients might have contracted the disease before they were inoculated with it. Better results were obtained in Australia, where a dengue-free zone existed. It had been noticed that daytime visitors to Brisbane contracted dengue, and suspicion fell heavily on day-biting mosquitos, with aëdes (*Aëdes aegypti stegomyia*) the primary candidate. The suspicion appeared justified when E. N. Bancroft managed to infect a volunteer with dengue using the aëdes mosquito, and in 1907, two other researchers, Ashburn and Craig, injected filtered blood from a dengue fever patient into a healthy person and brought on an attack. The causal agent was clearly a filter passer, or virus. In 1916, these conclusions were fully confirmed by epidemiological survey and in the laboratory, and they were reconfirmed in 1924 by a research team working in Manila. In 1945, Albert Sabin and his associates propagated dengue in mice, and in 1948 the dengue virus was cultivated in chick embryo.

Though dengue routinely produced large incidences, the appearance of the hemorrhagic variety has made the disease more threatening. However, little is known about it. In 1954, in the course of severe outbreaks in Thailand and the Philippines, dengue hemorrhagic fever was separated from dengue fever and a diagnostic profile established. The origin of the hemorrhagic type remained unknown. One theory suggested two sequential infections by different dengue virus strains; another argued for an abnormally virulent dengue virus. Neither theory is susceptible of proof at this time.

Since dengue mortalities are relatively small and, apart from the hemorrhagic variety, result most often from conditions of weakness or other illness, the social consequences of this disease are primarily discomfort, inconvenience, and the interruption of the routine of life. During an outbreak near Rio de Janeiro in 1846, for example, the entire work force on the haciendas fell ill at the same time, bringing everything to a standstill, while in the port "none of the principals and not always a half-crippled clerk was to be found, often for a whole week long. Ships were delayed in loading and unable to put to sea, and even the schools were deserted."

The economic costs of dengue epidemics can be very high in the short run, and for marginal or undeveloped economic systems, the cumulative losses are significant. In areas where conditions of health are poor, and the general disease level is high, dengue attacks add measurably to the continuing debilitation, and for the very young, the old, and the chronically ill, they become a threat to life. Controlling dengue is easiest for a stable, affluent society with well-developed public health facilities. But such a society is also better able to absorb the effects of an epidemic. Less-developed societies are both less capable of implementing effective controls and more susceptible to the epidemic's effects. Thus the prospects are excellent for dengue to continue to be a burden in the Philippines, southeast Asia, and east Africa, and throughout the Caribbean. It is less threatening for the southern United States and Australia. In no area, however, has dengue fever as a disease with epidemic potential been eliminated.

ADDITIONAL READINGS: William Beatty and Geoffrey Marks, *Epidemics*, New York, 1976, 184–189; Donald E. Carey, "Chikungunya and Dengue: A Case of Mistaken Identity?," *Journal of the History of Medicine* 26 (April 1971): 243–262; N. Joel Ehrenkranz et al., "Pandemic Dengue in Caribbean Countries and the Southern United States: Past, Present, and Potential Problems," *New England Journal of Medicine* 285 (December 1971): 1460–1469; August Hirsch, *Handbook of Geographical and Historical Pathology*, Charles Creighton (trans.), 3 vols., London, 1883, 1, chap. 2, 55–81; H. Harold Scott, *A History of Tropical Medicine*, 2 vols., London, 1939, 2, 808–819.

Diabetes Mellitus

Diabetes mellitus is a complex metabolic disorder which has been recognized for thousands of years but which is still only partially understood. The discovery and preparation of clinically safe insulin in 1921 and 1922 have made management of diabetes possible, and while there is no cure, millions of people are now able to live with the disease who in past years would have died. It is this dramatic reversal of diabetes' traditionally mortal prognosis that led Dr. Frederick M. Allen, a long-time student of the disease, to call the discovery of a purified and usable insulin "one of the greatest achievements of modern medicine."

Diabetes occurs when the nutritional system is unable to complete the process of breaking down and absorbing carbohydrates. Normal systems reduce carbohydrates to carbon dioxide and water, with glucose, a by-product of the process, absorbed into body cells. The diabetic is unable to absorb glucose, and sugars begin to accumulate in the blood. Increasing quantities of urine are secreted to flush out the glucose concentrations, causing the body to void profuse quantities of urine with substantial amounts of sugar in it. At the same time, to substitute for the energy lack from the inability to use sugar, the body begins to use up its fat stores, thus producing the physical wasting which with the sweet urine, is among the classic symptoms of diabetes. The individual suffering this syndrome becomes extremely hungry and thirsty, may eat huge quantities of food while rapidly losing weight, and has very low energy and stamina levels. As the disease progresses, wasting may be marked, and an extreme lassitude develops, with coma and death not far behind.

A large volume of glucose-laden urine, higher-than-normal glucose concentrations in the blood, fatigue, and body wasting typify juvenile or "thin" diabetes. This is much the most severe form which the disease takes, and without treatment it is invariably fatal. The second general classification, adult-onset diabetes, is more varied. It is most commonly diagnosed between the ages of 40 and 60, though it can occur at any time, and it produces a wide variety of conditions including atherosclerosis leading to heart disease, cataracts or other eye conditions, and severe circulatory problems which sometimes end in gangrene in the extremities. Obesity and gluttonous appetite have been associated with mature-onset diabetes as both premonitory symptoms and contributory causes, but the root problem, as in juvenile diabetes, is the failure of beta cells located in the pancreas, called the islets of Langerhans, to secrete sufficient insulin to metabolize glucose.

In juvenile diabetes, there are clear pathological signs of pancreatic disorder involving the beta cells, but this is not necessarily the case with mature-onset diabetes. Moreover, the triggering mechanism which starts both kinds of diabetic attack is not understood. Recent studies on diabetes refer to etiologies and pathogeneses of diabetic conditions, frankly disclaiming any definitive knowledge concerning causal mechanisms or the effects. It is clear, however, that susceptibility to diabetes is inherited, although one line of research indicates that bacterial infection sets off an immunological reaction in susceptible persons which can produce juvenile-onset diabetes. Other conditions which may indicate or trigger diabetes include pregnancy and menopause, trauma, emotional upheaval, glandular disorders affecting other hormones, and such specific conditions as pancreatic cancer.

Once it is established, there is no cure for diabetes. The general approach is to manage the disease, control the symptoms, and avoid crises. This is commonly accomplished by controlled diet, regular exercise, and insulin injections. The particular conditions generated in mature-onset diabetes have to be dealt with individually while carrying on control or management. Susceptibility to diabetes may be suspected for reasons of heredity, but such a predisposition is impossible to test. Active diabetes can, however, be easily diagnosed. The most reliable method is a glucose tolerance test. The patient ingests glucose, and tests are done over a three- or five-hour span to determine whether or to what degree the glucose metabolizes. The test for urine sugar can also indicate a developed condition or suggest the need for further testing.

Presumably the pool of diabetics was infinitely larger in the past than the extreme cases which came to physicians' attention, and reliable demographic data on the disease have only become available recently. One study on diabetes in the United States suggested an incidence for the disease of 2 percent, which, in a population of 200 million would mean about 4 million cases. Over half of these would be diagnosed. It is believed, however, that there are an additional 5.5 million people susceptible to diabetes who could become diabetic. This would suggest a population of between 9 and 10 million diabetics and potential diabetics. The United States is not, however, a reliable guide for general conditions, because diabetes is more prevalent in sedentary societies, and a high sugar intake contributes to a rising diabetic incidence. Advancing life expectancy also increases the number of persons with diabetic conditions. It would appear, therefore, that, while diabetes (especially in its extreme forms) was common enough to be readily recognized in the past, the conditions which favor its development have appeared in modern times; it would also appear that it is most prevalent in advanced societies.

History The existing medical record hints that physicians may have been aware of diabetes for nearly 4,000 years. What may be the earliest reference ot the condition appears in the Ebers papyrus (ca. 1550 B.C.), which summarizes a much older medical tradition. There we find various remedies suggested to control a too-copious flow of urine, a condition which can be symptomatic of diabetes. Vedic medical treatises from pre-Buddhist India describe conditions in detail which seem definitely to be diabetic. They mention two types of disease: one congenital, and the other coming later in life as a result of life-style. They identify the disease by the copious flow of urine, and while they describe many other urinary conditions, they set this one aside as incurable though susceptible of management. They also noted a hereditary disposition to the disease and connected it with obesity, indolence, lethargy, and overindulgence in sweets, rich foods, and milk products. Oddly enough, the vedic physicians implicated freshly harvested cereals, pulses, and meat of domestic animals as well. Dieting and purging were strongly recommended, and some drugs were suggested, especially a bituminous preparation from the Himalayas which contained benzoates and silica. A much later tradition (thirteenth century A.D.) also recommended zinc. Sushrut noted the sweet urine, an observation which does not appear in the western literature until the seventeenth century. These extraordinary medical sources were first obscured by Buddhist influence in the fifth and fourth centuries and finally obliterated by the Islamic invaders of the eleventh century A.D.

Greek medicine also contributed a description of diabetes. Aretaeus of Cappadocia, writing in the second century A.D. referred to diabetes as "a wonderful affection" which was not very frequently met and which he described as "a melting down of the flesh and limbs into urine." The disease took a long time to form, but once it was established, "the melting is rapid, the death speedy," which was just as well since "life is disgusting and painful," as victims suffer "nausea, restlessness, and burning thirst" before expiring. Though Aretaeus did not mention the sweet urine, he did notice that there was more urine voided than liquid consumed, and he showed a thorough familiarity with the course of the disease. He also commented on the word "diabetes," which signifies a siphon, speculating that this word was used "because the fluid does not remain in the body, but uses the man's body as a ladder . . . whereby to leave it."

Avicenna, the great Arab physician of the eleventh century whose works were widely known in Europe, may have introduced the idea of sweet urine to western observers. Paracelsus (Theophrastus Bombastus von Hohenheim) knew Avicenna's work very well, but his sixteenth-century comments on diabetes showed his iatrochemical approach, referring to the disease as caused by "a dry salt . . . lasting, permanent and fixed." He also included a variety of clinical details such as chronic thirst, vast quantities of yellow, acid urine, swelling fat, a rapid pulse, and pains in the thigh.

The beginnings of the modern approach to diabetes are usually traced to Thomas Willis, personal physician to King Charles II. It was Willis who stated unequivocally that diabetic urine is "wonderfully sweet as if it were imbued with Honey or Sugar" in consequence of which he added the Lation word *mellitus,* or "honey sweet," to the Greek *diabetes.* Willis was puzzled over the causes for the disease, though he noted the contemporary taste for imbibing huge quantities of sweet wine, and while he thought that early diagnosis and treatment could bring success, once the disease was established, it was rarely cured. Willis recorded that diabetics "piss a great deal more than they drink," while suffering from "persistent thirst and a low but continuing fever." About a century later (ca. 1775), Matthew Dobson confirmed the presence of sugar in the urine; but even more significantly, he found sugar in the blood, thus suggesting that diabetes was not a kidney problem but rather one of metabolism and digestion. Nothing further appeared to advance the understanding of diabetes until the later nineteenth century. The great French physiologist Claude Bernard showed that sugar was produced in the liver with the aid of an enzyme. In 1869, Paul Langerhans found the special cell construction in the pancreas that bears his name, but he had no idea of its function. And in 1874, Adolph Kussmaul provided clinical details on death from diabetes, and especially the sound of breathing in the final coma. These contributions were potentially important for understanding the disease, but until there was some further advance in physiology and biochemistry, their significance could not be appreciated.

In 1889, an accidental discovery pointed the road. Oskar Minkowski and Joseph von Mering explored the question of whether a dog could live without its pancreas. While von Mering was away from the laboratory, Minkowski removed a dog's pancreas. The animal lived but developed diabetes. Other experiments showed that only the total removal of the pancreas had that effect, and it was also clear that without the pancreas, dogs could not digest fat or proteins. Finally, Minkowski and von Mering tied off the excretory ducts of the pancreas, but even this "degenerated" pancreas did not produce diabetes. The disease was now associated with the pancreas, though 30 more years passed before the nature of the association was explained and put to use for diabetes control.

Several workers contributed to or approached the discovery of insulin before 1921. In 1901, a Johns Hopkins pathologist, Eugene Lindsay Opie, noted that in persons who had died of diabetes there was evidence of pathological changes in the islets of Langerhans. A Russian physician, Leonid Sobelev, reported similar findings from St. Petersburg the following year. In 1908, Dr. George Ludwig Zuelzer in Berlin made an extract of pancreas, which he tried on eight diabetes patients. The extract had some effect, reducing glycosuria and producing some improvements. It also had toxic side effects which were sufficiently threatening to force an end to its clinical use. The effort now was to purify the substance. E. L. Scott was working on a promising process in the United States in 1912 and 1913, while the Rumanian N. C. Paulesco developed a pancreatic extract which was effective in controlling hyperglycemia and glycosuria in dogs whose pancreases had been removed. When the Germans took Bucharest in 1916, his research was stopped, and he did not publish his results until 1921. In the meantime, Sir Edward Albert Sharpy-Schafer had established to his own satisfaction that the substance necessary for carbohydrate metabolism was produced in the islets of Langerhans, and he used the Latin for the word "island" (*insula*) as the root for the name of this new substance, "insuline."

The discovery of insulin and its purification for clinical use took place in the physiological laboratory of Dr. J. R. Macleod at the University of Toronto. The discoverers, Frederick (later Sir) Grant Banting and Herbert Best, had been given space in the laboratory, though neither received a stipend or had a research budget. Their assignment was to discover a method for making pancreas extract which would be effective and safe. Their work began where Minkowsky and von Mering's left off. Though aware of Scott's work, they were unable to appreciate what Zuelzer and Paulesco had published, owing to their weakness in reading German and French. Their results were similar; that is, they obtained a pancreatic extract which clearly reduced glucose levels in dogs whose pancreases had been removed. Macleod, who was skeptical originally, was impressed with the progress when he returned from three months in Scotland. Banting and Best summarized their conclusions in a paper for the local physiology society on November 14, 1921 and submitted a revised version to the *Journal of Laboratory and Clinical Medicine,* where it was published in February 1922. An abstract of their findings appeared in the December 1921 issue of the *American Journal of Physiology.*

When the Banting-Best pancreas extract was used clinically, toxic reactions appeared, and it seemed that the Zuelzer story was to be repeated. Macleod, however, recruited James B. Collip, a talented biochemist, to purify the extract. Using a 95 percent alcohol solution—he deemed absolute alcohol better—Collip solved the problem of purifying insulin in a matter of weeks. It was this purified version which made control of diabetes clinically possible. The first successful clinical use of insulin was initiated in Janury 1922, when an advanced and difficult case was brought under control, and the following year, the Nobel prize committee awarded the discoverers the prize in medicine.

Unfortunately, the Nobel committee botched the awards. Herbert Best, who had worked with Frederick Banting throughout the project's life, received no prize, but Macleod was named a discoverer despite the fact that he was away throughout the discovery period and played no part in the actual research. Collip, who completed the development of a clinically safe and usable substance, also received no prize. The vagaries of the prize committee were partially redressed when Banting shared his prize with Best, and Macleod did the same with Collip. This was not the end of controversy, however. There has been a continuing and occasionally acrimonious debate over what scientific debts Banting and Best owed Zuelzer and Paulesco, and there has been a claim of priority as well for E. L. Scott. None of this, of course, affects the importance of the discovery of insulin in 1921, which has made control over diabetes a realized fact.

ADDITIONAL READINGS: S. S. Alfgaonker, "Diabetes Mellitus as Seen in Ancient Ayurvedic Medicine," in J. S. Bajaj (ed.), *Insulin and Metabolism,* Bombay, 1972, 1–19; J. S. Bajaj, "The Discovery of Insulin: A Critique," in J. S. Bajaj (ed.), *Insulin and Metabolism,* Bombay, 1972, 35–48; Michael Bliss, *The Discovery of Insulin,* Chicago, 1982; A. P. Cawadias, "Diseases of the Endocrine Glands," in Walter Bett (ed.), *The History and Conquest of Common Diseases,* Norman, Okla., 1954, 204–219; Stephen S. Fajans (ed.), *Diabetes Mellitus,* Bethesda, Md., 1976; N. S. Papaspyros, *The History of Diabetes Mellitus,* London, 1952; J. H. Pratt, "A Reappraisal of Researchers Leading to the Discovery of Insulin," *Journal of the History of Medicine* 9 (July 1954): 281–289; L. G. Stevenson, *Sir Frederick Banting,* Toronto, 1940; G. A. Wrenshall, G. Hetenyi, and W. R. Feasley, *The Story of Insulin: Forty Years of Success Against Diabetes,* London, 1962.

Diphtheria

Diphtheria is an acute contagious disease dangerous primarily to children. Sporadically epidemic before the nineteenth century, diphtheria became pandemic as well as highly malignant in the middle nineteenth century. Thanks to the revolution in bacteriological and immunological studies at the end of the nineteenth century, the means to cure and control diphtheria were discovered, and in much of Europe and North America the disease is no longer a serious threat.

The Disease The causal agent for diphtheria is a nonmotile, rod-shaped bacterium with one or both ends appearing swollen. It varies in length and has been designated *Coryne bacterium diphtheriae.* There are three strains of this bacterium, a fact which accounts for the varying malignancy shown in diphtheria attacks. The strains are called gravis, intermedius, and mitis. The first two are thought to produce severe epidemic outbreaks with high mortality. Mitis appears to be responsible for endemic diphtheria, which is often mild and confers immunity. Death from the mitis strain is often from unrelieved blockage of the air passages.

The diphtheria bacillus can enter the body wherever an opening is provided, but it is most commonly inhaled to lodge in the nose, throat, or windpipe. Its primary mode for transmission is in the droplets of moisture from respiratory secretions. Once established, the bacterium reproduces and generates a poisonous exotoxin which the blood carries around the system to produce general symptoms. These include a moderate fever, general malaise, sore throat, and a hard cough. Swelling occurs in the mucous membranes of the upper respiratory tract as the membranes become coated with a layer composed of dead cells and bacteria. As the membranes grow thicker and the swelling spreads into the mouth, nasal passages, and trachea, swallowing and breathing become difficult, and victims may die of asphyxia. In the classic accounts, there was ulceration, pus, and blood discharged from the nose, a vile odor, and unless the stoppage of air could be relieved, death was common.

The exotoxin sometimes damages the heart and peripheral areas, bringing on temporary paralysis where the nerve system is involved, or inflammation of the heart muscle. Normally the body produces an antitoxin in reaction to the exotoxin, and in most cases this is sufficient to control the disease and confer future immunity. The only effective treatment for diphtheria has been to inject antitoxin to aid the body's efforts. Other treatments deal with symptoms and include tracheotomy (an incision in the throat to introduce a tube to facilitate breathing) and intubation (placing a slender silver tube in the windpipe). Antibiotics have no effect on diphtheria. Immunization by inoculating children with diphtheria toxoid, that is, exotoxin treated with formalin, has proved effective with an initial injection at about one year, a booster after two or three years, and another on school entrance. The Schick immunity test is used to identify children with low immunity levels. There is no effective method for mass immunization of adults. Treatment and immunization together have nearly eliminated diphtheria as a fatal disease in western countries, though it continues to appear in other parts of the world.

Early History Diphtheria is undoubtedly an ancient disease, though there is no basis for determining how extensive it may have been, nor is it really possible to separate diphtheria from other throat conditions which had serious consequences. The most common confusion is with scarlet fever. Classical medical writings refer to severe sore throat ending in death as *kynanchē* (Greek) and *angina* (Latin). What is meant is an acute inflammatory infection of the throat and larynx which produces difficulty in swallowing and breathing, and which is sometimes severe enough to kill. Some of the illnesses included under this rubric were probably diphtheria. The first clear description of a disease which was probably diphtheria appears in the second-century A.D. writings of Aretaeus of Cappadocia. Late Roman or Byzantine medical authorities who appeared to describe diphtheria include Caelius Aurelianus in the fifth century A.D., and Aetius of Amida in the middle of the sixth century. Sanskrit medical writings from the same period mention a disease which sounds very much like diphtheria. The record is unclear, but it would appear that diphtheria was endemic in the Mediterranean area from Italy east to Syria and south to Egypt, including Greece, and there may have been epidemic outbreaks. It was also present in northwest India.

The Medieval Experience There is no medical evidence on diphtheria from the European Middle Ages, but the chronicles contain hints that the disease was present and active. These hints gain support from positive literary evidence in the sixteenth century which shows familiarity with diphtheria. The chronicle of St. Denis recorded a "pest" (pestilence; plague) of "esquinancie" (*squintia*, a term later used for angina maligna) in the year A.D. 580; the ecclesiastical annals of Baronius cite a plague of mortal throat disease in 856 and again in 1004; there was an outbreak of kynanchē in 1039, according to the Byzantine chronicler Cedrenus; and William Short refers to an outbreak of angina in England in 1389 which killed many children. There is no mention of children, however, in the earlier references.

In the sixteenth century, the references multiply, and the descriptions become more detailed. This suggests an expanding experience with the disease. Hartmann Schedel, city physician for Nuremberg, describes a disease which struck in 1492 which was probably diphtheria, and Frank von Wörd recorded the outbreak of a disease in the Rhine region in 1517 which attacked the mouth and throat. There was a severe "angina maligna contagiosa" in Amsterdam in that same year, and this disease also appeared in the Rhine territories in 1544 and 1545, and again in 1564 and 1565. This latter epidemic of malignant angina was, according to Van Wier's contemporary description, very destructive for children. Finally, Guillaume de Baillou, a French physician noted for his epidemiological studies, described what seems amost certainly to have been a diphtheria outbreak in Paris in 1576. It would be unwarranted to call diphtheria a major disease problem in the Middle Ages, but it seems clear that the disease existed, and that it attracted serious professional attention in the sixteenth century.

The Seventeenth and Eighteenth Centuries The first absolutely trustworthy epidemiological information concerning angina maligna, or diphtheria, came from Spain and dealt with severe outbreaks in Iberia which reached their high point in the second decade of the seventeenth century. The disease was called "garrotilla" after the truncheon used by Spanish executioners to strangle their victims, and 1613 was called "l'año de los garrotillos" after the extremely high angina mortality. The epidemic was described in clinical detail by several physicians. Among those writers the most important were J. de Villa-Real, who published in 1611; J. Alonzo y de los Ruyzes de Fontecha (1611); C. Perez de Herrera (1615); and F. Perez Cascales (1611). J. A. Sqambatus, J. B. Carnevalis, A. Cletus, and F. Nola wrote on the concurrent outbreaks in Italy and published in 1628. All these treatises described the disease as contagious. There was little to be done for the stricken. Leeches were applied at the beginning of the illness, and scarification was used later together with such cauterizing substances as acids, alum, copper, and arsenic. Tracheotomies were frequently performed in Italy.

Although the most serious outbreaks occurred in Iberia and Italy, there were scattered incidents of angina maligna reported elsewhere. In 1614, diphtheria seems to have appeared at Cuzco, Peru. Cotton Mather, the great Puritan preacher, reported that in 1659 a "Malady of Bladders in the Windpipe" killed a number of children in the Massachusetts Bay Colony. He went on to record that "by Opening of one of them [the deceased children] the Malady and Remedy (too late for very many) were discovered." Tracheotomy was the remedy to which he referred. There were other reports of contagious throat infections from the colonies in 1673, 1686, and 1689.

Diphtheria spread more widely in the eighteenth century. There were new outbreaks in Spain in 1701, and later in the century it appeared in France, Italy, Holland, Switzerland, Germany, and Sweden. The first outbreaks in England were reported in 1734 and 1739 in Devon and Cornwall. A severe epidemic began in 1735 in New England which spread gradually into the mid-Atlantic region.

The malignancy of the disease differed from place to place, but it was now clear that children were the main victims. There are no general figures to provide a guide to incidence or mortality, but some local examples convey an impression of the disease's impact. In Hampton Falls, New Hampshire, for example, 20 families lost all their children. One thousand deaths were recorded in the entire region, and of these, 900 were children. Hampton Falls' population was about 1200. In one year during the epidemic, 210 deaths were recorded there, 95 percent of which were people below the age of 20. In Kingston, New Hampshire, of the first 40 cases reported, all died.

Such locally severe outbreaks occurred in Europe as well as North America, though there were many regions where the attacks were slight, and in most there were none at all. Probably the most famous adult victim of the eighteenth-century angina maligna was George Washington, who died at Mount Vernon on December 15, 1799, of asphyxia from a severely swollen throat. The description of his last illness makes a diphtheria diagnosis virtually certain.

The Nineteenth-Century Crisis In the early years of the nineteenth century, only France suffered from significant angina maligna outbreaks. Most of Europe and all of North America were essentially free from the disease. In France, however, the outbreaks were numerous and extensive, especially those at Lyons in 1810 and 1811, and in the Loire region between 1818 and 1821 and 1824 and 1825. The disease was most serious in France between 1825 and 1836. Though French medical writers concentrated on diphtheria in the early nineteenth century, interest in the disease and its epidemiology waned elsewhere, and writing on the subject virtually disappeared from the medical and scientific journals.

The period of remission was a false calm, and there were indications of new activity beginning even in the midst of it. Minor outbreaks of diphtheria occurred in Switzerland and Germany in the 1830s and 1840s, and by mid-century there had been new outbreaks in Scandinavia, England, Italy, and the United States as well as in France. Then the situation changed radically. Between

1850 and 1860, for the first time in recorded history, diphtheria became pandemic, exploding all around the world with a previously unknown intensity. August Hirsch noted in his classic *Handbook of Geographical and Historical Pathology* (1883) that this outbreak was "an absolutely new thing," and more recent authority agrees. The new virulence of the disease is explained either by an evolution of the diphtheria bacterium or by the introduction of more malignant types of diphtheria bacilli.

Statistics for the pandemic era are scattered and incomplete, but those that exist reveal relatively high mortalities. Holland, where the mortality was considered low, recorded 400 diphtheria deaths per annum from 1859 to 1863, and the number rose to 600 between 1866 and 1870. Scotland reported 151 deaths in 1861, and 478 two years later. In Russia, diphtheria was far worse. The disease reached epidemic proportions in St. Petersburg, Moscow, and Orel in 1858 and 1859, and then it spread to the southern provinces and Rumania in subsequent years. A contemporary report from the south stated that "the victims were numbered in every village by the hundred, and in every commune by the thousand. The children were exterminated." In the United States, diphtheria deaths in the city of New York averaged 325 per annum for the period 1866–1872; in 1873 the number went to 1151, in 1874 to 1600, and in 1875 to 2329. By 1887, diphtheria was active throughout the United States. The new outbreak also affected India, China (where 20,000 deaths were reported from Peking alone), Australia, Polynesia, and Tunis. By the end of the century, diphtheria girdled the world.

Diphtheria in Decline: 1890 to 1920 The pandemic began to decline in the 1890s. By the first decade of the twentieth century, death rates were falling substantially. In 1894, the rate in New York was 785 per 100,000 of population; in 1900, that figure was down to 300 and by 1920, it was under 100. Effective therapeutic techniques and immunization help to explain why diphtheria virtually disappeared from New York City by 1940, when mortality fell to just 1.1 per 100,000. The decline also was assisted by the disease's own cyclical pattern. The pandemic character of the outbreak in the second half of the nineteenth century probably owed something to rapid modern transportation as well as diphtheria's own characteristics. An endemic-sporadic disease pattern with large numbers of children immunized by mild infections could be seriously disrupted by the multiplication of more virulent strains as well as by a natural increase in disease activity. It seems that this is what happened in 1857 and 1858, combined with artificial extension of the disease to nonimmunized zones. The most significant developments to emerge from the pandemic period, however, were the isolation of diphtheria's causal mechanism and the subsequent discovery of how to cure and control the disease.

Diphtheria and Medical Science: The Discovery of Cause The revival of a clinical approach to disease in the sixteenth century, Thomas Sydenham's attempt to develop a disease taxonomy based on the classification of symptoms in the seventeenth century, and Giovanni Battista Morgagni's efforts to connect pathological conditions with clinical symptoms in the eighteenth century were the intellectual background for the nineteenth century's successful work on diphtheria. The new science of bacteriology provided the techniques to answer questions on cause, dynamics, and immunization. Pierre-Fidèle Bretonneau made the most important prebacteriological contributions. In 1818, while working as chief physician of the Hospice Générale in Tours, Bretonneau had the opportunity to study and compare outbreaks of scorbutic gangrene among soldiers and malignant angina in the town. His studies, which included 60 autopsies, led him to conclude that scorbutic gangrene and angina maligna were different manifestations of the same disease. He presented his arguments in 1821 before the Paris Academy of Medicine. It was Bretonneau who coined the word *diphtérite* from the Greek for "leather" (*diphtera*), a reference to the choking mucous tissue which developed in the throat, and at the very end of his career, in 1855, he revised the term to *diphtérie*. His classic study, *Special Inflammations of the Mucous Tissue,* published in 1826, established diphtheria as a single specific disease while doing away with such concepts as malignant angina and croup.

Bretonneau's doctrine was generally accepted in France, but it proved controversial elsewhere. The problem for the majority who accepted it was to find the unknown agent which caused diphtheria and the means by which it was communicated. The attack on these issues through the third quarter of the nineteenth century focused on Rudolf Virchow's concept of cellular pathology, the study of tissue changes in depth, on an attempt to produce the diphtheritic false membrane by artificial means in experimental animals, and on the effort to deduce diphtheria's etiology by studying patterns of communicability. None of this work produced satisfactory results. The central issue only yielded to bacteriological study following the assumptions, techniques, and ideas established by Louis Pasteur and Robert Koch. The bacterial cause for diphtheria was isolated in 1883 by Edwin Klebs, who informed the Congress for Internal Medicine which met that year in Wiesbaden that he had identified a rod-shaped bacterium, varying in size and in some cases clubbed or compressed on the ends, in diphtheria membrane. The bacillus did not appear in the blood or internal organs. The next year, Friedrich Loeffler, one of Koch's research team in Berlin, confirmed Klebs's findings. Loeffler also discovered the bacillus in a healthy child, thus raising the fundamental epidemiological issue of the unidentified carrier.

Immunization and Control Once the cause was known, the problem of how the bacterium worked in the human system had to be resolved in order for the means to control and cure the disease to be developed. The answers came with comparative ease. In retrospect, the diphtheria bacterium offered much less complex problems than those responsible for tuberculosis, syphilis, influenza, and poliomyelitis. Between 1888 and 1890, as a result of a series of brilliant laboratory investigations by Émile Roux, Alexandre Yersin, Karl Fraenkel, and Emil Behring (supported by his able coworker Shibasaburo Kitasato), the mysteries dissolved. Roux and Yersin showed that the diphtheria bacterium produced a poison (exotoxin) which, when separated from the bacteria and injected into animals, produced diphtheria symptoms. This discovery permitted definitive diagnosis. Within 24 hours of each other, on December 3 and 4, 1890, Fraenkel and Behrings–Kitasato published results of immunological research fundamental to resolving the problem of diphtheria protection and control. Fraenkel showed that attenuated cultures of diphtheria bacilli, when injected into guinea pigs, produced immunity to diphtheria infection, while Behring and Kitasato, working on tetanus toxins, revealed the principle underlying the creation of immune serums which could generate immunity when injected into another animal. Their work showed that "immunity of rabbits and mice ... treated with tetanus cultures, depends on the capacity of cell-free blood serum to render innocuous the toxic substances elaborated by the tetanus bacillus." On December 11, 1890, Behring published a further article applying the same principle to diphtheria, thus establishing the actual basis for serum therapy and prophylaxis against diphtheria and, by extension, against other communicable diseases. The first patient to receive the serum treatment was a child in the Bergmann Clinic in Berlin on December 25, 1891. Roux delivered a definitive survey of the principles and their application in September 1894, at the Eighth International Congress of Hygiene and Demography in Budapest. After 1894, the diphtheria antitoxin approach was employed generally.

The elaboration of the serum principle led directly to successful immunization in the first quarter of the twentieth century. In 1913 Behring, following similar work by Theobald Smith in 1909, used toxin treated with antitoxin to produce immunity; while in that same year, the Hungarian physician and bacteriologist Bela Schick developed the test which bears his name to identify the presence or absence of immunity. By 1923, G. Ramon had discovered the method for treating toxin with formalin to produce anatoxin (toxoid) which was much improved over antitoxin, especially as it was less likely to produce severe reactions. An alum-precipitated toxoid proved even more satisfactory. Large-scale immunization programs were now possible. In New York City, William H. Park and Abraham Zingher set up a program which immunized 500,000 schoolchildren by 1928 and 60 percent of preschool children by 1940. Other cities followed this example, and by 1940, diphtheria mortality had almost disappeared. An upsurge of the disease in Germany, Norway, and Holland during World War II underlined the importance of immunization and serum treatment. Since World War II, immunization for diphtheria as well as for whooping cough and tetanus is routinely given to children in their first year.

Though by no means eradicated, diphtheria has ceased to be a major disease problem. Although severe reactions to toxoids have made mass adult immunization impractical, immunization for children has been effective. Always allowing for problems of delivery and administration in disturbed areas of the world, it appears that diphtheria is in a stable state of control. The one unresolved problem concerns whether current procedures would continue to be effective if a new cycle of virulent and malignant infection were to occur. At the very least, it would appear that medicine is far better prepared to deal with such an eventuality now than it was 125 years ago.

ADDITIONAL READINGS: H. F. Dowling, *Fighting Infection: Disease Conquests of the Twentieth Century*, Cambridge, Mass., 1977; John Duffy, *Epidemics in Colonial America*, Baton Rouge, 1953, 113–137; Geoffrey Marks and William Betty, *Epidemics*, New York, 1976, 137–138, 167–170, 173–174; Medical Research Council (Great Britain), *Diphtheria: Its Bacteriology, Pathology, and Immunology*, London, 1923, 13–63: J. H. Parish, *History of Immunization*, London, 1965, 118–163; George Rosen, "Acute Communicable Diseases: Diphtheria," in Walter R. Bett (ed.), *The History and Conquest of Common Diseases*, Norman, Okla. 1954, 3–26.

Drug Abuse

The abuse of addictive drugs is a problem which has developed in the western world since the middle of the nineteenth century. The reasons for its growth are as complicated as the problem is widespread, and the question of what to do about it remains essentially unanswered. Drug addiction is seen in most cultures, though the United States has experienced it in a particularly acute form, and neither medicine nor law enforcement agencies have found the means to control it. Part of the reason for this failure is that while drug dependency, tolerance, and the withdrawal syndrome are all well-recognized phenomena, the physiological mechanisms which they involve remain stubbornly obscure. Without clear guidance on these issues, it has proved virtually impossible to develop successful treatments, and the relapse rates remain as high today as they were 75 years ago.

Medicine played a critically important role in the evolution of modern attitudes toward drugs by defining and exposing the dangers of drug abuse. Though other factors from economic interest to racial prejudice were also important, it was largely with warnings originating with the medical profession that the drive for regulating addictive substances began. This was only justice, since drug abuse in the west originated in the unrestricted use of opium for medical purposes.

History Before 1870, European medicine regarded opium as a virtual panacea. It appeared in various forms in the working pharmacopeia of the Middle Ages, but it was in the early modern period that it came to be considered the most useful drug in the entire *materia medica*. The great English clinician Thomas Sydenham won the nickname "opiophilos" for his enthusiastic advocacy of opium, and Sydenham's laudanum, a special compound in which opium was dissolved in sherry and the mixture flavored with cinnamon, cloves, and saffron, became a standard item. It was Sydenham's laudanum which captivated Thomas DeQuincey, who described its wonders in his classic *Confessions of an English Opium Eater* (1822). DeQuincey regularly consumed a pint and more a day, but this was not typical. One or two ounces of laudanum was nearer to normal consumption for a regular user.

Opium's uses were legion. It was universally prescribed as an analgesic, a specific for fever, a sedative, and a corrective for diarrhea. Its most valued functions, however, were to control pain and promote a sense of well-being. In this respect, injected morphia, the alkaloid derivative of opium, was even more successful than opium itself. Morphia became available commercially in the 1820s, but it was not until 1858 that Dr. Alexander Wood publicized his methods for subcutaneous injection of morphia with the hypodermic syringe, an instrument invented by Charles Gabriel Pravaz in 1853. Morphia injection was greeted as miraculous, "the greatest boon given to medicine since the discovery of chloroform," as one contemporary wrote in 1869. The realization that this boon was won at a major price came shortly after.

Opium use expanded steadily with the population through the middle of the nineteenth century. Then it rose sharply to crest just before the century's end. Medicine was primarily responsible for this growth. Opium was prescribed freely, it was available in a variety of popular patent medicines, and when morphia became the drug of choice, physicians not only injected their patients but even taught them the technique. Physicians were not unaware that opium had its dangers, but while they warned against them, they considered the dangers less significant than the benefits. Dr. George Wood, an eminent American physician who held a professorship at the University of Pennsylvania and was president of the American Philosophical Society, published his *Treatise on Therapeutics* in 1868, which exemplified medical attitudes. Dr. Wood recognized that opium was addictive and that in extreme cases addiction could result in "total loss of self-respect, and indifference to the opinions of the community." He also reported that for the truly addicted, "everything is sacrificed to the insatiable demands of the vice." Even so, he believed that opium addiction was only marginally dangerous to the individual and society, and that it was a lesser threat than alcohol because it could do no permanent physical damage. Moreover, opium addiction was easily corrected by gradual withdrawal of the drug.

By contrast, Dr. Wood's praise for opium and injected morphia was fulsome to the point of eloquence. Opium produced "a universal feeling of delicious ease and comfort," it brought about "an exaltation of our better mental qualities, a warmer glow of benevolence, a disposition to do great things . . . a higher devotional spirit," it raised "the intellectual and imaginative faculties . . . to the highest point," and it generated none of the destructive violence which alcohol unleashed but elevated "the imagination and the soul above the levels of reality." Nor were the aftereffects unpleasant. On the contrary, "exaltation sinks into a corporeal and mental calmness, which in a short time ends in sleep." Who, indeed, could resist?

Another sort of medical opinion reinforced opium's favorable image. Physicians and civil servants who had experience with the drug in India and China were inclined to see it as essentially benign. Their views need to be considered against the backdrop of Britain's lucrative traffic in opium with China, but there is little doubt that they reported what they thought they knew. Thus Sir George Birdwood, writing to the letters section of the London *Times* in 1881, entirely exculpated opium as a dangerous drug on the basis of years of experience with people who used it regularly. Smoking of opium, the preferred method of use in China, "is, of itself, absolutely harmless," he pointed out. So far as opium eating was concerned, "sound, hale people in comfortable circumstances who lead healthy lives, seldom or never suffer from the habitual use of opium"; and he reminded his readers that while they were obviously addicted to opium, "there are few finer people in the world than those of Goojerat, Kattywar, Crutch, and Central India." So influential was this sort of testimony that a Royal Commission on Opium, which published its findings in 1895, concluded that there was very little evidence from India or from England that opium had undesirable physical or moral consequences.

Medical literature from the eighteenth and early nineteenth centuries showed that many doctors were aware that opium created dependency, that regular and sustained use produced physiological consequences, and that to stop taking it suddenly provided symptoms of considerable discomfort. John Jones, an English physician writing in 1701, included sweats, frequent urination, loose bowels, melancholy or depression, rapid pulse, and itching as possible results of stopping regular opium ingestion. He also pointed out that the condition for which the opium was taken generally returned. At the end of the century, Samuel Crump recorded that opium users deprived of their drug even for a single day "became languid, dejected, and uneasy" at the time their dose was usually taken, and that only the usual amount of opium or "a large draught of wine would serve to arouse them." Sir Astley Martin expressed a similar view in one of his public lectures on poisons in 1824. At least two members of the Westminster Medical Society spoke out against opium's dangerous properties, including its addictiveness, when the issue was debated in 1840, though the majority considered alcohol the more serious problem. Jonathan Pereira, who claimed in the 1843 edition of his widely respected *Elements of Materia Medica and Therapeutics* that "opium is undoubtedly the most important and valuable remedy of the whole Materia Medica," noted in his 1850 edition that opium indulgence was physically and morally destructive, that it upset the digestive system, and that it damaged the nerves. He also indicated that addicts' children tended to be "weak, stunted, and decrepit," while addicted persons required progressively larger doses to gain the same pleasurable sensations or stave off the effects of withdrawal.

Morphia injection intensified drug reactions and raised further questions about addiction. Injections multiplied the quantities of drug which actually went into the system, and addicts raised the quantities of drug they were using. Many regularly injected 10 to 12 grains daily, while daily doses of 30, 40, or even 50 grains were not uncommon. In contrast it was estimated that a typical daily intake of laudanum was no more than 1 or 2 ounces. Injected morphia raised the problem to a new order of magnitude, leading Dr. Thomas Clifford Allbutt to wonder publicly in 1870 whether morphia injections did not create a clear dependency. If so, were not physicians themselves "incurring a grave risk in bidding people to inject whenever they need it, and in telling them that morphine can have no ill effects upon them so long as it brings with it tranquility and well-being"?

Though the English literature contained warnings and reflected a growing unease over drug abuse, German physicians led the way toward defining drug addiction as a specific disease with a definite symptomology, etiology, prognosis, and prophylaxis. The most important work was Eduard Levinstein's *Die Morphiumsucht*, which was translated into English as *The Morbid Craving for Morphia* (1878). Levinstein described morphia addiction as "the uncontrollable desire of a person to use morphia as a stimulant and a tonic, and the diseased state of the system caused by the injudicious use of the said remedy." He did not consider the craving for morphia to be psychological or a consequence of moral weakness. On the contrary, it resulted from "the natural [physical] constitution and not from a certain predisposition to its use." This meant that anybody could become addicted, and the best means of prevention was to close off all public sources of supply while severely limiting medical use. Since addiction was physiological, there was no way for patients to assist in their own cures; they were the victims of their own reflexes, of their own bodies, and one of the effects, according to Levinstein, was to make them clever liars, particularly where drugs were concerned. Consequently, Levinstein's cure was total withdrawal under medical supervision. He recommended that a patient be institutionalized and kept in isolation for from 8 to 14 days in a room from which all means of committing suicide had been removed. Nurses and a physician were to be in constant attendence. The withdrawal symptoms could be fought with hot baths, bicarbonate of soda, chloral hydrate, and unlimited quantities of brandy and champagne. Only the patient's complete collapse would justify injecting morphia, and then no more than ½ grain should be used. Levinstein originally believed that once a cure had been effected, there should be no relapse, provided that there was no further exposure to morphia. He was equally optimistic about the effect of controls. Once morphia was rigidly regulated by government decree and only physicians were allowed to possess and use the drug, he was certain that addiction would become a rare occurrence.

Levinstein's optimism died an early death as his own patients relapsed at a rate of 75 percent, but his approach was influential. In England, the Society for the Study and Cure of Inebriety, which was founded by Dr. Norman Kerr in 1884, took up and expanded Levinstein's theme. The society's interest was primarily in alcohol abuse, but it also dealt with opium, chloral hydrate, chlorodyne, and cocaine. Inebriety, as Kerr defined it, was a disease which resulted from "certain physical conditions . . . the natural product of a depraved, debilitated, or defective nervous organization" and which was fully comparable with "gout, or epilepsy, or insanity." The active agents which produced the physiological condition were drugs or alcohol, and persons who succumbed to their effects required treatment rather than punishment. Kerr was much less sanguine about drug cures than his German contemporaries. He claimed that while alcohol abuse was more dangerous because it fostered violence and physical degeneration, "opium transcends alcohol in the generation of a more irreclaimable and incurable diseased condition." He also recognized that hypodermic injection was the swiftest and most potent method of application.

Twentieth-Century Attitudes By the first decade of the twentieth century, a medical consensus on drugs was in place. It held that addiction, including alcoholism, was a disease, and that the narcotic drugs, though less damaging socially, were more dangerous for the individual user. Levinstein's "physicalist theory" of drug addiction remained central, with special emphasis on the "cerebro-spinal and sympathetic systems . . . [which] bear the brunt of opium excess, which induces changes which give rise to great nervous derangement, when the opiate is withdrawn." But psychological explanations which were coming into vogue as well called addiction a "form of Moral Insanity," or a "disease of the will," and with the advent of psychoanalysis, the concept of addiction acquired an entirely nonphysiological dimension. Psychoanalytic therapy was conceived as teaching "this otherwise normal drug addict to irradiate and sublimate this libido which he is so wantonly wasting on the fetish of drug addiction." Though "moral insanity" could be called a psychological concept, it also showed the persistence of an ethical etiology for addiction: that addicts were in some special fashion morally flawed, or, as Allbutt and W. E. Dixon put it, "nowadays whoso betakes himself to the morphia syringe does so of his own naughtiness."

There was also growing support for the idea that there was an addict type, a person with a predisposition to use stimulants, who would switch from one drug to another or combine them. Such persons were commonly considered "neurotic"; that is, they were believed to suffer from a defective nervous system, and with such persons all drugs were roughly equal. There was, therefore, nothing to be gained by distinguishing among addiction to morphine, cocaine, or heroin. Moreover, it was also agreed that most drug habits started with medical treatment. A patient given morphia and taught to inject himself or herself was already well launched, and people who suffered a "wearisome" rather than an acute disease were particularly susceptible to habituation.

There were some broader generalizations about addicts. Drug addiction was considered a modern disease, contracted by people seeking relief from the pressures of modern life, a condition to which professional people, intellectuals, and people in business were particularly prone. A high addiction rate among physicians was noted early. Creative people of artistic temperament were also considered to be prime candidates for addiction. In fact, however, little was known about drug abuse outside the middle class. Since few poor or working-class people could afford physicians' fees, they were not among the addicts whom physicians saw, and this was plainly reflected in the ideas about who became addicted and why. Chinese and Mexican workers and American blacks represented a drug threat of an entirely different sort. They were considered carriers who would infect otherwise innocent people, while as abusers they were considered to be dangerous. Racial and ethnic stereotypes involving drug abuse played an important part wherever there were significant concentrations of such minorities—urban centers, the rural American south, or the far west—and they found their way into an increasingly sensationalist popular literature. Though of minor significance in medical perceptions of drug abuse, such stereotypes were extremely important in promoting severe regulatory policies.

By the twentieth century, most medical authorities agreed that some drug addicts, if not deprived of their drugs, could function normally, but it was considered more likely that prolonged use and the inevitable increases necessary to achieve the desired result would generate physical, psychological, and moral decline. It was also generally believed that the only hope was for addicts to rid themselves of their habits, but the prognosis for cures was mixed. The earlier belief that withdrawal would eliminate a habit gave way to the certainty that many patients would relapse. This was no more than the result of accumulated experience with drug addicts. At the same time, relapse was not considered inevitable. T. D. Crothers, writing at the turn of the century, summarized the balanced view: "The prognosis in morphinism will vary very widely according to the condition of the patient, the length of time of the addiction, and the influence of heredity." The prognosis was especially doubtful for persons with well-established habits who suffered from a chronic disease, were neurotic, or had a second (beyond morphine) drug addiction. Even so, cures were to be attempted in all cases, and there was wide agreement on the best method. It involved isolation in an institution, gradual withdrawal of the drug, and management of the withdrawal symptoms. Substituting cocaine, cannabis, or heroin—procedures recommended as recently as three decades before—was considered fundamentally wrong. Though inclined to quarrel over the best way to ease the addict's passage back to health, physicians were in agreement on the fundamentals.

Once addiction was defined as a disease, medical opinion shifted relatively little. The modified optimism concerning cures which appeared in the early twentieth century had almost entirely disappeared by the 1920s. In part, the reaction was generated by the collapse of claims by asylum operators or monitors of so-called addiction clinics that they could, indeed, cure addiction. Charles B. Towns, one of the most flamboyant of those who peddled certain cures, even convinced the United States government that his method (once summarized as "diarrhea, delirium, and damnation") would significantly reduce the high level of addiction in the Philippines and held forth hope for China. But the Mayor's Committee on Drug Addiction for the City of New York came closer to the truth when, after reporting the treatment of 318 patients at Bellevue Hospital during 1928 and 1929, it concluded that there was no evidence to confirm any claims of cure, and that, in fact, the withdrawal of narcotics did not constitute a cure. Such hopelessness contributed directly to new emphasis on the doctrine of predisposition, though this was carried to a radical extreme. Dr. Lawrence Kolb, Sr., of the U.S. Public Health Service, a leading researcher on drug addiction, concluded on the eve of World War II that "normal" persons do not choose to become addicted; that addiction by choice shows a psychopathic personality; and that only psychopaths feel joy at morphine injections. With this outlook, strict regulation was essential to prevent accidental exposure of the predisposed, while the drug addict could be considered a potential if not an actual criminal because his or her predisposition to addiction included social ineptness and a penchant toward criminality.

Regulation and Control In the first quarter of the twentieth century, most western countries were moving toward regulation of addictive drugs. The general tendency was to restrict such substances to physicians' use, and in England, for example, the medical profession was accepted as the primary source of information, advice, and counsel on legislative approaches to the drug problem. The result was legislation which allowed physicians to prescribe drugs without interference. This proved to be a major barrier against criminalizing drug abuse. On the Continent, the tradition of stiff controls over compounding and dispensing pharmaceuticals made control of addictive drugs relatively easy and effective and achieved a result comparable to that in England. In the United States, on the other hand, nonmedical influences dominated the arguments over regulation, though medical opinion was used freely to justify or, more accurately, to dramatize the demand for ever stronger regulatory measures. There was relatively little interest, for example, in national regulatory statutes on addictive drugs until the United States took a stand against the opium traffic with China. The American position owed as much to the aim of winning favor with Chinese reformers to gain access to Chinese markets as to any distaste for addictive drugs. For the United States to be credible on issues related to the drug traffic, it was necessary for a drug control law to exist.

Economic advantage hardly stood alone. There was a powerful determination among progressives to use state power to protect society through antitrust legislation, statutory rules governing the composition and quality of drugs and food, rate regulations on the railroads, and laws controlling the production and distribution of alcohol and dangerous drugs. Congressional legislation in 1909 prepared the way for the more comprehensive Harrison Act of 1914 which, when interpreted by the Supreme Court, ended by making drug addiction a crime. This move was in phase with the Eighteenth Amendment to the Constitution and the Volstead Act (1919), which together prohibited and provided the measures to enforce the prohibition of the manufacture and sale of alcoholic beverages. But though the Prohibition was repealed in 1933, the rules governing drugs were further tightened by special legislation against the sale or use of marijuana in 1937.

The Marijuana Control Act marked the high tide of regulation. In the period after World War II, a growing body of American opinion criticized maximum legal sanctions against individuals for drug abuse. Involved in this reaction was the dramatic rise in the incidence of drug abuse and addiction and the mounting evidence that drug addiction was a major element in crimes against property. There was strong evidence that "criminalization" was not a successful approach, and while the conviction remained that police controls on the sale or distribution of drugs were essential, medical thinking brought up new hopes for control through treatment. The combined techniques of medical and psychiatric social work, the use of methadone as a substitute for heroin, and proposals for the controlled distribution of heroin itself announced a new era. In 1962 the Supreme Court took the position that addiction was in fact a disease and not a crime, and 10 years later the President's Commission on Drug Abuse recommended that criminal penalties for the private use of marijuana be eliminated. Even so, the situation under law has not changed significantly, though public opinion has. Despite legal controls, popular acceptance has sanctioned the use of marijuana, cocaine, and a number of other addictive substances. Medical opinion has contributed relatively little to this stage of the debate. Certainly nothing comparable to the influence of the concept of addiction as disease has surfaced, though medical pronouncements on drug-related issues are regularly cited. Medicine made its most important contribution to the problem of drug addiction between 1870 and 1920. During the last half century and more it has elaborated its opinions while improving aspects of its practice, but it cannot be considered a leading influence where drug addiction is concerned.

ADDITIONAL READINGS: Virginia Berridge, "Morality and Medical Science: Concepts of Narcotic Addiction in Britain, 1820–1924," *Annuals of Science* 36, 1979, 67–85; Virginia Berridge, *Opium and the People: Opium Use in Nineteenth Century England*, London, 1981; David T. Courtwright, *Dark Paradise: Opium Addiction in America Before 1940*, Cambridge, Mass., 1982; Brian Inglis, *The Forbidden Game: A Social History of Drugs*, New York, 1975; Norman Howard Jones, "A Critical Study of the Origins and Early Development of Hypodermic Medication," *Journal of the History of Medicine and Allied Sciences* 2(1947): 201–247; H. Wayne Morgan, *Drugs in America: A Social History*, Syracuse, 1981; H. Wayne Morgan, *Yesterday's Addicts: American Society and Drug Abuse*, Norman, Okla., 1974; David J. Musto, *The American Disease: Origins of Narcotic Control*, New Haven and London, 1973; Terry M. Parssinen, *Secret Passions, Secret Remedies: Narcotic Drugs in British Society, 1820–1930*, Philadelphia, 1982; Terry M. Parssinen and Karen Kerner, "Development of the Disease Model of Drug Addiction in Britain, 1870–1926," *Medical History* 24 (1980): 275–296; Glenn Sonnedecker, "Emergence of the Concept of Opiate Addiction," *Journal mondiale de la pharmmacie* 3 (1962): 275–290, 1 (1963) 27–34; Thomas Szasz, *Ceremonial Chemistry: The Ritual Persecution of Drugs, Addicts, and Pushers*, London 1974.

See also: PHARMACY.

Dysentery

Dysentery has been one of the most pervasive dangerous diseases in human history. Like cholera and typhoid, it is waterborne, and its incidence correlates specifically with societies' abilities to maintain water sources safe from contamination. Humans are the primary reservoir for dysentery, and human excrement is the main pollutant. Therefore, the maintenance of personal hygiene and the safe disposal of wastes are fundamental to controlling the disease. Contamination of foods by dysentery carriers provides another mechanism for communicating the disease, while various insects, most notably houseflies, can transfer the active dysentery agent to humans by carrying it on their bodies and depositing it on food. Unlike typhus or bubonic plague, however, there is no necessary insect vector, and the disease is transmitted by ingesting contaminated water or food. Dysentery, like typhus, typhoid, and cholera, is a disease of massed humanity. It has been the constant companion of armies throughout history, but it has also been active on shipboard, in jails, or wherever numbers of people are crowded together without adequate sanitary facilities.

The Disease There are two basic types of dysentery—bacillary and amebic—but the difference between them can only be determined with a microscope. *Entamoeba histolytica*, the causal agent for amebic dysentery, was first identified in St. Petersburg in 1875 by Frederick Lösch. The bacterium which causes bacillary dysentery was isolated in 1898 by Kiyoshi Shigu, a Japanese bacteriologist, and the genus was then named *Shigella*. The *Shigella* group has been broken further into four subgroups, according to fermentation characteristics and serological affinities. The most important of the bacilli are *Shigella dysenteriae*, formerly Shiga's bacillus, *Shigella flexneri* (named for Simon Flexner, 1863–1946, its discoverer), and *Shigella sonnei*. Mortality rates vary widely, depending on the bacillus involved. Overall case mortality from bacillary dysentery in adults before chemotherapy was probably no more than 5 percent, but Shiga's bacillus produced mortality as high as 50 percent, and mortality among babies, especially where nutrition was deficient, may have been higher still.

Famine or other causes of debilitation would raise death rates, and dysentery in its turn increased susceptibility to other infections and reduced resistance.

History Before 1875, dysenteries were lumped together, or at most distinguished according to whether they were endemic or epidemic. Moreover, there was no certain way to separate dysenteries from diarrhea, and without bacteriological analysis, it would appear that historical records also confused dysenteries with typhus and typhoid. It is virtually impossible, therefore, to state with any precision what proportion of illness should be ascribed at any given time to any one of these diseases. Nevertheless, medical sources from a very early period accurately describe dysentery's symptoms, while modern epidemiology provides reasonably precise evidence on current incidence and mortality. The latter gives a guide for determining relative incidence on the basis of what the written sources reveal.

There is ample evidence of dysentery for Europe, the Mediterranean, and western Asia. One of the earliest sources is the Ebers papyrus of Egypt (ca. 1550 B.C.), and there is an Egyptian tradition that Horus, the son of Isis and Osiris, sickened with dysentery. The best clinical description, however, comes from the Hippocratic writings of the fifth and early fourth centuries B.C., where the prolific blood- and mucus-streaked stool which provides a clear diagnostic image for dysentery was fully described. The sections of the Hippocratic writings which cover dysentery are judged to be among the finest in the entire work. Later Greek, Roman, Arab, and early medieval authorities continued to discuss dysentery, though in the second century A.D. Galen broadened the field to include other intestinal fluxes. This makes it difficult to know just what the secular medieval chronicler meant when he recorded severe "dysentery epidemics" in France, Germany, and Hungary in the sixth, eighth, ninth, eleventh, and twelfth centuries. Similar chronicle sources which tell the tale of European Crusaders in the Holy Land between the eleventh and thirteenth centuries indicate that dysentery, together with other fevers and fluxes, killed Christian knights far more efficiently than did Saracen warriors. The connection between dysentery and war was inescapable. England's warlike kings Edward I and Henry V both died of dysentery; Edward the Black Prince may also have been a victim; and so riddled with dysentery and its attendent infections was the English army at Crécy in 1346 that the French dubbed them "breechless" and "barebottomed." (For all that, it was the diarrheic English who won the field.)

Dysentery, or "campaign fever," plagued European armies into the nineteenth century. As one authority put it, "There has hardly been a single war of long duration, hardly a single seige protracted for several months, in which dysentery and diarrhea have not broken out." During the nineteenth century, when more accurate records were kept, the statistics supported the tradition. The Union army in the Civil War (1861–1865) lost 186,216 men to disease; of these, 81,360 were claimed by typhoid and dysentery. These numbers can be compared to the 93,443 killed in action. In the Russo-Japanese War (1904–1905), for the first time battle was more deadly than illness, and a relatively low score of dysentery casualties on the Russian side underlined improving military hygiene. The Czar had 709,587 men in action and only 7960 deaths from disease. The Japanese lost 21,802 men to disease with 5877 succumbing to dysentery and typhoid. The Russian military health record collapsed in 1917, and dysentery joined cholera, typhus, typhoid, influenza, and malaria in a horrible complex of epidemic outbreaks which lasted through 1923 and carried off millions of Russian victims.

A high incidence of dysentery is often an index of social distress. Ireland, for example, suffered severe outbreaks of dysentery in the famine years of the early nineteenth century and again during the potato famine of 1846 and 1847. That was also a year of shortage and dysentery in Belgium, Bohemia, and parts of Russia. On the other hand, dysentery has tended to decline with rising living standards and improving public health. From the early medieval period through the eighteenth century, dysentery appeared again and again throughout the western world. Endemic areas tended to be restricted to southern Europe, but there were repeated epidemics in England, France, Germany, and Scandinavia. Sweden was particularly susceptible, and dysentery was also a constant visitor in North America.

During the nineteenth century, the pattern changed. Dysentery was worldwide, but the most serious outbreaks were reported from Africa, India, and southern China, together with southeast

Asia, the coastal zones of South and Central America, the Caribbean, and the jungles of northern Brazil. Incidence declined in Europe, North America, and temperate South America. This decline was the product of a cultural process which gradually improved personal hygiene, sanitary engineering, and social control.

Dysentery in the Twentieth Century At the opening of the twentieth century, as the sanitary revolution advanced and the technology of public health improved, an enormous difference emerged which still divides the developed and less-developed nations. Sanitation, hygiene, and public health administration require expanding wealth, and most of the world where dysentery rules is poor. In India, one of the world's worst endemic foci, dysentery and diarrhea together accounted for up to 75 percent of the disease mortality in the middle of the nineteenth century. A century later, India was still suffering from dysentery, reporting 1,500,000 cases in 1938. This pattern remains unchanged. The main areas for dysentery infection in the late 1960s and in the 1970s have been the Middle East, parts of Asia, and sections of Central America. Severe outbreaks with high mortality were recorded, for example, in 1969 and 1970 in Guatemala, El Salvador, and Mexico. These outbreaks brought a sharp increase in dysentery cases in the United States in states bordering Mexico and in Los Angeles in the Mexican-American sections. A similar development occurred in England and Wales between 1972 and 1975, when heavy dysentery outbreaks in India, Pakistan, Bangladesh, and Afghanistan were mirrored in rising British incidence through importation into immigrant centers. Disease intelligence and control kept such outbreaks localized in the United States and the United Kingdom. Throughout the developing world, however, dysentery remains a critical problem which only economic improvement and continued progress toward safe water and controlled sanitary conditions can resolve.

ADDITIONAL READINGS: Frederick F. Cartwright, *Disease and History*, London, 1972; John Duffy, *Epidemics in Colonial America*, Baton Rouge, 1956; August Hirsch, *Handbook of Geographical and Historical Pathology*, Charles Creighton (tran.), 3 vols., London, 1883–1886, III, chap. X; 284–370; H. Harold Scott, *A History of Tropical Medicine*, 2 vols., London, 1939, II, chap. XVII.

See also PUBLIC HEALTH.

Egyptian Medicine

Medicine in ancient Egypt blended magic, prayers, spells, and sacrifices with empirical treatments and some surgery. The first written evidence appears in the medical papyri of the second millennium B.C., but these records refer to older traditions which in the more remote past were transmitted orally. The most important texts, discovered in the nineteenth century and named for the men who acquired them, are the Georg Ebers and Edwin Smith papyri, which have been dated to the middle of the second millennium B.C. The Ebers papyrus deals with diseases, prescriptions, and incantations. The Smith papyrus has been called a book of wounds and could have been an army surgeon's manual. In addition, the Kahun papyrus (ca. 1850 B.C.) treats gynecology and veterinary medicine, and the London papyrus (ca. 1350 B.C.) describes maternal care. Other sources include the Hearst (ca. 1550), Berlin (ca. 1250), and Chester Beatty (ca. 1200) papyri, which add to the information on prescription and treatment in the Ebers papyrus.

The papyri, supplemented by archaeological evidence, provide a picture of how Egyptian medicine was practiced, though many particulars remain obscure. Medicine was a trade organized hierarchically under state control. The court physicians (*iri*) stood at the head of the hierarchy and were led by the greatest physician, or chief physician, of Upper and Lower Egypt. There were also a superintendent of physicians and a chief of physicians. The physicians themselves (*swnu*) were specialists in particular diseases, and by the fifth century B.C., when Herodotus observed medicine in Egypt, it appeared that "every court physician was in charge of a single illness."

The *swnu* were one of three types of healers. The others were priests of Sekhmet and sorcerers. The pharoahs' armies probably had medical service from the temple priests or state physicians. There is no indication of a separate military medical service. Individual physicans are virtually impossible to identify, though a few are named. These include Hesy Re (ca. 2600 B.C.), who was chief of dentists and physicians to the pyramid builders; Peseshet, identified as chief woman physician or overseer, whose date is uncertain but is probably late; and the famous Imhotep, chief vizier to King Zozer (2980–2900 B.C.), who was known as an astrologer, priest, and pyramid designer as well as a physician. Imhotep became a cult figure similar to and sometimes confused with the Greek god Asclepius.

Beliefs and Practices Egyptian medicine assumed a balance between humanity's temporal and spiritual worlds. Illness meant imbalance, which could be restored to equilibrium by prayers, incantations, and rituals. Concomitantly, the physical conditions which cosmic disorder produced were treated empirically with palliatives. Conditions were closely observed, symptoms described, and effective treatments noted. The result was a burgeoning empirical practice based on an extensive pharmacopeia which paralleled the priests' and sorcerers' arts. Surgery was limited to repairing injuries and bone fractures, with occasional treatments for organic conditions such as abscesses, boils, or superficial growths. No identifiable surgical tools have been found, though it appears that Egyptian wound treatments were effective. Clamps, sutures, and cautery were used, a wound dressing which combined honey and grease or resin provided protection and promoted healing, and copper salts in eye paint and salves gave an antiseptic effect and lead to the conclusion that the Egyptians had some concept of infection.

Though the evidence is indirect, temple precincts appear to have served for hospitals, and the physicians may have received their training at a special institution called the House of Life, where medical texts were also compiled. Such knowledge as there was concerning anatomy came from food preparation and sacrifices. Bone structure and major organs were identified, but fine relationships and physiological function remained mysterious. Embalming, a highly developed art, apparently taught medicine very little. Embalmers formed a separate guild and were shunned by society. Moreover, since the embalmers wished to preserve the body intact, they removed the organs through small slits and avoided opening cadavers in any way that would facilitate observation. A speculative physiology developed which centered on the heart and postulated a system of vessels originating there which connected with all parts of the body. These vessels were thought to carry air, blood, urine, sperm, tears, and solid wastes. The vessel system was compared to Egypt's great river and canal system, and, like the canals, the vessels had to be kept clean and open. The waste and decayed material passing through were considered the seat of disease, and periodic purgings were considered effective preventive medicine as well as therapy.

Incomplete as the Egyptian record is, it reveals a medical practice of great complexity which appears to have been able to deal effectively with the commonplace conditions that disturb life. How far these comfort-giving efforts extended into society is unknown, though the high degree of organization which characterized Egyptian society suggests that there were channels available for regular care to reach the lowest classes. Culturally, Egyptian medical practices and ideas formed an important element in the reservoir of concepts which grew up around the Mediterranean and which shaped Hebrew and Greek medicine (q. v.). In this respect, Egyptian medicine, in common with that of Mesopotamia, contributed directly to the historical seedbeds from which scientific medicine ultimately developed.

ADDITIONAL READINGS: Darrel W. Amundson and Gary B. Ferngren, "The Forensic Role of Physicians in Ptolemaic and Roman Egypt," *Bulletin of the History of Medicine* 52 (Fall 1978): 336–353; J. H. Breasted, *The Edwin Smith Surgical Papyrus*, 2 vols., Chicago, 1930; P. Ghalioungui, *The House of Life* (*Per Ankh*), Amsterdam, 1973; Guido Majno, *The Healing Hand: Man and Wound in the Ancient World*, Cambridge, Mass., 1975, chap. 3; J. B. de C. M. Saunders, *The Transition from Ancient Egyptian to Greek Medicine*, Lawrence, Kans., 1963; Henry Sigerist, *A History of Medicine*, 2 vols., New York, 1951, I, chap. 3; René Taton, *History of Science: Ancient and Medieval Science from the Beginnings to 1450*, A. J. Pomerans (trans.), New York, 1963, pt. I, chap. 1.

English Sweating Sickness

The English sweating sickness, or English sweats, has puzzled historians for 200 years. The disease appeared in England at the end of the fifteenth century, recurred four times in the sixteenth century, attacked continental Europe once, and disappeared, seemingly forever. Modern medical historians point out that various ancient writers described "sweating diseases" which included the heart diseases described by Asclepiades, Celsus, and Galen, and which had some symptoms in common with the sweats. Historians have also been at pains to identify the Picardy, or Milary, sweat, which was widespread in eighteenth-, nineteenth-, and even twentieth-century France, with England's special sixteenth-century plague. Their efforts are inconclusive. Modern scholarship is no nearer to identifying the English sweating sickness with a particular family of diseases than contemporaries were, though there has been progress toward explaining how the disease may have produced the effects it did. It seems likely, however, that an exact identification of the disease will remain elusive, and that it is best viewed in the context of its own time.

History The sweats appeared at the very outset of the Tudor era. The first hints of a new and awful disease were rumored just before August 22, 1485, the day the Duke of Richmond, Henry Tudor, defeated and killed King Richard III on Bosworth Field. The disease appeared on the Welsh borders and spread to London, where its rapid onset and extraordinary mortality stunned contemporaries. It lasted for about five weeks and then disappeared, not to return until 1508. The first outbreaks were followed by epidemics in 1517, when London, Oxford, and Cambridge were severely hit; in 1528; and finally in 1551. The disease appeared in Europe in 1529, and it spread across Germany, reached Vienna (which was under Turkish seige), appeared in the Netherlands, Scandinavia, Lithuania, Poland, Livonia, and possibly Muscovy. It never reappeared in the form in which the sixteenth century saw it.

The first description of the English sweating sickness of 1485 and 1508 was written by Polydore Vergil, an Italian diplomat and scholar who came to London in 1501. His description, together with John Caius's account of the 1551 outbreak, provides a detailed picture. The disease was, in Polydore Vergil's words, "a pestilence horrible indeed, and before which no age could endure." The onset was as sudden as a blow. Healthy, well-fed men and women collapsed and expired, usually in 24 hours, and the violence of the disease was such that "not one in a hundred evaded it." The illness began without warning with a violent, soaking, pouring perspiration accompanied by wracking pains in the head and stomach and an insufferable sensation of internal heat. The sweat stank, and no measures gave relief.

John Caius, the celebrated physician and scholar who was master of Gonville and Caius College, Cambridge, from 1559 to 1573, produced a comprehensive summary of the English sweats which was published in 1552. His purpose was to "declare the beginning, name, nature, and signs of the sweating sickness," to explain its causes, and to report "how to preserve men from it, and remedy them when they have it." What John Caius observed of the disease pertained to 1551, though he summarized the preceding outbreaks, and his account of the symptoms and progress of the disease reinforces Polydore Vergil's earlier narrative. He laid the cause to an infection in the air and "impure spirits by repletion," a reference to the excessive consumption of beer among the English, which some authorities thought explained why the disease was largely restricted to them. Apart from beer, Caius deplored dirty rush floors, urged greater attention to a balanced and moderate life, and altogether showed himself, as Hecker put it, a follower "of the old Greek school throughout." Apart from temperance, John Caius had faith in purifying fires, fumigations, and a generally benign or gentle therapy. His favorite remedy was a preparation of pearls, sugar, and scented substances, called *manus Christi*. When perspiration started, however, he counseled an end to medicines and "trusted to aromatic vinegar and gentle succession alone for keeping off the lethargy." Polydore Vergil had held that the best one could do was to lie quietly in one's clothes, avoiding food if possible, and drinking no more water than was normal and none that was colder than normal.

No better treatments were found in subsequent outbreaks, though much worse ones were practiced. In at least one case in 1528, however, a treatment was found which gave immediate relief. A clyster, or rectal enema, was administered to the daughter of Sir Thomas More, and a remarkable recovery followed. Clysters were recommended for restoration of fluids and even nutrients in premodern times. Recent authorities suggest that whatever the causal agent of the sweats may have been, it produced a radical dehydration comparable to that in cholera or desert dehydration, which would account for coma and death. With oral administration of replacement fluids impossible, replacement by a clyster in the bowel could have had the effect recorded. Less happy methods for treating the sweats included intensifying the sweating process by closing patient's rooms, building up the fires, piling bedclothes over them, and even lying on top of them to add heat and to keep them down. At least one anonymous village physician released the victims and drove their tormentors away, but the use of these methods was apparently widespread and indiscriminate.

The English sweats was too short-lived to be significant demographically, though its specialized effects in certain localities may have been important. The 1517 epidemic, for example, struck Oxford and Cambridge where "the sciences, which then flourished, for they were never more zealously cultivated than in England at that time, suffered severe losses by death of many able and distinguished scholars." Moreover, the rich and wellborn were not spared, and though it would be an exaggeration to claim that the sweats killed the upper classes while sparing the poor, there is no doubt that merchants, gentry, and nobility all suffered, as did the common people. The actual extent and mortality of the disease remain vague, though it seems to have been widespread and deadly where it struck. On the other hand, the fear which the sweats inspired was sufficient to force cancellation of holidays, to send those flying who could flee, and to sharpen religious conflicts. Even so, the public responses were less violent, given the nature and extent of the disease and the disordered character of the times, than might have been expected. This may owe to the relatively short duration of the epidemic visits, the ferocity of their effects, or the contemporary presence of such pestilential killers as bubonic plague, typhus, malignant syphilis, and smallpox. Historians have studied reactions to particular diseases in the past, but there is as yet no systematic appraisal of the composite effects which such a variety of death-dealing infections had, though such a synthesis is clearly needed.

Since the English sweats has not reappeared in its sixteenth-century form, and modern efforts to isolate a bacterial cause for the Picardy sweats have failed, only speculation remains. Given the course of the disease and the dehydration thesis, the suggestion that a virus which generated immunity in its recipients and then mutated itself into the more benign forms recorded in the eighteenth and nineteenth centuries is a possible explanation. Influenza viruses, which are notably unstable, would be a possible candidate, and at least one authority on influenza, Major Greenwood, was prepared to accept an identification of flu as the disease called the sweats. The only thing which can be certain, however, is that the sweats, which existed as a positve epidemic disease for a brief time and in a reasonably limited area, proved as deadly an infection as the early modern world has known.

ADDITIONAL READINGS: J. F. C. Hecker, *The Epidemics of the Middle Ages*, B. G. Babbington, (trans.) 3d ed., London, 1859; R. S. Richards, "A Consideration of the Nature of the English Sweating Sickness," *Medical History* 9 (October 1965): 385–388; M. B. Shaw, "A Short History of the Sweating Sickness,"*Annals of Medical History* 5 (May 1933): 246–274; M. B. Strauss, "A Hypothesis as to the Mechanism of Fulminant Course and Death in the Sweating Sickness," *Journal of the History of Medicine* 28 (January 1973): 48–51; John A. H. Wylie and Leslie H. Collier, "The English Sweating Sickness *(Sudor Anglicus)*: A Reappraisal," *Journal of the History of Medicine and Allied Sciences* 36 (October 1981): 425–445.

Epidemiology

Epidemiology is a modern medical discipline which studies the occurrence of disease, infectious process, or any other abnormal physiological condition which appears in groups or communities. Epidemiological method may be applied to disease in any group, but as a medical discipline, it is concerned with human communities. Its purposes are to explain the way diseases develop, to correlate the occurrence of disease with group characteristics—age, sex, occupation, race—and with environmental factors, and to establish those relationships over time. Ultimately, epidemiology is concerned with disease causation and the factors which may predispose a population to a particular condition, and therefore with the means for lessening disease's effects or preventing it altogether. In this respect epidemiology is critical to the formation of effective preventive public health policies.

History Epidemiology has developed in the nineteenth and twentieth centuries, though medical classics contain speculations on disease causation, including various environmental theories. The Hippocratic writings called *Airs, Waters, Places* (*Epidemics* I and III) describe specific diseases, some of which seem identifiable, which are correlated with locations, seasons, and climates.

In the sixteenth century, Paracelsus connected fibroid phthisis with the environment in which miners worked. The great seventeenth-century English physician Thomas Sydenham used the Hippocratic idea of "constitutions" to explain the kinds of fevers which prevailed in given years. Such explorations, however, lacked both the mathematical tools and the quantitative data necessary to establish disease characteristics among groups.

The beginnings of modern epidemiology lay in population statistics and the study of mortality. This subject was first dealt with systematically in John Graunt's *Natural and Political Observations upon the Bills of Mortality* (1662), and toward the end of the seventeenth century, Edmund Halley, the noted astronomer, compiled a table of births and funerals for Breslau. Collecting statistics on population, trade, and natural resources became a matter of great importance in the eighteenth century, and one of the main tools for European statesmen. As a branch of political economy, statistics was a recognized discipline which was believed to provide the most accurate information available on society's composition, potential, and weaknesses. Population dynamics received close attention as increasingly detailed information on populations by age, occupation, sex, ethnic origin, and economic status made comparative statements on birth, death, and disease possible, and medicine used "social arithmetic" to assist in classifying diseases and to test the efficacy of treatments. Several studies on smallpox vaccination were made, including one statistically sophisticated review by Daniel Bernoulli, who also introduced the idea of a "life table," in which a population's mortality was presented with the number of smallpox deaths removed. Pierre-Charles-Alexandre Louis, the most influential nineteenth-century proponent of medical arithmetic, used statistics to explode once and for all the myth that bloodletting was therapeutically sound. Louis also laid down principles for an epidemiologically valid study of typhoid fever.

The statistical approach to disease required that diseases be viewed as specific entities, a concept which gained ground in the early nineteenth century. It required as well some method for determining the degree of randomness or chance in any given sample. Here the work on probability which Pierre Simon, the Marquis de Laplace, published in 1810 was particularly significant, though the normal curve, or the normal curve of error, was actually discovered in 1733 by Abraham de Moivre. Karl Friedrich Gauss and Adolphe Quetelet contributed refinements and applications to the use of the normal curve, but Sir Francis Galton's *Hereditary Genius* (1869) firmly established the normal curve as a scientific application of statistical methods. In the next 50 years, statistical methods were even further refined to permit more accurate and discriminating judgments, and in the twentieth century statistical analysis became an important tool for medicine in general.

Louis' influence was pervasive in early epidemiological work. His followers or students included Josef Skoda and Ignaz Semmelweis in Austria, William Farr, Francis Galton, William Budd, and John Snow in England, and Oliver Wendell Holmes, George C. Shattuck, Jr., and Edward Jarvis in the United States. French physicians were less interested in studying disease as a mass phenomenon than were either the English or the Germans. The first significant epidemiological results were recorded in Great Britain and in Germany, while epidemiological principles were given an even broader application in the environmental health movement.

The battle over contagion (q.v.) was at its height in England during the outbreaks of typhoid and cholera (qq.v.) before the middle of the nineteenth century. The weight of both medical and popular opinion was anticontagionist, and the prevailing view indicted bad water and unhealthy living conditions for generating a miasma or creating an epidemic environment. Contagionists and anticontagionists alike, however, suspected the public water supply of being a source of disease, and William Budd, who accepted Louis' doctrine that typhoid was contagious, made the argument that typhoid's "infective principle" was probably waterborne. Budd made the same arguments in 1849 concerning cholera. Dr. John Sutherland of Manchester held similar views, proposing pure water as the best answer to epidemic cholera. It was John Snow, however, originally an anticontagionist, who demonstrated that cholera was waterborne by comparing cholera incidence between customers of two London water companies who drew their water from different sources. Snow's further investigation of the Broad Street pump as the source for a particularly virulent cholera outbreak is an epidemiological classic, though it was not recognized as such when it was published in 1854.

The work which John Snow and William Budd did was field epidemiology. This type of work remains basic to the discipline. Historical epidemiology appeared at the same time. In this area, the intent is to identify disease outbreaks, locate them geographically, and, by correlating their appearance with climate and season, topography, soil types, and culture, arrive at an explanation for the disease and its epidemic occurrence. Historical reviews of epidemic disease go back at least to John Caius's account of the English sweating sickness (q.v.) in the sixteenth century, but the first systematic historical epidemiologist was the German scholar Justus Friedrich Karl Hecker, who wrote essays on the black death (1832), the dancing mania (1832), and the English sweats (1834). An English edition appeared in 1846 as *The Epidemics of the Middle Ages*. Heinrich Haeser compiled information on epidemic diseases in history, which he first published in a history of medicine in 1845. In the third edition of that work, which appeared in 1882, an entire volume was given over to the history of epidemic diseases. Monumental though Haeser's work was, it was less comprehensive than August Hirsch's *Handbook of Historical and Geographical Pathology*, the first volume of which appeared in German in 1859. An enlarged second edition was published in 1870 which was translated into English by Charles Creighton. This extraordinary work of scholarship deals with both epidemic and nonepidemic diseases throughout the entire world. Written just before the establishment of the germ theory of disease, it presents a broad environmental approach while using some basic epidemiological principles.

Bacteriology and the germ theory of disease have reduced the medical significance of historical epidemiology. Recent historical studies on epidemic diseases use current medical knowledge to correct historical misconceptions concerning how, where, and why epidemic diseases spread. Disease has come to be viewed as an integral and important aspect of human history, but the nineteenth-century conviction that historical epidemiology would contribute significantly to the understanding of disease has largely disappeared.

Modern Epidemiology The discovery that microorganisms caused infectious diseases sharpened diagnoses and refined the problem of how diseases spread. The life cycle of bacteria, the connections between causal organisms and their victims, the role of vectors, and the factors which influenced virulence as well as morbidity became elements in epidemiological analysis. Latency and carriers added to the complications, and while Theobald Smith epitomized infectious disease as part of a system of parasitism, laboratory methods which permitted the study of that phenomenon were in preparation. Laboratory epidemiology involved the study of infectious diseases in controlled groups of animals. Mice proved particularly adaptable. Tests run during the 1940s found, for example, that increased virulence had little or nothing to do with mutations of the infective organism but had a great deal to do with crowding and the influx of suceptibles, that is, animals with no previous exposures and immunities, into the population. Disease outbreaks died down as the number of immune survivors increased, but it was also noted that dispersal of the affected population into small cage units was helpful as well. Though hardly making a case for quarantines, such laboratory studies demonstrated the wisdom of flight, the dangers of close sequestration, the threat inherent in crowded living conditions, and the necessity for regular monitoring. Laboratory epidemiology offers a means for testing hypotheses concerning disease which it would be inconvenient or dangerous to set up in the field. In turn, the principles discovered can be tested in actual disease conditions.

Epidemiology is commonly connected with infectious disease, but in recent years it has won some of its most dramatic victories over noninfectious diseases. Epidemiological method has been applied to deficiency diseases, cardiac and circulatory problems, cancer, mental illness, alcoholism, and drug addiction. The conviction, for example, that cigarette smoking is dangerous rests on an enormous body of data correlating cigarette consumption with cancer and other pathological conditions. Science cannot explain the mechanism at work, any more than John Snow and his contemporaries could explain the causal mechanisms in cholera, but the data indicting the Bond Street pump and the cigarette are equally clear. Similarly successful studies have been made on respiratory problems and heart conditions, while environmental pollutants which are dangerous to health from chemical wastes, industrial effluvia, and automobile emissions to high noise levels have been identified.

Epidemiological studies are of major importance all around the world as public health departments and the World Health Organization look into the causes and consequences of disease. Beginning as a discipline which explained epidemic crises, epidemiology has become a method for studying disease wherever and under whatever circumstances it may appear. Periods of quiescence are as significant as the times of maximum virulence, and the epidemiology of noninfectious diseases underlines the critical importance of viewing disease in its environment while identifying the degree to which environmental differences may affect any condition's incidence. In this respect, epidemiology is a beginning point for public health planning and the basis for implementing strategies to control or eliminate health problems. Important though it is, however, and sophisticated as its methods have become, epidemiology remains essentially the application of quantitative and comparative techniques to determine the character of man's diseases.

ADDITIONAL READINGS: W. H. Frost, "Some Conceptions of Epidemics in General," *American Journal of Epidemiology* 103 (February 1976): 141–151; Major Greenwood, *Epidemics and Crowd Diseases: an Introduction to the Study of Epidemiology*, London, 1935; A. M. Lilienfeld, "Epidemiology of Infectious and Noninfectious Disease: Some Comparisons," *American Journal of Epidemiology* 97 (March 1973): 135–147; A. M. Lilienfeld, *Foundations of Epidemiology*, New York 1976; A. M. Lilienfeld (ed.), *Times, Places, and Persons: Aspects of the History of Epidemiology*, Baltimore, 1980; D. E. and A. M. Lilienfeld, "Epidemiology: a Retrospective Study," *American Journal of Epidemiology* 106 (December 1977): 445–449; George Rosen, *A History of Public Health*, New York, 1958; Charles Edward Amory Winslow, *The Conquest of Epidemic Disease: A Chapter in the History of Ideas*, Princeton, 1943, Madison, Wisc., 1980 (reprint); T. H. Work, *Tracing the Patterns of Disease: The Role of Epidemiology and Biometry*, Bethesda, Md., 1977.

See also CONTAGION; PUBLIC HEALTH; and specific disease articles.

Epilepsy

The history of epilepsy is a dramatic instance of the modern change in western attitudes toward disease and the evolution of a rational, empirical way of thinking about illness. Until the modern period, conceptions of epilepsy, and the treatments afforded it, existed in a state of tension between the acceptance of supernatural, magical, or religious forces and a rational weighing and classification of symptoms and behavior. This was not so much a confrontation of opposites as a succession of syntheses in which the empirical, the supernatural, and the rational combined in differing proportions. All this changed in the second half of the nineteenth century, when neurology (q.v.) provided a basic scientific context within which to study epilepsy as a medical phenomenon. From that time on, effective methods for diagnosing and treating epileptic conditions arose out of and contributed to basic research on brain functions.

The Condition Epilepsy is now understood to be a condition resulting from the dysfunction of cerebral nerve cells manifested in sudden and repeated mental disturbances, alterations in the state of consciousness, disordered sensory activity, or convulsive physical movements. Generalized convulsions, loss of consciousness, falling down, shaking limbs, and spontaneous evacuations of bowels and bladder are characteristics of grand mal epilepsy. A second type, petit mal, involves momentary lapses in awareness, while focal seizures produce localized movements or sensations in particular parts of the body. Epileptic attacks also may include bizarre or uncoordinated automatic behavior, nightmare memories, illusions or hallucinations, and unexpected mood changes.

Epilepsy is a complex of symptoms rather than a specific disease, and its causes may include anything which produces excessive or exaggerated action in the brain cells. In some instances, lesions resulting from head injuries or other external causes correlate with the onset of epilepsy, but epileptic seizures also occur when there is no apparent pathological evidence. Epilepsy brings about changes in brain wave patterns. Therefore, electroencephalograms (EEGs) have proved to be invaluable for diagnosing epilepsy and for locating the areas in the brain which generate seizures.

Though not a common disease, epilepsy has been present in all cultures. Where statistics are maintained, the modern incidence approximates 0.5 percent of the population, with men somewhat more likely to be affected than women, and with 70 percent of cases arising before the age of 20. Though damage which may produce attacks is irreversible, modern physicians tend to be optimistic about the prognosis for epileptic patients. Some children outgrow the condition, and medication can reduce the number and the frequency of attacks. In some cases surgery can eliminate the condition entirely or significantly weaken its effects. Yet the disease poses serious problems of care and training. Though it is not degenerative, severe epileptic seizures may make normal living impossible, and massive medication can reduce both motivation and capacity to learn. For the worst-afflicted, therefore, epilepsy can be seriously incapacitating and can require institutional care. Modern treatment has reduced this problem to a minimum, and the majority of epileptics live within society.

Early History There is no definitive way to judge epilepsy's incidence in prehistoric times, though there are interesting remains which show primitive efforts to deal with problems of brain dysfunction. Stone age cave paintings suggest that primitive peoples knew about convulsive seizures and tried to cure them by trephining skulls, presumably to permit the malign influences causing the convulsions to escape. Of course, the extensive physical evidence of trephining does not suggest the extent of epilepsy alone since the operation served a variety of purposes.

The earliest written evidence concerning convulsive seizures which might be epileptic connected the condition with supernatural forces. An Akkadian medical text (ca. 2000 B.C.) describes a convulsive attack in terms which suggest epilepsy while identifying the onset of the condition with demonic powers and reporting on the exorcism of the cause. The Greek tradition identified convulsive seizures with religious, magical, or divine causes and called epilepsy the "sacred illness." This tradition persisted until the seventeenth century, though the effort to counter it with rational explanations also began very early. One of the Hipprocratic writers in the fourth century B.C. denied that epilepsy was sacred in any sense, asserted that its seat was in the brain, and, as a humoralist, diagnosed its cause as an excess of phlegm. Another writer in the same tradition ascribed seizures to a mixture of blood and air.

Clinical observations led ancient authorities to the conclusion that epileptic seizures were different from other convulsive illness in that they produced a convulsion of the entire body as well as imparing the body's leading functions. They came to recognize three types of attack: convulsion, sleep, and convulsion followed by sleep; they were able to identify such premonitory symptoms as stupor, dizziness, or slurred speech; and they distinguished them from such symptoms of an attack's onset as visual hallucinations, ringing in the ears, bad odors, or a creeping sensation in the extremities moving toward the head. They also recognized the epileptic scream as well as the danger of tongue biting and suffocation during an attack.

If Greek medicine was effective in describing and classifying convulsive seizures, the remedies proposed showed the coexistence of magical or religious explanations for disease, with conclusions drawn from a rational medical philosophy. Recent authority identifies 45 different remedies for epilepsy from Greco-Roman practice, most of which are strongly marked by magical influences. Human blood, livers, bones, or ground and powdered skulls (preferably unburied) were among the specifics recommended, and Pliny the Elder reported in the first century A.D. that gladiator's fresh-spilled blood applied to an epileptic's lips was thought to be particularly efficacious.

Epilepsy in the Middle Ages and Renaissance. Galen's second-century synthesis of classical medicine revived the Hippocratic view of epilepsy and proposed humoral treatments, including bleeding. Over the next 1500 years, the Galenic system in one form or another combined with a strong element of religion and the supernatural to shape approaches to epilepsy, or the "falling sickness," as medieval Europe knew it. Epilepsy was commonly ascribed to demonic possession, and a number of saints were called upon to cleanse the sufferers. Epileptics were shunned and feared, as they had been in the classical world, and there was a strong conviction that it was possible to be infected by observing or having contact with an epileptic. Treatments showed a combination of folk cures, classical medicine, and sorcery. John of Gaddesden, in the fourteenth century, for example, recommended reading the Gospel over an epileptic patient as well as decking him with amulets of peony, chrysanthemum, or the hair of an all-white dog. His contemporary, Arnold of Villanova, favored Galenic bleedings and dietary regimens, while Jean Fernel, a sixteenth-century Parisian physician responsible for what has been called the first original work in physiology since Galen, recommended a mixture of mistletoe, powdered human skull, and male peony seeds or roots gathered by the light of the waning moon.

As the shift away from Galen and toward empirical observation developed, new schools of medical interpretation grew up, each of which explained epilepsy according to its particular chemical, mechanical, or vitalist orthodoxy. They contributed no more to understanding the disease than Galen or the medievalists. One exception, a man who was well in advance of his time, was Jan Marek (Johannas Marcu Marci, 1595–1667), rector of Prague's Charles University. Jan Marek rejected humoralist and mechanistic theories to call attention to the role of external stimuli in bringing on attacks and to define "absences" or losses of awareness. Marek's work is the bridge between traditional approaches to epilepsy and the modern view.

Modern Approaches The nineteenth century produced a transformation in thinking about the brain and neural system. Studies of epileptics contributed to that revolution, and a better understanding of epilepsy followed. Early in the century, epileptics in both France and England began to be segregated from the insane, and in 1815, E. Esquirol, the prominent French psychiatrist, organized a special hospital for epileptics. Esquirol feared that they would infect the mentally disturbed, who might "contagiously" become epileptic. By 1860, special hospitals had been founded in France, Britain, and Germany, and in 1891, the first hospital exclusively for epileptics in the United States was established in Gallipolis, Ohio. Segregation meant greater concentration on epilepsy, and substantially more clinical data became available. Esquirol himself produced an improved description of petit mal, L. F. Calmeil described "absence," distinguishing between passing mental confusion and the onset of a grand mal attack, and W. R. Gowers clarified the "aura." Efforts to establish a pathology for epilepsy were less successful, though a beginning was made when K. F. Burdach identified nearly 2000 postmortem brain abnormalities, with 476 coming from the epileptic population. W. J. West, whose infant son suffered the condition, described the so-called salaam convulsions. There was a therapeutic step forward in 1857 when Sir Charles Locock reported on the successful use of bromides for reducing the frequency of attacks.

At mid-century, Charles Edward Brown-Séquard initiated a period of intensive research on epilepsy which, though it produced no definitive discoveries, heightened interest in the condition. Brown-Séquard recruited John Hughlings Jackson, who became one of the leading neurologists in Europe and the man who put the study of epilepsy on its modern footing. It was Jackson who broke with the conventional wisdom that cortical functions were undifferentiated, identifying local symptoms with specific foci in the brain. This work interacted with that of Paul Broca and Carl Wernicke on aphasia, which precisely located speech function in the cortex. Jackson also defined the epileptic neuron, that is, nerve cells giving excessive discharges which brought on convulsions. Localization of function was a concept which opened the way to brain mapping for surgical purposes. This was followed up by Gustav Fritsch and Edward Hitzig in 1870, and in 1876 by David Ferrier, who used electrical stimulus to identify particular brain control points for physical functions. With these methods, a brain tumor was diagnosed and removed in 1884, after which V. A. H. Horsley used the same techniques for operating on focal epilepsy.

A further and more important therapeutic step was taken in 1912, when phenobarbital, which began life as an anesthetic, was found to be effective in suppressing epileptic seizures. It remains, as one authority wrote in 1970, "the most widely used, the cheapest, and the most potent of the antiepileptics." It is supplemented by diphenylhydantoin (Dilantin), which was first found in 1908 but was put to use for epilepsy in 1938, trimethadione (1946), and primidone. Preventing seizures or controlling their frequency is the most effective method available for dealing with epilepsy, and between 1912 and 1974, 18 different compounds were introduced for that purpose. The development of effective medication paralleled further progress in surgical techniques, especially the improvement in diagnostic insight provided by the electroencephalogram (EEG), which Johannes Berger developed between 1929 and 1938. Wilder Penfield of Montreal and Hubert H. Jasper have become the leading authorities on surgical treatment for epilepsy since World War II.

Although epilepsy continues to be a serious problem, medicine has made substantial progress with it. Its clinical symptoms have been systematized, its location identified, its nature clarified, and with effective medication and occasional surgery, its effects can be brought within bounds. Most epileptics are able to function adequately in society. The ancient stigmas which attached to epilepsy are fading, though the problems of helping epileptics to adapt to society remain severe. Epilepsy is now a medical issue which can be approached directly without diminishing the dignity or threatening the life of the person suffering from it.

ADDITIONAL READINGS: James L. O'Leary and Sidney Godring, *Science and Epilepsy: Neuroscience Gains in Epilepsy Research*, New York, 1976; Owsei Temkin, *The Falling Sickness: A History of Epilepsy from the Greeks to the Beginnings of Modern Neurology*, 2d rev. ed., Baltimore and London, 1971.

See also NEUROLOGY.

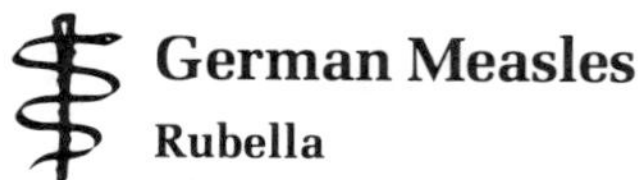

German Measles

Rubella

German measles, or rubella, is a mild eruptive disease of childhood whose cause is a filterable virus. The disease is of indeterminate antiquity, though the first description of it as a disease entity came in the seventeenth century. In 1619, a German physician, Daniel Sennert, identified "röteln" as a variation of morbilli or measles (q.v.); but while similar in that it began with fever and coughing and produced a rash, it appeared to be less dangerous. The name, "röteln," or "rubella," was a colloquial expression which described the red color of the slightly elevated papular eruptions which attended it, which helped to distinguish it from a true measles. It was also differentiated from scarlet fever.

Though rubella was recognized in the seventeenth century, it was not systematically separated from measles until the nineteenth century, when David Hosack observed it in epidemic form in New York in 1813 and dubbed it "rubeola sine catarrho" ("measles without catarrh"). "Rubeola" and "rubella" were the common designations for this disease in the nineteenth century, though in the English literature "German measles" began to be used in the second half of the century in recognition of the interest and effort German medical science had given to the disease. The so-called Koplik spots, which appear only in the mouths of measles patients, were identified in 1896 by Henry Koplik, an American physician, and provided a clear diagnostic test for measles. They also provided a basis for differential diagnosis between measles and rubella. In 1938, two Japanese physicians, Y. Hiro and S. Tanaka, successfully transferred the disease to children by inoculation. It has also been transferred to rhesus monkeys (1942).

German measles had a worldwide distribution and reached epidemic extent on occasion. But it was not considered a dangerous disease and so did not attract much attention until 1941, when N. McAlister Gregg, an Australian ophthalmologist, showed a correlation between children born with congenital defects and mothers who had rubella during their pregnancies, especially in the early months. Subsequent studies in the United States, Great Britain, and Australia have confirmed Gregg's hypothesis, and in at least one instance, epidemic incidence of deafness in children has been correlated with rubella outbreaks. The most common rubella-induced birth defects include deaf-mutism, cataracts, heart malfunction, and microcephaly.

Until recently, relatively little was known concerning the rubella virus. Since 1969, however, acceptable vaccines have been established and vaccination programs instituted. Selective immunization of school-age girls has become the accepted approach, with the goal of controlled exposure to rubella before the childbearing age. Because rubella contracted during pregnancy is almost certain to affect the fetus, though the effects may not appear for some years after birth, termination of the pregnancy is a recognized and accepted option.

ADDITIONAL READINGS: Kenneth J. Hammond et al., "Rubella Immunization," *Journal of the American Medical Association* 235 (1976): 2201–2204; George Rosen, "Acute Communicable Diseases: German Measles," in Walter Bett (ed.), *The History and Conquest of Common Diseases*, Norman, Okla., 1954, 45–47.

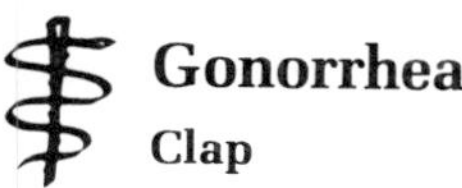

Gonorrhea

Clap

Gonorrhea is the oldest and most common of the venereal diseases. Its causal agent is a gram-negative diplococcus, *Neisseria gonorrhoeae*. The gonococcus is related to meningococcus, with which it may well have shared areas in the nose, throat, and genitourinary tract. At some point the gonococcus invaded the tissues of the genitourinary tract, producing a disease specific to the urethra whose symptoms included a burning sensation during urination and purulent discharges. These symptoms, which led the French to call gonorrhea "chaude pisse" ("hot piss"), could appear 36 hours to five days after exposure to an infected person. In males gonorrhea is self-limiting, and if the infection remains in the front of the urethra, it tends to subside in four to six days. If the back of the urethra becomes infected, the disease may also affect the tubes which carry sperm from the testicles (epididymis). In the case of such infection, the disease may remain active for months, with sterility a possible consequence.

Ninety percent of the women who contract gonorrhea show no symptoms of the disease, or only transient ones, and therefore act as unknowing reservoirs and carriers. Women appear to be at least three times more susceptible than men. There are some special problems for women with gonorrhea. When the infection is serious, it moves into the cervix or fallopian tubes, where it may persist for a long time. In both men and women, when the gonococci overwhelm local defenses, they enter the bloodstream and can attack joints, eyes, or the endocardium. Children born to mothers with gonorrhea often contract the disease in their eyes and can lose their sight, though washing the eyes of the new born with silver nitrate helps eliminate this danger. Since infection does not confer immunity, individuals who recover from one attack are subject to reinfection on exposure. James Boswell, Dr. Samuel Johnson's biographer, reported 19 episodes of urethritis in his journals, about a dozen of which appear to have been fresh gonorrheal infections. In general, though gonorrhea can have serious consequences, its most common effect is interference with sexual functions and urination, thus contributing to discomfort and inconvenience.

The gonococcus has been well adapted to its human host for thousands of years, and gonorrhea can be recognized in the earliest Egyptian, Chinese, Japanese, and vedic sources. One ancient Chinese manuscript refers to a disease which is "different from all others," whose symptoms include infection of the urethra and vagina at the same time as the bladder and "the drainage of corrupt materials white or red by the urethra or vagina." An Assyrian tablet speaks of thick or cloudy urine, and the Hippocratic writers at the end of the fifth century B.C. refer to "strangary," that is, the blockage of the urethra. In the second century A.D., Galen was familiar with gonorrhea and is credited with naming it. (The term refers to a flow of seed.) Biblical references suggest that Hebrew medicine knew and feared gonorrhea. Chapters 12 and 15 of the Book of Leviticus recommend washing after copulation and refer to an "unclean discharge from the body"; the word "issue" recurs as a term designating gonorrhea; and Moses warned against "carnal knowledge of strange women," for, as it was argued in Proverbs, strange women should be avoided lest flesh and body be consumed.

The medieval world was also concerned about gonorrhea. A decree in 1162 by the bishop of Winchester directed that "no stewholder keep no woman within his house that hath any sickness of brenning [burning]." In the fourteenth century, Henri de Mondeville and John of Arderne provided the first detailed diagnostic picture of gonorrhea which stressed "chaude pisse."

Until 1493, gonorrhea and soft chancre were the dominant venereal diseases in Europe, and gonorrhea was readily recognized. After the great syphilis (q.v.) epidemic began in the last decade of the fifteenth century, gonorrhea was regularly confused with it, and eventually gonorrhea came to be viewed as the onset stage of syphilis. As syphilis moderated, physicians had even more reason to confuse the two, and in the eighteenth century, John Hunter, the eminent Scottish surgeon who practiced in London, argued that the cause for the two diseases was the same. He believed that their different effects were conditioned by the location of the disease. In 1767, Hunter infected himself with what he thought was gonorrhea and got syphilis. The chancre which developed bears his name, and the influence of his mistaken conclusion remained strong for at least 30 years. Benjamin Bell was one of a group of medical men who resisted Hunter's dictum, and in 1793, Bell argued for separating gonorrhea from its more deadly rival. In 1838 Philippe Ricord, working at l'Hôpital du Midi in Paris, replicated Hunter's experiment and reached the correct conclusion, asserting that gonorrhea was a separate disease from syphilis. His conclusions were confirmed in 1879 when the Breslau bacteriologist Albert Neisser identified the gonococcus which causes gonorrhea. The causal agent in syphilis was found 26 years later.

Though gonorrhea is neither a killing disease nor even one that cripples extensively, it severely reduces the capacities of those who have it to function effectively in society, and its very pervasiveness, both in the past and in the present, underscores the need for control. Most ancient treatment for gonorrhea was symptomatic and palliative, seeking to reduce the evidence of infection by instillations, irrigations, antiseptic lotions, and herbal concoctions. In the nineteenth century, sandalwood oil was a highly regarded therapeutic agent that was not displaced until potassium permanganate was introduced in 1892. At base, however, the disease was thought to be self-limiting. There was no effective cure for gonorrhea until 1937, when sulfonamides became available, and it was discovered that sulfanilimide killed gonococcal infection and could dispose of a case of gonorrhea in just five days. The new cure was short-lived, however, for sulfa-resistant strains of gonococci began to appear. Penicillin was then introduced, but it has become increasingly apparent that the gonococcus has developed resistance to penicillin as well. The problem is serious. One recent authority concluded that up to 40 percent of the prostitutes active in the Philippines carry penicillin-resistant strains of gonorrhea. This factor, which threatens to leave society without effective treatment and hence control, is undoubtedly influential in the sudden upsurge in reported cases of gonorrhea in recent years.

Though modern statistics on the incidence of gonorrhea are not reliable, it is apparent that the disease has been increasing rapidly worldwide. The 0.5 million cases which the United States reported in the early 1970s could, by conservative estimate, have been nearly 2 million, and the correct figure may have been closer to 5 million. Increased sexual activity at a younger age, nonbarrier forms of contraception (most notably the birth control pill), and less effective public health administration contribute as well. Modern control policies rely on identification and treatment to extirpate infection, but resistance to sulfa and penicillin leaves the system weak at its center. Just as gonorrhea is one of the oldest and most pervasive diseases in human history, so it has become the most extensively reported disease in the contemporary world, and its future control is becoming a matter of pressing concern.

ADDITIONAL READINGS: H. F. Dowling, *Fighting Infection*, Cambridge, Mass., 1977; Theodore Rosebury, *Microbes and Morals: The Strange Story of Venereal Disease*, London, 1972.

Gout

Gout is a metabolic disease resulting in an excessive concentration of uric acid in the blood from improperly metabolized protein. It produces swollen and painful joints, especially in the feet and great toe. Gout accompanies recurrent attacks of acute arthritis and uric acid stones in the kidneys. Since heavy meat eaters have been particularly prone to gout, the disease has been most prevalent among the affluent. Upper-class European eating habits before the twentieth century, which combined vast quantities of sweet or fortified wines with a diet which was heavy in protein and starch, generated a high incidence of gout. Gout, painful as it was, became a symbol of success and social status. And since the predisposition is hereditary, the disease was sometimes considered one of the burdens of nobility. It was also believed that stress, whether from overwork, dissipation, or sexual overindulgence, brought on gout, an assumption which, by a curious association of ideas, tied gout even more firmly to the privileged.

Many people of historical importance were gouty. Such distinguished physicians as Thomas Sydenham and the great sixteenth-century French surgeon Ambroise Paré were gout sufferers, as was the fifteenth-century Florentine banker and humanist patron Cosimo di Medici. For such men gout was a painful inconvenience. The condition was much more than an inconvenience for the emperor Charles V, whose gout so tormented him that it contributed to his decision to abdicate in 1556; and for his son and successor, Philip II of Spain, who suffered such crippling attacks of gout that in his later years he governed from his bed. The political personalities of both men were undoubtedly affected by their suffering. The same was true of the contemporary Tudor statesman William Cecil, Lord Burghley, whose prostrating attacks regularly interfered with the performance of his duties under Henry VIII and Elizabeth I.

What was true in the sixteenth century was even more true in the eighteenth, which might be termed the golden age of gout, particularly in England. Among politicians, both the elder and the younger William Pitt were gouty, while Dr. Samuel Johnson, Benjamin Franklin, and John Wesley, the Methodist reformer, epitomized an intellectual society in which gout became a common denominator for believers and unbelievers, scientists, preachers, and writers. In the case of politicians like the Pitts, whose gout attacks can be set against political crises and decisions, the disease could take on some significance as an influence. For the rest, it was as much a part of the cultural scene as rhymed couplets, sedan chairs, and Adam ceilings.

By the middle of the nineteenth century, changes in nutritional emphases toward a balanced diet were making inroads on gout's incidence. Nevertheless, gout has remained to the present time a significant fact of life for millions of people, though it is no longer the badge of a high-living established class.

Although early medical observers confused gout with several similar afflictions, there is evidence that some authorities recognized its special character. The Hippocratic writers differentiated between acute gout (which they called *podagra*) and acute arthritis. They considered the former the "most violent of all joint affections," long lasting, chronic, and with "the pain . . . fixed in the great toes." The primary Hippocratic therapy for gout was a diet whereby "the humors may be kept in healthy balance and disease obviated." In intractable cases, heroic therapies involving purging with white hellebore were prescribed, because "the best natural relief for this disease is an attack of dysentery." Where persistent pain continued in specific joints, a counterirritant was introduced by burning the veins above the affected joint with raw flax. There were also three Hippocratic aphorisms concerning gout, all of which implicated sexual function. The connection between gout and sexuality remained close, so much so that castration was proposed as one remedy for the condition.

Gout was a familiar subject in Roman medical literature, but there was very little change in point of view from the Hippocratic writings. Galen, the greatest of the Hippocratic disciples and the author who shaped the intellectual history of medicine for more than 1000 years, differed from the tradition only on matters of detail, particularly in recommending more violent purgatives and the extensive use of bleeding. Galen held closely to the Hippocratic dietary recommendations.

The post-Galen era added one new item to the armory of weapons against gout: the use of colchicum (hermodactyl) as a purgative. Though known by the ancient Greeks, this extract from the corm of a crocuslike plant which grew near ancient Colchis in Asia Minor brought positive relief to gout sufferers. Earlier writers considered it a poison, but Alexander of Trolles saw its properties for dealing with a certain kind of "arthritis." It became a favored specific until the end of the seventeenth century when Thomas Sydenham criticized its use and sent it into obscurity again.

The Hippocratic authors had believed that gout arose from a disordering of the humors, and their view obtained essentially unchanged until the nineteenth century. But there were some skeptics. In the sixteenth century, for example, Paracelsus, one of the most imaginative of the early modern medical writers, postulated a chemical cause for gout—but his arguments remained in a traditional humoral frame. Indeed, the word, gout was derived from the Latin *gutta* ("drop") and referred to the idea that the disease resulted from an excess of one of the four humors settling in a previously weakened or damaged joint. Throughout the classical and medieval worlds, the tendency was to lump gout and rheumatism together. It was not until 1642 that Guillaume de Baillou (Ballonius) once more distinguished the two clinically; and Thomas Sydenham made the distinction definitive.

Apart from good advice on diet, medieval medicine offered little to the growing number of gout sufferers but remedies which competed with one another in grotesquerie and sometimes danger. A particularly dismaying instance was a sixteenth-century prescription for a roast goose stuffed with, among other things, chopped kittens. Basic treatment, as a recent authority has pointed out, was still the same in the eighteenth century as that employed in Greek and Roman times. One major development, as important for social as for medical history, was the rise of hydrotherapy, in which sufferers bathed in mineral waters and drank the waters for a natural purge. Such watering places as Bath in England and Baden-Baden in Germany became centers for a rich society intent on improving its health and quieting the pains of gout.

Medical science was able to do relatively little with gout until late in the nineteenth century. Sir Charles Scuddamore studied the condition clinically, to find means for its relief. In 1848, Alfred Garrod identified uric acid as "the specific morbid humour which inflames all joints in which it enters" and devised a simple bedside test for excess uric acid. In 1859, Garrod established the difference between rheumatoid arthritis and gout. Professor Emil Fischer of Berlin and J. J. Berzelius of Sweden worked on the structure and synthesis of purine protein, a critical step in grasping the processes which contributed to the development of gout. Fischer's work won the Nobel prize for medicine in 1902 and marked the opening of the modern era of gout studies.

A further diagnostic breakthrough occurred in 1913 with the introduction of the colometric system for estimating uric acid levels. It was not until 1948, however, that a satisfactory modern specific for treating gout, caranamide, was found as a by-product of penicillin research. Diagnosis and treatment for gout have continued to advance during the last 30 years, but understanding of the disease and its mechanisms is still incomplete.

ADDITIONAL READINGS: W. S. C. Copeman, *A Short History of the Gout and the Rheumatic Diseases,* Berkeley and Los Angeles, 1964.

See also ARTHRITIS; RHEUMATISM.

Greco-Roman Medicine

Greek medicine, which was deeply indebted to the medical practices of western Asia and Egypt, was established in the first millennium B.C. Its influence subsequently moved westward where it dominated Roman medicine, and the resulting synthesis formed a substantial part of the medical inheritance of medieval and early modern Europe. Modern scientific medicine has taken over the Greek tradition as an ideal appropriate to its own values and claims Hippocrates, the best-known physician of the classical age, as its symbol and moral inspiration.

Though it is imperfectly documented, more is known about Greco-Roman medicine than about any other ancient medical tradition. For the period before the sixth century B.C., the main sources are the literary tradition, especially the Homeric cycle, mythology, religion, and archaeology. The best evidence for Greek medicine's golden age, the period from the sixth through the fourth centuries B.C., is found in the compendious Hippocratic writings, while knowledge about subsequent developments, including the Alexandrian school, owes primarily to Galen of Pergamum, writing in the second century A.D.

Beliefs and Practices Ancient Greek medicine was rooted in religion. The Greek tradition abounded in gods and heroes who were identified with health and curing disease. The most important of these was Asclepius (Aesculapius in the Roman tradition), the offspring of Apollo, the god of medicine, and Coronis. According to legend, Coronis exposed Asclepius on a mountainside, where he was rescued and nurtured by a goat and a herd dog until the shepherd recognized his divine attributes. Asclepius was thought to cure diseases and to have the power to raise the dead. A different tradition appears in Homer, who portrays Asclepius as a mortal, a tribal chief who was also a skilled healer of wounds. His sons, whom he trained, were called Asclepiads and physicians. Asclepius became an important medical cult figure who embodied the qualities of Homer's blameless physician and who became the physicians' patron. His temples were found throughout the Mediterranean, and medical communities formed around them. The best known were at Epidaurus and at Cos, but at least 200 other sites have been found.

Along with Apollo and Asclepius, there was Hephaestus, the god of fire, who was believed to confer medicinal qualities on the earth where he fell. Hera and Eleithyia were patronesses of matrimony and childbirth, while Athena's wisdom also extended to healing. Castor and Pollux, the twin sons of Zeus and Leda, were considered healers. Introduced late, they carried over into the Christian era as saints Cosmos and Damian, the patron saints of physicians and pharmacists.

Ancient Greek medicine began as a skill but evolved as a trade with some of the trappings of a learned profession. According to the Homeric legends, warrior-heroes cared for each other's wounds, and some were noted for their healing skills. Women also nursed the sick and the wounded. The practice of medicine prior to the sixth century B.C. appears to have been a mixture of common-sense treatments and fanciful ideas. There were no medical books. Greek physicians were itinerant craftsmen, and the medical tradition was oral.

In the course of the sixth century B.C., a rational approach to medicine appeared which combined observation, reasoning, and philosophical assumptions. Special centers for study and treatment developed which became known for their contributions to medical knowledge. The most important were in the eastern Aegean and on the coast of Asia Minor, for Greek medicine, like philosophy and science, was born in the Ionian colonies where the cultures of Greece and the orient met. These medical communities were free associations of physicians and teachers, students and apprentices. Among the best known were those at Cyrene, Cos, Cnidus, and Croton in Italy. The school at Croton was Pythagorean, an aristocratic religious order which was both mystical and scientific. Cos was the seat of Hippocratic medicine, while Cnidus was a rival.

The school of Cos and the Hippocratic tradition represent the core of classical Greek medicine, and the *Corpus Hippocraticum,* the so-called Hippocratic writings, provide the substance of that tradition. These writings, compiled into some 60 books, were not only the work of many authors but were set down at different times and reflect different medical emphases. Several of the major Greek medical communities are represented. The famed Hippocratic oath, for example, has been identified as Pythagorean; there are Sicilian and Cnidian as well as Coan doctrines; and the concept of breath, the one idea closely associated with the historic Hippocrates, is only mentioned.

Hippocrates of Cos was a historical figure who is mentioned in Plato's *Protagoras* and whose approach to medicine is discussed in the *Phaedrus.* It is doubtful, however, that he occupied the dominant position in Greek medicine in his own time that tradition has ascribed to him. Hippocrates appears to be the most senior of three well-known physicians, Praxagoras and Chrysippus being the other two, who developed the dietetic system introduced by Herodicus. It is speculated that, because he was the senior physician, it was Hippocrates's name which stood first in compilations of this medical system. When the later Alexandrian physicians attempted to separate his work from that of his colleagues, more and more titles were ascribed to him. Thus his name became better known than any other individual physician's, and as the Romans honored the fifth century B.C. as the golden age of Greece, so they came to accept Hippocrates as the medical hero of that age. Hippocrates's reputation grew further as first Galen and then Avicenna systematized the Hippocratic writings into a full-blown medical philosophy. Hippocrates became a hero, the possessor of all medical virtues, and the ideal physician: devoted to his patients, kind, pure, patriotic, and skillful. In the modern period he has been invoked as the patron of clinical medicine (q.v.), and, less justifiably, as the founder of scientific medicine.

The Hippocratic collection reveals a radical practice based on naturalistic rather than religious explanations. Thus *On the Sacred Disease,* a book dealing with epilepsy (q.v.), develops the argument that despite its name, the sacred disease is a consequence of natural causes, not the gods' intervention, and that this is true of disease in general. The theory of the humors (q.v.), which was derived from contemporary cosmological speculations, provided an interpretive framework for explaining why diseases attacked and what could be done about them. Particular diseases were given detailed descriptions, an attempt was made to connect diseases with seasons of the year, and in *Airs, Waters, Places,* the Hippocratic writers produced the first classic of medical geography. Similarly, the *Epidemics* contains carefully observed case records which the authors seek to correlate with weather conditions and other environmental factors. Though weak on anatomy and employing all-encompassing philosophical explanations in place of an experimental physiology, the Hippocratic writings reveal wide experience of diseases and a naturalistic approach to their causes and cures.

The theory of humoralism led Greek medicine to stress diet and the prevention of disease rather than its cure. The physician's purpose was to aid nature in reestablishing a patient's health. Surgery, which was used primarily to repair damage rather than to correct imbalances, was not emphasized, but purging and bleeding were considered useful in restoring harmony and balance among the humors. Apart from the Asclepian temples and the physicians' shops (*iatreia*), there were no hospitals, but communities employed a physician to minister without charge to those who needed his services. People who could afford their own physician paid at the outset of the treatment. There was no regulation of fees, though the Hippocratic writings warned against overcharging. It is virtually impossible to judge the health and well-being of golden age Greek cities, but all the evidence indicates a persistent concern for health, and a major effort to accumulate information concerning disease causes, prognoses, and cures.

In the fourth and third centuries B.C., new schools of medical thought took shape which built on the classic traditions, and in 331 B.C. a major center for medical study, research, and teaching was founded at Alexandria in Egypt. Knowledge of these developments rests on works written in the first and second centuries A.D. which include Pliny's *Natural History,* the medical compilations of the encyclopedist Aurelius Cornelius Celsus, and the collections made by Soranus and Rufus of Ephesus, Aretaeus of Cappadocia, and Galen of Pergamum.

Practically speaking, post-Hippocratic medicine added little to what was already known about disease and its treatment. Ideas were elaborated upon, and the schools of medical thought grew increasingly dogmatic and exclusive. At Alexandria, the most important medical center in the Mediterranean until its destruction in the second century A.D., Greek medical and scientific philosophies from Hippocrates and Aristotle through Democritus were represented, and some new work developed as well. In the fourth century B.C., Herophilus and Erasistratus began anatomical experimentation, with the latter beginning to study physiological questions. A new empirical school was established at the end of the third century by Philinus of Cos and Serapion of Alexandria. This school believed in an exclusively experimental method, with all general propositions to be derived from experience. So radical a break with the traditional approach was unable to stand for long, and a partial reconciliation with theoretical concepts followed. The resulting synthesis, which included a strong Hippocratic strain, reemphasized the importance of observation and proved a major component in training many of late antiquity's leading physicians.

Two other schools developed after the Alexandrian empiricists and in part were a reaction against them. These were the Methodics, or Methodists, founded by Themison of Laodicea in the second half of the first century B.C., and the so-called pneumatic school created in the first century A.D. by Athenaeus of Attalia. The Methodics, strongly philosophical in outlook, viewed disease as a disarrangement of atoms in the body, and their practice involved manipulating the body by exercise, massage, or bathing to restore order. Their theories were never well-developed, and some Methodics ended by denying medicine entirely and concentrating on the techniques themselves. Others slipped back to a kind of simple empiricism.

The pneumatic school stressed breath (*pneuma*) as the stabilizing influence in the human system. This doctrine, which followed the ideas of Stoic and dogmatic philosophy, also had a long and respectable tradition in Greek thought. One of Athenaeus's pupils, Agathinos of Sparta, moved from pneumatism to an eclectic or episynthetic approach which picked and chose among the various doctrines and practices available. It was essentially this version of medicine which Galen practiced.

Galen of Pergamum was born about A.D. 129, studied at Smyrna, Corinth, and Alexandria, and at the age of 28 returned to Pergamum, where his practice included dietetics and surgery. He acted as physician to a gladiatorial school. He went to Rome in A.D. 161 and 162, where he won fame as a physician and a teacher. He was away from Rome during the Antonine plague and was summoned by the emperor, Marcus Aurelius, to serve the army. He became Commodus's personal physician. Until his final departure in A.D. 193, Galen devoted himself to scholarship, anatomical studies, and medical practice. He wrote voluminously, producing more than 500 works covering philosophical, rhetorical, and philological subjects in addition to the entire range of medical disciplines. His main work on therapy, the *Ars Magna,* became the bible for medical practice for centuries.

Galen's work formed a vast and complicated whole, a system of medical thought resting on general postulates which particular evidence demonstrated or fulfilled. Philosophically, Galen followed Aristotle, though elements from both Plato and the Stoics were also present; the medical tradition he most vigorously espoused was that of Hippocrates, which he reinterpreted to fit his own conceptions. Galen was a polemical writer whose violent diatribes reconstructed his opponents' arguments in order to demolish them. These essays in scientific abuse are extremely valuable to historians, because in many areas his reconstructions of these opponents' works are their only remaining traces.

Galen himself was a brilliant scholar and scientist who excelled in comparative anatomy and whose physiology was entirely adequate for the system he proposed. His anatomical studies were done with animals, particularly apes, rather than with human subjects, and this accounted for some of the variations in his findings with those of the Alexandrians, who dissected humans. His most important weakness, however, was his philosophical approach, particularly the teleology he took over from Aristotle, which tended to determine what his researches would discover.

Galen approached disease in terms of a complex physiology which was basically humoral and called for maintaining a balance in the system among elements, humors, and qualities. *Pneuma* ("breath," or "air") was critical in his system, environmental influences were considered important, but the very center of it was digestion and nutrition. As the system was a complex one, it was also closed. Everything could be explained in terms of the way the system functioned, and the system determined what treatments would be necessary. This totality of explanation was a major reason for Galen's appeal, for he made the functioning of the human organism comprehensible.

Philosophical speculation and medical treatment interacted in Galen's work. His therapeutics built exactly on his physiology. Pharmaceuticals were classified according to their affinities for humors, elements, or principles, and *theriac,* the famous panacea which he concocted, contained some 70 ingredients beyond the opium base. Given the humoral physiology, bleeding, purgatives, and diuretics were central to his methods. At base, however, and consistent with the Hippocratic tradition, Galen held that it was better to maintain health by dietetic and prophylactic measures than to try to restore health therapeutically. Ultimately, Galen's vast influence owed to his extraordinary versatility, to the consistent, systematic character of his medical philosophy, to his own moral character, and to his outspoken support of Christian values. He summarized what had gone before; he provided a stable, satisfying, and complete medical system; and his work affirmed and reinforced what was to become the dominant order of religion and authority. Until the sixteenth century, there was no viable alternative to Galen's synthesis and method.

Conclusion The main medical tradition in the Greco-Roman era stretched from the Hippocratic writings through Alexandria to Galen. The view of medicine which this tradition embodied was rational, philosophical, and naturalistic. Mystic religions abounded in the Mediterranean, but after the sixth century B.C., mysticism and medicine separated. Medical thought stressed natural, if speculative, causes, offering both explanation and specific treatments. Some explanations were simply fantastic, and most, in the light of later discoveries, were wholly or at least partially wrong. But the close observation of disease symptoms, the correlation of diseases with time, place, and season, and the identification of disease with disorder or dysfunction within the physical system revealed a developing mode of thought that pointed toward the hard tests of empirical proof. The Alexandrian anatomists, the empiricists, and Galen himself multiplied factual observations and recognized their value even though they were unable to move effectively from what they observed in particular to what they knew in general. Neither Hippocratic medicine nor Galen's system was the source for modern medicine. Entirely sufficient to the cultures which generated and used them, they had little to offer substantively to the future. What they did contribute to modern medical thought were the principles of natural explanation, rational perception, and empirical proof. The reaction to Galen has actually arisen from reapplying the rational and empirical principles which originally permitted the construction of his system.

ADDITIONAL READINGS: L. Cohn-Haft, *The Public Physicians of Ancient Greece,* Northampton, Mass., 1956; E. V. Edelstein and L. Edelstein, *Asclepius,* 2 vols., Baltimore, 1945; Werner Jäger, *Paideia: The Ideals of Greek Culture,* New York, 1944, III; W. H. S. Jones and B. T. Withington (trans.), *Hippocrates,* 4 vols., Cambridge, Mass., and London, 1923–1931, 1959–1967; Guido Majno, *The Healing Hand: Man and Wound in the Ancient World,* Cambridge, Mass., 1975, chap. 4; M. T. May, *Galen: On the Usefulness of the Parts of the Body,* 2 vols., Ithaca, N.Y., 1968; E. D. Phillips, *Greek Medicine,* London, 1973; G. G. Sarton, *A History of Science: Hellenistic Science and Culture in the Last Three Centuries B.C.,* Cambridge, Mass., 1959; J. B. de C. M. Saunders, *The Transition from Ancient Egyptian to Greek Medicine,* Lawrence, Kans., 1963; J. Scarborough, *Roman Medicine,* London, 1969; R. E. Siegel, *Galen's System of Physiology and Medicine,* Basel, 1968; Henry E. Sigerist, *History of Medicine,* 2 vols., New York, 1951, 2; Charles Singer and E. Ashworth Underwood, *A Short History of Medicine,* 2d ed., Oxford, 1962; Wesley D. Smith, *The Hippocratic Tradition,* Ithaca, N.Y., 1979; René Taton (ed.), *History of Science: Ancient and Medieval Science from the Beginnings to 1450,* A. J. Pomerans (trans.), New York, 1963, pt. II, passim; Owsei Temkin, *The Double Face of Janus,* Baltimore, 1974; Owsei Temkin, *Galenism: The Rise and Decline of a Medical Philosophy,* Ithaca, N.Y., 1973.

See also HOSPITAL; PUBLIC HEALTH.

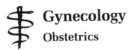

Gynecology

Obstetrics

Gynecology deals with the anatomy, physiology, pathology, therapy, and surgical repair of the female reproductive system. Problems related to pregnancy, birth, and the physical consequences of birth fall under the general heading of gynecology but have become the subject of obstetrics, itself a modern medical specialty. Traditionally, midwives advised women on questions which are now covered in obstetrics and some aspects of gynecology. Midwifery (q.v.), however, continues to be important throughout the world, and in European countries, Great Britain, and Japan, licensed midwives deal with the majority of births. The United States is a major exception to this pattern.

As a scientific medical discipline, gynecology is less than 200 years old. The subject matter, however, is as old as humankind. Female sexuality is the basis of many ancient religious rituals and customs, while women's problems are prominent in the earliest extant medical texts. Several Egyptian medical papyri touch on gynecological questions. The Kahun papyrus (ca. 2000 B.C.) is divided between female medical problems and veterinary subjects, a combination which remains puzzling, while the Ebers papyrus (ca. 1550 B.C.), the best known of the Egyptian medical papyri, includes gynecology as one of many medical subjects. The ayurvedic medical books from Hindu India date between 1200 B.C. and 500 B.C. and reveal a sophisticated medical culture. Though anatomical conceptions appear to be formalized and imaginative, the vedic writings describe a wide range of surgical procedures, including cesarean section, and there are indications that the vedic physicians studied uterine anatomy and may have identified the fallopian tubes.

The Mesopotamian civilizations lying between India and Egypt also possessed a substantial medical tradition, but almost nothing pertaining to gynecology has been preserved. The Hebrews, however, who drew heavily on Egyptian sources, particularly the teachings of the Alexandrian school in the third and second centuries, show both a very rich medical heritage and considerable gynecological knowledge. Much of their knowledge appears as references in nonmedical works, particularly the so-called Pentateuch (Genesis, Exodus, Leviticus, Numbers and Deuteronomy), and in the Talmud. The books of the Pentateuch are roughly contemporary with the early vedic writings and contain evidence on ritual practices and behavioral norms which involve sexual functions. There are references to contraception, abortion, midwifery, menstruation, virginity, and venereal diseases. The Talmud, which was set down between the second and seventh centuries A.D., is similarly informed on the cultural aspects of female sexuality, but it also contains medical information which reveals familiarity with the anatomy of female genitalia as well as recommendations for avoiding infection. The Hebrew tradition has been particularly strong in promoting hygiene and personal cleanliness.

Greek medical writings contributed relatively little to gynecology, though five books in the Hippocratic writings treat the subject and include a notable warning against puerperal fever. The Alexandrian school, which flourished in Ptolemaic Egypt in the third and second centuries B.C., practiced human dissection and apparently could have added to gynecological knowledge. Unfortunately, most of what was discovered or taught at Alexandria was lost, and even the works of the most important investigators are known only by fragmentary citation or quotation. Significantly, the two leading classical authorities on gynecology, Rufus and Soranus of Ephesus, were trained at Alexandria, and substantial fragments of Soranus's work survived in Latin and Byzantine compilations.

Soranus of Ephesus worked in Rome in the late first and early second centuries A.D. Called by some the most important figure in gynecology in the ancient world, Soranus combined scholarship with anatomical observation. He was a firm opponent of abortion, except in those cases where the mother's health was threatened; he believed that it was best to prevent conception naturally; and he prescribed numerous medications for that purpose as well as an ingenious version of coitus interruptus. He also was known to have recommended podalic version (turning the baby to bring it out feet first) in difficult deliveries. This idea surfaced again with Ambroise Paré in the middle sixteenth century. Soranus's work on obstetrics has been called the greatest prior to that of François Mauriceau in the late seventeenth century, while his summary on gynecology may well have been the most valuable contribution to the subject until Jean Astruc's book on women's diseases appeared between 1761 and 1765.

In the centuries following Soranus, gynecology gradually declined. The Byzantine and Arab systematizers recorded portions of what had been done, but there was no basis for further development as the west broke down politically and culturally. In the major medical centers of the Islamic world, gynecology withered as a result of Moslem prohibitions on male examination of female genital organs, and it remained to Jewish physicians to continue the older Alexandrian traditions. In fact, in most of Europe and throughout the Mediterranean world, gynecology all but disappeared as a discipline, and when recovery began in the fifteenth and sixteenth centuries, only fragments of the ancient knowledge could be recovered.

The knowledge of gynecology in the first century A.D. was clearly superior to what was known in 1500. In 1513, Euchärius Röslin published a small book at Worms entitled *Rosengarten.* This book, which was based on fragments of Soranus, was, as one writer put it, "the first obstetrical textbook in thirteen centuries." The book was important enough to be plagiarized in 1545, and it was then translated and published in London as the *Byrthe of Mankynde.* Other ancient texts which were recovered and published in the sixteenth century included Caspar Wolff's edition of *Gynaeciorum*, which appeared at Zurich in 1566, which Caspar Bauhin then enlarged and reissued 20 years later. Modern gynecology, in fact, began with the recovery of ancient texts. It developed with progress in anatomical studies.

Though precursors did exist, modern anatomy (q.v.) began in earnest with Andreas Vesalius and his school at Padua. Vesalius's classic work, *De fabrica corporis humani* (1543), provided the first accurate descriptions of female internal reproductive organs and disproved the ancient teaching that the pelvic bones separated during labor. His contemporaries and students elaborated on what he did. Bartolommeo Eustachio accurately drew the uterus for a series of anatomical plates; these, however, remained in storage in the Vatican and went unpublished for a century and a half. Gabriel Fallopius, who succeeded Vesalius as professor of anatomy at Padua, contributed descriptions of the ovaries, fallopian tubes, round ligaments, the vagina, and the placenta. Ambroise Paré, the leading French surgeon of the period, was a follower of Vesalius who contributed a number of procedures to gynecology and obstetrics, including induced premature labor in uterine hemorrhage, amputation of the cervix (an operation which was not performed until the next century), and podalic version.

From the middle of the sixteenth century to the opening of the nineteenth century, obstetrics and midwifery were more active fields than gynecology. The recovery of ancient obstetrical works provided the basis for modern summaries to guide contemporary midwives, while new publications emphasized obstetrical themes. William Harvey, whose classic work on circulation of the blood was published in 1628, contributed to this literature. His *Concerning Animal Generation* (1651) contained a chapter on labor which was the first original study in obstetrics by an English writer. Gynecological surgery was fairly common in the seventeenth century, particularly in repairing damage caused during deliveries. Hendrik van Roonhuyze firmly supported cesarean section, a procedure which had been outlawed in Paris as too deadly to be tried, and he performed several successfully. Another Dutch surgeon, Johann Weyer, treated amenorrhea from an imperforate hymen by incision of the membrane, while the famed Tulpius (Nicolas Tulp) of Amsterdam carried out a successful amputation of the cervix in 1652. More complicated operations, including ovariotomies and treatment of vesico-vaginal fistula, waited for the nineteenth century.

Medical midwifery dominated gynecological work in the eighteenth century, though Jean Astruc's *Treatise on the Diseases of Women* (1761–1765) was a clinical landmark. Beginning in the late seventeenth century with the work of Hendrick Vandeventer of the Hague, sometimes called the father of modern midwifery, and François Mauriceau of Paris, medical midwifery attracted some of the leading minds in European medicine. Great Britain was particularly rich in this field, with William Smellie and William Hunter in London, and Charles White in Manchester. William Smellie established an extremely successful school which trained hundreds of students in a naturalistic and unforced approach to birth and in the use of his improved obstetrical forceps (q.v.). William Hunter was his pupil and successor. The two together are credited with establishing the principles of scientifically based obstetrics and gynecology in Britain. Charles White is best known for his stress on cleanliness as the best defense against puerperal fever and for his extraordinary record of safe births.

Where the eighteenth century was rich in developments for midwifery and obstetrics, the nineteenth century produced a notable expansion in work on women's diseases, advances in gynecological surgery, and a growing separation of gynecology from midwifery. These developments were part of broader social changes. The nineteenth century was a period in industrializing, urban societies in which many groups found a basis for claiming rights to education, economic opportunity, and social status. Middle-class women were among these groups, and the medical literature treating women's diseases provides interesting insights into cultural attitudes which inhibited women's success.

Nineteenth-century medical literature portrayed women as weak, nervous, chronically ill, and entirely the prisoners of their sexual system. William A. Alcott, a Boston physician who wrote on women's health, noted in 1850 that half of America's women suffered from "nervousness," which he called a "real disease," and his opinion was shared by colleagues on both sides of the Atlantic. The consensus was that women suffered as much as they did, and the way they did, because they were women. Pelvic disorders, sick headaches, nervousness, and related physical or emotional problems were said to stem from malfunctions in the female sexual organs, specifically the uterus, an organ unique to women which exercised a "paramount power" over the entire female physical and moral system. More broadly, the rhythms of women's reproductive lives, beginning with the onset of the menstrual cycle at puberty and ending with menopause, were considered to be the controlling influences. Naturally, marriage and motherhood were the social functions determined by this physiological reality.

Nineteenth-century gynecology focused its attention on women's sexual organs, specifically the uterus, as the key to curing their indispositions. This was neither entirely fanciful nor irrelevant. Uterine, cervical, and menopausal problems were common, and childbirth was a dangerous and difficult procedure which often left behind conditions requiring extensive repairs. Unfortunately, since the uterus was considered the fulcrum of female physiology, it was also blamed for conditions which had little to do with it. The normal course of treatment for supposed uterine illnesses could be fierce. What was called "local treatment" was applied to a whole range of problems from *prolapsus uteri* after childbirth to cancer, menstrual problems, nervousness, and backache. Local treatment contained elements of heroic therapy and was invoked most commonly between 1830 and 1860. It began with manual manipulation to correct positional problems but could escalate through applying leeches internally to cauterizing with powerful astringents such as nitrate of silver or hydrate of potassa. An exceptionally resistant infection might be treated with a white-hot iron. Cauterizing, whether with the iron or with caustics, had to be repeated several times to be effective. The results, while sometimes successful, were excruciatingly painful and were acknowledged to be dangerous. Advances in surgery and the establishment of the germ theory of disease helped to eliminate local treatment by 1880.

There can be little argument that the stereotype of feminine weakness based on innate female sexuality affected women's self-image in the nineteenth century and inhibited them in important areas of social action. Nor can there be much doubt that an overwhelmingly male medical profession promoted this idea to preserve established social patterns and cultural values. However, this complex of ideas arose from generations of medical thinking; from that perspective, the parallels between gynecology and all other fields of medicine are important. By the opening of the twentieth century, a new kind of medicine built on bacteriology, cell theory, and biochemistry reoriented medical practice. As gynecology shared in the errors, misplaced emphases, and even cruelty of earlier medical methods, so also it participated in the development of the new order and its particular problems.

Gynecological surgery moved ahead dramatically in the early nineteenth century. Its achievements came before the general use of anesthesias and in advance of antiseptic or aseptic surgery. American surgeons were responsible for the most important advances, with the work of Ephraim McDowell and James Marion Sims leading the way. Ephraim McDowell studied under John Bell of Edinburgh in 1793 and 1794. In 1795, he established a successful surgical practice in the small frontier town of Danville, Kentucky. In 1809, he performed the first successful ovariotomy on a 47-year-old widow who not only survived but lived 31 more years. The ovariotomy had had no place in surgical practice before McDowell. He, however, performed the operation on 13 patients, and 8 of these recovered. His paper on the first operation was sent to John Bell, who was living in retirement in Italy. Bell apparently died without seeing it, but it reached an associate of his, John Lizars, who published it in his *Observations on Extractions of Diseased Ovaria* in 1825. Lizars had little success with the operation, but the Atlee brothers in Pennsylvania made it very nearly routine. John Attlee did 78 ovariotomies between 1843 and 1883, with 64 recoveries, while William reported 387 in the same period. By mid-century the operation was done regularly in England by Sir Spencer Wells (London) and Charles Clay (Manchester). In France, it was performed successfully in 1862 by Eugène Koeberlé, and in 1864 by the celebrated Auguste Nélaton and by Jules Peau.

James Marion Sims was responsible for a second dramatic achievement, a successful treatment of vesico-vaginal fistula. Sims was a South Carolinian who graduated from Jefferson Medical College in Philadelphia in 1835 and settled in Alabama. He built a strong practice and a reputation for surgical skill and imagination. In 1845, he attended a woman who suffered a uterine displacement in a riding accident, and while he was carrying out a digital examination, he put the patient into a lateral position which greatly facilitated examinations. "Sims's position" and a special curved speculum which he invented permitted him to see vesico-vaginal fistula "as no man had ever seen it before." He also developed a silver wire suture to avoid sepsis and used a catheter to empty the bladder. It took Sims four years to develop his technique, and a black slave girl named Anarcha underwent 30 attempts before Sims attained success. It might be thought that she and two other black girls, known as Lucy and Betsey, deserve a memorial for their part in what Sims, with characteristic lack of humility, called "one of the most important discoveries of the age for suffering humanity." Sims published a description of his work in 1852, but his colleagues were skeptical, and when he moved to New York in 1853, the operation still had not been tried there. Sims performed it successfully. In 1855, he established the Women's Hospital, which became a major gynecological center, and he went abroad in 1861. He demonstrated his operation in Germany and France, where he was very well received, and he published his *Clinical Notes on Uterine Surgery* in 1866.

There were other gynecological developments in the course of the nineteenth century. Gustav

Adolf Michaëlis at Kiel in Germany began the systematic study of pelvic architecture, founding a school which culminated in the work of Carl Conrad Theodore Litzmann, who published a study in 1861 which was the basis for the modern clinical classification of pelvises. Sir James Y. Simpson of Edinburgh, an outstanding gynecological surgeon who rejected Lister's theories on the bacterial causes of infection, introduced a variety of improvements in surgical procedures during the 1840s and 1850s, which included using iron wire for abdominal sutures in ovariotomies, using a sponge tent for dilating the cervis, and listening for a particular uterine sound to diagnose retroposition of the uterus. He also introduced chloroform as a general anesthesia for women in labor in 1847, just two months before N. C. Keep of Boston used ether. The controversy over general anesthesia and that between ether and chloroform went on for many years. T. Gaillard Thomas published his *Practical Treatise on the Diseases of Women* in 1872, a standard work which was translated into four European languages and Chinese.

With the introduction of general anesthesia and antiseptic surgery, gynecological operations became routine and increasingly sophisticated techniques were then possible. Lawson Tait, in Birmingham, one of the most successful gynecological surgeons of his day, performed literally thousands of ovariotomies and other abdominal sections. Indeed, there was concern that gynecologists, like other medical men, were becoming too quick to employ surgery, and when Robert Battey began in 1872 to remove ovaries for reasons other than the extirpation of cysts or tumors, many practitioners believed the pendulum had swung too far. The controversy continued into the twentieth century.

The development of gynecology as a specialty led to intensified efforts to separate it from obstetrics in the twentieth century. The obvious relationship between the two fields, however, blunted the most radical attacks, with the result that for general purposes the two fields live together, accepting their areas of common interest as well as their different emphases. Progress in endocrinology and the understanding of hormone function have greatly enlarged the physiological significance of gynecology and have given the field psychological and social significance as well. The use of hormonal substances in manipulating or controlling both emotional and physical disturbances carries far beyond the boundaries of gynecological concern in one sense. On the other hand, operations to bring about sexual change from male to female, which first gained wide publicity in the Christine Jorgenson case in the 1950s, show the strikingly new dimensions of gynecology in its most recent phase. The primary development of the field, however, has remained within the confines of treatment for women's problems, with prevention and treatment of cancer occupying a central role. The degree to which the women's movement has affected gynecology, apart from increasing the number of women in the field, is not clear. Gynecologists have contributed relatively little to the debate on abortion, tending to remain within the guidelines established by state and federal regulations as well as their own profession. On the whole, this has made their influence a conservative one.

ADDITIONAL READINGS: Audrey Eccles, *Obstetrics and Gynecology in Tudor and Stuart England*, Kent, Ohio, 1982; Harvey Graham, *Eternal Eve*, London, 1950; Mary Hartman and Lois W. Banner (eds.), *Clio's Consciousness Raised: New Perspectives on the History of Women*, New York, Evanston, San Francisco, and London, 1974, 1–71; Edwin Jameson, *Gynecology and Obstetrics*, New York, 1936; Richard A. Leonard, *History of Gynecology*, New York, 1944; James V. Ricci, *The Genealogy of Gynaecology: History of the Development of Gynaecology Throughout the Ages, 2000 B.C.–1800 A.D.*, Philadelphia, 1943; James V. Ricci, *One Hundred Years of Gynecology, 1800–1900*, Philadelphia, 1945; Sarah Stage, *Female Complaints: Lydia Pinkham and the Business of Female Medicine*, New York, 1979.

See also MIDWIFERY.

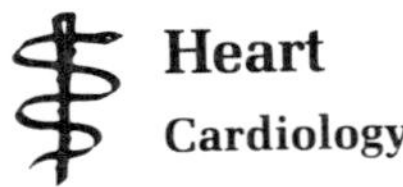

Heart
Cardiology

The heart is a powerful hollow muscle which plays an important part in the respiratory-circulatory system. Together with the lungs, arteries, veins, capillaries, and blood, the heart assists the system in its most important function: the delivery of oxygen throughout the body. Failure in any of the system's parts produces either severe illness or death, depending on the extent and the location of the malfunction. The heart's failure, however, stops the entire system and is synonymous with death. In that sense, the heart is the body's primary organ.

Paleopathology gives very early evidence of heart disease, and the heart figured significantly in religious practices throughout the ancient near east. Early Greek religio-philosophic ideas identified the heart as "the seat of the soul" and "the vital principle of life," and these ideas, systematized in the early fifth century B.C. by Alcmaeon of Croton, were repeated in the fourth century by Aristotle and the Hippocratic writers. In this tradition, the heart was second in importance to the brain, which was the seat of consciousness, and there seems to have been no perception that the brain depended in any organic sense on the heart. Nevertheless, though the Hippocratic school was not strong on anatomical detail, there is an early description of the heart in the Hippocratic writings portraying it as a strong muscle with two ventricles. The author knew about the auricles and was able to describe the structure and presumed function of the valves. Such information undoubtedly came from animal dissections. Much more data became available in Alexandria, where human dissections were done routinely. Unfortunately, the Alexandrian work was lost, and what little is known about it is what was preserved by commentators and critics. It does seem, however, that the two leading anatomists of fourth-century Alexandria, Erasistratus and Herophilus, had a clear and generally accurate understanding of the heart. Herophilus seems to have extended his studies to the blood vessels and the pulse as well and to have developed an early four-stage account of respiration.

In the second century A.D. Galen of Pergamum synthesized the Hippocratic, Aristotelian, and Alexandrian traditions with his own extensive observations and experience to form a comprehensive medical system. Galen was a notable anatomist who practiced animal dissection and vivisection. He had wide medical experience which included acting as gladiators' physician, and he was extraordinarily well-read. Yet on questions related to the heart, Galen perpetuated a number of critical errors, including the supposed fact that blood passed from one side of the heart to the other through the septum. He denied that the heart was a muscle on the grounds that muscles by definition were fibers which engaged in voluntary action, whereas heart movement was involuntary; and he remained convinced that the vascular system originated in the liver, while the heart itself was located at the body's center rather than off to the left.

The most serious weaknesses in Galen's system, however, were not the result of inadequate, incorrect, or misinterpreted information. They arose rather from his approach, for, despite an asserted reverence for demonstrable fact, Galen's work was always dominated by what he believed. Thus while Galen described the valves in the heart, distinguished veins from arteries on structural grounds, and conceived of a connection between the heart and the lungs, he missed discovering basic heart function and blood circulation.

Relatively little was added to the anatomy or physiology of the heart until Andreas Vesalius led the sixteenth-century reformation of anatomy, and William Harvey, building on the work of the anatomists, described the circulation of the blood (q.v.) and the heart's role in it. Harvey considered the heart to be a pump whose sole purpose was to send arterial blood out into the system to return through the veins. His contribution was to describe the entire mechanism for this procedure, heart included, in precise detail. But Harvey's demonstration had surprisingly little influence. Scientists postulated grand principles to explain the body's functioning in ways analogous to the way Newton's laws explained the universe. The systematizers explained how the body functioned either by treating it as a machine responding to particle action or the flow of fluids, while noting such factors as vessel size, or by positing characteristics inherent in different body structures. Albrecht von Haller argued that all tissue had the inherent qualities of irritability (a disposition to involuntary contraction) or sensibility and could be classified accordingly. The heart, whose involuntary motion was one of its primary characteristics, was deemed to be the "most irritable" tissue in the body. It was "irritated" by the flow of blood through it. Other scientists refined von Haller's views in the direction of allowing both irritability and sensibility to be present in a single organ, pointing to the different kinds of fibers which composed the heart muscle. The idea that muscle tissue contained a quality or potential which could activate the muscle, a vital principle, was very near to conceiving of the heart as a self-running, self-regulating organ.

Cardiology, the modern medical discipline devoted to studying the physiology and pathology of the heart and to devising means for diagnosing and treating its diseases, first appeared as a unified field with a specialized organ focus in the middle of the eighteenth century.

In 1749, Jean Baptiste de Sénac published a specific descriptive work on the heart which summarized what was known to that time. This was the most detailed study on the anatomy, physiology, and diseases of the heart then available, and it remained the standard work for several decades. Sénac's work was also the starting point for new research. The basic questions concerned the heart's role in respiration and how heart function was controlled. Working on these problems led to unexpected discoveries of diagnostic and therapeutic techniques as well as a variety of instruments for measuring heart function. By the beginning of the twentieth century, the control mechanisms involved in heart function were coming to be understood, and the heart's place in the body's physiology was growing clearer. This gave meaning to the idea that the heart was at the center of life and inspired the discovery of further and more discriminating methods for diagnosing and treating heart conditions.

The heart's role as a pump had become well understood. What was not clear was why the heart worked at all, and what conditions were responsible for its malfunction, why the heart ran more swiftly at some times than at others, and how the heart's function related to changes in the veins and arteries. It was noticed as early as 1777 that arteries contracted and dilated in phase with heart action, but it was not until 1831 that Ernst Weber showed that these were controlled by the same type of nerves. Alfred Volkmann suggested in 1837 that the vagus nerve had the power to inhibit heart action, a suggestion which Ernst Weber and his brother Edward confirmed in 1845. Shortly after the middle of the nineteenth century, Claude Bernard, the greatest of the French physiologists, followed up studies on the role of sympathetic nerves in regulating metabolism and body temperature to identify the regulatory function of vasometer nerves; and in 1852 Charles Brown-Séquard demonstrated that cutting the sympathetic nerve produced vasodilation, while stimulation of peripheral sympathetic nerve endings induced vasoconstriction. Early in the twentieth century understanding of the mechanisms involved in neurocontrols over involuntary movements (as in the heart) was further refined when T. R. Elliot of Cambridge suggested that adrenalin or a similar substance might be released at the sympathetic nerve endings. Sir Henry Dale followed this work with demonstrations that acetylcholine was the substance released at the parasympathetic nerve endings and by the sympathetic vasodilator nerve fibers. The nerve endings which controlled constriction secreted an adrenalinlike substance. Sir Henry Dale received the Nobel prize for this work in 1936.

The study of nerve control systems applied to all involuntary movement thoroughout the body, but of course it was of major importance for understanding the heart. Diagnostic techniques, most notably the methods of percussion developed by Joseph Leopold Auenbrugger and revised by Jean-Nicolas Corvisart in the eighteenth century, and René Laënnec's stethoscope (q.v.) in the early nineteenth, were important for chest conditions in general. In the hands of such early-nineteenth-century practitioners as James Hope, they led to diagnoses of cardiac aneurism or abnormal dilation while the patient was still living. Previously these conditions were only known postmortem. By the middle of the nineteenth century, listening for sounds in the chest had become an accepted diagnostic practice in heart cases.

A more sophisticated diagnostic approach identified the presence of electricity in the heart and then used it to monitor heart action. This process began with the competing experiments of Luigi Galvani and Alessandro Volta on electricity in the muscles of frogs' legs at the end of the eighteenth century. Interest in electricity led to the development of the galvanometer to measure it, and in 1838 Carlo Matteucci was able to show that the heart muscle generated a measurable electrical charge. An instrument for measuring the electrical impulses from animals' hearts was in use by 1875, and in 1903 William Einthoven modified a string galvanometer to record heartbeats. This was the origin of the electrocardiograph (EKG), which has become fundamental to heart practice. It was an early version of this instrument which permitted Sir James MacKenzie to identify the irregular action known as heart block and to treat it by influencing ventricle action with drugs. More recently, such irregularities have been controlled by implanted, battery-charged pacemakers which deliver an electrical impulse directly to the heart. For many years the electrocardiograph was the single most important diagnostic tool for coronary heart disease, though recently it has been complemented by chemical analysis of the blood and regular temperature surveys.

Understanding the regulatory mechanisms in heart function was significant physiologically and opened key areas for diagnosis and therapy. The most important pathological advances for the heart, however, resulted from exploration of the conditions which develop in the veins and arteries or which follow bacterial or viral infections. James Herrick's classic essay on coronary thrombosis, published in 1912, opened an era of research which still continues. Research on coronary heart disease (q.v.) has shown the conditions of venous and arterial degeneration which lead to significant heart damage. The critical issues of concern here are less involved with direct damage to the heart than with the discovery of causes for degeneration in blood vessels. Many causal mechanisms remain unclear, but epidemiological studies combined with laboratory research have identified smoking, obesity, high-fat diets, emotional tension, and lack of exercise as factors contributing significantly to the incidence of heart disease. Raising public awareness on these matters has proved to be an effective response to a major medical problem. Similarly, work on virology, bacteriology, and immune response has produced a better understanding of the way infection may affect the heart, while the use of penicillin and other antibiotic substances has significantly reduced the incidence of rheumatic heart disease from streptococcal infection. This achievement has been most notable since 1945.

Surgery (q.v.) has provided cardiology with its most visible and dramatic achievements, culminating in the well-publicized heart transplants pioneered by Dr. Christiaan Barnard of South Africa in 1967. Open-heart surgery to repair tissue damage and a variety of operations intended to improve blood flow to the heart, though less dramatic than transplants, have added measurably to the ability to treat heart conditions effectively. This entire class of operation has been greatly facilitated by advances in surgical techniques which have made it possible to work directly on the heart.

Twentieth-century advances in understanding heart function and disease underscore the interconnectedness of modern medical science. In the eighteenth and nineteenth centuries, the questions asked concerned the heart's own structure and function. By the first quarter of the twentieth century, most of the physiological information on the heart was in place, and the most important work relevant to heart problems concerned related structures. Moreover, modern understanding of how the heart works, what conditions of disease it is subject to, and how it relates to the total organism is a major accomplishment of empirical investigation. The ancients identified the heart as the seat of vital powers, and early modern authorities recognized it as the working source for maintaining life. Modern studies have been able to show how those wonders are performed, and why they sometimes fail.

ADDITIONAL READINGS: P. E. Baldry, *The Battle Against Heart Disease*, London and New York, 1971; Louis P. Bishop and John J. Neilson, *History of Cardiology*, New York, 1927; C. R. S. Harris, *The Heart and the Vascular System in Ancient Greek Medicine from Alcmaeon to Galen*, Oxford, 1973; James B. Herrick, *Short History of Cardiology*, Springfield, Ill., 1942; Saul Jarchow (ed.), *The Concept of Heart Failure from Avicenna to Albertini*, Cambridge, Mass., 1980; H. A. Snellen (ed.), *A Disorder of the Breast: A Collection of Original Texts on Ischaemic Heart Disease*, Rotterdam, 1976.

See also CORONARY HEART DISEASE.

Hebrew Medicine

The early Hebrew medical tradition can be traced to the Bible and the Talmud. The Bible was compiled between 1500 B.C. and 300 B.C.; the Talmud, a book of rules and precepts, was completed between 70 B.C. and the second century A.D. There are two versions of the Talmud—the Babylonian and the Palestinian, or Jerusalemic. These sources reveal indigenous medical practices, but they are a record as well of the many influences which affected Hebrew medicine. In ancient times, the Hebrews shared medical ideas with Egypt and Mesopotamia, while during the Hellenistic period, Persian, Greek, and Alexandrian influences gave the old medicine a new look. It was through this tradition and later through contact with Islam that Hebrew medicine became an important influence in the medieval world. This development began with the dispersion of the Hebrew people following the second conquest of Jerusalem (A.D. 70) which carried Jewish physicians wherever there was a community to serve.

Beliefs and Practices The medical practice of the Hebrews emphasized preventive measures and gave therapy a low priority. It was believed that only God could heal; hence those treating the ill were considered helpers, and they concentrated on symptoms rather than the causes of illness. Most physicians among the Jews were Jews themselves, though some foreigners appeared, including Egyptians, and it was acceptable to have an Egyptian embalmer. The *rofé*, or "foreign healers," however, were not held in high regard.

With the exception of a brass serpent invoked against snakebite, the Hebrew approach to therapy was rational. Herbal medicines, ointments, salves, and baths were basic to treatment, and there was an extensive *materia medica*. The excremental pharmacopeia popular among neighboring peoples was not acceptable. Magic, incantation, and mystical experience appear to have been less significant than in other ancient cultures, though in his earliest appearances the Hebrew physician was priest, sage, and sorcerer. In the late biblical and talmudic periods, the religious and medical remained firmly joined in rabbi-physicians; but medical treatment was separated from religious practice when the religion itself became more legalistic and temporal. One important exception was the Essenes, a group which splintered from the Pharisees in the second century B.C., who combined the mystical with herbalism, stressing amulets and incantations. Considered the group from which Christianity arose, the Essenes held views similar to those of the Persian and Chaldean magicians and the Hindu sect known as gymnosophists.

Biblical physiology held that blood was the vehicle for the soul, but that life was in breath. This pneumismatism was qualified during the talmudic era as the rabbis collected information and ideas, first in Persia and Alexandria and later from Greece. Practical anatomy and pathology flourished among the Hebrews thanks to animal sacrifice and the ritual slaughter of animals to be eaten. Examining carcasses for evidence of disease or blemishes which made them unfit for consumption contributed to anatomical knowledge, and it appears that experiments were performed on animals before and after slaughter. There were also postmortem examinations on human cadavers.

The talmudic rabbi-physicians held to a solidary rather than a humoral pathology, but they did their most valuable work on matters related to public health. They formulated rules for disease control based on the belief that some diseases were communicable by foods, bodily discharges, clothing, beverages, water, and air, and that plagues in particular were spread by contaminated water. In epidemic periods they proposed isolation of those infected, fumigation, disinfection of clothes, and avoidance of flies. No well was to be dug near a cemetery or a dump. Water should be boiled for drinking, while water left standing uncovered was considered unfit to drink. They knew the effects of opium and cautioned against abusing it. In the conviction that "physical cleanliness is conducive to spiritual purity," they developed rules applicable to city planning, personal hygiene, social relationships, and agriculture. People were forbidden to live in cities which had no physician or public bath, kissing on the lips was not permitted, and food was to be clean, fresh, and cooked enough to destroy parasites. Some of these rules appeared later in Europe during epidemic periods, though without the emphasis on everyday cleanliness.

With so complex a social medicine, the physician was extremely important. The talmudic tractates urged the people to consult "their own" physician, that is, the physician in their own community and not an alien. Physicians performed many public roles, including assessing damage to accident victims and determining whether persons condemned to be flogged could stand the punishment. A local court of justice would license physicians to treat the sick, and they were often consulted in their own homes. There were no clinics or hospitals, though there were hostels to provide shelter and care for the foreigners. Native sick were permitted to stay in the halls of the synagogue, and operating space for surgery was assigned, though just where is uncertain. There were "houses set apart" for lepers, and in the temple at Jerusalem there was a special section where priests could be examined for physical fitness. Finally, the Jewish physicians of Palestine and Babylonia appear to have been organized. Their emblem was the *haruta*, a branch of palm or peach, and a special ointment was made from the *haruta* which was thought to be effective in slow-healing wounds.

During the Diaspora (period of dispersion), Hebrew medicine became increasingly Greek, and eventually, in common with the medical culture of both western Asia and Europe, it accepted the prevalent Galenism. The empirical tradition remained alive, but the anatomical knowledge which marked earlier talmudic medicine was submerged in newer medical ideologies. During the Middle Ages, Jewish physicians, like their Byzantine and Moslem counterparts, acted as repositories for the classical heritage and played an important part in transferring classical medicine to western Europe. The rich community and empirical medicine of biblical and talmudic times, however, contributed relatively little to the evolution of modern practice, though traces appear in plague regulations and epidemic control.

Traditional Hebrew medicine had been most notable for its preventive and social dimension and for its integration into the personal and public life of the community. The breakup of Jewish community life produced cosmopolitan physicians, indistinguishable from their Christian or Moslem colleagues, who abandoned their ancient medical heritage. The practices of Jewish communities were restricted in their influence by their isolation from the cultures which surrounded them. In the end, the influence of traditional Hebrew practice outside the Jewish community was limited to what non-Jews were able to learn from the Old Testament. This was by no means inconsiderable, but it was also much less than the contribution of Jewish medical men to the development of medical thought.

ADDITIONAL READINGS: Harry Friedenwald, *The Jews and Medicine: Essays,* Baltimore, 1944; S. S. Levin, *Adam's Rib: Essays on Biblical Medicine,* Los Altos, Cal., 1970; Julius Preuss, *Biblical and Talmudic Medicine,* Fred Rosner (trans.), New York, 1978; Fred Rosner, *Medicine in the Bible and the Talmud: Selections from Classical Jewish Sources,* New York, 1977; Henry E. Sigerist, *History of Medicine,* New York, 1955, II; René Taton, *History of Science: Ancient and Medieval Science from the Beginnings to 1450,* A. J. Pomerans (trans.), New York, 1963, pt. I, chap. 3, pt. III, chap. 6.

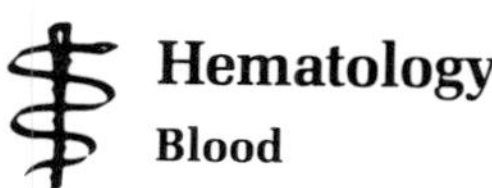

Hematology

Blood

Hematology is a modern discipline which studies the structure and function of blood. It is scarcely 100 years old, though its scientific antecedents appeared in the sixteenth century, and the conviction that blood and life are inseparable appears in some of man's earliest cultural artifacts. Cave paintings in northern Spain which date from 20,000 years ago appear to identify the hearts of animals as the source of life and blood, and therefore as the point of greatest vulnerability at which the successful hunter will strike. In later religious practices, ritual sacrifices gave blood pride of place together with the liver and the heart, while traditional therapies endowed blood with magical healing powers. Early medical references to blood combined an appreciation of its vital function with sensitivity to its magical properties. The earliest of such references is probably in the ritual formulas of the Egyptian Ebers papyrus (ca. 1550 B.C.), and for at least 1000 years the magic and medicine of the ancient near east gave blood a special standing.

As medicine separated from magic, blood retained its central role, and nowhere more significantly than in the Greek Hippocratic writings of the fifth and fourth centuries B.C., which identified blood as one of the four humors (q.v.) controlling health and disease. It has even been suggested that the four humors themselves (blood, phlegm, yellow bile, and black bile) can be derived from the separation of blood standing in a vessel into its component parts: Blood poured rapidly into a tall container first appears to be a uniform red fluid; when it is left alone, however, the upper part becomes a transparent yellow fluid, while at the bottom there is a dark red, almost black, jelly; on the surface, a thin layer of bright red blood appears, while the presence of diseases will separate a greenish white layer from the dark red fluid. In effect, the blood humor (the thin layer of bright red blood) rises to the top, overlaying the yellow bile and the black bile, with phlegm separating itself from the black bile. As A. H. T. Robb-Smith argues, it was "this separation of an apparent excess of phlegm in disease which was to dominate pathology for over two thousand years" and which has returned in recent times to play a significant part in modern physiology and pathology. Over the centuries, phlegm, the greenish-white layer separated from the dark red mass, was called the *crusta sanguinis, inflammatoria,* or *phlogistica;* the "buffy coat," "inflammatory pellicle," or "sizy blood." In modern times, hematologists refer to this phenomenon in terms of raised sedimentation rates and "the interplay of fibrogenesis and fibrinolysis in health and disease."

Humoral doctrines dominated western medical thought from the Hippocratic era through the seventeenth century. The primary version was that propounded by Galen of Pergamum in the second century A.D., a synthesis of Hippocratic teachings, Aristotelian doctrines, certain Alexandrian ideas, and Galen's own observations and arguments into a vast and comprehensive system in which blood played a central part. The Arab interpreters of Galen preserved and extended his doctrines, and their texts became fundamental to the revival of medicine in the west in the high Middle Ages. Bleeding (see Bloodletting) and purging were basic to Galenist therapies, and the first direct challenge to Galen's authority actually concerned the best place to open a vein for bleeding. Avicenna's version of Galenist doctrine was to make the incision as far from the lesion as possible. But Peter Brissot, a member of the Paris faculty of medicine, claimed in 1514 on the authority of Hippocratic texts that this was mistaken and that bleeding should be done as near the lesion as possible. His argument engendered a violent controversy which led to his banishment. He fled to Spain, where he died, but his posthumously published *Apology* kept the controversy alive. The Arabist supporters of Galenism compared Brissot's doctrine with Lutheranism as an assault on legitimate authority, but their arguments failed when the emperor Charles V, who had lost a relative treated according to the Arabist doctrine, ruled in favor of Brissot's ideas. A synod convened at Bologna under Pope Clement VII took the same position.

Humoral pathology and bleeding remained influential into the nineteenth century, while blood played a critical part in both mechanistic and vitalist physiologies. But the Brissot controversy caused anatomists to give greater attention to veins and arteries, setting in train a series of observations and discoveries which led through Vesalius and the anatomists of the sixteenth century to William Harvey and his description of the circulation of the blood (q.v.) in the seventeenth. Harvey's monumental treatise *The Motion of the Heart and the Blood* (1628) was less influential in his own time than later, but it did foster a mechanistic approach to physiology which was then strongly reinforced by Newton's work on planetary movement and gravitation. Harvey himself was certain that blood was the primary life-giving and life-bearing element in the body and that it was also a part that was "generative" and "endowed with soul," and he called it "the hearth, the Vesta, the household deity, the innate heat, the sun of the microcosm, the fire of Plato . . . because it preserves and nourishes and increases its very self by its perpetual wandering motion." More than two centuries elapsed, however, before it was possible to demonstrate what blood actually was and how it worked the wonders which Harvey desribed.

Modern hematology began with a series of random observations, and the discipline has retained a significant element of the fortuitous and the nonsystematic up to the present day. Structural studies on blood began with the first microscopists in the second half of the seventeenth century. Both Marcello Malpighi, who found the capillary system which confirmed Harvey's circulation theory, and Antonjvan Leeuwenhoek, the masterly Dutch lens maker and amateur observer, saw and described red corpuscles. Malpighi outlined his findings in two letters to Giovanni Borelli which were published in 1661; Leeuwenhoek published his observations in 1673 and 1674 in communications to the Royal Society, London. Jan Swammerdam, who died in 1680, had observed red corpuscles in frogs' blood in 1658, and he referred to the "blood particles" of human blood in 1662. His observations were not published until 1737, though when they were, they proved to be superior to all previous descriptions in accuracy and anatomical discrimination.

Studies on blood function also had roots in the seventeenth century. Harvey's exposition on blood circulation gave impetus to studies of respiration. Robert Boyle, who was also interested in the chemical properties of blood, was able to demonstrate that air was necessary to life; while Richard Lower, who is better known for his successful efforts at blood transfusion (q.v.), showed that contact with air changed the color of venous blood to that of arterial blood. There the matter rested until the eighteenth-century revolution in chemistry and Joseph Priestley's discovery of oxygen (1775). Antoine Lavoisier's definitive experiments followed, showing the processes which took place during oxidation and applying the same concept physiologically. By 1793, Lavoisier had connected respiration with oxidation, demonstrated that people used varying amounts of oxygen depending on how active they were, and established that chemical processes were at work in respiration and blood circulation. Lavoisier's discoveries were the starting point for modern metabolic studies.

Experiments with the mechanics of blood transfusion also began in the seventeenth century, but the interest was short-lived, and the subject was not considered seriously until the second half of the nineteenth century. Studies on blood components fared better. In the early eighteenth century, Hermann Boerhaave was impressed by Jan Swammerdam's descriptions of red corpuscles, and while arranging their posthumous publication, he began studying the chemical properties of blood. He performed similar tests on egg whites and whole blood, coming to the conclusion that the two substances had similar elements in them. Though the concept of proteins was still a century in the future, Boerhaave had taken an important step toward understanding blood chemistry. His work was paralleled by that of William Hewson, an English anatomist and surgeon who published on blood properties in 1771. Hewson followed and worked with John Hunter. He was interested in the coagulable lymph, and his studies on coagulation permitted him to describe fibrinogen and defibrinated blood. He also worked on white corpuscles. Though they had been previously described, Hewson was the first to study them systematically. He was able to connect them to the lymph system and assign them a role in pus formation.

By the end of the eighteenth century, there was a substantial body of information on blood available to scientists. A *Dictionary of Medicine and Surgery Practice* (1835) contained an article on blood which was the work of Forget and Gabriel Andral. They pointed out that the constituents of blood were derived from the respiratory and digestive tracts, and that blood was the source of materials from which all the other tissues were built up. They discussed the components of normal blood: water, albumin, fibrin, "coloring matter," fatty crystallizable matter, oily substances, water- and alcohol-soluble substances, iron salts, chlorides of sodium and potassium, and carbonates of calcium and magnesium. Additional substances which derived from other secretions were noted as well, nor was this considered to exhaust the list. There were still other, undetected materials to find. The authors explained blood coagulation by chemical and physical laws without reference to vitalistic processes, variations in the character of blood during the presence of disease were noted, and differences in blood composition under different physiological conditions, for instance, sex or age, were described. The essay also explored the way alterations in the blood affected other tissues as well as the possibility that blood could serve as the medium for communicating disease. This summary showed a thoroughly empirical approach and a rather sophisticated understanding of the subject.

There were further developments in the early nineteenth century. Alfred Donné identified platelets, the third physical element in blood; and in 1830, François Magendie identified and described the "large white globules" known as leukocytes and worked on techniques for measuring the diameter of red corpuscles. He also suggested a method for counting red cells. This idea was elaborated by Karl Vierordt in 1852. The following year Hermann Welcher developed a method for counting white corpuscles. The modern "counting chamber," or hemoglobinometer, was devised by Sir William Richard Gowers in 1878. As the understanding of blood changes under pathological conditions advanced, such techniques took on critical importance for diagnostic purposes.

Studies on blood pathology expanded through the second half of the nineteenth century. In 1864 Sir Samuel Wilkes collected and published Thomas Hodgkin's observations from 1832 on neoplasms of the absorbent glands and spleen, and Henri Vaquez established true erythremia in 1892. Thomas Addison's seminal work on anemia, first presented in a paper to a London medical society in 1849, marked the beginning of two generations of dispute and progress. Addison opposed microscopy and in other respects failed to value the contribution his contemporaries made. However, his clinical descriptions of the condition later known as pernicious anemia were excellent. Work by other investigators between 1870 and 1885 produced a classification for anemias and a better understanding of pernicious anemia. The latter disease was considered infallibly mortal until the discovery of raw liver treatment (1926) and the synthesis of vitamin B_{12} (1948).

Paul Ehrlich, the most protean of late-nineteenth- and early-twentieth-century scientists, made several major contributions to blood studies. His early work at Strasbourg with aniline dyes and staining techniques led to the development of the triacid stain for blood films. This permitted differentiation of blood particles and revolutionized hematological research. Ehrlich developed a differential blood count, studied bone marrow and its relation to blood, distinguished the megaloblast of pernicious anemia, and contributed his "side-chain effect" to immunological studies—specifically to the concept of immunohematology. This work and more led one recent writer to suggest that Paul Ehrlich was the father of modern hematology as well as immunology and chemotherapy.

Recipient reactions made blood transfusion a dangerous procedure. The reason was shown at the opening of the twentieth century, when Karl Landsteiner found that when certain blood samples were mixed, the cells clumped together. The clumping resulted from the presence of two antithetical antigens, which he labeled A and B. Landsteiner was able to show that all human blood could be classified according to the presence or absence of these antigens. Using O for the absence of antigen, he found that A and O accounted for 41.8 percent and 46.4 percent of all people; B appeared in 8.6 percent and AB in just 3 percent. The ABO system made it possible to match donor and recipient blood types. Landsteiner's work brought him the Nobel prize in 1930. In 1940 another grouping, called Rh, was found. This factor has severe effects when used in transfusion and is responsible for hemolytic diseases in newborns. Its discovery on the eve of the United States' entry into World War II forestalled a serious problem, since blood transfusions were used extensively in treating battle casualties.

Hematology's development in the eighteenth and nineteenth centuries owed a great deal to advances in chemistry and microscopy. Continuing improvements in the technology and techniques of scientific research made increasingly precise measurements and distinctions possible. The structure and composition of the blood were revealed, nutritive and immunological functions were identified, measurable changes in blood characteristics under specific disease conditions were established to serve as diagnostic tools, and a number of diseases particular to the blood itself were identified. The most important among these were the various anemias, qualitative deficiencies in the blood which produced marked pathological results, and leukemias, identified with the overproduction of white cells. The extremely important role of proteins, first noted in the eighteenth century and developed in some detail in the nineteenth, emerged as a major factor in the twentieth century with broad implications for biology in general, while the development of plasma and blood-grouping techniques made transfusions both common and safe. Modern hematology remains empirical and eclectic, though protein and plasma studies undertaken at the Harvard Medical School have reopened the possibility of a unitary approach to hematology and possibly to physiology in general. Whether this happens or not, the fact remains that hematology numbers among its achievements some of the most important advances in modern medical science.

ADDITIONAL READINGS: Camille Dreyfus, *Some Milestones in the History of Haematology*, New York and London, 1957; Earle Hackett, *Blood: The Paramount Humour*, London, 1973; Richard Hardwick, *Charles Richard Drew: Pioneer in Blood Research*, New York, 1967; S. M. Lewis, *History of Haematology*, London, 1956; R. G. Macfarlane and A. H. T. Robb-Smith, *The Functions of the Blood*, London, 1961; L. J. Rather, *Addison and the White Corpuscles: An Aspect of Nineteenth Century Biology*, London, 1972; A. H. T. Robb-Smith, "Unravelling the Functions of the Blood," *Medical History* 6 (January 1962): 1–21; Charles Singer and E. Ashley Underwood, *A Short History of Medicine*, 2d ed., Oxford, 1962; M. L. Verso, "Some Notes on a Contemporary Review of Early French Haematology," *Medical History* 5 (July 1961): 239–252; Maxwell M. Wintrobe, *Blood Pure and Eloquent: A Story of Discovery, of People, and of Ideas*, New York, 1980.

See also Bloodletting; Blood Transfusion; Circulation of the Blood; Clinical Medicine.

Hospital

Origins The hospital as an institution offering care to those who need it is of great antiquity. The modern word is derived from the Latin *hospes* ("host"), which is also the root for the words "hotel," "hospice," and "hospitality." The earliest examples approximating the institutions we call hospitals, however, were the Egyptian temples of 4000 years ago. The association of religion and medicine was a natural one in many ancient cultures. In Greece, the temples dedicated to Asclepius were noted for their cures. Here treatment involved a mystical experience. If the person seeking help were admitted to the temple (not all supplicants were), he or she was made comfortable until the god appeared in a dream to suggest what treatment the patient ought to follow. The temples of Asclepius were numerous and popular. The best known were at Epidaurus and at Cos, which was also noted as the seat of the Hippocratic school, but there were at least 200 other sites, including one at Rome.

Greek surgeons saw their patients in offices or surgeries called *iatreia;* but while medical treatment was offered there, these institutions were not used for caring for the ill. The idea of an institution created specifically to care for the sick appeared in Hindustan in the third century B.C., and in first-century Rome. In Hindustan, a certain king, Asoka, is credited with establishing some 18 centers for treating the ill. There were physicians and a nursing staff, and the expense was borne by the royal treasury. These institutions may have been forerunners of the elaborate Byzantine and Moslem hospitals which attained their zenith between the eighth and the twelfth centuries A.D. Hospital-style institutions appeared in China in the first millennium A.D. as part of a state-supported care system, while in Rome, there were special institutions for slaves, gladiators, and soldiers. The best-authenticated of these *valetudinaria* were those constructed as parts of frontier military camps. Comparable facilities were built in provincial towns to serve administrators and their families, while excavations at Pompeii show that Roman physicians maintained rest or convalescent homes for their wealthy patrons.

The Byzantine/Moslem Hospital In the latter part of the third century A.D., the Roman emperor Diocletian moved the political center of the empire to the east; and in the fourth century, Constantine the Great converted to Christianity and founded the eastern capital of Constantinople near the ancient fishing village of Byzantium on the Bosphorus. Christianity became the official faith of the Roman empire in the course of the fourth century. It was the Christian commitment to care for the sick, to comfort the lonely, and to feed the hungry which motivated the prodigious growth of hospices, orphanages, old-age retreats, and hospitals proper throughout the medieval world. In A.D. 325, meeting at the behest of the emperor Constantine, a formal church council commanded the construction of a hospital in every cathedral town. This commitment was subsequently renewed and expanded. One of the first results for which there is documentation was the hospital of St. Basil at Caesarea in Cappadocia, which was completed between 368 and 372. This hospital accepted and treated the sick and infirm as well as providing shelter and help for the indigent and for travelers. There was a separate section for lepers. A regular staff lived in the hospital, and financing was provided by income from lands granted to the church at Caesarea. Other hospitals were built at Constantinople and Alexandria in Egypt, in Syria, and in Asia Minor. In 540 a Byzantine-style hospital was erected at Gondishapur on the Persian Gulf. It became a model for subsequent construction in Sassanian Persia, in central Asia, and ultimately in China.

During the seventh century, the rise of Islam led to the Moslem conquest of west Asia, Egypt, north Africa, and Spain. Islam inherited a rich medical tradition, and by the ninth century it had established a sophisticated medical system. Hospital complexes were constructed at Baghdad in the ninth and tenth centuries which employed up to 25 staff physicians, which maintained separate wards for different conditions, and which gave medical instruction. Nor was this an isolated phenomenon. Thirty-four such hospitals have been identified in Moslem cities from Moghul India to Spain. One of the best known was built in Cairo in 1283 and was still in use at the end of the eighteenth century. It had a permanent staff of physicians under a director, male and female nurses, and special wards for women, fever cases, eye diseases, and mental patients. The wards for the insane were particularly famous for the luxury of their appointments and the kindness of their care. Islam, like Christianity, emphasized the community's responsibility for those who needed help. The hospitals they built reflected this commitment as well as a high level of medical and administrative skill.

Byzantium's political resurgence under the powerful Macedonian dynasty in the ninth and tenth centuries brought further hospital construction which continued under the weaker Comneni and Angeli rulers of the eleventh and twelfth centuries. Hospitals were built in Anatolia and at Constantinople, including the world-famous Pantocrator, which was begun by John II

Comnenus in 1136. Built as part of a complex of buildings which included a sumptuous church, tombs for the ruling dynasty, and a monastery, this hospital was the greatest achievement of the long Byzantine tradition. The hospital comprised 50 rooms which were divided into five departments. There were 5 rooms for surgical cases, 8 for acute illnesses, 10 each for men and women with various complaints, and 12 for gynecological cases. The remaining 5 were available for miscellaneous use, including emergencies. Each department had a staff of two physicians, five surgeons, and two nurses or attendants. The hospital also trained students. There were also an outpatient department for ambulatory cases, a pharmacy, baths, a mill, and a bakery.

Hospital building reached its peak in the east in the thirteenth century and then declined. There was a brief resurgence following the Ottoman conquest of Constantinople in 1453, but that ended by the seventeenth century. The extent to which the hospitals of Byzantium and Islam affected western medieval and early modern development is uncertain, though the Moslem role in the revitalization of western medical thought is an established fact. It is also true, however, that it was not until the late Middle Ages that the concept of the hospital as an institution essentially for medical purposes reappeared, and it was only during the eighteenth century that that idea became accepted as an operating principle. In effect, society's needs, economic potential, and cultural values in the medieval west fostered different emphases in providing care, and parallels with Byzantine or Moslem hospital development had to wait for a similarly centralized, urbanized, and medically oriented civilization.

The Latin West In the medieval west, as in the east, the church bore primary responsibility for developing institutions of care. Hospices for pilgrims and merchants, orphanages and almshouses, leprosaria, and pesthouses as well as hospitals were built in considerable numbers. Among the hospitals was the Hôtel Dieu, founded by the Bishop of Paris in the seventh century, which today is the oldest working hospital in existence. Medieval hospitals cared for the poor, but they offered little more than shelter and nursing.

Monasteries played a particularly important part. Built in remote areas for the better contemplation of God's goodness, they were often the only facility for miles around which offered refuge for weary travelers and care for the sick. At the Abbey of St. Gall in Switzerland, which was built between 816 and 830, one entire section of the monastery grounds was given over to medical facilities. For people arriving from the outside, there was a Hospice of Pilgrims and Paupers, and there was a House of Distinguished Guests. The former was a large common room with no sanitary facilities. The latter contained separate quarters for parties of travelers and was equipped with latrines, or *necessaria*. There were separate infirmaries for monks and novices. The monks' infirmary was divided into three sections, one for the sick, including a room for dangerous illness, one for the infirm, that is, superannuated or aged monks, and a special section for those who had been bled and purged. These last were allowed relief from the difficult routines of monastic life and received a more nourishing diet. In the House of the Physicians, one room was provided for very ill lay people. It is thought that this was to serve the monastery's own lay community, though it is possible that it was also used in emergencies for sick paupers or pilgrims. Distinguished guests could eat and rest in their own quarters. Class distinctions apart, such facilities as there were at St. Gall were essentially for the monastic community, while visitors were offered shelter and hospitality.

Hospital facilities expanded radically from the eleventh through the fourteenth centuries. The Crusades were in part responsible, and crusading orders including the Knights of St. John of Jerusalem (later the Knights of Malta), the Knights Templar, and the Teutonic Knights built hospitals in Germany and throughout the Mediterranean world. Nonmilitary brotherhoods such as the Order of St. Anthony and the Order of the Holy Spirit were also noted for their contributions to hospital work. The latter order specialized in administration and by the fourteenth century was directing hospitals from Alsace in the west throughout Germany and Austria to Poland in the east. The Order of St. John of God appeared in Spain in the sixteenth century, building hospitals for the insane. This order was also active in northern Italy and southern France, but it made its largest contribution overseas, founding some 200 hospitals throughout the Spanish empire in the Americas.

Royal and noble families also contributed to

the growth. England's first hospital was built at York in 937 by Athelstan, a grandson of King Alfred the Great. Duke William of Normandy, who conquered England in 1066, founded hospitals at Cherbourg, Bayeux, Caen, and Rouen in France. Henry II was responsible for renovating the hospitals at Caen and Rouen and for promoting new building in and near Angers. Henry's work included some of the most beautiful hospital buildings of the Middle Ages.

Many specialized institutions were founded. Hostels for merchants and other travelers had been built since Roman days, but in the Middle Ages hordes of pilgrims passing to such holy shrines as Santiago de Campostela, Mont St. Michel, and St. Michael of Gargano required additional facilities. Hostels were built at crossroads and river fords, at bridges, and at the openings of mountain passes as well as in large towns. Some of these hostels became major hospitals, such as the Hôtel Dieu in Lyons.

In the twelfth and thirteenth centuries, when Europe was in the grip of a vast leprosy epidemic, hundreds of leper asylums, or leprosaria, were built. It has been estimated that in 1225 there were 19,000 leprosaria in Europe. These too were built on main roads or in major towns. A high wall would separate the leprosarium from the community, while small huts within provided accommodation for the lepers. As leprosy declined, the leprosaria were used for persons suspected of carrying infectious diseases, the insane, and even the indigent. Some thereby became hospitals. Thus the Hôpital des Petits Maisons near the monastery of St. Germain de Près outside Paris on the Sèvres road, which began as a leprosarium, was used later for indigent syphilitics and mentally disordered pilgrims. St. Giles-in-the-Fields, a hospital at the gates of London, was originally a leprosarium, as were the hospitals for incurables built between 1239 and 1327 on the four roads leading out of Nuremberg, Germany.

When the bubonic plague (q.v.) struck Europe in the fourteenth century, the leprosaria were the first plague hospitals. Lazarettos, or pesthouses, began to be built in the later years of the century, first as a measure for protecting trade and later to guard the city populations. The first documented pesthouse was built at Dubrovnik (Ragusa) on the Adriatic in 1377, and it was followed by the infirmaries of Marseilles in 1383. Venice built two lazarettos on islands in its lagoon, the first in 1423, the second in 1468. Milan completed a pesthouse 20 years later which was much studied and imitated, while the hospital of St. Sebastian, built in Nuremberg in 1498, became the model for other German plague hospitals, notably those at Augsburg and Ratisbon.

The common practice when medieval hospitals were endowed was for them to become church property and to be entirely administered by the church. In the thirteenth and fourteenth centuries, however, as guilds and town corporations took responsibility for financing hospitals, merchants and guild members retained powers of decision. In addition to showing the increasing strength and confidence of the merchant classes, secularization began a shift in the ideology of hospital care. The conviction grew that secular communities should provide health facilities, not because that was the road to salvation, but because it was essential for their stability and prosperity. Trading communities in particular found hospitals a necessary investment and built them in increasing numbers in the fourteenth and fifteenth centuries. Among the cities doing so were Venice, Pisa, Genoa, Augsburg, Ratisbon, Regensburg, Lüneburg, Lübeck, and in the east, Novgorod. There was also increased concern over medical staffing. Frankfurt-am-Main appointed a municipal surgeon in 1377 and a physician in 1381. Both were attached to the Holy Ghost Hospital and gave free treatment to city employees. In 1439, Holy Roman Emperor Sigismund issued a plan for hospital reform, the *Reformatio* Sigismundi, which recommended that a municipal physician be appointed in every town to attend the poor without charge. In 1486, Nuremberg used private donations to employ a hospital physician, and Strasbourg did the same in 1515. Finally, each of the five royal hospitals in London at the middle of the sixteenth century had a surgeon and a barber for "professional and technical attention."

European Hospitals to 1700 By the end of the sixteenth century, monarchs and municipalities had become the prime movers in hospital development. The problems they were to solve still concerned the poor, the displaced, the indigent, and the insane, but they had become vastly larger than three centuries before, and the spirit in which they were attacked was very different. Wars and rebellions, changes in land tenure, the rapid growth of towns, inflation, political instability, and religious conflict all contributed to uprooting thousands of people who became victims as well as bearers of a variety of diseases, and the institutions needed to deal with them had to be created.

The problem of the destitute was particularly acute in England, where Henry VIII's expropriation of monastic lands and church properties had destroyed the entire charitable system, including hospitals. From 1536 to 1544, there was no help of any kind in the city of London for indigent people. In desperation, the lord mayor and corporation petitioned the king to reestablish the city hospitals which the crown had taken. If the king would do so, the city would administer and support the institutions. The king agreed, and the royal hospitals were restored. In 1569, the City of London issued a declaration which asserted its determination to round up "all Idle, Begging people, whether Men, Women, or Children or other masterless Vagrants . . . to take them all up to dispose of them in some of the four Hospitals in London by the sixteen Beadles belonging to the same." Vagabonds and "sturdy beggars" went to Bridewell; the "aged, impotent, sick, sore, lame, or blind" went to St. Bartholomew's or St. Thomas', while children under 16 went to Christ's Hospital. St. Mary's of Bethlem, which had had a ward established for mental cases in the fifteenth century, was reserved for the insane. Ultimately St. Bartholomew's and St. Thomas', both of which had been built in the twelfth century, became the main refuge for the sick poor and remained so for 175 years.

England's development was peculiar in its emphasis on local solutions to the problems of the sick and indigent. In France, as in most continental European states, the central government took responsibility. In 1656 Cardinal Mazarin created the Hôpital Général in Paris. This, like the London hospital system a century earlier, was conceived to meet a whole family of social problems and was furnished with virtually unrestricted coercive powers. The general hospital was actually a governing board with several institutions available to it. Its clientele were old people, sufferers from venereal diseases, epileptics, and the insane. But the general hospital also dealt with able-bodied boys to the age of 25 who refused to work, with debauched girls, and, after 1690, with girls who were in danger of being debauched. Soon after its establishment, the general hospital had taken in some 6000 people, 1 percent of the contemporary population of Paris, and it remained active until the revolution. Its functions were only incidentally medical. Its stated purposes were to increase manufactures and provide productive work (there was a factory workshop); to punish willful idleness; to rid Paris of beggars and restore public order; to provide relief to the needy ill; to counter immorality and antisocial behavior; and to provide Christian instruction.

The London hospitals and the general hospital of Paris showed the evolution of the medieval concept of care into the secularized one of the sixteenth and seventeenth centuries. Though much larger and more administratively complex than their medieval predecessors, these institutions were similar in that social functions were fundamental, while treatment was of minor importance. A further change, however, was coming. Vesalian anatomy, William Harvey's circulation theory, and a growing interest in clinical medicine were giving hospitals a new significance. It was there that the actual sick could be observed, that medical applications of scientific discoveries could be made most conveniently, and that students could be taught. Bedside observation and teaching began in 1626 at Leyden and Utrecht, won support from leading English scientists including Sir Francis Bacon, and through the work of Hermann Boerhaave, the Leyden clinician and one of Europe's greatest teachers, gained a European following. Even so, the transformation of the hospital into a medical institution was not completed for another century and a half.

Origins of the Modern Hospital to 1850 Between 1700 and 1850, the foundations of the modern hospital system were established. The number of hospitals increased, the quality of medical practice improved, specialization advanced, and the emphasis shifted from care toward treatment and cure. The process was most rapid in England, whose eighteenth-century development was phenomenal, but by the middle of the nineteenth century most European societies as well as the United States had established a basic hospital system. The further development of the hospital into an institution which society accepted as fundamental to its health needs and the realization of the hospital's potential as the institutional catalyst in modern medical treatment occurred between 1850 and the outbreak of World War II.

Throughout the entire period of development, two contrasting systems for planning and financing hospitals appeared. In England and America, private funds and independent boards were the norm. On the Continent, central governments and public funds led the way. In the German states outside Austria, local princes and their administrations dealt with hospital development until 1871. After Germany's unification, a federal system was established in which the state governments played a leading role with the oversight of the central government.

The English private, or voluntary, hospital appeared in the early eighteenth century to provide care for people who either did not qualify for parish help or were aliens in English society. French Huguenots organized a private hospital on City Road, London, in 1718, just a year before the Charitable Society in Westminster was formed to offer care and shelter to those of London's sick poor and indigent who were ineligible for poor law assistance or who could not find places in the crowded wards of St. Bartholomew's and St. Thomas'. Other voluntary hospitals followed soon after. In 1724, Guy's Hospital was established under a bequest by Thomas Guy, a successful merchant and former governor of St. Thomas' Hospital who was concerned over the fate of the chronically ill and the incurable who were not accepted at either of the city's hospitals. He endowed his hospital to serve incurables, but the board of governors soon took advantage of ambiguities in his will to admit acute cases. Before the century was out, Guy's Hospital was refusing the incurables for whom it had been founded. Other hospitals established in this period included St. George's (1733), the London Hospital (1744), and special hospitals for smallpox, venereal diseases, women, and children. The voluntary system also produced hospitals outside London at Bristol (1733), York (1740), Exeter (1741), and Liverpool (1745). By 1760, there were 16 new hospitals outside London, and by 1800 most of the cities and large towns in Britain were furnished with a hospital.

In the American colonies, the first general hospital was founded in Philadelphia in 1751. Benjamin Franklin, who was pressed into service to encourage private subscriptions, found people reluctant to give, and the Pennsylvania General Hospital only became possible when the Assembly agreed to match £2000 from private subscription. Franklin appears to have invented the matching grant. The New York Hospital was established in 1773, burned down, was reconstructed, and then was used to quarter British troops. It was finally reopened in 1791. The Massachusetts General Hospital was founded in 1811, though it did not open until a decade later. These hospitals catered to the sick poor. Franklin's arguments for establishing the Pennsylvania hospital included the need to clear deranged persons from the street for their own good and the public's safety and the need to return workmen to a condition of vigor in order to gain their productive labor. The American hospitals served a social need, but their staffing with trained physicians as both house physicians and consultants showed an orientation from the beginning toward treatment and cure. The American hospitals reflected advanced English thinking and, in the case of the Pennsylvania hospital, exerted a critical influence on the development of American medicine in the late colonial period and after.

The brilliance of French medical scientists both before and after the revolution was unconnected with the state of hospitals or other institutions. Throughout much of the eighteenth century, the hospitals of Paris, notably the Hôtel Dieu, were in dreadful condition, but despite extensive damage by fire on two occasions, no significant reformation was undertaken. At the same time hospital reformers, activated by a humanitarian concern over the real suffering of those unfortunate enough to be hospitalized and convinced that an enlightened age had the means to relieve it, began to agitate for changes. John Howard, an English prison reformer who became interested in hospitals, was probably the person who did most to popularize reform ideas on the Continent. He was particularly emphatic about the need for cleanliness and fresh air to combat the deadly miasmic vapors which were thought responsible for illness, infection, and high mortalities.

When Louis XVI asked the French Academy of Sciences to look into hospital reform, one member, Jacques Tenon, not only read the English literature but visited England. He was particularly impressed with the Royal Naval Hospital at Plymouth and with the pavilion style of construction which permitted thorough ventilation. His plan for an entirely new hospital complex for Paris, completed in 1788, was founded on the English style. A more traditional plan had been presented two years earlier. Neither was realized. The revolution stopped all building projects, though the national assembly set up a commission to review French health services. Its report in 1794 stressed home care and ignored hospital development. Both the revolutionary governments and Napoleon made the ancient stock of buildings serve their needs, and no serious hospital program was begun until after 1815. The building which then took place, first in the provinces and finally in Paris, closely followed Tenon's prerevolution plans, culminating between 1846 and 1854 in one of the great hospitals of Europe, the Hôpital Riboisière.

Probably the most important eighteenth-century continental hospital was Vienna's Allgemeine Krankenhaus (general hospital), built by order of the emperor Joseph II in 1784. This hospital epitomized the Enlightenment absolutists' approach to medical care and public health through administrative centralization and rationalization of function. It also showed the growing conviction that hospitals were primarily institutions for treating sick people, while its provision to accommodate both the poor and paying patients struck a modern note. By far the largest part of its facilities, however, was for the poor. The hospital was planned for 1600 patients. It was divided into six medical, four surgical, and four clinical sections. Clinical facilities for teaching comprised 86 beds, divided among medicine, surgery and wound repair, and studies of the eye. The administration of the hospital was carried on by a director supported by an assistant director and a physician in charge of teaching functions. There were 6 physicians, 3 surgeons, 13 assistant physicians, and 7 assistant surgeons. This hierarchy did not evolve but was established by decree. In subsequent years, of course, it expanded.

The Allgemeine Krankenhaus was the centerpiece in a plan for hospital construction for the Hapsburg lands. The most important of the provincial hospitals was built at Prague (1789), with others at Laibach and Brünn (1786), Olmütz (1787), Linz (1788), and Lemberg (1789). Vienna's influence was also significant throughout other parts of Europe, appearing in a series of 100- to 200-bed hospitals built between 1784 and 1850. Among these, the Juliusspital at Wurzburg (1789–1793) was especially notable for its superb operating room using full north light. Padua's Ospedale Civile, itself of considerable importance for later hospital construction, was built on the Vienna model in 1798, as were hospitals in Zagreb (1804) and Trieste (1833–1841).

Vienna's influence was less important in the north. Berlin's Charité Hospital, which had a staff of practicing physicians and one of Europe's first operating rooms, was built in 1768, 14 years before the Allgemeine Krankenhaus. In the next century, Prussia's romantic monarch, Friedrich Wilhelm IV, attempted to embody the medieval ideal of loving Christian care in a modern hospital. The result was the crenelated and turreted Krankenhaus Bethanien in Berlin (1845–1847) in which nursing was provided by a semicloistered order under the aegis of the Lutheran church. This new gothic or romantic hospital style was also used at Aachen (1848–1855).

Hospital building in Russia in the eighteenth and early nineteenth centuries followed Vienna and Paris. The ideas of royal absolutism and centralized administration fitted the Russian autocratic tradition, and both public health in general and hospital development in particular remained primarily state matters. Catherine II (1762–1796), who was herself of German origin, promoted hospital construction, completing the famed Obuchov Hospital the same year that the Allgemeine Krankenhaus was finished. Here it was hospital organization which showed French and Austrian influence, while the building's architecture was modeled on an early-seventeenth-century plague hospital in Hamburg. Hospital construction expanded in the first half of the nineteenth century, especially under Nicholas I, and there was a substantial increase in institutions for special conditions, particularly eye problems. Though firmly rooted in European science, Russian medical development was limited by slow economic growth. Thus, despite having the largest population in Europe, the Russian empire was last among the major European states in both the number of hospitals and the number of beds per capita at the midpoint of the nineteenth century.

The Modern Era: 1850 and After By the middle of the nineteenth century, the institutional characteristics of the hospital were fixed. Architectural styles differed, but the insistence on maximum ventilation as the main defense against miasmal infection made the pavilion form the choice of progressive, reform-minded hospital builders. Their views were powerfully supported by Florence Nightingale's advocacy, based on her heroic work during the Crimean War (1854–1856). Florence Nightingale made her most important contribution in nursing (q.v.), but the dramatically low mortalities in her temporary barracks hospitals at Scutari made her a nearly irresistible influence on questions of hospital organization and architecture as well.

The Civil War (1861–1865) was also an important influence. Both sides built large temporary military hospitals which were considered models of organization and further proof for the "fresh air" thesis. Prussia and Russia took serious note of the American military hospitals and used the experience to good effect in the wars they fought between 1866 and 1878. The Prussian military hospitals were especially noteworthy in the Franco-Prussian War (1870–1871). Rudolf Virchow, the founder of cellular pathology and one of Germany's most influential scientists, was deeply impressed by American military hospitals, and he used their example to promote the open pavilion style and maximum fresh air for civilian hospitals. The Rudolf Virchow Hospital (1899–1903) in Berlin, the last of the major pavilion-style hospitals, is a memorial to the role he played.

The influence which British and American military hospitals exerted on hospital design had no comparable effect on hospital use. In the United States, hospital construction virtually halted with the last shot of the Civil War, and there was no attempt to apply the lessons learned about inexpensive hospital construction or efficient hospital management for nearly two decades. Society believed that hospitals were essential in wartime, but that their peacetime use, teaching and research apart, was to offer low-cost or free care to the poor. The hospital was still considered dangerous, and while the terrible sights and sounds which made eighteenth-century hospitals notorious had been moderated, a stay in the hospital remained an experience to be avoided. For those who could afford it, home care was considered safer and more comfortable, and the achievements of British, American, and German military medicine did little to change those attitudes.

The Hospital in Modern Times The reorientation of social attitudes toward hospitals and the hospital's movement to the center of modern medical practice resulted from scientific advances and rapid economic growth. The maturation of the European industrial economy in the middle and later nineteenth century and the formation of new industrial systems in the United States, Russia, and Japan provided the economic base. Concurrently, proofs for the germ theory of disease and the introduction of antiseptic methods reduced and finally ended the dangers of cross-infection and the terrible epidemics of hospital fever which had decimated patient populations before the middle of the nineteenth century. By the early twentieth century, anesthesias and antisepsis were turning surgery into a routine treatment for literally hundreds of conditions, but it was medical technology that made the hospital a necessity. Modern surgery requires an operating room; x-ray technology, which developed first as a diagnostic tool, has become a form of therapy requiring special instrumentation and facilities; while advances in biochemistry opened a wide variety of treatments and diagnostic tests which only a fully equipped laboratory could perform. In much the same way that manufacturing technology shaped the factories and shops necessary to its efficient use, medical technology influenced the development of the modern hospital.

In the early twentieth century, hospital facilities underwent a revolutionary expansion. This growth was nowhere more dramatic than in the United States. In 1873, the United States had only 178 hospitals and fewer than 50,000 beds, even including mental institutions. By 1909, these numbers jumped to 4359 hospitals with 421,065 beds; and in 1939 there were 6991 hospitals with 1,186,262 beds.

As hospital care expanded, the necessity for giving it public support and for introducing public controls grew as well. Most European hospitals were under some form of state control. The nationalization of British hospitals as part of the National Health Service after World War II brought public control to the country which originated the private hospital. Even in the United States, it has been estimated that two-thirds of the 1,670,000 beds available in 1965 were supported by city, county, state, or federal funds. On the other hand, in the United States, public authorities have relatively little control over hospital matters. Medical and health professionals have protected their rights of decision even where the hospitals are public.

Scientific medicine administered through hospitals has proved to be very costly. Publicly funded insurance and compensation plans and state-funded free medical care have helped to ease this problem in Europe. In the United States, private health insurance has been the favored method. It was estimated in 1962 that 141 million Americans had some form of health insurance, with at least 38 million Americans carrying major medical expense coverage. In addition, the Social Security Administration estimated in 1961 that one-third of the population, possibly 56 million people, were eligible for some medical or hospital care at government expense. The introduction of medicare in 1965 to provide hospital insurance for people 65 and over further enlarged the number of people eligible for help.

In the course of the 1970s, it became clear that private insurance protection against high hospital costs was inadequate, and the creation of a further national health insurance program has become a political issue. It is also widely believed, however, that insurance programs have underwritten the rising costs of hospital medicine while promoting unnecessary use of hospital facilities. At the same time, rising costs have produced cutbacks in hospital services as well as hospital closures, raising again the problem of accessibility to care for the poorest groups in society. Finally, the very size of modern hospitals, their increasingly bureaucratic organization, and the impersonal, technologically sophisticated treatments which they have developed have contributed a dehumanizing element to hospital care. Hospital medicine in the latter decades of the twentieth century has been responsible for major medical achievements, but it has also become part of important social and economic problems which require resolution.

ADDITIONAL READINGS: Brian Abel-Smith, *The Hospital: 1800–1948*, Cambridge, Mass., 1964; P. S. Codellas, "The Pantocrator, the Imperial Byzantine Medical Center of the XIIth Century A.D. in Constantinople," *Bulletin of the History of Medicine* 12 (July 1942): 390–410; Henry F. Dowling, *City Hospitals: the Undercare of the Underprivileged*, Cambridge, Mass., 1982; Eliot Friedson, *The Hospital in Modern Society*, New York, 1963; George E. Gash and John Todd, "Origins of Hospitals," in E. A. Underwood (ed.), *Essays on the Origin of Scientific Thought and Medical Practice Written in Honor of Charles Singer*, London, 1953; Grace Goldin, "Building a Hospital of Air: The Victorian Pavilion of St. Thomas' Hospital," *Bulletin of the History of Medicine* 49 (December 1975): 512–535; Louis S. Greenbaum, "Jean-Sylvain Bailly, the Baron de Breteuil, and the Four New Hospitals of Paris," *Clio Medica* 8 (Fall 1973): 261–284; Louis S. Greenbaum, "Measure of Civilization," *Bulletin of the History of Medicine* 49 (January–February 1975): 43–56; Sami Harmaneh, "The Development of Hospitals in Islam," *Journal of the History of Medicine* 17 (July 1962): 366–384; George Rosen, "Hospital," *Encyclopedia Americana* 14, New York, 1977, 439–443; George Rosen, "The Hospital: The Historical Sociology of a Community Institution," in *From Medical Police to Social Medicine: Essays on the History of Health Care*, New York, 1974; George Rosen, "Hospitals, Social Policy, and Medical Care in the French Revolution," in *From Medical Police to Social Medicine: Essays on the History of Health Care*, New York, 1974; Charles E. Rosenberg, "Inward Vision and Outward Glance: The Shaping of the American Hospital, 1880–1914," *Bulletin of the History of Medicine* 53 (Fall 1979): 346–391; David Rosner, *A Once Charitable Enterprise: Hospitals and Health Care in Brooklyn and New York, 1885–1915*, New York, 1982; Henry E. Sigerist, "An Outline of the Development of the Hospital," *Bulletin of the History of Medicine* 4 (July 1936): 573–581; John D. Thompson and Grace Goldin, *The Hospital: A Social and Architectural History*, New Haven, 1975; Morris Vogel, *The Invention of the Modern Hospital: Boston, 1870–1930*, Chicago, 1980; William H. Williams, *America's First Hospital: The Pennsylvania Hospital*, Wayne, Pa., 1976.

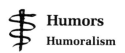

Humors

Humoralism

The doctrine of the humors was central to premodern European medicine. It originated in Greece at the end of the sixth century B.C., was first expressed systematically in the Hippocratic writings, took philosophical form with Aristotle, and became a definitive medical system with Galen's works in the second century A.D. Humoralism spread with Galen's influence throughout the Mediterranean world, Mesopotamia, and western Europe. The doctrine only began to decline in Europe in the late sixteenth or early seventeenth century, and it remained an influential mode of medical thought through the eighteenth and into the nineteenth century. Even today, doctrines emphasizing body fluids and their actions are often called humoral, and it has been suggested that ancient humoralism contained foreshadowings of such modern concepts as endocrine function and immune reaction.

The humoral pathology which appears in Hippocrates and Aristotle had a dual origin. Pre-Hippocratic physicians observed that the expulsion of body fluids often preceded a patient's improvement. There was also considerable interest in food and digestion. The idea followed that the by-products of digestion trapped within the body created some illnesses, while others, such as catarrh, resulted from organ discharges. These observations led to assigning such qualities as acid, salt, and sour to body fluids and linking those qualities to disease conditions. The second source of humoralism was Greek cosmology. All existence was thought to be composed of four basic elements: earth, air, fire, and water. Each element was endowed with a dominant and a subordinate quality. The qualities were hot, moist, cold, and dry. Thus fire was hot and dry; air was hot and moist; earth was cold and dry; while water was cold and moist. These elements and their qualities were found throughout nature, and in humans as well, where they were represented in four humors: blood, phlegm, black bile, and yellow bile. The humors probably derived from medical observations on body fluids. But to systematize those observations while making them compatible with the cosmology, the number of fluids was reduced to conform to the four elements and their qualities, a process entirely in harmony with the philosophical approach to physiology, pathology, and medicine.

The system was treated differently by different writers. The Hippocratic writers took the position that health and illness were functions of the balance among the elements, qualities, and humors. They argued the need for considering the particular balance which was most effective in each case, resisted any attempt to schematize diagnosis and treatment, and held that nature would attempt to restore balances where imbalances appeared. The physician could aid nature's action. Imbalances which ran contrary to nature, which reversed the idea of counterbalancing influence, were incurable. Cancers were a primary example of the latter. The Hippocratics were close enough to the older tradition of practical observation to stress the importance of correct diet. There are also indications that they viewed bodily fluids and humors as essentially the same thing.

The Hippocratic tradition synthesized an earlier generation's views with its own. Aristotle elaborated on the now-established humoral concept, stressed the purposiveness in the system, and created a philosophy for it. Galen and his successors continued in the Aristotelian direction while claiming to follow Hippocrates. Between Aristotle's writings in the fourth century B.C. and those of Galen in the second century A.D., humoralism emerged as a full-scale system of physiology, pathology, and therapeutics. Blood came to be considered the primary humor and a composite of all the humors. It was thought that a healthy mixture of elements, qualities, and humors was maintained by body heat, which was generated from the bloodless left ventricle of the heart. *Pneuma* ("air") together with *fuel* ("food and drink") were necessary for combustion, while the whole body system was penetrated by an all-embracing *physis* ("nature"), which directed body functions according to nature's laws. Disease occurred from imbalance in the humors, which thus became the main concern for therapy. The physician, as the Hippocratic writers said, was to aid nature in correcting such imbalances. Diet was very important. All foods were thought to contain elements which corresponded with the humoral qualities. They could be watery, phlegmatic, bilious, or blood elements. But Galen and the Moslem interpreters who followed him added a further idea of degrees, so that it was possible to assign a numerical designation to the potential effect of any edible substances on humoral qualities. Sugar, for example, was held to be cold in the first degree, warm in the second degree, dry in the second degree, and moist in the first degree. The system was used for compounding specifics to treat particular conditions, and it was widely followed in the Middle Ages. Paracelsus' "chemiatry" followed precisely the same reasoning in the sixteenth century, using chemical elements and qualities.

Organs with cavities such as the uterus, the heart, the bladder, and the kidneys were thought to attract and trap humors. Spongy structures such as lungs, spleen, and mammaries were believed to absorb humoral fluids from the surrounding tissues. Blood was not only the primary humor but the nutritive element which contributed to the formation and growth of organs, while the brain (Aristotle argued for the heart) was considered the center of the system and the agent of the soul. Humoral balance affected all aspects of life, including temperament. Personalities were defined as sanguinary, choleric, splenetic, or bilious, depending on which humor was ascendant.

Humoral theory provided a total view of the human being, human nature, and human ills. The system was complete, vigorous, and authoritative. As such, it paralleled medieval European and Islamic religious thought. Moreover, it provided approved and acceptable answers to questions concerning health, sickness, and physiological function. There was no basis for challenging this system until the work of sixteenth-century anatomists was absorbed and applied. Paracelsus' attack on Galen's authority suggested a chemical-empirical approach to body fluids, and William Harvey's description of how blood circulates proved Galen wrong. Humoralism was too deeply rooted to be overcome by one discovery, however major, and even when the system ceased to be used specifically, the vocabulary and many of humoralism's treatments remained in vogue. Nevertheless, humoral doctrine as it has been known earlier was transformed, and in the nineteenth century it was destroyed by basic studies on blood composition and the chemistry of body function, the establishment of cell theory, and the discovery of bacterial causes for disease. Descriptions of gland functions and hormonal secretions, studies on nutrition and deficiency diseases, and the problem of allergies and immunities invite a new humoral vocabulary. The content of that vocabulary would be very different, however, for while modern medicine knows the importance of body fluids, it does so in a radically changed physiological context from that of traditional humoralism.

ADDITIONAL READINGS: L. J. Rather, *The Genesis of Cancer: A Study in the History of Ideas*, Baltimore, 1978; Margaret S. Ogden, "Guy de Chauliac's Theory of the Humors," *Journal of the History of Medicine* 24 (July 1969): 272–291; R. Siegel, *Galen's System of Physiology and Medicine*, Basel, 1968; Owsei Temkin, *Galenism: Rise and Decline of a Medical Philosophy*, Ithaca, N.Y., 1973.

Hypnosis

"Hypnosis" is the term coined in 1842 by a Manchester surgeon, James Braid, to describe artificial somnambulism induced by scientific means. The word displaced "mesmerism" (q.v.) and "mesmeric trance," which had unfortunate associations with occultism and sensational popular science. Nevertheless, hypnotism developed directly out of mesmerism, and in the early nineteenth century both "mesmerism" and "animal magnetism" were terms used by writers referring to artificially induced trance states or sleep.

The mesmeric trance appeared as an early and accidental phenomenon in Dr. Franz Anton Mesmer's therapeutic practice, but it became centrally important. It was essential to the realization of his theory of "crisis," and since it was under the operator's control, it introduced an element of direction into the treatment. Two of Mesmer's leading French disciples, Charles Deslon and the Marquis de Puységur, recognized early that the trance state provided unique opportunities to mobilize the patient's will to aid his or her own cure, and that it was a psychological rather than a physiological phenomenon. Puységur induced trances, first accidentally, later intentionally, with no reference to the grotesque properties connected with "concentrating" animal magnetism; and even before Mesmer abandoned his practice after 1785, Puységur was collecting data on what he called "somnambulism." Puységur and later J. P. F. Deleuze developed a therapy which involved putting patients into a state of somnambulism and then encouraging them to act out their troubling symptoms. These men recognized that the "magnetized" (hypnotized) patient was susceptible to probing of the subconscious memory, but they considered such a procedure to be an intolerable invasion of the patient's "innermost self." Hence they promoted a relationship in which patients carried out their own treatment. This approach involved defining the subconscious probings and their results as a "masochistic catharsis," reinforced by a "sadistic" control over their magnetizer, which was achieved by the magnetizer's making himself available any time the patient demanded it to induce the trance condition.

The evolution of mesmerism into hypnotism took a considerable step forward in the work of a Portuguese monk, Abbé Faria, who wrote *On the Cause of Lucid Sleep* (1819). His theme was Puységur's somnambulism and the best methods for inducing it. Abbé Faria used Puységur's idea of concentration on a single idea or command which produced both boredom and fatigue while disposing the mind to rest on command. He was particularly interested in recalcitrant subjects, experimenting with different motions and objects to overcome their resistance. He induced hallucinations, experimented with posthypnotic suggestion, and devised hypnotic treatments for paralysis and blindness. Much of what Faria wrote is now part of hypnosis' received wisdom. His book was not widely disseminated in the early nineteenth century, however, and it was not rediscovered until the century's end. Alexander Bertrand, whose *Treatise on Somnambulism* (1823) was less advanced, was better known.

Though the specific issues were different, the history of hypnotism in England in the nineteenth century recapitulated mesmerism's history in France before 1789. While struggling unsuccessfully for scientific respectability, it achieved substantial popular success as part of spectacular medical-scientific demonstrations which were really public shows. Scientists quarreled furiously, reputations were ruined, the reading public was vastly entertained, but in the end, hypnotism failed to establish itself with the medico-scientific fraternity.

As popular science, hypnotism in England developed with phrenology, the "science" of reading character from the conformation of the skull. It was carried forward by John Elliotson, a respected physiologist who held an appointment at University College Hospital. Elliotson introduced phreno-mesmeric demonstrations into the hospital wards, published articles concerning his findings, and finally was forced to choose between his professorship and phreno-mesmerism. He chose phreno-mesmerism. Elliotson, like Charles Deslon in the previous century, gave the movement scientific respectability while influencing others who carried it along the scientific path. The most important of these followers was James Braid, whose *Neurypnology, or the Rationale of Nervous Sleep, Considered in Relation with Animal Magnetism* (1843) stressed the themes developed by Puységur, Faria, and Bertrand, especially those of concentration and suggestion. Braid argued that "hypnosis," this artificially induced sleep, could have an important therapeutic and diagnostic effect on nervous diseases and the study of psychological dynamics.

Hypnotism occurs in the mind. The hypnotist could induce a trance by having his subject concentrate on a single object, but Braid found that he could also hypnotize the blind, and he concluded that "it is not so much the optic as the sentient motor and sympathetic nerves and the mind, through which the impression is made." It was this aspect which was carried back to France by Ambroise Auguste Liébault, whose work built on that of Braid. Liébault trained Hypolyte Bernheim, and these two clinicians established the Nancy school of hypnotic study. Its rival was Charcot's clinic in Paris.

Though the word for hypnotism came from England, and James Braid greatly advanced the subject, modern scientific hypnotism was defined by Liébault and Bernheim. Hypnotic sleep was like ordinary sleep. It meant no special powers, it opened no doors into a magical or occult world, it generated neither clairvoyance, precognition, nor telepathy. It did mean, however, control over the subject which, though hardly absolute, enabled the hypnotist to direct the subject's behavior in the trance and after it. Suggestion was the key. The mind was thought to be passive and under the hypnotist's control. In the trance state, the mind was thought to know only what the hypnotist placed there, and his last suggestion dominated. The subject was thought incapable of taking any action until the hypnotist provided the idea.

Jean Martin Charcot, at the Salpêtrière clinic in Paris, challenged the views of the Nancy school, arguing that the hypnotic state was abnormal. He called it "an artificially caused morbid condition," and in his *Lessons on Illnesses of the Nervous System* (1880–1883) he identified this disease as possessing three stages: lethargy, catalepsy, and somnambulism. The last found the patient in a state of suggestibility. It was Charcot's conclusion that only potential or actual hysterics were susceptible to hypnosis. Bernheim successfully rebutted Charot's views in his own *Suggestive Therapeutics: A Treatise on the Nature and Uses of Hypnotism* (1888), in which he drew on a mass of recorded clinical observations of hypnotics. The Nancy view that hypnotic sleep was not pathological and was not analogous to hysteria prevailed, even at the Salpêtrière.

It also revealed a more complex idea of the mind and its functioning than had been known hitherto. Different levels of personality appeared, as under hypnosis persons behaved differently than in their waking lives. This led Pierre Janet to describe in his *Mental State of Hystericals* (1892) a concept which he called "dissociation." He envisaged aggregates of "ideas" clustered around some dominant idea yet dissociated from the conscious mind. Such dissociated ideas could create maladjustments while remaining below the level of consciousness. Janet used hypnotism to uncover and treat such dissociated phenomena. In this same area, hypnotism helped to reveal multiple personalities. Morton Prince, in his *Dissociation of Personality* (1906), recorded one woman who had four clearly defined personalities. He identified and attacked the problem with hypnotism. Sigmund Freud, the founder of psychoanalysis, had studied with Charcot and Bernheim and translated the *Suggestive Therapeutics* into German. Freud used hypnotism in his early work, but he shifted to free association as a more effective approach.

Hypnotism developed over the nineteenth century from roots in mesmerism. By the end of the century it was firmly established in the burgeoning field of psychological studies, with special affinities for psychoanalysis. Yet hypnosis never entirely escaped its origins. Its associations with occult practices on the one side and the carnival sideshow on the other, have rendered it suspect and limited its development as a modern tool. People's fears that the hypnotist could force them to commit acts which their conscious minds reject have added to the difficulty of using hypnosis in any general way. Its value as an anesthetic which permits control over physical shock is recognized, but it is only sparsely used this way. Most, though not all, therapists prefer other methods. Thus while hypnotism developed at the same time as other major medical and scientific ideas, its potential for medicine has never been developed.

ADDITIONAL READINGS: Vincent Buranelli, *The Wizard from Vienna: Franz Anton Mesmer,* New York, 1976; Robert Darnton, *Mesmerism and the End of the Enlightenment in France,* Cambridge, Mass., 1968; Eric J. Dingwall, *Abnormal Hypnotic Phenomena: A Survey of Nineteenth Century Cases,* 4 vols., London, 1967–1968; Henri F. Ellenberger, *The Discovery of the Unconscious,* New York, 1970; Fred Kaplan, "The Mesmeric Mania: Early Victorians and Animal Magnetism," *Journal of the History of Ideas* 35 (October–December, 1974): 691–702; Maurice M. Tinterow, *Foundations of Hypnosis: From Mesmer to Freud,* Springfield, Ill., 1970; Lancelot Law Whyte, *The Unconscious Before Freud,* New York, 1978.

See also MESMERISM; PHRENOLOGY; PSYCHIATRY.

Immunology

Immunology, the systematic study of the way living bodies protect themselves against invasion by other bodies, is a discipline scarcely a century and a quarter old. It was born with bacteriology in the second half of the nineteenth century, and it has only achieved maturity as a body of scientific knowledge in the last four decades. The idea that the body has powers to protect and cure itself is much older, reaching back to the earliest medical writing, while the reality of immunity goes to the beginnings of life itself. Natural defense against disease-causing microorganisms was a necessary condition for successful survival. Humankind, in common with other life forms, possesses such a system, but we have only begun to understand it.

The idea that immunity from certain diseases could be induced long antedated the discovery of the immune system, and it was very limited in application. Inoculation against smallpox is the most obvious example. Following success with smallpox, the inoculation principle was tried with other diseases, notably syphilis, but to no good effect. Interest in the procedure then languished until Louis Pasteur, who was familiar with it, made some accidental observations which led him to study specific immune reactions. Pasteur's work on chicken cholera, anthrax, and rabies contributed directly to the development of immunology.

Anthrax is an acute infectious disease in animals, particularly cattle and sheep, which causes septicemia and produces very high rates of mortality. It affects human beings as a kind of skin disease, characterized by malignant pustules. It can occur in the lungs (wool-sorters' disease) and occasionally in intestines. In the nineteenth century, anthrax was epidemic in agricultural France and Germany, producing heavy annual losses. Preliminary steps toward controlling this disease began with a review of the cowpox-smallpox issue, and at least one person, Henri Toussaint of the Veterinary School at Toulouse, worked on a vaccine for sheep from anthrax-infected blood. Pasteur was familiar with the debate and this work, and he later used some of Toussaint's methods in his preparation of cultures.

In 1879 and 1880, Pasteur was working actively

to find the cause for chicken cholera, a disease very nearly as damaging economically as anthrax. The two campaigns became related when, by chance, Pasteur used a colony of cholera-causing microbes which was two weeks or more old to infect healthy birds. There was no disease. He then, for reasons still unclear, injected some healthy birds with a new culture and treated other birds with both the old and the new. Those injected only with the new culture fell ill; those injected with both remained healthy. Without being able to explain the phenomenon, Pasteur had found the means to protect chicken flocks against cholera. He then applied the same principle to anthrax. Using Koch's recently isolated anthrax bacillus, he began to experiment with different time periods and environments to identify the means to attenuate the bacillus effect and finally succeeded in producing an effective vaccine. In May 1881, he arranged a public demonstration. On May 5, he injected 24 sheep, 1 goat, and 6 cows with living attenuated vaccine, leaving a similar number of like animals without injection. He gave the test animals a further and stronger injection on May 17, and on May 31, all animals were given a highly virulent anthrax culture. By the night of June 2, all the control sheep and the goat were dead; the cows were bloated and ill. The vaccinated animals had no symptoms, though one died the next day. The cause was a complicated pregnancy, not anthrax. The experiment was a complete success, but more importantly, it suggested the possibility of preparing effective vaccines against all so-called infective diseases by attenuating the infective agent.

Pasteur's discovery of a vaccine for rabies (q.v.) greatly strengthened that conclusion. Centers for rabies protection sprang up throughout Europe and Latin America, and while variations on the Pasteur method were used widely to prevent a rabies attack, rabies vaccination for pets became a standard preventive practice.

Pasteur's critically important work was followed almost at once by the discovery of the toxin-antitoxin reaction in diphtheria and tetanus (qq.v.). Friedrich Loeffler's thesis that the diphtheria microorganism produced a diphtheria toxin was proved by Pierre Paul Émile Roux in 1888. Carl Fraenkel showed not only that heat-killed diphtheria bacilli could be injected without harm into susceptible animals but also that animals so treated would resist wild diphtheria infections. Fraenkel was one of Robert Koch's assistants, as were Emil von Behring and Shibasaburo Kitasato, who found a toxin-antitoxin reaction in tetanus (q.v.). Von Behring and Kitasato used the word "antitoxin" in describing what occurred, and their findings, together with Fraenkel's, were published on December 3, 4, and 11, 1890. The greater range of von Behring's and Kitasato's work justifies their designation as the discoverers of antitoxic immunity.

Important as this work was, it would have remained a series of highly successful adventures if comparable developments in physiology and biochemistry had not occurred to provide a context. The basic question was why immunization actually worked, but that question opened the larger puzzle of immunity in general. Was the body capable of protecting itself, and if so, what were its defenses? The answers offered began with the circulatory system and divided into a "humoral" school of interpretation and a "cellular" school. The humoral school held that there was resistance to disease within the body, and that there were bactericidal properties in the blood. This thesis was propounded in 1888 by George Nuttall, who was able not only to show bacteria-killing properties but also to demonstrate the limits on their action.

Élie Metchnikoff began working in 1884 on a cellular theory which he published in "Lessons in the Comparative Pathology of Inflammations" (1892). Metchnikoff's career had begun in Russia, but he became subdirector of the Pasteur Institute in Paris in 1887, and he remained there. He developed the idea that there were special cells in the blood, which he called phagocytes (cell eaters), which attacked foreign matter. There were two types of cell: the macrophages, which were large, mononuclear cells in blood and tissue; and the microphages, which were polymorphonuclear leukocytes in the blood. Metchnikoff showed not only that one special kind of macrophage, the white cell, or granulocyte, ate bacteria, but also that the number of these white cells increased when infection occurred anywhere in the body. Metchnikoff's views were clearly a beginning point for explaining immune response.

By 1900, scientists had identified both a cellular and a serum system. Robert Koch's work on tuberculin brought up a third: a group of smaller, light-staining white cells which were clearly different from the larger, dark-staining white granulocytes. These were called lymphocytes. In fact, it was becoming apparent not only that there was an immune system, but also that it was composed of several elements which worked together. For example, granulocytes of immunized animals were more efficient as bacteria killers than those of nonimmunized animals. Moreover, immunization made blood, without any white cells, able to "clump" bacteria together, thus making them more vulnerable to white cell attack. At the same time, some types of immunization set off violent antagonisms, demonstrating that the immune system would react to anything which appeared to be incompatible. The reasons for this lay with the chemistry of immunization, an area which Paul Ehrlich was exploring.

One of the truly seminal minds of the early twentieth century, Paul Ehrlich was a man whose work, as Robert Muir has said, found its core in "the question of the relation of chemical substances, natural or synthesized, to animal cells." Ehrlich made his primary contributions to immunity theory between 1891 and 1903, elaborating a view which, though qualified, remains fundamental to immunology today. One technical problem Ehrlich worked on was that of establishing a system for standardizing dosages of diphtheria antitoxin. Wide variations in effectiveness brought the entire procedure of immunizing against diphtheria into question, especially in England. Ehrlich found the problem in the unstable character of diphtheria toxin, which could lose virulence rapidly. Since standards were set by measuring the amount of antitoxin necessary to neutralize toxin, instability introduced a variable which resulted in enormous differences in the effectiveness of the antitoxins. In solving this problem, Ehrlich laid down a series of important assertions. He pointed out that each molecule of toxin combines with a single and inalterable amount of antitoxin and therefore a standard definition is possible. Moreover, the toxin-antitoxin connection involves complementary groups of atoms whose fit is similar to that of a key in a lock, while the cells' production of antibodies involves the "enhancement of a normal cell function" rather than the production of any new molecules. Nonlethal toxin doses stimulate and intensify the normal defensive reaction. Tetanus toxin seeks out and becomes bound to the cells of the central nervous system, attaching itself to the chemical "side-chains" on the cell protoplasm, thus blocking the side-chains' physiological function. This blockage leads the cell to produce fresh side-chains to compensate for what is blocked, but the production is more than what has been destroyed, and the excess is sloughed off. These are the antibodies produced by toxin action, or as Ehrlich defined them, "side-chains of the cell protoplasm which have been produced in excess and therefore thrust off." He also noted that there was no necessary relationship between toxin's neutralizing power and toxicity. Tetanus toxin which was wholly harmless still energized the production of antitoxins which rendered the injected animal immune to large doses of wild toxin. He called the combination of a modified toxin with antitoxin "toxoid," a substance giving protection against a possible inoculation infection as well as generating immunity.

Though Ehrlich's side-chain effect was the product of laboratory study, he held it as a theory and spent years arranging new evidence to fit it. Jules Bordet, the Belgian scientist whose studies on hemolysis were a further major contribution to early immunological studies, sharply criticized Paul Ehrlich for taking theory, even hypothesis, for fact, and for vastly overcomplicating the explanation of how the system functioned in the name of working out the side-chain theory. Bordet believed, for example, that there was a single complement which clumped or agglutinated bacteria, whereas Ehrlich postulated a complement for each separate invasive toxin. In fact, on this as on much else, Ehrlich was partially though not entirely right, as the complement factor in the immune system actually involves nine different complements. Ehrlich's basic ideas concerning bonding and chemical affinity, including the recognition of foreign or dangerous entities, have remained as conceptual foundations for modern immunology, though new evidence has forced substantial changes in particular aspects of his doctrines. His contribution was such, however, that he deserves to be called the originator of modern immunology, as he is the founder of modern chemotherapy. Ehrlich's immunology studies won him a Nobel prize in medicine in 1908.

At the beginning of World War I, immunology had developed to the point where the complexity of the defense was coming to be clear. The role of phagocytes had been clearly demonstrated, with granulocytes, leukocytes, and lymphocytes all identified. Serum defense was clearly indicated by research on both bacteriolytic and hemolytic functions, while the role of complement in agglutination added a further dimension. Successful antitoxins for diphtheria and tetanus had been created, while vaccines for controlling a variety of diseases were in process of development. Preventive vaccination was successful against cholera, bubonic plague, and typhoid; rabies vaccination was coming to be accepted; and the search for further protective substances moved on. Among the most enthusiastic supporters of inoculation therapy was Almroth Wright, in whose Inoculation Division at St. Mary's Hospital, London, treatment vaccines were prepared for each patient from the patient's own infective bacteria. At the very least, Wright's work spurred studies in bacteriology; at the best it provided relief for hundreds of patients. Opinion remains divided on the actual value of this work.

One further area of fruitful work came through the efforts of Theobald Smith at Harvard and Charles Richet in Paris, who called attention to the dangerous reactions which the immune system fostered. Smith noticed that guinea pigs being used for testing diphtheria antitoxin often became ill when long periods intervened between injections. Richet, following up on work begun by François Magendie earlier in the nineteenth century, injected dogs with protein from another animal. The first injection produced hypersensitivity, and a second foreign protein injection would kill the animal. Richet called this reaction "anaphylaxis." It was valuable for explaining certain human reactions to injections with various serums. Serum sickness and the sensitivity it suggested were important for broadening understanding of allergies.

In the years between World War I and World War II, immunology became a modern science. The controversy over priority in effect among different elements in the defense system was settled. In 1925, Hans Zinsser showed conclusively that any infection would mobilize the whole of the defense system, and it became clear that phagocytes, serum factors, antibodies, and complements were interactive and reinforcing rather than competitive. Twelve years later, the disease-resistant element in blood serum was identified and classified. The active elements were found to be proteins whose varying electrical characteristics permitted them to be separated and classified according to the speed of their reactions to electrical impulse. Three groups were found, which were called alpha, beta, and gamma globulin. This classification was further refined in subsequent years. The immune reactions concentrated in the gamma globulin fraction; none appeared in alpha or beta. The serum factor in gamma globulin was produced in response to attack by foreign elements and was called "antibodies," which were now separable from all other blood proteins. It was then established (1948) that antibodies were produced by special cells in bone marrow and the lymph nodes called plasma cells, and this was further refined by the conclusion that they arose from lymphocytes. By 1962, the full character of antibodies was known, including what they are, of what they are made, how they work, and especially how they improve the efficiency of granulocytes and lymphocytes.

Throughout much of its history, the immune system has been viewed piecemeal, with the system being the sum of its parts. Each major structure could be located: granulocytes and macrophages came from bone marrow; the liver was the source for complement and properdin; plasma cells produced antibodies; lymphocytes derived from lymph nodes. Robert A. Good showed that there was an integrative factor which linked the whole together: the lymphocytes. This interpretation only became possible when radioactive tracking techniques permitted the lymphocytes to be labeled and followed. Their course was not random; it was a specific route traveled at high speed, in the course of which foreign bodies (antigens) would be recognized and an immediate response started by contact with the nearest lymph node. Lymphocytes live for years (in some cases as long as the body), and they come, as Good showed, from the few primitive cells lining the embryonic yolk sac at the start of embryonic development. Antigens are recognized by surface characteristics—it makes no difference whether they are alive or dead. Once the structure has been recognized, the immune response is triggered. The body responds to antigens in foreign cell walls. Immunity is conferred by the presence of antibodies following an attack, and by their being present to destroy the same type of attacker before it has the opportunity to develop and cause disease.

Immunology contributes significantly to disease control, to study of allergies, and to understanding of hypersensitive responses to foreign proteins and conditions generated within the body itself. Such reactions are significant for rheumatic heart disease, arthritis, and rheumatism and may offer a new and vitally important approach to cancer. Sir Frank Macfarlane Burnet has suggested an immune surveillance failure as a factor in cancer. The argument is still in its hypothetical stage, but there is some suggestive evidence. Aging is destructive of immune reaction, a demonstrated fact, and cancers occur most frequently in the older population. Moreover, young people who have had their immune systems suppressed in order to tolerate organ transplants contract cancer at a rate over 100 times higher than the expected rate for their age group, and the cancers which occur are precisely the types which occur in older people.

The importance of the immune system has been recognized by cancer specialists, and steps have been taken to enlist its aid in future cancer therapies as well as in preventive measures. Correlations have been established between severe bacterial infections which activate a strong immune response and cancer regression, while the use of bacillus Calmette-Guérin (BCG) injections, which stimulate immune response, has had some positive effect on cancer. Immunology has by no means achieved a definitive understanding of the defensive system with which the body protects itself, and an important key to the current riddle of cancer may well yet be discovered.

ADDITIONAL READINGS: William R. Clark, *The Experimental Foundations of Modern Immunology,* New York, 1980; H. F. Dowling, *Fighting Infection: Twentieth Century Conquests,* Cambridge, Mass., 1977; W. D. Foster, *A History of Medical Bacteriology and Immunology,* London, 1970; Ronald J. Glasser, *The Body Is the Hero,* London, 1977; Margaret J. Manning and Rodney J. Turner, *Comparative Immunology,* New York, 1976; Sir Peter Bryan Medawar et al., *An Introduction to Immunology,* New York, 1977; J. H. Parish, *History of Immunization,* London, 1965; Charles Singer and E. Ashley Underwood, *A Short History of Medicine,* 2d ed., London, 1962; 409–445; 731–740.

See also ALLERGY; CANCER; INOCULATION; RABIES.

Influenza

Influenza is an acute infectious respiratory disease caused by viruses. There have been regular worldwide outbreaks of influenza involving millions of people, and the years 1918 and 1919 saw high mortality rates as well. The reasons for that unusually virulent epidemic are still debated, and though the causal agents which produce influenza have been identified, there is a great deal concerning its etiology and epidemiology which is still obscure. In its usual forms, influenza is briefly incapacitating, debilitating, and uncomfortable. It is most dangerous for predisposing its victims to pneumonia, and mortality in influenza epidemics is greatest in older age groups with a lower capacity to resist pneumonia and among people with chronic respiratory problems or weakened hearts. Though not especially significant demographically, influenza epidemics in modern societies are disruptive and cause substantial economic loss.

The Disease Several viruses cause influenza. Influenza virus A (1933) and B (1940) account for most known flu outbreaks. Virus C, which is not related immunologically to A or B, is still relatively unknown. Virus A is associated with highly infective epidemics recurring in two-year cycles. The A strain, which is related to the virus causing influenza in swine, is commonly thought to have been responsible for the 1918 pandemic. B virus is more likely to be found in sporadic, localized outbreaks which occur at irregularly longer intervals. It also spreads less rapidly in a community. Influenza viruses are unstable and prone to mutation and vary greatly in virulence. Moreover, they are RNA viruses composed of eight "pieces," each of which is separately coded. The pieces rearrange themselves in response to each other and to the host cell in which they lodge. This means that influenza viruses will produce at least 160 different antigenic combinations, a fact which by itself makes the production of an effective general vaccine extremely unlikely.

The first strain of A virus to be identified was called WS, the initials of the researcher studying it. Within a year, the WS strain gave way to a strain called PR8, which then remained the dominant A strain from 1934 to 1946, when the strain called A-prime (A1) appeared. This strain is still important, but it shares ground with the Asian strain (A2), which was identified in 1957. One major variant on influenza virus B was isolated on Taiwan in 1962. The varieties are significant because the reactions in the host are always specific to the particular infecting virus, and immunity to one type of flu virus does not confer immunity to the others. Moreover, the duration of any given immunity is unpredictable.

Flu virus may be communicated from person to person in droplets of moisture from the respiratory tract. However, direct communication cannot account for simultaneous outbreaks of influenza in widely separated places. It is thought that chains of mild infections, or possibly animal reservoirs, may explain what happens to the virus during interepidemic periods. There are no definitive data on this point, nor on the related point of what activates the virus. It has been argued that cold, inclement weather or a shock to the host's system may play a part. A further explanation will undoubtedly be found in the complex relationships among viruses, bacteria, and hosts. Those relationships are only partially understood at present.

Most authorities agree that influenza recurs in periodic waves which vary with the viral strains involved. Influenza epidemics usually begin with a rise in the number of sporadic cases, followed by a mild general infection, and then by a period of severe infection, which finally gives way to a period of decline. The pandemics of the period 1889–1893 were preceded by nearly 40 years of relative quiet and were followed by another trough of disease activity before the onset of the devastating outbreaks of 1918 and 1919. A similar period of decline set in after 1920, and though epidemic peaks were reached in 1957, 1971 and 1972, and 1975, it is generally agreed that the world is still in a quiescent period after the peak of 1918 and 1919.

There is no specific treatment for influenza, though antibiotics are effective against secondary bacterial infections, and two promising synthetic drugs are in the experimental stage. Amantadine and its derivative rimantadine have shown antiviral characteristics, while a third, isoquinoline, is the first drug known to affect influenza virus B. The World Health Organization's Influenza Center has been effective in diagnosing and charting influenza outbreaks and consulting on the preparation of vaccines. Specific groups in limited areas have been protected against influenza, but there is no general immunizing procedure, and there is no way to halt a developed influenza outbreak. The most important achievements in the influenza field have been in virology and epidemiology, though it is also there that the most pressing questions remain to be answered.

History Influenza is difficult to trace in history because it lacks a well-defined diagnostic image. Its clinical symptoms are similar to those of many other common diseases, and before its causal agents were identified the existence of an epidemic was essential to justify giving the name "influenza" to an outbreak of disease with fever, aching joints, cough, and respiratory involvement. Influenzalike conditions are described in the medical classics, but the descriptions are too general for specific attribution.

Most authorities consider sixteenth-century accounts to be the first to give sufficiently precise information to identify influenza certainly, though August Hirsch dated a recognizable influenza outbreak in 1173 and claimed to find sources describing influenza in the fourteenth and fifteenth centuries. There were at least 20 influenza epidemics in sixteenth-century Europe, with particularly widespread outbreaks occurring in 1510, 1557, and 1580. The 1580 outbreak became the world's first recorded pandemic.

Influenza reached the new world in the seventeenth century. In 1647, John Winthrop described the first influenzalike epidemic in the North American colonies. This outbreak moved from the mainland to the islands of St. Christopher's and Barbados in the West Indies, where it was far more severe than in New England, killing between 5000 and 6000 people. Reports of the disease continued in the eighteenth century. During the epidemic of 1732 and 1733, Dr. John Huxham introduced the word "influenza," Italian in origin, into the English medical vocabulary. Influenza previously was popularly known under literally dozens of names, ranging from the "jolly rant" and the "new acquaintance" to "febrile catarrh" and "la grippe."

Despite occasionally severe epidemics, none of influenza's names suggested a particularly dangerous disease. Death tolls were commonly light, and though the disease was ubiquitous, before

1918 influenza lacked the terrible associations of the great killer plagues. The people who died of flu were usually the old or the very young, and because both groups were extremely vulnerable in high-mortality societies, their deaths had only a minimal impact. Thus, though influenza continued to be active through the eighteenth century and into the nineteenth, administrators and physicians made little of it. Even the epidemic outbreaks in the last two decades of the nineteenth century aroused little interest or concern. Other diseases were more important. Against this background of complacent acceptance, the deadly Spanish influenza of 1918 and 1919 was as unexpected as it was unwelcome.

Pandemic: 1918 to 1920 The influenza epidemic which exploded around the world in 1918 and 1919 was uncharacteristic both in its high mortality and in the radical change in mortality profile which it created by claiming large numbers of victims among young adult males. The epidemic appeared in three waves. The first was mild and attracted little attention. The second, which began in the latter part of August 1918, was very different. The first outbreaks came in places separated by thousands of miles: Freetown, Sierra Leone; Brest, the French port of debarkation for the American expeditionary forces; and Boston, Massachusetts. It was estimated that two-thirds or more of Sierra Leone's population contracted flu, and more than 1000 people died in Freetown and its environs alone. Hospital records from Brest show 1350 flu admissions between August 22 and September 15, and 370 people died. In Boston, the incidence may have been as high as 10 percent of the city's population; and of those reported to be influenza patients, between 60 and 70 percent died. Influenza spread rapidly among American soldiers at bases in the United States and abroad. At Camp Devens, Massachusetts, for example, the first influenza diagnosis was made on September 12. Six days later there were 6674 cases, and on September 23, the number had reached 12,604.

Epidemic influenza was a familiar disease. What made the 1918 outbreak so terrible was the rapidity with which influenza developed into pneumonia and the secondary complications, and the mortality that followed. At Camp Devens, Massachusetts, when the influenza count passed 12,600 cases on September 23, there were already 727 cases of pneumonia, and by the time the records were brought up to date four days later, the total had passed 1900. Pneumonia developed rapidly, with death coming often within 48 hours of the first signs of illness. Eyewitnesses described men wrapped in blankets waiting for medical treatment who were turning blue as their lungs filled; in the camp morgue, bodies "the color of slate" were scattered about the floor or "stacked like cordwood." Postmortem examinations showed swollen blue lungs filled with "thin, bloody, frothy fluid." These victims had died so rapidly that there had been no time for the degeneration of lung tissue into a heavy, liverlike texture. William Henry Welch, a leading pathologist and physician who had been sent to Camp Devens to manage the outbreak, could find no consolidation of lung tissue; yet the lungs were so abnormal that when pieces were placed in water, they sank instead of being buoyant. The most notable aspect of these cadavers was the vast quantity of thin, bloody fluid, which oozed from sectioned lungs, mixed with air in the passages leading to the throat to produce a bloody froth, and poured from the nose or soaked through body wrappings. Still living victims, apart from displaying the blue color and feverish aches associated with flu, coughed bloody sputum and bled freely at the nose.

Better preparation could have avoided the chaos which greeted Colonel Welch, but the disease which attacked Camp Devens repeated its depredations over the next several months on a rapidly increasing scale. This pneumonic influenza—some authorities thought it similar to pneumonic plague—was as deadly a pestilence as any western society had suffered in the modern era, and its effects on the most advanced societies were notable. By October 1918, some 20 percent of the U.S. Army was ill. By the time the epidemic ended, 24,000 soldiers had died of flu. Battle casualties were 34,000. Twenty-eight percent of the civilian population in the United States contracted influenza. This estimate corresponds with military figures on incidence as well as with reports from Scandinavia and Great Britain. The mortality in the United States for the epidemic period stood at 527 per 100,000. For England and Wales, the comparable figure was 680. Death rates in American cities were higher. Using 1000 of population as the base, the rates went from New York's low of 60 to Philadelphia's high of 158. Boston (100), Washington, D.C. (109), and Baltimore (148) fell in between.

Mortality statistics are more reliable than figures on incidence, but even mortality figures are subject to distortion. The flu struck a world prostrated by war, and for many major countries, there are no reliable figures at all. The extent to which influenza contributed to social disorder at the end of World War I needs systematic study; on the other hand, political and social instability brought about the collapse of public health administration in many countries and significantly reduced their capacity to deal effectively with disease. As a result, the impact and the consequences of the influenza pandemic at the end of World War I are epidemiologically and historically obscure in many parts of the world. The record was further muddled because in many countries influenza was not a reportable disease, and deaths from pneumonia were tabulated separately.

The net effect of these considerations was a considerable underreporting of influenza deaths. How serious or significant underreporting was remains uncertain, and the effort to compensate for it has undoubtedly produced distortion and exaggeration. Even so, some points stand out. Notable among these is that India suffered more heavily from influenza than any nation in the world. The mortality rate there approached 4000 per 100,000 of population, and the absolute number of deaths has been conservatively estimated at 12 million, though numbers as high as 30 or 40 million have been suggested. The worldwide death toll for influenza has been set at 22 million, but this figure is undoubtedly low. American mortality figures for the epidemic period are relatively reliable. They show a total of 675,000 influenza deaths. Normal mortality for the period would have been 125,000; hence influenza was responsible for an excess of 550,000 deaths.

While influenza's social effects in a period of massive upheavals have yet to be studied, it does not appear that the disease was of major military consequence. General Lüdendorff was inclined to blame the first influenza wave at least in part for Germany's failure to reach the English Channel in July 1918. There is as yet no detailed evidence to support his conviction, but it does seem clear that all armies were affected in some degree by the disease. In May, 10 percent of the complement of the British Grand Fleet reported ill with flu, and a month later, the British command postponed an offensive at La Becque because of influenza. At the epidemic's peak, the French were evacuating between 1500 and 2000 flu cases a day from their positions at Soissons and Rheims. At Belleau Wood, flu was widespread among German forces, while the Americans, though not reporting flu, were affected by severe diarrhea. In none of these instances, however, did influenza become a determining factor, though it surely added to the misery of already miserable men.

Governments considered flu a minor obstacle, a problem to be solved in the course of winning the war. In the United States, despite flu's acknowledged contagiousness, mass bond rallies, parades, and demonstrations were held. The war effort had priority. On the other hand, flu appears to have produced little of the hysteria associated with other deadly epidemics. People seemed to ignore influenza while putting their energies into patriotic demonstrations and war work.

Influenza epidemics similar to the outbreak of 1918 and 1919 recurred during the 1920s, though with a declining virulence, and by the end of the decade, the Spanish influenza appeared to be finished. Swine flu, which appears first to have showed itself in the epidemic, returned annually to kill thousands of hogs in the American middle west; and after the first influenza viruses were isolated in 1933, several broad periods of infection were charted over the 1930s and 1940s. Flu has continued in broad outbreaks since World War II, but nothing comparable to the Spanish influenza epidemic has appeared. In 1975 and 1976, public fears were aroused in the United States that a swine flu outbreak was imminent which threatened a recurrence of the influenza outbreak of 1918 and 1919. The U.S. government under President Gerald Ford attempted to develop a vaccination program to ward off the threat, but the program collapsed under overwhelming immunological and logistical problems. Fortunately, the anticipated epidemic did not materialize.

The Study of Influenza Influenza was among the diseases attacked by the first generation of bacteriologists in the late nineteenth century. In 1890, R. F. Pfeiffer, using Robert Koch's techniques, identified a bacillus called *Haemophilus influenzae*, and in 1892 he announced that he had isolated the causal agent for influenza. Pfeiffer was a careful worker, and his claims for his discovery were more modest than the publicity he received, but despite stubborn problems, he was firmly convinced that he had found the cause for influenza. Most medical opinion agreed, though everyone, Pfeiffer included, found it troubling that it was not yet possible to generate influenza consistently under laboratory conditions. This also meant that Pfeiffer's work could not lead to a successful vaccine. It was thought that the problem with Pfeiffer's bacillus was one of laboratory technique rather than causal agent, but during the summer outbreak of 1918 skepticism about the bacillus itself began to spread when it did not appear until after the disease was well-established. *H. influenzae* retained some credibility as the cause for influenza for over a decade, but it could not be considered the final answer, and research began to move toward a nonfilterable virus as the cause. This line of thought also very nearly failed since the most commonly used laboratory animals did not react to influenza virus, while efforts at human experimentation gave inconclusive results.

Fifteen years passed before a team composed of Wilson Smith, C. H. Andrews, and Patrick Laidlaw recovered influenza virus A from throat washings of infected patients and was able consistently to reproduce flu symptoms under laboratory conditions. The accidental discovery that ferrets were susceptible to influenza infection considerably advanced the work. The experiments done in 1933 were definitive, and C. H. Stuart-Harris, a major authority on influenza epidemiology and virus research, was able subsequently to declare that "there is no longer any possible doubt that this virus alone, and without any bacterial accompaniment, is the causative agent of the majority of country-wide epidemics of influenza and of most pandemics since 1933."

Although influenza virus B was found in 1940 in New York by Thomas Francis, Jr., and T. P. Magill, the problem of what caused the 1918 epidemic was still unsolved, and despite enormous efforts, it remains so. One theory which has gained a wide following is that the 1918 epidemic arose from a synergistic effect involving flu virus and a bacterial cause, possibly Pfeiffer's bacillus. This theory rested on work which R. E. Shope did with swine flu between 1929 and 1944. Shope was able to show that Pfeiffer's bacillus, acting with an influenza virus, produced annual epizootics among pigs which had the pneumonic involvement and which showed the high mortality characteristic of the 1918 epidemic. Shope successfully explained the complex life cycles of bacteria and viruses in swine and showed a causal connection between the onset of fall weather and the activating of the infective agents. But his hypothesis concerning the way the 1918 epidemic came about, though highly regarded, has not been susceptible to proof.

The currently accepted view is that human influenza is a virus-caused disease, and the critical factor in the outbreak of 1918 and 1919 was the virulence of the virus strain involved. It is thought likely that the causal virus was one which had been present before 1918 but which developed its greater virulence through mutation. Even so, the Shope thesis is acknowledged to offer a reasonable alternative explanation and to demonstrate points important for influenza epidemiology. One notable aspect of the Shope thesis is the connection between human and animal influenza which he established, which suggests that the influenza virus may remain in animal reservoirs between epidemics. This hypothesis gained support from the experience of the Hong Kong flu epidemic of 1968, which infected both people and animals, especially pigs. The Hong Kong flu virus also appears to be related to the virus which causes "cough" in horses. The answers to the cause of the 1918 epidemic and the dynamics of influenza generally undoubtedly lie in the relations among bacteria, viruses, humans, and animals, though *what* the answers are remains unknown.

ADDITIONAL READINGS: William J. B. Beveridge, *Influenza: The Last Great Plague: An Unfinished Story of Discovery* New York, 1977; Richard Collier, *The Plague of the Spanish Lady,* London, 1974; Alfred W. Crosby, *Epidemic and Peace 1918: America's Deadliest Influenza Epidemic,* Westport, Conn., 1976; Thomas Francis, Jr., "Influenza: The Newe Acquayantance," *Annals of Internal Medicine* 39, 2 (August 1953): 203–219; Major Greenwood, *Epidemics and Crowd Diseases,* London, 1935; A. A. Hoehling, *The Great Epidemic,* Boston, 1961; Edwin D. Kilbourne (ed.), *The Influenza Viruses and Influenza,* New York, 1975; C. H. Stuart-Harris, "Influenza," in Walter Bett (ed.), *The History and Conquest of Common Diseases,* Norman, Okla., 1954, 71–83; C. H. Stuart-Harris, *Influenza: The Virus and the Disease,* Littleton, Mass., and London, 1976.

Inoculation

Vaccination; Variolation

Inoculation, or variolation, was an early form of inducing immunity to smallpox by directly infecting a person with matter from an active smallpox pustule. Vaccination is the procedure invented by the English physician Edward Jenner, which he described in 1796. This procedure, also intended to induce immunity against smallpox, used material from cowpox lesions to infect a recipient. "Variolation" has dropped out of the modern vocabulary, while "inoculation" and "vaccination" tend to be used synonymously. Where a distinction is maintained, it is that vaccination (in deference to Jenner) is specifically associated with smallpox, though Pasteur called inoculation with killed cultures "vaccination." Inoculation remains the more general term.

Inoculation against smallpox was very nearly a universal practice. It was reported in India and China and throughout west Asia to the Mediterranean. Modern anthropology suggests that it was used among African tribes, and there is direct evidence that to "buy the pox" was an accepted practice in the west and north of England, in Wales, and in Scotland. Though the principle involved in all cases was the same, the techniques varied. Some infected in the nose; others on the hand or arm; still others at the hairline. The practice was common in the Ottoman empire, where the wife of the British ambassador to Constantinople, Lady Mary Wortley Montague, saw and reported it in 1718. Lady Mary had herself and her children inoculated and did much to popularize the practice among the English aristocracy. Condemned felons at Newgate and orphan children were used to test the safety of inoculation before it was used to protect the English royal family.

Early English inoculation differed from that practiced by their Turkish tutors. The Turks scarcely broke the skin while introducing minute quantities of infective material. Their tool was a needle which pricked and raised the outer skin layer. English physicians evolved a complicated technique beginning with a long preparatory period during which the patient was purged and bled. The inoculation was performed with a lancet which was used to open a substantial wound which went well through the outer skin. The infective agent was often bound into the wound. Infected limbs and occasional cases of smallpox resulted.

Since there was a large demand, with a minimum of regulation, inoculation became a lucrative business in which nonmedical practitioners were often superior to the medical. Robert and Daniel Sutton, father and son, were among the most successful, both in their inoculation results and as businessmen. The Suttons rejected the deep wound method in favor of a technique which was very similar to the original Turkish procedure. It involved two parallel pricks or tiny breaks in the skin which were then infected with only as much material as was caught on the point of the needle. This tiny wound was left unbound. There was no preparation.

Since the Sutton method was easy, safe, and effective, it became very popular, and the Suttons' effort to keep it to themselves failed utterly. When Thomas Dimsdale carried variolation to Russia in 1768, it was the Sutton method which he introduced. The empress Catherine II had first asked Daniel Sutton to come, but he had refused. Dimsdale became a baron of the Russian empire and received the princely sum of £10,000 for successfully inoculating the empress, the grand duke Paul, and members of the court. Ultimately, some 2 million Russians received inoculations. Nothing comparable to Catherine's program was undertaken by her continental contemporaries.

By the time Edward Jenner began publicizing vaccination, the "light" inoculation was in general use and had been employed successfully for nearly 50 years. It was gradually supplanted by Jenner's method in the nineteenth century. Russia apart, inoculation never had the acceptance in continental Europe that it did in England, and vaccination came to be the preferred approach to conferring immunity. This meant, of course, that the reduction in smallpox mortality which inoculation conferred did not begin in Europe until the nineteenth century.

Since inoculation required the use of live smallpox virus, it is thought to have been the more dangerous procedure, with the possibility always present of starting an epidemic. The Jenner vaccination was considered safer because immunity was achieved with no possibility of contracting true smallpox. The alleged difference between the two operations has been questioned on historical grounds. The argument is that inoculation involved a measure of attenuation of the smallpox virus and was inherently safe. Eighteenth-century reports of smallpox from inoculation can be explained by natural infection during the period of preparation; confusion of smallpox with chickenpox and the use of the latter for inoculation, which would confer no smallpox immunity at all; and the method of inoculation practiced in England until the middle of the eighteenth century. The last was the most serious of the three. The other aspect to the argument is that there is evidence that the cowpox preparations Edward Jenner used and distributed in the late eighteenth and early nineteenth centuries were contaminated with true smallpox, though in attenuated form. The conclusion is that the difference, in historical fact, between inoculation and vaccination was less significant than the definition of these terms would lead us to expect, or than contemporaries believed. The argument is still open, if not moot; but there is little question that the methods of variolation practiced in England, including the long preparatory period, contributed to the danger of the procedure. Inoculation and vaccination together substantially reduced mortality from smallpox in England and in the English colonies in North America.

ADDITIONAL READINGS: Genevieve Miller, *The Adoption of Inoculation for Small Pox in England and France*, Philadelphia, 1957; Peter Razzell, *The Conquest of Small Pox: The Impact of Inoculation on Small Pox Mortality in Eighteenth Century Britain*, Firle, Sussex, 1977; K. B. Roberts, *Small Pox: An Historic Disease*, St. Johns, Newfoundland, 1978; Ola Elizabeth Winslow, *A Destroying Angel: The Conquest of Small Pox in Colonial Boston*, Boston, 1974.

See also IMMUNOLOGY; SMALLPOX.

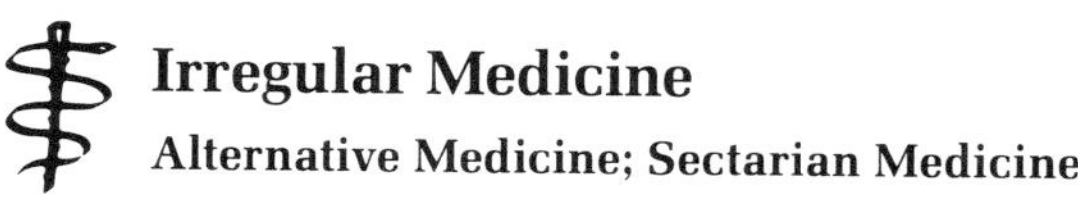

Irregular Medicine

Alternative Medicine; Sectarian Medicine

The development of scientific medicine was accompanied by a variety of competing medical ideologies and a considerable incidence of quackery (q.v.). As professional standards based on scientific principles grew firm, however, and allopathic medicine became the standard practice, there was less tolerance for doctrines which did not conform. The new medical establishment believed that its status was rooted in medicine as science, and it attacked alternative medical philosophies as threatening its hard-won professional image. The therapeutic revolution of the second half of the nineteenth century gave scientific medicine tools of unprecedented effectiveness and forced alternative medical practices either to submit to legislated limitations or to institutionalize training requirements comparable to those of regular medicine. In some cases, sectarian techniques were absorbed into regular medicine, while the irregular forms that remained took on characteristics of scientific medicine.

Alternative medical systems offered a radical simplification of disease theory and therapeutics. They showed strong naturalist tendencies and commonly rejected accepted treatments, especially excessive bleeding and heavy drugging. The sectarian systems usually established schools where their principles were taught together with basic anatomy and supporting scientific work. Through the middle of the nineteenth century, sectarians in the United States received training comparable in quality to that of most regular practitioners, and notably better than some. In Europe, sectarian movements tended to pass into the hands of regular physicians who then made them a part of established curricula and institutions. In the United States, alternative practices had a better opportunity to grow independently of established medicine, though osteopathy, the most successful sectarian therapeutic system in America, quickly internalized diagnostic methods and supplementary therapies from regular medicine.

Thomsonianism and Homeopathy The Thomsonian movement, named for its originator, Samuel A. Thomson, was an early alternative medical system which peaked before the middle of the nineteenth century. Thomson, who was born in New Hampshire in 1769, was an outspoken critic of "book doctors" and developed a therapy based on vegetable compounds. Though unschooled, Thomson called himself "doctor," and he organized a network of Friendly Botanic Societies throughout New England. Thomson's interests were at least in part commercial. Any person who was interested in his therapeutic system could buy it for $20. The societies provided an institutional structure for the movement and a base from which to confront the medical establishment. Because the core of Thomsonianism lay in its vegetable cures, however, the movement lacked ideological structure, and its followers soon began to modify the master's teachings. Thomson himself was indicted for murder after a patient on his regimen died, and though he was never convicted, the publicity attending the trial undermined the movement's credibility. By the middle of the century, Thomsonians were entering the regular medical system, which they then criticized. But the movement had lost its identity, and it disappeared by the end of the century.

Homeopathy was contemporary with Thomsonianism, though much longer lived, and shared its natural approach to cures. It differed in that it was built on a positive medical philosophy which gave its application a clear rationale. Homeopathy originated in Germany in the late eighteenth century in the work of Samuel Christian Friedrich Hahnemann, but it won its largest following in the United States. Originally a true alternative to allopathic medicine, by the twentieth century homeopathy had become a complement to regular medical practice.

The basic work on which homeopathic medicine was built was Hahnemann's *Organon der rationellen Heilkunde* (*Principles of Rational Medicine*), published in 1810. Hahnemann revived Paracelsus' doctrine of "signatures," which held that the symptoms of diseases provided the key to effective cures. Drugs which produced pathological effects similar to the effects of a disease could be expected to cure that disease since, in nature, "like cures like" (*similia similibus curantur*). All drugs, therefore, had first to be tested on a healthy person to determine what pathological effect they had. Only when the effect was determined was it possible to prescribe for someone who was ill. One difference between homeopathy and Paracelsus' system was that Hahnemann treated symptoms and to that extent was empirical; the Paracelsian approach sought only to identify and treat causes.

A second basic principle in homeopathy flatly contradicted contemporary practice. Hahnemann recommended infinitely small drug doses on the grounds that this allowed the most concentrated effect. His approach provided an alternative to the overdrugging prevalent in the early nineteenth century, and as homeopathy's influence spread, it modified abusive drug practices. The parsimony in drug use found a parallel in diagnosis and prescription. Each case required separate handling, and no prescription was to be made until all symptoms were understood and a comprehensive treatment could be undertaken. In this respect, the homeopathic approach was holistic. A third principle concerned chronic diseases, which early homeopathy ascribed to a suppressed itch, or *psora*. This idea was quickly dropped. In the end, the movement's identifying themes were "like cures like," mild dosages, and the holistic approach to diagnosis and treatment.

Homeopathy was a by-product of eighteenth-century medical theorizing which won a large following in part as a reaction against heroic treatments. Its emphasis on painstaking case studies to find the best fit between condition and treatment for each individual corresponded with the clinical tradition which gave regular medicine its greatest effect. The idea of combining with and assisting nature rather than fighting it reasserted a long-standing Hippocratic principle and underlined a major theme in alternative medical philosophies. Homeopathy became a popular movement, developed schools for training its practitioners, and emerged as the most complete of the alternative systems in the nineteenth century. Its influence has been greatly diminished by the transformation in medical treatment and technology during the past century.

Hydropathy Dissatisfaction with allopathic medicine's basic treatments led to other therapeutic experiments in the nineteenth century. One of the most significant was hydropathy, the use of water treatments to cure disease. Here there was a direct connection with other movements. Water cures involved cleansing and purifying the physical system according to the same principles which held that cleanliness, fresh air, and clear water were the best answer to infection and disease. The hygiene movement, which crested on the eve of the discovery of germ theory, was widespread and offered a welcoming environment for a therapy based on the cleansing and vivifying effects of water, country air, and simple foods. In common with other alternative systems, hydropathy was also a reaction against heroic therapy, and in particular the indiscriminate use of powerful drugs.

Nineteenth-century hydropathy originated in Germany with Vincent Priessnitz, a sort of rural prophet who became convinced of water's healing powers and established a spa at Gräfenberg in Austrian Silesia, where he accepted patients for extended cures. Priessnitz believed that health was the body's natural condition, that ill health resulted from introducing foreign matter into the body, and that acute disease was the body's attempt to expel diseased matter. The only element which could assist this process was water. Priessnitz rejected regular therapy entirely. Drugs, purges, and bleeding not only could not assist the body back to health, but could be expected to change acute conditions into chronic ones. He said a water treatment was the only way to reverse this process, bring an acute condition to a crisis, and expel the destructive matter from the system. Priessnitz's techniques included withdrawing all drugs, promoting sweat followed by a cold bath, and wet bandages and special baths designed for every part of the body. His patients drank no less than 12 glasses of water a day and gave up alcohol and rich food to live on coarse brown bread, butter, and milk for breakfast and supper, with meat and vegetables at noon. The mountains where the spa was located provided clear, bracing air and the opportunity for healthful exercise. The mountain location was an essential part of the treatment.

There was some question in the beginning whether Priessnitz was practicing medicine without a license. The representatives of the imperial government who investigated him were so favorably impressed, however, that the regulations covering medical practice were set aside in his case, and Priessnitz was given a free hand. His establishment grew from a modest 45 patients in 1829 to 1400 ten years later, and by the time of his death in 1851, his reputation had spread throughout Europe. His clients were the rich and wellborn, including royalty as well as leading nobles, and the medical establishment began to take note. When hydropathy reached England, crusaders for scientific medicine and professional standards led by the *Lancet* attacked the therapy as a fraud. Practicing physicians were impressed, however, and they began to introduce hydropathy into their treatments. Some visited Gräfenberg and came away convinced that they had witnessed remarkable cures of long-standing conditions from fistulae and hemiplegia to deafness. Hydropathy, as one physician writing to the *Lancet* averred, was clearly not quackery but rather an "extra-professional" method of treatment. Skepticism remained, but regular physicians took over and ran hydropathic institutions, and in the second half of the century, hydropathy achieved some measure of professional acceptance.

The merger with professional medicine was realized most fully in the work of Wilhelm Winternitz, who was a professor of medicine at Vienna, the director of a famous hydropathic spa at Kaltenleutgeben, and the founder of a journal for clinical hydropathy. Winternitz also initiated clinical and experimental research on hydropathy and published a major treatise on the subject in 1877–1880. By the twentieth century, the movement initiated by Priessnitz had been absorbed into professional medicine, where it ceased to be significant. Bathing fads and water cures continued to appear, but they failed to gain the standing hydropathy achieved, though the underlying concept of nature's benign and creative power remained influential in popular health movements.

Osteopathy and Chiropractic In the second half of the nineteenth century two related alternative systems of treatment appeared in the American middle west. Osteopathy, the more comprehensive of the two, was originated by Dr. Andrew Taylor Still in 1874. Dr. Still established a College of Osteopathy at Kirksville, Missouri, in 1892 which remains the traditional center for the movement, though many other institutions have grown up, and osteopathy has become a recognized practice across the United States. The second movement was chiropractic, a method of treatment established by Daniel David Palmer in 1895, when he reportedly restored the hearing of a Davenport, Iowa, man by adjustment of vertebral articulation. Palmer was a "magnetic doctor" before he became the founder of chiropractic. His method was systematized, he founded a school to teach it, and it has come to be accepted as a legitimate practice in many states.

Osteopathy asserted the body's inherent capacity to resist disease and to repair itself. It also accepted the interrelationship of all portions of the body and laid disease to "structural derangements" or "somatic components of the disease processes," which were also called osteopathic lesions. Slight strains or dislocations anywhere in the skeletal system were believed to affect the body's structural integrity and result in disease symptoms. Treatment involved discovery of strain or dislocation points followed by manipulation to correct them. Dr. Still himself gave a narrow interpretation to osteopathic practice, emphasizing spinal lesions, but his followers extended the principle of manipulation beyond the spine to the entire skeletal structure and even to certain organs. Similarly, they enlarged their arsenal of techniques to include electric and water treatments, massage, and eventually surgery. This flexibility made a merger with regular medicine possible, and the schools accredited by the American Association of Osteopathy to grant the degree of doctor of osteopathy now offer a course of instruction in traditional medicine as well. Accredited osteopaths are licensed to prescribe drugs, perform surgery, and practice medicine, though some tend to concentrate on conditions responsive to osteopathic manipulation. Osteopathy has maintained its identity as an alternative to regular medicine. By accepting and building on scientific medicine's basic principles, osteopathy has come closer to being a form of regular medicine than its founder envisioned.

Chiropractic began from the assumption that a flow of energy from the brain was the essential life-giving force in the body, and that interference with this force produced disease. The doctrine was revised in 1953 to refer to nerve impulses, though the idea that interfering with impulses or the flow caused disease remained constant. The spine was considered the area most commonly responsible for interfering with flow or nerve function, and spinal manipulation by hand (the word "chiropractic" derives from the Greek for "doing by hand") was and is the basic method for treating the spine, though modern chiropractic uses some diagnostic equipment, including x-ray. Unlike osteopaths, chiropractors are not licensed for surgery, prescribing, or general medical practice, and they have remained closer to the spirit of their founder. Chiropractic was also slower to win approval of its status, though colleges of chiropractic have existed and trained students from the beginning of the century. Though approval was delayed, chiropractors are now licensed throughout the United States and in some countries abroad.

Conclusion Irregular medical systems developed to meet needs that conventional medicine failed to fill, or as a reaction against established medical practices. In most cases, convergence with regular medicine permitted the sectarian versions to continue, though not without alteration. (Chiropractic is a partial exception.) Nevertheless, the contemporary vogue for acupuncture (q.v.) and interest in nonwestern medical systems suggest that scientific medicine has cultural and social limitations, and that, in fact, healing has more flexible boundaries than those imposed by medical orthodoxy in the last century.

ADDITIONAL READINGS: Linn J. Boyd, *The Simile in Medicine*, Philadelphia, 1935; Noel G. Coley, "Cures Without Care: 'Chymical Physicians' and Mineral Waters in Seventeenth Century English Medicine," *Medical History* 23 (1979): 191–214; Russell W. Givens, "Physicians-Chiropractors: Medical Presence in the Evolution of Chiropractic," *Bulletin of the History of Medicine:* 55 (Summer 1981): 233–245; Wayland D. Hand, *Magical Medicine: The Folklore Component of Medicine in the Folk Belief, Custom, and Ritual of the Peoples of Europe and America*, Berkeley, 1980; Martin Kaufman, *Homeopathy in America: The Rise and Fall of a Medical Heresy*, Baltimore, 1971; Phyllis H. Mattson, *Holistic Health in Perspective*, Palo Alto, Cal., 1981; Ronald L. Numbers *et al.*, *Medicine Without Doctors: Home Health Care in American History*, New York, 1977; Robin Price, "Hydropathy in England, 1840–1870," *Medical History* 25 (July 1981): 269–280; Richard Shryock, *Medicine in America: Historical Essays*, Baltimore, 1966; Andrew Taylor Still, *Autobiography of Andrew Taylor Still with a History of the Discovery and Development of the Science of Osteopathy*, New York, 1897, 1972.

See also QUACKERY.

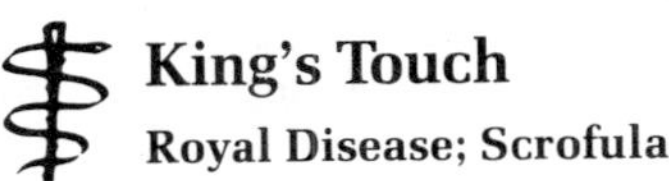

King's Touch

Royal Disease; Scrofula

The king's touch was a ritual performed by monarchs in France and England to cure tubercular adenitis, or scrofula, which was known from this ritual as the king's disease or the king's evil. Touching subjects for scrofula began to be done on a regular basis by the French kings after Louis IX's return from the Crusades in 1254. The English began between 1259 and 1272, possibly on St. Edward's Day, October 13, 1269. Earlier monarchs in these lines were said to possess healing powers, most notably England's Edward the Confessor (1002?–1066) and Robert the Pious (996–1031) of France. There is no evidence, however, that either touched subjects for scrofula.

Diseases called the king's evil are mentioned in various medieval sources, but the belief that these were scrofula is incorrect. The king's evil referred to in the classic or humoral tradition appears to have been jaundice, while that originating in the patristic (Judaic) sources was a degenerative disease, probably leprosy. In none of these cases was the king's disease scrofula, though scrofula was mentioned among gland and skin infections. Scrofula only came to be called the royal disease or the king's evil when royalty began to touch for it in the high Middle Ages. It was not until then that the ability to relieve scrofula came to be considered an attribute of royalty.

It has been suggested that scrofula became the object of the French and English monarchs' attention because it was an affliction which their intervention might seem to cure. It was a common condition, highly visible, which produced swellings and open sores on the neck and face. Scrofula was almost never fatal, but it was uncomfortable, and the suppurations were unsightly. In advanced stages, they became putrid. Left to itself, scrofula often was arrested or even disappeared. Such natural remissions in one touched by royalty would be laid to the king's influence, and success of this sort would strengthen the conviction that the treatment worked. Scrofula sufferers who improved were inclined to talk about their cure, and since they were more likely to be helped than other persons who also received the king's blessing, it was not unnatural for the royal healing power to be identified exclusively with scrofula.

The English adoption of the French ritual reflected the Plantagenets' need to buttress their position with their subjects and may also have reflected their ambition to rule France as well. Edward the Confessor, the last Saxon king of England, was considered a saint, and his healing powers were believed to arise from his holy character. The Plantagenets appropriated the healing tradition and linked themselves with Edward. They regularly touched for scrofula, and since alms were given (the king's penny), there is quantitative evidence to show how widespread the practice was. In three different years, for example, Edward I (1272–1307) touched 983, 1219, and 1736 scrofulous subjects; in other years, the numbers ran from a low of 197 to a high of 725.

Popular acceptance of the ritual was reinforced by other authorities. Though papal reformers condemned it, the ecclesiastical establishment in both France and England supported it, thus identifying the touching ritual with a national or antipapal point of view. Similarly, medical authorities in the two kingdoms accepted the ceremony as a legitimate therapy, often recommending it before, and in preference to, a visit to the surgeon. Such acceptance of the royal touch was consistent with a medical outlook in which both astrology and alchemy were influential, and magic was appreciated. Not all medical authorities were enthusiastic. The famous Arnold of Villanova, one of the leading physicians of the fourteenth century, makes no mention of the king's power to cure scrofula, though he devoted a chapter in his *Breviarum Medicinae* to the disease. A certain Jan Yperman, a surgeon resident in Yprès, who was either more courageous or simply farther removed from the reach of royal authority, asserted that the touch was not always efficacious. These men, however, were a minority.

By the eighteenth century, the medieval world view had shattered, and a rational skepticism eroded faith in the royal power to heal. The Stuarts kept the practice alive only as evidence of their divine right. William III considered touching a useless superstition, and he performed the ceremony only when forced to. Queen Anne (1702–1714) was the last English ruler to touch for scrofula. The ceremony lasted somewhat longer in France. Louis XV touched more than 2000 scrofula victims at his coronation in 1722, but the king himself later discredited the ceremony by failing to appear for it on three separate occasions. Though the populace retained some faith in touching, the educated classes largely rejected it, and Louis XVI abandoned it entirely after 1789. Following the restoration of the Bourbons, romantic conservatives tried to revive touching in the vain hope of strengthening Charles X (1824–1830) on the throne. It was he who performed the ritual for the last time on May 31, 1825.

ADDITIONAL READINGS: Frank Barlow, "The King's Evil," *English Historical Review* 95 (January 1980): 3–27; Marc Bloch, *The Royal Touch*, J. E. Anderson (trans.), London and Montreal, 1973.

Leprosy

Hansen's Disease

Leprosy has inspired fear and loathing throughout history. Though modern attitudes are neither so violent nor so unforgiving as those of the past, there is considerable misunderstanding over the disease and its effects. Today's leprosy specialists give public education about the disease top priority. Many fears about leprosy are baseless, and the more severe measures which societies have invoked to protect themselves against it have been as useless as they have been inhuman. Yet leprosy is a dangerous disease which, once contracted, can cripple, grotesquely disfigure, and sometimes kill. Today, leprosy can be managed, in many cases cured, or its effects alleviated. Treatment, however, is measured in years, and in the most serious form, it continues for life. There is as yet no quick cure, nor is there any consistently reliable method for prevention.

The Disease The causal organism for leprosy is *Mycobacterium leprae*, a bacillus which was identified by the Norwegian scientist and physician Gerhard Henrick Armauer Hansen in 1873. The disease is contagious in a limited and partially understood way. Most adults have a natural immunity to *M. leprae*, but children are susceptible, and possibly 10 percent of the population may have weakened immunities or no immunity at all. It is they, together with the children, who contract leprosy. Leprosy has a relatively long incubating period. From exposure to the appearance of clinical symptoms may take from two to seven years, or even longer. The type of disease which develops depends on the degree of immunity, where the bacteria lodge, and the character of the immunological response.

Leprosy shows two clearly defined forms, and two that are less well defined. The latter two have the potential of polarizing to one of the two more clearly defined syndromes. Lepromatous and tuberculoid leprosy are the most serious forms. The less developed forms are dimorphous, or intermediate, and indeterminate, or mild. Of the four, only lepromatous leprosy involves a dense bacterial concentration and is communicable. The mode of communication is through nasal or laryngeal droplets. Physical contact, whether a fleeting touch or sexual intercourse, does not communicate the disease. Leprosy is not hereditary, though susceptibility may be, and the infective agent does not pass through the placenta. A leprous mother can bear a normal healthy child, though the child may become infected after birth.

In tuberculoid leprosy, the number of bacilli is relatively small, and the damage is done by immunological response. This version follows the nerve system, producing loss of sensation in the hands and feet, which become swollen or deformed, in part as a result of persistent injury stemming from loss of feeling. The tuberculoid form is self-limiting, though severe damage can occur before the disease ends. In lepromatous leprosy, there appears to be no resistance to the bacillus, or at most a very slight one. The bacillus seeks out the cells most attractive to it, multiplies in great numbers, and produces severe cell destruction. Swelling in the face and a yellowish cast produce the grotesque lionface of the leper; the eyes are attacked, with blindness following; the nose may collapse inward as the underlying structures are eaten away; and severe throat damage and nasal destruction alter the voice to a hoarse whisper and eventually will affect breathing. Nodules break out all over the body; men's testes are affected; high temperatures (106° or 107° F) occur; and there are severe nerve pains. Though difficult to diagnose in early stages, lepromatous leprosy is easily recognized in advanced forms by the damage which it does.

It is estimated that there are between 10 and 15 million lepers in the world today. The heaviest populations are in tropical and subtropical areas of Africa, Asia, and Latin America. Climate is not a limiting factor, however, because leprosy was common in central and northern Europe during the Middle Ages, and in central and northern China as well. Its current distribution shows a predilection for depressed or backward areas with compacted populations living in squalor and lacking rudimentary health facilities. In this respect, leprosy is similar to a number of diseases which are more serious in underdeveloped regions than they are in richer, more technologically advanced societies. There are racial factors as well. Dark-pigmented people appear to have stronger immunity to leprosy than the more lightly pigmented. White people are highly susceptible and are most likely to develop the lepromatous form. Darker-pigmented people also seem to be more responsive to treatment.

In itself, leprosy is not a killing disease, though it creates dangerous conditions. The most common cause of death is kidney failure, although in some advanced cases where facial collapse has occurred, death may come from asphyxia. Leprosy's debilitating effects, however, make lepers more vulnerable to other infections. One explanation for leprosy's decline in Europe since the fourteenth century is that lepers, whose disease defenses were substantially weakened, were killed off by the virulent plagues which swept Europe in the early modern period.

Origins and Early History It is impossible to identify leprosy's point of origin, nor can it be said with any certainty where the earliest record of encounter with it may be found. Egyptian sources from as early as 2400 B.C. contain referenes to a skin disease which has been interpreted to be leprosy; 900 years later, the Ebers papyrus offers a prescription for treating boils and pustules, while mentioning a skin disease which is often said to be leprosy. One explanation for Ramses II's expulsion of 90,000 Jews from Egypt is that they were harboring "a disgraceful disease," and the tradition has come down that the disease was leprosy. Finally, a University of Pennsylvania expedition digging in 1925 and 1926 at Tel El-Hasn in Israel found a jug in the form of the dwarf god, Bes, whose facial features in this case seem to show the ravages of leprosy. Such evidence, however, is inconclusive.

The earliest dating for leprosy in Asia is similarly obscure. There are several references to the disease in the Chinese medical classic, *Huang di nei jing su wen (The Yellow Emperor's Classic of Internal Medicine)*, but modern scholarship suggests that this work be dated about 250 B.C., a period for which there are already other sources. A case can be made that these references reflect a much older tradition, but there is no way to know. The picture is somewhat clearer in India. Indian vedic medicine contains clinically recognizable descriptions of leprosy which were probably compiled between 600 and 400 B.C. Because the method of compilation was to record the teachings of past masters, these descriptions could reach back to the late second millenium. The vedic writings probably contain the oldest known descriptions of leprosy, though this would not justify identifying India as the point of origin for the disease. Too little is yet known concerning the origin of life forms to permit speculation on that point.

Assuming that leprosy was active in China and India during the second and first millennia, it was probably carried into Persia along the major trade routes leading to the west. Later sources, including the Old Testament, place disease syndromes which could be leprosy around the eastern rim of the Mediterranean during the first millenium. It is thought possible that Xerxes' armies, invading Greece in the fifth century B.C., carried leprosy into Europe, while both Roman legions and Phoenican traders have been implicated in its further spread. But even here there is uncertainty. Greek sources only refer to "elephantiasis," a condition thought to be tuberculoid leprosy, but the identification is subject to debate. Translators of biblical sources intruded later ideas, including the concept of leprosy as a punishment for sin, and especially for excessive sexuality.

Premodern Attitudes Toward Leprosy There is a strong presumption that true leprosy probably existed in the eastern Mediterranean from biblical times or earlier. Leprosy, however, has never been a mass disease, and it is equally certain that the term came to be used to describe a variety of conditions which produced suppurating sores and ulcers, and in their most severe forms, disfigured and crippled their victims. Positive evidence of true leprosy in medieval Europe appears in the work of Theoderic of Cervia, who lived and practiced in the thirteenth century, and who provides a recognizable account of leprosy, including the intermediate variety. The descriptions suggest considerable experience with the disease. The insistence on leprosy's venereal character has led some scholars to conclude that the term may cover a pre-sixteenth-century syphilis (q.v.)—it has been noted further that the medieval European image of leprosy, which included clearly marked spots or blotches, was transferred to pictures of syphilitics in the sixteenth century.

The view of leprosy as corruption, the consequence of sin, or even God's will led to excluding the leper from society. Lepers were considered to be unclean and dangerous. A Chinese story relates how a village protested violently when a leper was buried facing the village, although his grave was three miles or more away. As unclean persons, lepers lost rights of participation in religious rituals, rights of inheritance, and even the protection of the community. There are also tales of lepers banding together to extort money and food from villagers by threatening to walk among them and infect them.

Prohibitions against lepers in medieval Europe were particularly strict. They were forbidden all normal social contacts. Lepers could not marry if they were single, and they could not remain with their families if they were married. They were forced to dress in a distinctive way, covering their bodies with enveloping garments and wearing gauntlets which prevented contact with other people. They were ordered to sound a bell or clacquer to warn people against their approach, and they were even prohibited from sharing a narrow walk or lane with nonlepers. Later in the Middle Ages, lepers were segregated in special houses called lazarettos, which were set in isolated spots well away from the towns. There was also a leper mass which was said with the victim in attendance, which declared him to be "dead among the living."

The church took the lead in enforcing restrictions on lepers until the Crusades, which began in 1096, forced a change in attitude. Crusaders contracted leprosylike conditions in the Holy Land, and when they returned, the church was loath to turn them into social outcasts. There was some rethinking of basic attitudes toward sin and suffering as well. Christ's compassion was recalled, and there was a reinterpretation of the Annunciation in the book of Isaiah which led to the position that leprosy was a "holy disease" and that lepers were "Christ's poor." In this same period, secular society expanded facilities to care for the sick. Hospitals were founded, and the towns enlarged their segregated housing for lepers. The church dropped the leper mass, and the Third Lateran Council declared that leprosy was no longer grounds for divorce. The Order of St. Lazarus was sanctified to provide people whose duty it was to look after lepers, and the Franciscan order also began its work, which included ministering to lepers.

While the Church moderated its views, the leper remained an object of fear. During the mass hysteria generated by the black death, lepers were accused of poisoning wells before suspicion fell on the Jews, and even as their numbers declined in Europe, they were still firmly separated from society. As the modern period dawned, lepers remained in isolation, not because they were unclean and bore the marks of sin, but for fear of the infection which they bore. No change in this basic approach appeared until effective treatments for leprosy were discovered in the twentieth century.

Leprosy in Modern Times The modern study of leprosy began in Bergen, Norway, with the work of Daniel C. Danielssen, a marine biologist and zoologist who became director of the Lungegarden Hospital in Bergen in 1849. Danielssen worked with the dermatologist Carl Boeck, and their book *On Leprosy* (1848) became the starting point for all further explorations. Though both tried, neither Boeck nor Danielssen was able to infect himself with leprous material. This led Danielssen to the incorrect conclusion that leprosy was a hereditary disease. Danielssen also searched unsuccessfully for a leprosy cure. He tried mercury, phosphoric acid, creosote pills, arsenic, and iodine, and when all these substances proved either dangerous or ineffective, he reaffirmed segregating lepers, especially to avoid breeding leprous children.

Gerhard Hansen was also from Bergen. He began his studies in 1868, became fascinated with leprosy, and after working in Bonn and Vienna, returned to Bergen to work out his ideas. He analyzed the family histories of leprosy cases, and he noticed that leprosy died out when families broke up and lived apart. This fact significantly weakened the hereditary interpretation of leprosy's cause, and Hansen, who was already convinced of the germ theory of disease, turned to the microscope to search for a causal organism. He was partially successful. In 1873, he spotted *M. leprae,* and he sent some nodule scrapings to Henry V. Carter, surgeon-major of the English Bombay army, noting his conviction that they contained the causal organism responsible for leprosy. Carter mentioned the hypothesis in a government white paper which appeared in 1874. Hansen also sent a paper on leprosy etiology to the medical society in Christiana (now Oslo). The difficulty was that while Hansen himself was certain that

M. leprae caused leprosy, he was unable to prove it. Although he found the microorganism in the blood of lepers and not in that of healthy people, he was unable to culture the bacillus, and he failed to establish the chain of infection. In his desperation to prove what he thought he knew, Hansen injected the eye of a leprous woman with material from another leprosy case. The experiment landed him in court, where the decision went against him, and he was barred from hospital practice for the rest of his life. Though incomplete, Hansen's work convinced the government that leprosy was contagious and that lepers should be segregated. Hansen became director of the Bergen Museum and involved himself in organizing scientists interested in further leprosy studies. His own research was at an end.

While Hansen worked on leprosy's cause, Father Damien de Veuster of the Sacred Hearts of Jesus and Mary was opening a personal campaign to humanize the treatment of lepers. Father Damien was a Belgian priest working in Honolulu, Hawaii, who volunteered to serve the leper colony on the island of Molokai. He went there in 1873, to remain for the rest of his life. The contemporary approach to lepers was to segregate and ignore them. Living useless, hopeless lives, the inmates of Molokai were dirty, diseased, sexually promiscuous, and alcoholic. Father Damien fought moral decay inside the colony while pressing the government to recognize lepers' rights to schooling, decent living conditions, and modern medical care. His campaign to publicize the leper's cause brought reforms and foreshadowed the more recent struggle to restore social status and political rights to people institutionalized for mental illness. After 13 years, Father Damien finally contracted leprosy, and he died on Molokai in 1889.

Wesley C. Bailey, a Presbyterian missionary in India and head of the Presbyterian Mission School and Hospital at Ambala, carried out a different sort of campaign. He too became interested in the plight of lepers, and when he moved to Dublin, Ireland, he began to give public lectures on lepers' needs and to organize a fund-raising program for their support. By 1900, his Mission to Lepers had founded a hospital at Chamba and was providing food, clothing, and shelter to some 3000 lepers in India. Other branches developed, the organization expanded, and new missions and hospitals were built.

Managing Leprosy: The Twentieth Century Many remedies were used against leprosy, but none successfully. Chaulmoogra, a product of the kalaw tree, gave some relief, and until the discovery of sulfonamides, it was the main substance used in leprosy treatment. Other treatments reflected local customs. In Ireland, leprosy was treated with whiskey, and in Portugal with turtle soup. The Chinese used arsenic, which had therapeutic value, but they also tried snakes and scorpions, to say nothing of acupuncture and moxa medicine. The moxa method was considered very strong; it involved stimulating the system in which leprosy lodged by burning a pinch of wormwood leaves on the skin, thus raising a small blister. Acupuncture achieved a similar end by pricking the skin with gold or silver needles at the acupuncture points.

Treatments for leprosy were only palliative. The relapse rate using chaulmoogra was approximately 80 percent, and no further progress was made until work on azo dyes produced prontosil and the sulfonamides (q.v.) in the mid-1930s. Then diaminodiphenylsulfone (DDS) was found as a contaminant of sulfanilamide at the Wellcome Research Laboratories, and tests were begun to see what the substancce would do. It proved to be far stronger than sulfanilamide, and much more toxic. A variant of DDS called promin was tested in 1937 at Washington University in St. Louis, Missouri, against rat leprosy, a condition which seemed closer to tuberculosis than to leprosy. The results were promising. Other tests were begun in 1940 at the Mayo Clinic in Rochester, Minnesota, by Dr. W. H. Feldman, a specialist in tuberculosis and comparative pathology.

Guy H. Foget, medical officer in charge at the U.S. Marine Hospital in Carville, Louisiana, which had been a leprosarium since 1896, also began testing DDS in 1940. Foget first tried oral administration of DDS but was deterred by the violence of the drug's side effects. The injection method was hardly more successful, bringing on anemia as well as severe discomfort. On the third attempt, however, the course ran six months, and at the end of that period, patients began to show signs of improvement. Promin reduced acute laryngitis, made tracheotomies to prevent asphyxia unnecessary, and began to clear nose ulcerations. Lesions on lips and tongue disappeared, and patients could hear normally. By 1943, Foget could report that 5 of the 22 cases treated had become entirely negative: the bacilli were gone. Ten patients improved, 6 remained static, and 1 declined. The work continued, and a further report in 1946 stated succinctly that "the use of promin in the treatment of leprosy results in improvement in all major chronic manifestations of the disease" while pointing out as well that clinical improvement was "accompanied by improvement in bacteriological and histopathological studies."

What has been called the Carville miracle was confirmed in a steady stream of reports from leprosy centers all over the world, and the development of an inexpensive dapsone (DDS) pill made administration of the drug far easier and more efficient, especially under field conditions. Nevertheless, leprosy continued to be an active disease with an expanding incidence. Epidemiologists are divided on the issue, but the consensus seems to be that there is no hope in current circumstances of eradicating the disease, and even control is difficult. Vaccinating with BCG (bacillus Calmette-Guérin) has given far from satisfactory results, even with supporting chemotherapy, and at present, identifying cases, treating them, and developing public awareness concerning the real character of leprosy appear to be the most important areas for preventive action. Moreover, treatment with sulfones does not kill the bacteria; the sulfones are growth inhibitors, and it has been found that viable bacilli can lodge deep in the human system where sulfone treatment does not reach them. This helps to account for relapses, even in patients showing negative bacteria count for several years. Moreover, in regions where it is difficult to monitor treatments, relapses are very common.

Since the high-incidence areas for leprosy are also areas with low income and poorly developed public health, leprosy control can be marginally effective at best. According to the World Health Organization, a third or less of actual cases are found and registered, and less than half of those have regular treatment. Finally, the evidence of the 1970s shows that strains of leprosy resistant to the sulfone treatment are beginning to appear, while the number of regressions is increasing, even in controlled conditions. Though hardly a mass disease, leprosy affects a large number of people, especially in underdeveloped societies, and the present prospect is that it will continue to do so, expanding somewhat more rapidly than the rate of population growth in those areas.

ADDITIONAL READINGS: Chapman H. Binford, "Leprosy," in H. Franklin (ed.), *Communicable and Infectious Diseases*, 4th ed., St. Louis, 1960; S. W. Brody, *The Disease of the Soul*, Ithaca, N.Y., 1974; R. G. Cochrane and T. Frank Davey (eds.), *Leprosy in Theory and Practice*, 2d ed., Bristol, 1964; Michael W. Dols, "Leprosy in Medieval Arabic Medicine," *Journal of the History of Medicine and Allied Sciences* 34 (July 1979): 314–333; Patrick Feeny, *The Fight Against Leprosy*, London, 1964.

See also SULFONAMIDES; TUBERCULOSIS

Malaria

Malaria is a parasitic disease whose origin probably antedates that of human beings. Though normally associated with tropical and subtropical regions, malaria has been active throughout Europe, including Russia, and in the United States and Canada. Both the disease and the means to control it are now well understood, and less than 20 years ago, it was firmly believed to be declining toward extinction. Its powerful resurgence in the last 10 years has reestablished malaria as a major disease problem, while its presence over vast areas of the civilized world for much of that world's history makes malaria a formidable component in humanity's historical ecology.

Etiology and Epidemiology The causal agents for malaria are a group of plasmodium parasites whose only vector from host to host is the female anopheles mosquito. The four species of plasmodia known to infect humans are *Plasmodium vivax*, *Plasmodium ovale*, *Plasmodium falciparum*, and *Plasmodium malariae*. The different intensities which malaria exhibits are determined by which one of the plasmodia is responsible for a particular infection, but since these infections are not mutually exclusive, it is possible for individual cases to involve more than one plasmodium. Where malaria is endemic, this situation is common. *P. falciparum*, which produces what used to be called malignant tertian malaria, is also the agent which causes the deadly black water fever, and *P. falciparum* has been estimated to be responsible for 50 percent of the world's malaria cases and 90 percent of the deaths. It has been especially active in Africa. *P. vivax*, which causes benign tertian malaria, generates 43 percent of the world's cases and is altogether less formidable. The other plasmodia are of negligible effect.

The anopheles mosquito acts as both a host and a vector. The primary reservoir of infection, however, is the human. The plasmodia develop in the stomach of the mosquito, in the liver tissue of the human host, and in the bloodstream. The plasmodia which become established in the bloodstream and liver of a human host go into a process of multiplication and reinfection which causes the cycle of malarial symptoms. The plasmodium parasite lodges in the red blood cells and feeds on hemoglobin. As reproduction occurs, the cell envelope bursts, releasing toxins which have been generated by the parasites' digesting the hemoglobin. It is the toxins which bring on the malarial attack stages of chill, fever, and sweat. There must be both a reservoir of infection and a vector to establish an endemic malarial system or to start an epidemic. When epidemics of malaria occur, it is because conditions have favored mosquito development. If there is rapid mosquito multiplication, a relatively small reservoir of plasmodium parasites is all that is necessary for a major outbreak to occur.

Malaria moves from infected to uninfected zones with its human host. It confers a limited immunity in areas where it is endemic; hence children will suffer more from it than adults. Malaria also affects pregnancies adversely, producing severe demographic effects in endemic areas. When newly introduced or reintroduced into a previously infected zone where the infective chain has been broken, malaria can have a devastating impact. Its mortality on the whole, however, is less than that of bubonic plague, typhus, cholera, or smallpox. What has made malaria the most significant single disease for world civilization over the past three centuries has been its prodigious geographical extent and its high incidence in infected areas.

Clinical Features Malaria occurs in waves in the individual patient, beginning with premonitory symptoms of headache, a heavy feeling in the limbs, and aching in the joints. The onset begins 10 days after infection and may last for 2 or 3 days. The victim then falls into the toxin-generated three-stage malaria pattern: First comes shivering cold, an ague with rapid pulse, and possibly some vomiting of blood. Young children may convulse. This stage lasts 45 minutes to an hour. The second or hot stage reverses the chills. The patient seems to be burning up and is wracked with fever pains. In the third stage, the fever breaks, sweating starts, vomiting stops, the headache passes, and the exhausted patient sleeps. This stage may last two to four hours, and then the cycle starts over again.

If the disease is untreated, the paroxyms will recur at regular intervals. The spleen swells and is palpable by the eighth to the twelfth day, and anemia develops, as does jaundice with liver damage. The symptoms may continue for 6 to 10 weeks, then disappear for an extended period, sometimes up to 28 weeks, after which, depending on the virulence of the infection, they may recur. Recurrence is likely in seasonal climates, usually in the spring following the attack, but other factors such as an operation or exposure to another disease can also bring on an attack. *P. vivax* has been known to persist for four years after the patient left an endemic region, but generally the infections wear out in two years.

Untreated quartan or tertian ague rarely was a sole cause for death. Its effect was to weaken the individual through destruction of hemoglobin and debilitation, thus making the victim susceptible to other conditions. Infections involving *P. falciparum* are a different matter. The symptoms are the same, but greatly exaggerated, with temperatures which reach 107° to 110° F, and cerebral responses similar to sunstroke. Delirium, convulsions, and death often come quickly with so violent an attack.

Both intermittent and continuous fevers were treated by purging, starvation, and bleeding. Bleeding was disastrous in malaria since the plasmodium destroyed hemoglobin and induced anemia. There was no effective specific until the seventeenth century, when cinchona bark which contained quinine was found. Cinchona did not affect all fevers, and so there was a tendency to classify fevers according to whether they responded to it or not. Quinine has been the major specific for preventing, managing, and controlling malaria in individuals.

Malaria: Early Historical Development The word "malaria" is derived from the Italian for "bad air," and it entered the English vocabulary in 1740 in a letter from Horace Walpole which was quoted by John MacCulloch in an English textbook in 1829. It was not used widely in English until the latter part of the nineteenth century, the common word for this type of fever being "ague." The disease, however, appears to be as old as medical writing itself. References to an intermittent fever accompanied by enlargement of the spleen are found in ancient Chaldean, Sanskrit, and Chinese sources, a fact which indicates its broad geographical spread in ancient times, while the frequency of reference suggests familiarity and an established historical personality for the disease. The Hippocratic writings give the first clinical descriptions, noting the different periods of onset—quotidian, tertian, and quartan—and calling attention to the enlarged spleen. The fever appeared to be a new one in Greece, and it is impossible to get a clear view of the disease's incidence. Some modern scholars believe, however, that malaria contributed to the decline of Greek culture after the fourth century B.C.

Early in the first century of the Christian era, Aulus Cornelius Celsus included a detailed account of malaria in his encyclopedic *De re medica* (ca. A.D. 30). Intermittent fevers were a serious problem in and around the city of Rome, in the Roman Campagna and the Pontine marshes, and along the west coast of Italy. These areas suffered a severe depopulation during the later years of the Roman empire in which malarial fevers were an important factor. They remained empty throughout the medieval era, and some spots were not occupied again until the antimalaria campaigns of the twentieth century.

Malaria has been a persistent rather than a dramatic disease, and its effects have been cumulative in the cultures where it has been active. Though debilitating, the less virulent malarial forms can be absorbed by civilizations, and populations have been able to adapt to them but often at great cost. Malaria can be an effective barrier against cultural contacts, as it was in Africa during the nineteenth century. It can also be extremely destructive when imported into newly settled areas, as was the case in the Americas.

Distribution of Malaria Outside the Americas While there is incontrovertible evidence that malaria existed on a world scale in ancient times, there is no reliable evidence detailing either its endemic incidence or its role as an epidemic disease until the sixteenth century. In the modern period, however, a world profile for malaria emerges, including information on intensity of infection. Coastal Africa, both east and west, was heavily malarial, as were the river basins, including the Congo and the Niger. Indigenous populations in west Africa developed a genetic characteristic, the so-called sickle cell, which gave them immunity against the extremely virulent and malignant *P. falciparum* which infested the region. This type of adaptation suggests a very long history for humanity and plasmodium in that region. Aliens penetrating the area, such as nineteenth-century European explorers or others of European origin, were decimated by malarial disease which left the indigenous population untouched.

India was a second major area for malarial infection. Indian art and medical classics make it clear that malaria had a long history on the subcontinent, while nineteenth-century British military medical statistics give some indication of the intensity of infection. In Bengal, Bombay, and Madras, over the periods 1847–1854 and 1860–1875, of 1,110,820 British soldiers, 457,088, or 41.1 percent of the total, were reported as malarial cases. While malaria was a major problem for the military, its effects on the civilian population can only be guessed, but if the same proportions held for native civilians as for the military, 20 million cases would not be an exaggeration. Twentieth-century figures support this idea with new case incidence in recent years passing the 30 million mark. Ceylon (today, Sri Lanka) was similarly infected, and malaria was serious throughout southeast Asia.

China has been a third major malarial region, though detailed information is lacking. Tropical and subtropical China was one of the most intensely infected malarial regions in the world. The coastal cities from Macao, Hong Kong, and Guangzhou to Tianjin and Shanghai were known for their malarial incidence. It is thought that China's interior may well have rivaled India for malarial infection, especially in the great river valleys, but detailed evidence is lacking. Australia, on the other hand, has been almost entirely free of malaria, and in the region, only the New Guinea coast has a serious malaria problem.

Malaria was important in the Mediterranean basin in classical times, and its incidence extended north into Europe. To the east a belt of malarial infection stretched from the Asian steppes across the Caspian region and the Black Sea littoral into the Balkans. The disease in the European east was known under several names, including the Dacian, Taurian, Crimean, Wallachian, and Hungarian fever. There were pockets of malarial infection in the west Russian (Pripet) marsh region, but also near Tula to the south, Yaroslavl and Kasan to the east of Moscow, and Orenburg in the southeast. The Hungarian and Danubian plains had the disease as well. In Italy in modern times the two main malarial regions were the plain of the Po across the north, and the Roman Campagna and Pontine marshes area. The information on malaria in Spain is sparse, but there appears to have been somewhat less there than in Italy or the Balkans, while in France, there were limited malarial areas in the west and south. Germany had scattered endemic areas, especially in marshy regions adjacent to the Rhine and Danube, and in the basins of the Weser, Oder, Elbe, and Vistula across the north. Schleswig and Holstein were among the worst areas for malaria, and there were malarial provinces in both Holland and Belgium. The British Isles were largely free of malaria in the west and north, but there were malarial centers on the east coast, particularly in the fens, and London was notably fever-plagued until after the Thames embankment was built and flooding controlled in 1864.

One of the worst centers for endemic malaria, comparable to Africa or India, was on the east coast of South America, particularly Guiana, while the northern coastal regions of Brazil were dangerously infected. Malaria also appeared on the pampas of Paraguay and in Bolivia. Moving toward the south, however, the incidence declined. The same was true of North America. The worst fever zones were subtropical and coastal, though malaria was active in the middle Atlantic region. Finally, malaria was a severe problem throughout central America, though notably worse on the Atlantic side.

Malaria epidemics were first recorded in the middle of the sixteenth century throughout Europe, and the second epidemic outbreak was noted in the seventeenth century (1678–1682). The eighteenth century recorded four epidemic periods between 1718 and 1783, and then another in the period 1806–1812. Additional epidemic outbreaks occurred in the periods 1823–1828 (very severe), 1845–1849, 1855–1860, and 1866–1872. The last outbreak affected most of Europe, India, and North America. With expanding agriculture and drainage programs, malaria's decline began to be noted in the later nineteenth century in the temperate regions of Europe and North America. Intensive public health campaigns were required to control the disease in the rest of the world in the twentieth century.

Malaria in the Americas European conquerors and explorers in the sixteenth century probably introduced malaria into the western hemisphere. Since the disease was endemic in the Mediterranean basin and in Africa, Spanish colonizers and black slaves account for the transfer. By the early seventeenth century, not only was there evidence of malarial fevers in the new world, but the Jesuits were extolling a native Peruvian remedy for fever. "Fever tree bark," or as it became known, "Jesuit powders," contained quinine (q.v.), which was effective against intermittent fevers and proved to be a valuable preventive as well as a therapeutic agent.

Malaria became endemic in the North American colonies in the seventeenth century. The Spaniards visited and attempted to settle on the Atlantic coast from Florida to Cape Fear, North Carolina, ascended the Mississippi as far as modern St. Louis, Missouri, and roamed through the southwest. By the second half of the seventeenth century, fevers showing malarial characteristics were reported throughout North America, Canada included, and the disease figured significantly in the journals of Father Jacques Grevier, who followed the Mississippi from what is now Illinois to its mouth in 1701 and 1702. Malaria appeared in seventeenth-century New England, but it disappeared from there by the end of the eighteenth century. It remained active, however, in the Middle Atlantic colonies and throughout the south.

After the American Revolution, new lands were opened in the west, and waves of settlers poured in. Those in the territories along the Mississippi found themselves plagued with agues and fevers, and the reports of such malarial incidence persisted into the second half of the nineteenth century. Malaria in the Mississippi valley may have been reintroduced with the migrations, since there are no reports of it between the first decade of the eighteenth century and the end of the French and Indian Wars (1763). Then, however, the incidence began to increase rapidly, so much so that a former governor of Illinois Territory said in his memoirs: "In 1800 to 1805, the idea prevailed that Illinois was a graveyard." A settler near Edwardsville, Illinois, summed up conditions and the problem when he wrote in 1819: "The principle [sic] objection I have to this Country is its unhealthiness." August and September were especially bad, and he had suffered fever and ague for nearly two months. This man gave himself one more season for his health to improve before moving out.

Central Illinois had its last major malaria season in 1872, and by the end of the 1880s, malaria had disappeared from most of the upper middle west. But it remained a continuing problem in the southern states. The 12 states of the old south had 1 million malaria cases annually from 1912 to 1915. The disease began to decline as modern agriculture spread. Preventive campaigns had local success, especially in cities, but in the rural south malaria remained a problem until after World War II when DDT became available for spraying. Then malaria in the southern United States fell precipitously. By 1960, it had effectively disappeared.

Cultural Effects Malaria's effects on history and culture have never been clear-cut or sharply defined. The less virulent endemic forms of the disease have relatively low death rates and very broad incidence. The disease has an adverse effect on birthrates in endemic areas, and because of its weakening, debilitating effects, it leaves populations open to other infections and with reduced physical strength to resist them. In places where malaria has been controlled, mortality rates have fallen significantly more than the rate which malaria alone could explain. This has led to the conclusion that extensive malarial infection depresses population growth and has distinctly adverse demographic consequences. Since many areas where malaria has been most active have also been areas of serious overpopulation—India and China are examples—the long-term effect on population may not have been as damaging as in less well-developed areas. Where populations are thin or in decline, malaria may well have serious long-term negative effects. Moreover, the effect of malaria is such that people will leave an area where it is active if they can. The abandonment of agricultural lands near Rome and on the Italian coast is a classic example. Demographic effect will be heightened by emigrations from malaria-ridden areas, and it is entirely possible that a region where malaria is widespread will be emptied of its people.

The debilitating effect of malaria may have farther-reaching consequences. If sufficiently persistent and widespread, it is thought to affect a society's capacity to function creatively, destroying the will to act and reducing the ambition and ultimately the capacity of the population to the point where the society's energies go entirely into providing for existence. Some classical scholars, using modern demographic models and applying social psychology, have argued that the cultural transformation of Greece, beginning with the decline of the fourth century, may have resulted from the enervating effect of endemic malaria.

Malaria's most important modern role has been as a barrier against Europeans in tropical or subtropical zones. Malaria was the most widespread and dangerous of the diseases which made Africa "the white man's graveyard." It held up the exploration of that vast continent until the second half of the nineteenth century, and it remains a serious problem for modern African governments. In Panama, malaria proved less amenable to control than yellow fever and was a major factor in Ferdinand de Lesseps' failure to complete a canal in the area. De Lesseps lost 5627 men from fever between 1880 and 1889. Not all, of course, were malaria cases. William Gorgas took over the sanitary administration of the Panama Canal Zone in 1904. By 1906, yellow fever had largely been stopped, but of 26,000 workers, 83.6 percent had to be treated for malaria. The following year, the percentage was cut in half (to 42.9 percent), and in 1911 and 1912 it had fallen to 17 percent, and there were just 32 deaths. Nevertheless, of 40,000 workers, 7000 had to have malaria treatment. The disease is stubborn, difficult to control, and expensive to keep under surveillance.

Malaria management has concentrated in recent years on eliminating anopheles mosquitoes. But societies lived with malaria long before control programs were considered. Quinine, quinine derivatives, and chemically created products producing quinine action have contributed to this achievement. Fever powders, imported in quantity, helped control fever's effects in seventeenth- and eighteenth-century Europe, while the quinine action was essential for Europeans seeking to live and work in the tropics. Malaria's historical significance is as a long-term ecological factor. It is an influence nearly as difficult to measure as the disease had been difficult to eradicate.

Malaria Discoveries The discovery of the mechanisms by which malaria was transferred took place in the last quarter of the nineteenth century and the first years of the twentieth. An association between mosquitoes and malaria had been made centuries earlier in Sanskrit writings, but there was no scientific basis for the idea until 1880, when a French army surgeon working in Algeria, Charles Louis Alphonse Laveran, saw the malaria plasmodium in its first stage of sexual reproduction. His observations were confirmed by Camillo Golgi, an Italian physician who added a great deal of detailed observation on plasmodium behavior. The next piece in the malaria puzzle was provided by Dr. (later Sir) Patrick Manson, who found filariasis growing in mosquito stomachs when fed with blood from filariasis patients. This observation correlated with current work on ticks and tsetse flies as carriers of cattle and horse diseases. It was Manson who then suggested that the mosquito was both the vector and the intermediate host for malaria, and he discussed these ideas with a young British army surgeon named Ronald Ross. Ross was captivated by the idea, and he returned to India where he tested it and proved it to be true. By 1898, Ross had established the mosquito's vector role and had worked out experimentally the entire plasmodium life cycle. His work was supported and confirmed by Giovanni Batiste Grassi, who further showed that only the anopheles mosquito was dangerous to humans.

Malaria Control The basic discoveries concerning malaria corresponded with those on yellow fever (q.v.), and the techniques which William Gorgas used in Havana and later in Panama influenced antimalarial compaigns as well. The mosquito vectors rather than the human reservoirs became the focus for control. The most successful measures included spreading oil or kerosene on ponds to prevent mosquito hatching, using copper sulfate to exterminate mosquitoes and their larvae, and planting fish which feed on mosquito larvae in ponds. In addition, screening windows and doors and, in badly infested areas, using bed nets to prevent night-feeding mosquitoes from biting humans while they slept were essential. In Malaya, Sir Malcolm Watson had already begun a malaria control program, which included ditching and draining and which dropped the overall death rate among his Tamil and Chinese workers from 368 per 1000 to 45. On one estate in Watson's jurisdiction, not one Tamil woman had had a live birth in six years; under his malaria eradication program, babies again began to be born.

These successes, together with those in Panama and Cuba, opened the possibility of a worldwide assault on malaria, but the question was whether disease control was possible at costs which a community could afford. The U.S. Public Health Service believed that it could be done, and, under Henry Rose Carter and Rudolph von Ezdorf, this organization set about an antimalaria program for the southern United States. The Rockefeller Foundation offered support and the cooperation of its International Health Division, but the administration of the program was carried on by the U.S. Public Health Serivce, working with state and local health departments. The first program was carried out in Arkansas, and the results were astounding: Malaria incidence dropped 50 percent in three years at costs ranging from $0.38 to $1.09 per capita. Pilot projects to test the preventive powers of quinine and the effects of drainage programs gave firm evidence for planning further work. When Paris green dust (copper arsenic) was introduced, a cheap and effective method for killing mosquito larvae was available. Paris green remained the basis for mosquito control until after World War II. The antimalaria program in the United States was most successful in towns and cities, where malaria was largely eliminated by 1927. The disease remained, though much reduced, in rural America until after World War II.

Although malaria was brought under control in the United States, severe endemic areas continued to exist in Europe, Asia, and Africa. During World War I, resistance to malaria control measures in Macedonia by line officers of both the Allies and Central Powers, who considered hygienic exercises a waste of time in war, resulted in massive malaria outbreaks which immobilized troops and established a reservoir of infection from which the disease spread through southern Europe and the Levant. Eventually, malaria moved into northern Europe and Russia. By 1923, the malaria incidence in the Soviet Union was around 18 million cases, with mortality in some areas running up to 40 percent.

Italy had had endemic malaria for centuries, but the war brought on new activity. By 1922, there were 2 million cases per year. The government decided to act, and the Italian National Health Department was given responsibility for organizing a campaign. The Rockefeller Foundation–sponsored International Health Division cooperated. New research and control measures were undertaken. The unpredictable behavior of Italian mosquitoes led researchers to the fact that there were six types of anopheles mosquito, three of which were dangerous as malaria vectors. Disease control plans were then adjusted to the various living and mating habits of these different strains. This permitted more effective specialized mosquito control programs.

The American type of antimosquito campaign was followed, and between 1924 and 1929, a radical reduction in malarial infections was achieved in the Portotorres test area. During the 1930s the campaign was carried into the country at large. These campaigns were carried on despite growing criticism of the American method. A League of Nations commission which investigated malaria suggested that the success of the program could be explained by declining virulence in the disease agent. Even so the campaign continued. By 1940, the worst malarial regions in Italy were under control, and in the previously uninhabitable Pontine marshes, 50,000 new settlers had opened and were farming 200,000 acres of new farm land.

Malaria control program successes in the United States, Italy, and the Caribbean led to further attempts in Brazil, Africa, and south Asia. Brazil had a major outbreak of malaria in 1931 and 1932 and another in 1938 and 1939. The latter was a particularly virulent epidemic with more than 100,000 cases, and 14,000 to 20,000 deaths. The area was one which had been free of malaria, and there were no natural immunities. The government of Brazil decided on an all-out eradication campaign. The mosquito in this case was *A. gambiae,* which had been imported from Africa within the preceding two decades. Despite enormous logistical problems, the campaign was completed between May 1939 and November 1940. Paris green was used to saturate breeding grounds, while every house interior in the malarial zone was sprayed with pyrethrum.

Malaria was an important problem during World War II, but once the cooperation of the military was won, the means for controlling the disease were implemented effectively. In the Pacific, where the threat was most serious, Gen. Douglas MacArthur accepted the need for systematic disease control and cooperated fully with the medical corps. The introduction of DDT as an insecticide during the war made control procedures more effective. DDT (dichlorodiphenyltrichloroethane) had first been synthesized in 1874 from chlorine, alchohol, and sulfuric acid. Its insecticidal powers were discovered in the middle 1930s. DDT was no more fatal to insects than pyrethrum, and it lacked the latter's swift killing properties. Its special quality was that it remained active for weeks or even months. DDT eliminated the need for repeated respraying. By the end of World War II, eradication of malaria appeared to be a feasible goal.

The Current Scene Malaria control measures have fallen far short of the hoped-for eradication of the disease, and after a period of great optimism around 1960, the statistics on malaria incidence and mortality have risen sharply. At the beginning of World War II, according to one estimate, malaria would have annually infected 300 million people. At the opening of the 1960s, in a more populous world, the annual incidence was estimated to stand below 100 million. In 1961, the director general of the World Health Organization pointed out that whereas malaria mortality in the 1950s had reached 3.5 million annually, the number by the mid-sixties would be under 1 million, while the economic, social, and cultural consequences of freeing millions of people from malarial infection were simply incalcuable.

Less favorable data have appeared more recently. During the late 1960s and early 1970s, there has been a dangerous recrudescence of malaria in areas where it had been endemic, and where the campaigns against it had been most intense. It was found that maintaining the intensive surveillance necessary for control is too costly of time and energy, especially for societies whose productive economies are weak. The surveillance system itself proved inadequate, at least in part due to human failures. The latter ranged from ignoring isolated villages which were difficult to reach to shortages of microscopic slides or careless readings of blood smears. The cost of DDT, which has a petroleum base, soared in the first oil crisis (1974), and the only substitute for it, malathion, is more costly still. Subsequent rises in petroleum prices, particularly in the spring and early summer of 1979, have only made the problem more intractable. Moreover, evidence of DDT's poisonous effects in the food chain have forced severe restrictions on the use of the compound. There is also evidence that *A. culicifacies,* the main malaria vector in India, is becoming DDT resistant.

In consequence of these developments, endemic malaria in India climbed from its low point in 1961 of less that 100,000 cases to 350,000 cases in 1969, and by 1974 there were fully 2.5 million malaria cases recorded. In 1975, that figure doubled, and by 1977, estimates of malaria case incidence in India had soared above 30 million. A similar resurgence has occurred in Sri Lanka (Ceylon), while the situation in Southeast Asia as a whole has become such that a World Health Organization official concluded in 1976: "The entire population living in the original malarious areas is now at malaria risk."

In other parts of the world, there are achievements as well as failures. Countries certified as having accomplished eradications since 1956 have held that status. Taiwan gained eradication in 1961 and was certified in 1965, while Cuba had eradicated malaria by 1973. Venezuela, Argentina, and much of Brazil and Paraguay are now clear of malaria, and Brazil is working on the final stages of an eradication campaign. Other areas are making no gains, however, and the situation has deteriorated in El Salvador and Guatemala. The Middle East, which had made great strides against malaria, lost ground again during the 1970s as a result of war and social upheavals. Iraq, Syria, Jordan, and Lebanon, all of which had made substantial progress, have been reinvaded, and malaria has returned to areas where it was nearly eliminated in Turkey, Iran, and Tunisia. Cyprus and Greece have had new malarial infections, though they appear to be under control. Malaria is still a problem in many Pacific islands, and there has been almost no progress at all against the disease in sub-Saharan Africa. It now seems plain that only an extended period of prosperity, peace, and economic growth will provide the needed base for a renewed antimalarial campaign in much of the third world. The world at the beginning of the 1980s offers little hope for such a revival.

ADDITIONAL READINGS: E. H. Ackerknecht, *Malaria in the Upper Mississippi Valley, 1760–1900,* Baltimore, 1945; Sir Robert W. Boyce, *Mosquito or Man? The Conquest of the Tropical World,* 3d ed., London, 1910, chaps. VI–IX; Leonard Jan Bruce-Chwatt, *The Rise and Fall of Malaria in Europe: A Historico-Epidemiological Study,* Oxford, 1980; Mary Schaeffer Conroy, "Malaria in Late Tsarist Russia," *Bulletin of the History of Medicine* 56 (Spring 1982): 41–55; M. Gelfand, *Rivers of Death in Africa,* Oxford, 1964; Lewis Wendell Hackett, *Malaria in Europe: An Ecological Study,* London, 1944; Gordon Harrison, *Mosquitoes, Malaria, and Man: A History of the Hostilities Since 1880,* London, 1978; Norman Levine (ed.), *Malaria in the Interior Valley of North America: Daniel Drake's Systematic Treatise,* Urbana, Ill., 1964; Sir Malcolm Watson, *African Highway: The Battle for Health in Central Africa,* London, 1953; Greer Williams, *The Plague Killers,* New York, 1969; Clive Wood (ed.), *Tropical Medicine: From Romance to Reality,* London, 1978, 27–114.

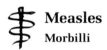

Measles

Morbilli

Measles is the most infectious of all common fevers. The disease is found throughout the world, and while its identification early in history is difficult, what we know suggests that it has played a significant role. In the modern world, measles is a children's disease which occasions little concern. For previously unexposed populations, however, measles has been a deadly scourge, as destructive as any in history. Even in modern terms, measles' side effects are such as to warrant caution, though medicine now has the means to prevent the disease and to manage it effectively.

Disease Characteristics Measles is a highly contagious febrile disease caused by a virus infection which takes place in the upper respiratory tract. The virus is communicated directly from person to person by droplets since the virus is present in large quantities in the secretions of the nose and mouth. Articles soiled by these secretions, such as handkerchiefs, will be very infectious. The measles virus has its most serious effects as it reduces resistance in the respiratory and gastrointestinal tracts to bacterial infection. The most common complications are laryngitis, tracheitis, and bronchopneumonia, the latter being the most common cause of death where measles occurs. Other complications include lobar and interstital pneumonia and emphysema.

Since the measles virus apparently does not vary, the fluctuations in result from infection relate to previous infection levels, general health conditions, and prevalent bacteria. Measles infection confers a permanent immunity. Therefore, where previous infections have occurred, only those young enough not to have had the disease will become infected, and, on the whole, measles has been a children's disease. It rarely occurs in infants under three months, owing to the transmission of antibodies to the fetus from a mother who has had the disease. In populations not previously infected, however, infection can be nearly total. This occurred in southern Greenland in 1951, when of 4000 previously uninfected susceptibles, only five persons escaped infection after the primary case appered. In tropical countries, measles generates very high mortalities from pneumonia and enteritis, while in developing countries, the disease's effect may be to disturb the already precarious nutritional balance, bringing on symptoms of vitamin deficiency and protein-energy malnutrition.

Improved standards of living, adequate diet, and effective nursing care have reduced the effects of measles significantly in developed industrial societies. The discovery of effective vaccines and the mounting of mass vaccination campaigns in the 1960s in the United States, Great Britain, and west and central Africa have shown that measles is susceptible to direct control in both developed and undeveloped regions. Political instability in Africa and a consequent breakdown of the vaccination delivery system in the 1970s demonstrate the problems in effecting medically sound programs in underdeveloped countries, while public apathy and financial problems have substantially reduced the effectiveness of the vaccination program in the United States.

Early History Most authorities agree that the so-called eruptive fevers, that is, measles, smallpox, scarlet fever, and rubella, probably became established in the Mediterranean world in the first millennium of the Christian era. They do not figure in the Greek classical texts, nor is there firm descriptive evidence concerning them in Roman or early medieval sources. Smallpox (q.v.) was known much earlier in Asia, and it has been speculated that smallpox entered the Roman empire as a new disease which generated the terrible pestilences of the second and third centuries A.D. It is also thought that one of these plagues may have established smallpox, while the other may have been measles. There is no direct evidence to support these ideas, though the virulence of the late Roman plagues is consistent with the introduction of new disease strains into virgin populations. The reputed high mortalities would correspond with the relatively low level of nutritional and living standards for the mass of the population.

The first unequivocal description of eruptive fevers which distinguished between measles and smallpox was written by al-Razi (al Rhazes) a Persian physician working in Baghdad. In about A.D. 910, al-Razi, citing the authority of a Hebrew physician, El Yehudi, identified measles as an affliction of the young, while smallpox was suffered by the mature. A basic change in the character of the blood was thought to account for the two afflictions, and while al-Razi distinguished between the two, he saw them as products of a common cause. The association between smallpox and measles remained in vogue into the eighteenth century. Al-Razi also gave a detailed account of the symptoms of the two diseases, including the rather different signals which announced the onset of each. His was the first "unambiguous clinical description of these afflictions," and the description showed a long and substantial familiarity with the disease.

No comparable tradition existed in Europe, though Gregory of Tours chronicled the outbreak of an eruptive fever in A.D. 580, and the word "measles" does not appear in an English treatise on medicine until the fourteenth-century *Rosa Anglica* of John of Gaddesden. There was a persistent semantic confusion concerning measles throughout the Middle Ages which further complicated disease identification. *"Morbilli"* meant "little disease," to distinguish it from *"il morbo,"* ("plague"). Neither term was particularly discriminating. In Chaucer and Langland, "mesel" meant leprosy, while throughout the sixteenth century, smallpox and measles were considered variants of the same disease. Moreover, the words "measles" and "morbilli" were frequently used to describe scarlatina (see Scarlet Fever), and the term "scarlatina" was often applied to what we know now was diphtheria (q.v.). In the seventeenth century, the semantic confusions began to clear, and in 1629, measles appeared as a separate category in the London bills of mortality. Even so, there was no clear diagnostic standard to follow until Thomas Sydenham established it in 1670. Sydenham's description, however, was complete, covering all the essential clinical features of measles.

Measles and Demography: 1500 to 1900 Though far older in Asia, measles became demographically significant in Europe at the close of the Roman period, and it remained so to the twentieth century. The disease was very active in the eighteenth and nineteenth centuries, especially the latter, when epidemics occurred nearly every other year. Almost no European child escaped infection, and measles came to be considered one of the most common causes of child mortality. The decline in measles' incidence and mortality in the twentieth century resulted from improving social and economic conditions rather than medical discovery.

Measles' influence outside Europe in the modern period was felt in the new world from the sixteenth century onward, and throughout the Pacific islands in the eighteenth and nineteenth centuries. European diseases had terrible effects on previously uninfected native populations, but the early historical sources are such that it is difficult to identify specific diseases. Smallpox, typhus, and syphilis have been set out as the most deadly, but there is little doubt that measles contributed as well. The earliest measles outbreaks were in 1519 (Santo Domingo), 1523 (Guatemala), and 1531 (Mexico). Repeated epidemics occurred in the seventeenth and eighteenth centuries, some of which were deadly. In 1785, for example, measles struck Ecuador, with 2400 deaths reported in Quito alone.

Measles repeatedly attacked the North American colonies, beginning in Canada in 1635. Because of thin population density, the epidemic pattern was dominant. Measles would be introduced into and would run through a community. It would then disappear and not return until several years later when a fresh infection would break out among a new crop of nonimmune susceptibles. Some outbreaks were very serious, Boston was hard hit in 1740 and again in 1772, when some 800 children died in the Charlestown section. Boston had other notable outbreaks in 1657, 1687, 1713, 1729, and 1739. In 1747, measles reached epidemic proportions in South Carolina, Pennsylvania, New York, Connecticut, and Massachusetts. New York and Philadelphia were visited in 1788, while outbreaks began to be reported from the Mississippi valley, Kentucky, and Ohio. As population grew and transport improved, measles in the United States settled into the European pattern of an endemic disease primarily of children with occasional epidemic outbreaks.

In 1846, an important measles epidemic occurred in the Faeroe Islands, where of 7864 people, 6100 became ill, and 102 died. The Danish government sent Dr. P. L. Panum to observe, and it was his work which laid the basis for modern measles epidemiology. The devastating effects which measles could have on a primitive population appeared when the British annexed the Fiji Islands in 1874, and the cruiser H.M.S. Dido arrived there with measles on board in 1875. The disease ran riot. In three months, some 40,000 islanders had died, that is, between 20 and 25 percent of the Fiji population, and when measles spread to neighboring island groups, the same result followed. Sheer panic and a total inability to cope with the disease symptoms contributed to the high death rates as the terrified sufferers immersed themselves in the sea to cool the effects of fever. European contact proved as devastating to Pacific island cultures as it was to the Amerindians, and one recent authority suggested that the combined effects of measles, tuberculosis, and syphilis carried off up to 90 percent of the island populations.

Immunization and Control: The Twentieth Century Since measles was identified with smallpox, it was natural, even after the diseases were separated, to try a form of variolation called "morbillisation" to induce immunity. Francis Home of Edinburgh had some success in 1758 in inducing measles by soaking cotton in the blood of patients in the acute stage and putting the soaked cotton on scarified areas of the arm in persons with no previous history of measles. Home infected 7 children out of 15 that he tried, and though the procedure was very uncertain and unpredictable, it was hailed by contemporary authority as "the most powerful means of alleviating the common sequences of measles." Such optimism was hardly warranted by the results, and it was not until 1905 that Ludwig Hektoen of the University of Chicago was able to carry out the first unequivocally successful measles transfers. Six years later, John F. Anderson and Joseph Goldberg of the U.S. Public Health Service for the first time produced measles in an animal other than a human by injecting monkeys with cell-free blood filtrate from a measles patient. This suggested that measles was a virus infection, a conclusion which was confirmed in 1914 when C. Hermann infected infants from three to five months with filtered nose and throat washings from infected persons. Though the viral point was proved, this method was dropped as too dangerous for maintaining or enhancing immunity. It was not until the period 1938–1940, however, that the virus was first cultivated, in a tissue culture by Harry Plotz, and in chicken embryos by Geoffrey Rake and Morris F. Shaffer.

During World War II, the availability of large quantities of blood plasma led to an expanded use of gamma globulin for passive immunization against measles. Though measles virus could be cultivated in chick embryos, production of an acceptably safe vaccine was blocked because there was no efficient way to measure the quantity of virus which developed in the embryos. In 1954, John F. Enders and Thomas C. Peebles of Harvard University removed this barrier when they discovered that measles virus produced visible changes in host cells when they were cultivated in tissue from human or monkey kidneys. Cytopathogenic effects, as such changes were called, provided a key to the quantity of virus working, and this made vaccine standardization possible.

The United States licensed a measles vaccine in 1963. Mass immunization began immediately in the United States and Europe, and an African pilot program was introduced in 1966. The effects were dramatic. In 1962, there had been 482,000 cases of measles reported in the United States. By 1968, the number had fallen to 22,000. By 1971, however, the number of cases was up again to 75,000. This correlated with a drop in 1969 in the number of children actually receiving the vaccine. This decline was particularly notable among low-income-family children where cuts in appropriations for immunization and public health programs were felt first. Redoubled efforts to reach the nonimmune have only partially redressed the balance.

In Great Britain, measles has been reduced to an insignificant problem. The World Health Organization program for immunization in Africa, however, after showing promising results, fell victim to political upheavals, though Gambia reported effective eradication of the disease. Medically, measles is no longer a significant problem, but social, political, and economic problems affect control plans directly and show the kind of future effort that will be required to establish and maintain immunities to measles virus.

ADDITIONAL READINGS: Frederick F. Cartwright, *Disease and History*, London, 1972; Barbara Gastel, "Measles: A Potentially Finite History," *Journal of the History of Medicine* 28 (January 1973): 34–44; J. H. Parish, *A History of Immunization*, London, 1965, chap. 30; George Rosen, "Acute Communicable Diseases," in Walter Bett (ed.), *The History and Conquest of Common Diseases*, Norman, Okla., 1954, 38–45.

Medical History

Medical history is a modern academic discipline which appeared in the eighteenth century but whose major period of growth came after 1890. German scholarship gave the field its classic definition, but after World War II, intellectual leadership shifted to the United States and Britain, while in terms of institutional support and volume of work, the Soviet Union became a major center. Soviet medical historiography has had relatively little influence beyond eastern Europe, however, owing to its inaccessibility to scholars who do not read Russian, its heavy emphasis on Russian medical history, and western resistance to its narrowly Marxist historical philosophy.

The main subject matter for medical history has traditionally been the ideas shaping medical practice, the evolution of specialized medical disciplines, and the diseases with which mankind has been afflicted. Until the middle of the twentieth century, general historians paid little attention to most of these subjects, while medical historians tended to be men trained as physicians who used historical data to explain or to enrich contemporary medical understanding. Their methods belonged to cultural history, and a great deal of attention was given to establishing, analyzing, editing, and commenting upon classic medical texts. The history which they wrote was biographical and intellectual, and after the nineteenth-century revolution in medical science, current knowledge provided the standards for historical significance. Ancient writings were scanned for ideas foreshadowing modern truths, and the history of medical science came to be conceived of in terms of progress toward a modern ideal. These tendencies remain a significant influence on modern medical historiography and are particularly strong in amateur and popularized accounts.

Institutionally, medical history developed as part of university programs for educating physicians. The universities at Würzburg (1743) and Göttingen (1750) charged their professors of medical theory with lecturing on the history of medicine, and in 1794 a joint chair for legal and medical history was established in Paris. By the early nineteenth century, most German universities offered lectures for beginning medical students which included the history of medicine, while specialized courses on the history of anatomy and physiology, ancient medical systems, pathology, surgery, obstetrics, medical police, and even psychiatry were available. The purpose of these offerings was, as a distinguished anatomist wrote in 1832, "to give physicians a clear insight into the present state of medicine, and the relation of the branches of medicine to each other and with other sciences." Similar developments occurred outside the German states. In Hapsburg Austria, an important chair of medical history was established in Vienna in 1808 which lasted to 1938, and which was occupied by three of the most distinguished medical historians of the era: Romeo Seligmann (1833–1879); Theodore Puschmann (1879–1899); and Max Neuberger (1904–1938). Medical history also flourished in medical school curricula in Hungary, Italy, Spain, and Russia.

Between 1850 and 1890, the scientific approach to medicine temporarily reduced medical history's role in medical education, but by the end of the century, a strong reaction against utilitarianism and academic pragmatism revived interest in history as a humanistic discipline. In medicine, where the physician's professional and social standing had come to be defined by his education, history's integrative and cultural role was particularly important. Moreover, as Theodore Puschmann argued in 1889, "Anyone who wants to have a complete and thorough understanding of scientific facts must study the history of their origin." Mastering a field meant controlling its history as well as its current substance. Sir William Osler, a Canadian who taught medicine at McGill, the University of Pennsylvania, and Johns Hopkins before he became regius professor at Oxford in 1904, exemplified the blend of classic culture with scientific knowledge which became the professional ideal. Oster was broadly read in the history and science of medicine, and his informal Socratic teaching methods and published writings all combined past knowledge with present perceptions to create a special synthesis. The method was vastly influential and reinforced the importance of both medical history and history as culture in physicians' training. It was also, however, an approach which invited imitation but defied systematization and so sustained an ideal while marking an unclear road to reach it.

Between 1900 and 1910, medical history was reestablished in Europe's medical schools, and the process was repeated in the United States between 1926 and 1939. The German Society for the History of Medicine and Science was founded in 1901 with Karl Sudhoff as president. That same year, a similar society was established in France, and others followed in Holland (1903) and Italy (1908). In 1905, funded with a large bequest from Theodore Puschmann's widow, an Institute for the History of Medicine was created at Leipzig with Karl Sudhoff as director. The Leipzig Institute, in George Rosen's phrase, "determined the objectives and directions for the investigation and teaching of medical history, during the first half of the twentieth century." By 1910, specialists in medical history were promoting research, offering courses, and training students at Berlin, Bonn, Budapest, Edinburgh, Erlangen, Geneva, Jena, Lemberg, Leyden, Vienna, and Würzburg. Courses were given at eight other German universities as well as at the University of Basel, while as a result of a private gift in 1903, the Royal

College of Physicians, London, had established a lectureship in the history of medicine.

In the United States, where medical education was entering on a period of significant reform, full-term courses in medical history were given in 1904 at the universities of Pennsylvania, Maryland, and Minnesota, and some instruction in the field was offered at several other schools. This record gradually improved to 1914, but the next major step was not taken until 1926 when Johns Hopkins created a chair of medical history for William H. Welch and established an Institute for Medical History in 1929. The German example was of primary importance, with the Leipzig Institute serving as a model. This connection became even closer in 1932 when Henry E. Sigerist, director of the Leipzig Institute from 1925 and a student of Karl Sudhoff, left Germany to take over the new institute at Hopkins. By 1937, 54 American medical schools were teaching medical history, 28 of these required the course, and 22 had medical history as a required examination subject.

The high point for medical history in American medical education was reached on the eve of World War II. Following the war, though the University of Wisconsin established a chair which Erwin Ackerknecht came to hold, the discipline fell precipitously from favor. The conviction that medical history was an essential part of the physician's intellectual equipment gave way in the face of expanding demands for new courses in medicine itself together with a further emphasis on clinical training. Appeals based on the social and ethical significance of medical history won little support as the opinion gained ground that medical history, while interesting, should not command a place in the required medical curriculum. As a result, while physicians remain fascinated by their history, and amateur historical writing by doctors continues to be a significant genre, the history of medicine has developed into an independent field of historical study producing a constantly growing literature of broad significance.

The first half of the twentieth century comprised the classic period of medical historiography. Building on nineteenth-century source collections and specialized studies, medical historians explored medicine as culture while adding further detail to the intellectual history of the profession. The Greek heritage, so critically important to the nineteenth-century view of European civilization, received special attention, as did the Renaissance, while studies of men and ideas dominated the writing. The intellectual-biographical approach fitted with a strong bias toward cultural history. Hippocrates and Galen, Paracelsus, Vesalius and Harvey, Paré and Sydenham were studied in the context of their times with their ideas compared against or explained in terms of the culture's religious, philosophical, scientific, and literary traditions. The systematic development of archaeology, numismatics, and art history provided new evidence and clues to reinterpreting older data. Toward the middle of the twentieth century, new disciplines added their methods and conclusions to medical history, with sociology and anthropology proving to be particularly influential. Though framed largely in cultural and intellectual terms, the classic era of medical history writing developed an approach which viewed medicine as an integral part of culture and a phenomenon which demanded to be understood in terms of the historical environment in which it lodged. Though naive positivism and a breathless wondering at the catalog of great discoveries in medicine run through twentieth-century amateur and popularized works, the mainstream of medical-historical writing has developed in the direction of methodologically sophisticated cultural history. Unfortunately, the image of twentieth-century medical history has been formed in popular works which emphasize adventure and the dramatic, and in general histories of medicine which are primarily chronological descriptions of people and their discoveries. The cultural treasures of modern research on medical history have largely escaped the reading public and have only begun to be synthesized into general history.

The most important recent shifts in medical-historical work have been toward medicine as social history and the entrance of nonmedically trained professional historians into the field. This latter trend has precipitated a soul-searching debate over what medical history is and what qualifications are necessary to study, teach, and write it. The more significant development, however, is the shift toward viewing medicine as social history. Embedded in this view, especially as expressed by a generation of young historians, is the rejection of medicine as exclusively a phenomenon of high culture, and, for the more radical, a rejection of high culture as such combined with the affirmation of a modernized democratic populism. What this has meant in historical terms is a search for correlations between medical ideas and class interests, and the study of medical functions where conflicting values identify competing groups. Professional standards, licensing and education, the history of midwifery and nursing, the development of hospitals, the story of drugs and drug abuse, the evolution of national health care programs, and a host of similar subjects have engaged a growing number of young historians. Since most of these people have little contact with medical schools, their work goes directly into the stream of contemporary historical thinking and the particular character of medical history as such is lost.

Several bridges connected traditional medical history with the developing emphasis on social history. Henry Sigerist, for example, was an outspoken proponent of medical history's social relevance, while Erwin Ackerknecht explored the interaction among medical ideas, society, and politics, while arguing for a history of medicine that dealt with what doctors did rather than what a few physicians thought. One of the most important figures in this connection was George Rosen, who followed a basic history of public health published in 1958 with a series of studies on the social hygiene movement, the history of hospitals, cameralism, medical police, and the evolution of national health policies, and, on quite another level, the study of madness in terms of socially defined phenomena. Both medically and historically trained, George Rosen connected the cultural-intellectual and social-historical traditions, and his work is seminal for contemporary medical historians.

Another powerful impetus to medicine and social history came from interest in epidemic diseases. This was an area in which nineteenth-century medical historians were active, led by classic works of August Hirsch on historical-geographical pathology, J. F. K. Hecker on medieval epidemics, and Heinrich Haeser on epidemics in general. Hans Zinsser's entertaining and medically sound *Rats, Lice and History* (1935) stirred general awareness of epidemics' historical significance, but it was only after World War II that serious and systematic study of epidemic phenomena began. In December 1957, William L. Langer addressed the American Historical Association on "History's Next Assignment," which he defined as studying the structural dynamics of social development. Demography was a central issue, with special attention recommended for epidemic diseases. Subsequent studies on plague, cholera, and yellow fever have explored the social ramifications of disease, the effects of epidemics, and, even more important, what can be learned about the character of societies by detailed study of their experiences with epidemics. The bulk of this work has been done by nonmedically trained historians whose primary interest has been in exploring social and cultural rather than medical questions as such. The same is true of William A. McNeill's *Plagues and Peoples* (1976), which stands out as a significant attempt at historical synthesis and generalization concerning the dynamic role of disease in human history.

Medical history today is a growing field of enormous potential. The conviction recently expressed in an editorial in the *Journal of the History of Medicine and Allied Sciences* that medically trained historians are essential to maintain the field's integrity has been widely approved, but as the field has expanded far beyond the limits of technical medicine, it is equally apparent that nonmedical historians increasingly will explore the socioeconomic, cultural, and political boundaries of the field. This movement has already brought medical phenomena into the historical arena and promises a further and deeper understanding of the dynamics shaping historical societies as well as the nature of medicine itself. In the long term this can be of inestimable importance in molding contemporary attitudes toward medicine and its role in modern life.

ADDITIONAL READINGS: E. H. Ackerknecht, "A Plea for a 'Behaviorist' Approach in Writing the History of Medicine," *Journal of the History of Medicine and Allied Sciences* 22 (July 1967): 211–214; John B. Blake (ed.), *Education in the History of Medicine*, New York, 1968; Edwin Clarke (ed.), *Modern Methods in the History of Medicine*, London, 1971; Iago Galdston (ed.), *On the Utility of Medical History*, New York, 1957; Fielding H. Garrison, *An Introduction to the History of Medicine*, 4th ed., Philadelphia, 1929, 663–667; F. Marti-Ibañez (ed.), *Henry Sigerist on the History of Medicine*, New York, 1960; George Rosen, "Health, History, and the Social Sciences," in *From Medical Police to Social Medicine*, New York, 1974, 39–59; George Rosen, "Levels of Integration in Medical Historiography," *Journal of the History of Medicine and Allied Sciences* 4 (Autumn 1949):

460–467; George Rosen, "People, Disease, and Emotion: Some New Problems in Research for Medical History," *Bulletin of the History of Medicine* 41 (January–February 1967): 5–23; George Rosen, "The Place of History in Medical Education," in *From Medical Police to Social Medicine,* New York, 1974, 3–35; Charles Rosenberg (ed.), *Health and History: Essays for George Rosen,* New York, 1979; Charles E. Rosenberg, "The Medical Profession, Medical Practice, and the History of Medicine," in Edwin Clarke (ed.), *Modern Methods in Medical History,* London, 1971, 22–35; Owsei Temkin, "Historiography of Ideas in Medicine," in Edwin Clarke (ed.), *Modern Methods in the History of Medicine,* London, 1971, 2–21.

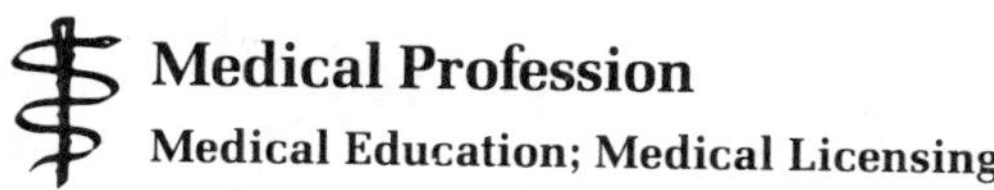

Medical Profession

Medical Education; Medical Licensing

Foundations The profession is a modern social institution whose roots are in the European Middle Ages, but whose development belongs to the nineteenth and twentieth centuries. Medicine, divinity, and law were the first learned occupations to be called professions, and the evolution of medicine and that of law provide the two basic models for histories of professionalization. Medicine developed the attribute of a profession by creating an independent body of knowledge which could be communicated systematically. This was the contribution of the medical school which grew up at Salerno between the ninth and the eleventh centuries and of the universities founded at Bologna, Montpellier, and Paris in the twelfth century. The university became the vehicle which disseminated medical knowledge and the authority which designated and approved the recipients of that knowledge as its legitimate practitioners. The medieval masters *(magistri)* were trained in Hippocratic and Galenic medicine to serve as diagnosticians, prescribers, advisers, and prognosticators rather than healers. They were also scholars, thinkers, and teachers, and their position in society was substantial.

Throughout the Middle Ages, medical services were provided by a variety of specialists who had learned to perform a particular medical function or trade. The most important of these, the surgeons, barber-surgeons, and apothecaries, or pharmacists, were organized in guilds and used an apprentice system. The guilds established rules governing training, practice, fees, and related matters. Some surgeons were educated beyond the common level of their trade, and a few, such as Guy de Chauliac or Bruno di Longoburgo, were learned, even erudite. The majority, however, were tradesmen or artisans who envied the special status of physicians and scrambled, largely unsuccessfully, to attain it.

Beyond the guild-organized specialties were popular practitioners: midwives, herb gatherers and compounders, bonesetters, hernia specialists, cataract couchers, stonecutters (lithotomists), and itinerant barber-surgeons who tended baths, cut hair, pulled teeth, bled, purged, and lanced boils. As in classical antiquity, popular medicine was a practical affair carried on according to market principles and with no effective regulatory oversight. Advances in medical education, licensing procedures, and regulatory agencies did not eliminate this sort of practice until the twentieth century.

State regulations governing medical practice were slow to develop in the west. By the first century A.D., both India and China had defined and applied standards for admission to medical practice. In the tenth century, the Caliph Al-Muqtadir required certification of competence for physicians in Baghdad. The first European laws appear to have been those laid down in 1140 by Norman king Roger of Sicily, who ruled that all who wished to practice medicine had to be approved by the masters of Salerno to ensure "that our subjects are not endangered by the inexperience of the physicians." In the next century German emperor Frederick II went further. In his *Constitutiones Imperiales* he reaffirmed the Norman statutes while requiring that for medical practice, a physician had to have three years of logic (i.e., humanistic training), five years of medicine, and one year of practical work. Examination by the candidates' academic mentors with a representative from the imperial court present led to a license issued in the emperor's name. These rules, which only applied in the emperor's Italian and Sicilian holdings, framed a pattern for education and licensing which came to be accepted throughout medieval Europe.

The Transition to Modern Times The *Oxford English Dictionary* ascribes the earliest use of the word "profession" to the sixteenth century. During the next 200 years, the concept of a medical profession developed smoothly to produce the research-trained, clinically experienced medical savant who eventually became a model for the American profession. The medieval tradition was modernized, the stress on university preparation was maintained, and the state took an increasingly active part in defining and enforcing curricular requirements. In Prussia, for example, candidates for the *magister medicinae* were required to take anatomy and to discuss a clinical case (*casus medicopracticus*) before the Collegium Medicum and the *medicochirurgicum,* or state board of health. Austrian requirements were similar. Licenses to practice were conferred by the universities of Vienna and Prague. In 1749, a state official was appointed with responsibility for overseeing the curriculum and the administration of examinations, though the examinations themselves were given by the university faculties. In France after 1789, full control over medical licensing and education was vested in the central government, and the same was true in Russia.

In France, Germany, and imperial Russia, medical practitioners held state appointments, and there was a heavy emphasis on research. In Russia, however, doctors were mere bureaucrats of a very inferior status and subject to galling limitations. Inevitably, Russian physicians considered bureaucratization a major evil and campaigned for greater autonomy as part of their struggle for professional standing. The Pirigov Society, Russia's national medical association, organized in 1881, became a reformist, politically active organization involved in contemporary social and political issues. In Britain and America, on the other hand, medicine developed with relatively little direct political control. Corporate traditions inherited from the Middle Ages influenced English medical development until the twentieth century, while in the United States, the national government had almost no part at all in controlling or directing medicine's growth.

The Profession and Society Between 1650 and 1850, the traditional content of academic medicine was revolutionized. Clinical training forced the reorganization of medical schools, and experimentation with a variety of therapeutic systems challenged the status of conventional allopathic medical practice. The highly structured European systems most easily absorbed these innovations and, in the case of clinical medicine, promoted them. This kept the bond linking the universities, the state, and the medical hierarchy largely intact. In England, on the other hand, the new medicine found no home at Oxford or Cambridge, though the universities retained their licensing powers, and it was the University of Edinburgh which became the leading academic center for medical education. In London, where the Royal College of Physicians retained the power to license, medical training was offered in private or proprietary schools, often organized and run by leading physicians, and in the hospitals which provided opportunities for clinical or ward teaching. Until the foundation of the University of London in 1836, there was no institution in England which offered basic scientific medicine in conjunction with clinical study.

English licensing procedures stressed definition of function rather than type or content of training. The universities and the royal colleges licensed physicians and surgeons, while apothecaries, who were actually general practitioners, were approved by their guild. Regulations drew lines between occupations—wrongful appropriation of a title could bring a fine, and performance of a function not permitted under a particular license could result in a prosecution—but that apart, there was a little differentiation in actual medical practice. There were, however, clear social distinctions. The well-to-do, who could afford the fees, generally sought a university-trained physician who was respectable and a gentleman. Such physicians had a vested interest in maintaining their social standing.

In the first half of the nineteenth century, as the middle class expanded, so also did the variety of medical practitioners who claimed their custom. University and hospital-trained physicians defended their positions and their claims to respectability by asserting that responsible medicine was scientific medicine, and that this was the only answer to "quacks and charlatans." Bruising battles were fought over hydropathy, mesmeric medicine, homeopathy, and other nonregular medical systems. The *Lancet,* established by Thomas Wakley in 1823, became an outspoken advocate of strong professional qualifications and scientific probity in medicine. The system, however, changed slowly. A medical reform bill in 1858 left licensing in the hands of guilds and universities and pointedly refused to identify impermissible medical doctrines. It did, however, establish a national medical register of regular practitioners, that is, persons approved by traditional bodies and considered medically respectable. Nor was this an empty designation, since only persons in the medical register were permitted to enter government service or sue for fees.

The assumption that physicians treated the better class of patients while apothecaries or other types of practitioner treated the working classes and the poor was not limited to England. Partially trained paramedics or medical orderlies called *feldshers* (Russia), *officiers de santé* (France), or *sekundär Ärzte* (*Germany*) were considered adequate to perform most medical services for the common people. The highest levels of medical training were only available to the affluent. In Europe, some of these practices were modified after 1850. Increased therapeutic effectiveness supported the superiority of scientific medicine, while a growing emphasis on egalitarianism—and a concomitant fear of organized political resistance from the working classes—promoted the idea of a single standard of medicine for all. Germany led the way, with Prussia legislating uniform educational standards during the revolutionary year of 1848; the other German states followed Prussia's lead in 1852. The resulting rise in medical costs eventually was covered by the German national insurance plan.

The United States to 1850 American medicine took shape during the eighteenth and early nineteenth centuries without guild or university guidelines and in a rural rather than an urban setting. A few "reputable men in medicine" who had trained abroad or who were otherwise familiar with European standards organized the earliest American medical societies and even promoted regulatory legislation. Local medical groups began to form between 1730 and 1760, and there were occasional warnings against untrained practitioners. In 1765 the first native American medical school was founded at what was to become the University of Pennsylvania. During the American Revolution, its founder, Dr. John Morgan, promoted qualifying examinations to ensure minimum standards of performance for military medicine; after the war, pride in American accomplishments brought popular support for medical reform by identifying progress in medical science with national progress.

Despite all this, the basic problem in America was that most medical practitioners had had little or no formal preparation. Moreover, physicians who hoped to establish minimum standards comprised a small minority, and they were swimming against an egalitarian tide. As additional medical schools were founded, there was a move to grant them licensing powers. The question first arose when the Harvard medical school was established in 1783, and 20 years later it was agreed that either a Harvard diploma or a qualifying examination would serve to license. A similar rule was adopted in Connecticut in 1810 and in South Carolina in 1817.

With no firm substantive standard against which to measure the quality of preparation, and with no agency prepared to enforce curricular requirements, medical schools were free to do as they pleased, and the states cooperated. In 1812, the Maryland legislature began to charter proprietary medical colleges, private institutions connected with neither a university arts faculty nor a hospital. The precedent spread. By 1840, 26 new medical schools had been established, and another 47 appeared between 1840 and 1875.

Students looked for the quickest and least costly course that would produce a license, and in the competition for students, standards evaporated at established and proprietary schools alike. In addition, sectarian colleges of homeopathic, eclectic, and botanic medicine proliferated. Until the second half of the nineteenth century, these schools had as much to offer intellectually as any other medical school, and, when questions concerning their right to exist were raised, the issue was contested as an invasion of religious freedom and personal rights. These arguments, when combined with a fierce laissez-faire commercialism and the populist conviction that anyone could tell competence from incompetence, cut the legs from under regulatory efforts. The newly forming western states wrote no licensing laws, regulations were repealed where previously they had been enforced, and by mid-century only New Jersey and the District of Columbia required a license to practice.

The American Medical Association, organized in 1847, claimed to speak for professional standards, but in fact its membership included many with a vested interest in nonregulation. A survey of physicians practicing in eastern Tennessee in

1850 showed the dimensions of the problem. Of 201 physicians serving 164,000 people, only 35 had graduated from a regular medical school, and 42 had had a course of lectures but had not graduated. Twenty-seven had trained at an irregular or sectarian school, and the remaining 97, virtually half of the total, had had no formal instruction at all. In the second half of the nineteenth century, when European (including English) standards and qualifications were rising, these conditions remained uncorrected. American medicine moved away from professional criteria toward the idea of medicine as a craft or occupation. This condition was widely deplored, but little was done about it until the closing decades of the century.

Science, Education, and Medical Professionalism In the last quarter of the nineteenth century, medical scholars with close European contacts provided the impetus for licensing reform. Their efforts were seconded by the newly founded philanthropic foundations. The catalyst for change, however, was the therapeutic revolution which followed the introduction of anesthesia and antisepsis, the establishment of the germ theory of disease, the discovery of immune response, and the introduction of x-ray technology. Scientific investigation and medical treatment were flowering together, and there was a mounting body of evidence to support the conviction that high standards of medical performance required consistent, systematic training in both basic science and clinical work. Between 1875 and 1914, an estimated 15,000 American physicians went abroad to study. They were exposed to systematic clinical teaching, the close coordination of hospitals and medical schools, professional specialization, salaried professorships, and the transforming influence of research on teaching and practice. Though opposition was heavy, European-trained American physicians came to lead a growing movement to reconstruct the medical profession in the United States according to European standards.

The drive to raise professional standards appeared in the work of the Illinois Board of Health. Established in 1877, this board began to review the licenses under which new doctors practiced and then expanded its investigations to include physicians of long standing. The board carried its review to medical schools outside the state of Illinois and in 1880 began to publish a list of the schools the board considered to be in good standing. Between 1883 and 1889, the board issued five separate surveys whose standards came to be widely accepted. According to the surveys, a candidate for medical school should be of good moral character and have earned a high school diploma; the medical course should comprise at least 10 subjects, with two courses in dissection and two terms of hospital instruction, the program should take at least three years; and the school should require regular attendance, two quizzes per week, and outside examiners for the finals. During the same period, the Association of American Medical Colleges, which was founded in 1876, abandoned in 1883, and revived in 1890, called for similar standards, with particular emphasis on the three-year curriculum. Its Nashville convention in 1890 attracted representatives from 65 regular medical schools. The following year a National confederation of State Examining and Licensing Boards was formed to promote strengthened curricula and to encourage the weaker schools to strengthen their programs. The Illinois example gained a national footing.

Economic factors also favored reform. The nineteenth-century proliferation of schools and students flooded and depressed the market for medical services, and both doctors and medical students had a poor public image. They were considered riotous, brutish, untrustworthy, and anything but gentlemen. Introducing curricular reforms based on scientific medicine could be expected to drive all but the most firmly grounded medical schools to the wall, while enhanced standards for admission and performance could only reduce the number of practitioners. In a numerically smaller profession, the public image could improve as higher standards were expected to attract a "better" sort of person, and the social status of the profession would rise. All this would substantially increase the economic value of a medical degree.

As the twentieth century opened, the American Medical Association (AMA) entered the campaign for improved professional standards. The AMA established a Council on Medical Education that in 1905 joined representatives of licensing boards and the Association of American Colleges to create a model program for training and licensing. In 1906, the council began to publicize the poor scores which candidates from weak medical schools made on state board examinations. It also began a comprehensive review of standards in medical schools across the country.

Backing for the reform campaign came from the Carnegie and Rockefeller foundations. In 1909, the Carnegie Foundation for the Advancement of Teaching took over the AMA's survey of medical schools and appointed Abraham Flexner to lead the investigation. His report, published the following year, was an outspoken (some have said exaggerated) indictment of American medical education and the standard of competence in the American medical profession. The Flexner report advocated a medical education which began with the liberal arts, including basic science, to be followed by specialized scientific instruction, clinical training, research, and internship. The model was consciously European, especially German, and the American example was the Johns Hopkins Medical School, which was established in 1893.

The equation of good health with scientific medicine won overwhelming support from the articulate, increasingly educated American middle class, and an effective public relations campaign maintained public enthusiasm. Major achievements in identifying and controlling epidemic diseases combined with the steady expansion of a sophisticated medical technology to strengthen the belief that modern medicine was scientific and demanded the highest possible standards for recruitment and training. The pressure generated was immediate and powerful. Private, fee-supported proprietary medical schools could not compete and were forced to close their doors. Other institutions were reorganized or merged. Financing shifted. Foundation grants supplemented public tax funds as medical schools lost their commercial character to become centers devoted to teaching and research. By 1928, only 74 regular medical schools remained out of the 154 counted two decades earlier, and this number declined further in the next five years. Quality, as measured by the AMA rating system, clearly improved, while the ratio of physicians to population declined. Medicine attracted more applicants for fewer places, and when Duke University Medical School opened in 1932, there were 3000 students competing for 68 openings. Medicine was on its way to becoming an elite profession, recruited from the best of the nation's college graduates. It was predominantly white, middle-class, and male, a profile which has only partially been modified in the years following World War II.

Conclusion During the first half of the twentieth century, "scientific medicine" established itself as the prototype of the modern profession. High entrance standards, a demanding course of study, effective licensing, a high average standard of living, social prestige, a strong national organization, and a more-than-favorable public image were among its characteristics. Rapid economic growth and the transformation of agrarian and mercantile societies into modern urban industrial complexes created the markets for modern medicine and the capital to build medical schools, research centers, clinics, and hospitals. In this sense, scientific medicine is an integral part of the modernization of societies.

The social and intellectual elitism explicit in the modern medical profession and the high costs of modern treatments have created the next generation of problems which the profession must resolve, ones which could force fundamental changes in the profession itself. Increasingly, the basic issues in modern medicine are social rather than scientific and involve making the preventive, supportive, and therapeutic powers of medicine available to growing numbers of people who need help but who are excluded from it economically. Voluntary and compulsory health insurance, nationalization of health services, and every variation on those themes have proved incapable of providing adequate care for whole societies. The core of the problem may well be found in the bases for medical professionalization and the extraordinary costs which scientific medicine entails. The medical profession advanced to its present position of leadership and respect through science and economic development. But modern societies appear to be reaching the limits of what their productivity can provide for all their members, and it may prove necessary to revise medical expectations. In that case, the profession's historical identity will become a part of the problem which the profession must solve to promote its future utility.

ADDITIONAL READINGS: H. P. Bayon, "The Masters of Salerno and the Origins of Professional Medical Practice," in E. Ashworth Underwood (ed.), *Science, Medicine, and History*, 2 vols., London, 1953, New York, 1975, I, 203–219; Joseph Ben-David, *Centers of Learning: Britain, France, Germany, United States*, New York, 1977; E. Richard

Brown, *Rockefeller Medicine Men: Medicine and Capitalism in America*, Berkeley and Los Angeles, 1979; Vern L. Bullough, *The Development of Medicine as a Profession: The Contribution of the Medieval University to Modern Medicine*, New York, 1966; A. M. Carr-Saunders and P. A. Wilson, *The Professions*, Oxford, 1933; Nancy M. Frieden, *The Russian Medical Profession, 1855–1904*, Princeton, 1981; Eliot Friedson, *The Profession of Medicine: A Study in the Sociology of Applied Knowledge*, New York, 1970; Eliot Friedson, *Professional Dominance: The Social Structure of Medical Care*, New York, 1970; Martin Kaufman, *American Medical Education: The Formative Years*, Westport, Conn., 1976; Joseph E. Kett, *The Formation of the American Medical Profession: The Role of Institutions, 1780–1860*, New Haven, 1968; Ronald L. Numbers (ed.), *The Education of American Physicians: Historical Essays*, Berkeley, 1980; Jeanne M. Peterson, *The Medical Profession in Mid-Victorian England*, Berkeley, 1978; Henry E. Sigerist, "The History of Medical Licensure," *Journal of the American Medical Association* 104 (March 30, 1935): 1056–1060; Richard Shryock, *Medical Licensing in America*, Baltimore, 1967; Paul Starr, *The Social Transformation of American Medicine*, New York, 1984.

See also CLINICAL MEDICINE; IRREGULAR MEDICINE.

Medicine in Ancient India

A rich medical culture flourished in ancient India from at least the second millennium B.C., and probably earlier. The pre-Aryan urban cultures of the northwest which were uncovered at Harappa and Mohenjo-Daro show an advanced system of hygienic engineering which included bathing pools, drains, and sanitary facilities. Since there is no contemporary literary evidence, however, there is no way to know on what hygienic principles the systems were built, and there is relatively little known about the medicine that was practiced. Hartshorn, cuttlestone, and bitumen apparently were used for medical purposes, but little else has been found. It is assumed that the Aryan invaders who overran the northwest around 1500 B.C. destroyed whatever formal medical tradition existed, though it is possible that elements in Aryan-Hindu medicine were acquired at the time of conquest.

Between about 1500 B.C. and the first century A.D., Indian medicine passed through three stages of literary and religious development. The first stage was an Aryan medical scientific tradition introduced from Iran and codified in the Sanskrit Vedas, or texts. Though transmitted as collections of sacred writings, the Vedas contained material on diseases, drugs, and the stars. The vedic literature was allusive, indirect, and ritualistic, and it invited commentary. This produced the second level of writing, the so-called Brahmanas, which were ritual commentaries on the Vedas. The period for the Brahmanas was from about 1000 B.C. to 400 B.C. There was no contradiction between the Brahman commentary and the vedic tradition. They shared a common outlook. The third stage was Buddhist medicine, which appeared in the fifth century B.C. and remained vital into the first millennium A.D. Brahmanism and Buddhism flourished side by side. Brahmanism produced the technical development and practical study of medicine at the same time that Buddhism was refining conceptual foundations and carrying Indian medical philosophy into China.

The two most important Brahmanic compilations for medical practice were the *Susruta-Samhita* (ca. 750 B.C.) and the *Charaka-Samhita* (ca. A.D. 150). Susruta and Charaka were physicians who, though widely separated in time, followed the ideas of Atreya, a physician from the northwest who was an older contemporary of Susruta. *Susruta-Samhita* and *Charaka-Samhita* together form the Aryan Veda, the medical portion of the *Atharva Veda,* including the spells and incantations of the Atharva priests for warding off trouble. Ayurvedic medicine combined such ritual incantations, omens, and sorcery with precise directions for handling wounds, diseases, and many surgical procedures. The magical and the empirical were entirely integrated in this system.

The physiology proposed in ayurvedic medicine rested on an ancient principle also found in Iranian tradition that the world is governed by a cyclical law called rta, meaning "normal," or "true," which requires a predetermined order of things in nature and morality. Irregularity and disorder cannot be tolerated, and in the body they are synonymous with disease. The body, which must maintain a normal order, is made up of the five elementary substances which compose the universe: earth, water, fire, wind, and space. In the body those substances are represented respectively by firm tissue, humor or mucus, bile, breath, and the organic cavities. The three active principles, wind, fire, and water, appear in the body as breath, bile, and mucus—which together form a triad called tridhatu, sometimes referred to as tridosha, or the triad of troubles. Each element in the triad has five principal forms. Bile, or pitta, for example, has an "igneous principle" and helps to "cook," that is, digest, food. It also acts to give color to the vital fluid resulting from digestion and to turn it into blood. In addition, bile "kindles the desires of the heart," shines from the eyes, governs vision, and glistens on the skin.

The succession of the seasons, climatic conditions, and the state of hygiene can accelerate or slow the action of these vital principles, and their relation to one another will determine the state of health at any given moment, while the dominance of one or the other in a particular constitution will define its character. Disequilibrium among all three elements was thought to produce very complicated disease conditions, but most diseases were associated with imbalances in one or another of the principles, or between two of them. The analogy with the Greek doctrine of the humors (q.v.) is striking, and historians continue to be fascinated by the possibility of a link between these contemporaneous physiologies.

Indian medicine classified diseases in three ways: by cause, by anatomical location, and by symptoms. There is abundant evidence of careful observation for diagnosis and classification. All the senses were employed to identify critical symptoms leading, for example, to the discovery of "sweet urine" and an early ayurvedic description of diabetes mellitus (q.v.). Classification by cause connected particular conditions with a failure in one of the three active principles. Failures in muscular coordination, convulsions, contractions, and paralysis were thought to be diseases of "the breath." "Anatomical location" meant no more than specifying where the disease was, for instance, on the head, on the skin, or in the eyes. Classification by symptoms required particular descriptions of the disease condition, beginning with such obvious manifestations as fever or tumors and continuing through deviations from the normal, wherever they appeared and whatever they might be. The *Susruta-Samhita* gave particular attention to local or surgical conditions such as piles, anal fistulas, erysipelas, and ulcers. The *Charaka-Samhita* dealt with fevers, hemorrhagic diseases (conditions of blood and bile), internal tumors, urinary problems, skin diseases, consumption, psychological conditions, and epilepsy. The approach to classification, like the etiology on which it built, had many parallels with the Hippocratic tradition.

Treatments described in the Indian classics combined omens and incantations with a naturalistic empiricism. Omens contributed to prognosis, but the accumulation of experience was equally important. With only a primitive grasp of anatomy, the significance attached to the location of a wound or a particular condition was established by a system of marmas, or vital points. Somewhat similar to acupuncture points (see Acupuncture), *marmas* were 107 anatomical locations which were critical or deadly. A wound at one of those points might produce hemorrhage, paralysis, or death. The ayurvedic physician, like the Greek or even the Egyptian, would refuse to treat someone with a clearly mortal wound. Where such a problem did not exist, treatments were gauged to assist the flow of vital principles and employed purges, diet, and bleeding to that end.

The Hindu pharmacopeia, which showed Chinese and Iranian influences, was extensive and leaned to vegetable substances. Minerals appeared in the early Christian era. There was an elaborate surgery. *Susruta-Samhita* contained extensive recommendations for wound management, including explicit directions for dealing with arrow injuries, suggesting that there was a considerable experience with military surgery. There was a wide variety of instruments and recommendations for embryotomies, cataract couching, and lithotomies. Hindu surgeons developed an ingenious, nonirritating suture for intestinal wounds. Large ants pinched the edges of the wound together, and their bodies were then clipped off, while the heads with mandibles were left in place. The opening in the abdominal wall was closed with ordinary sutures. Arab physicians learned this technique and carried it to the west. Today, the ant suture is still in use on the Somali coast in Africa.

Hindu surgeons were adept at cosmetic operations, in particular, at replacing a nose or an ear. Since having the ear or nose cut off was an accepted form of punishment as well as a common battle injury, this operation was in no way unusual. What was unusual was the high degree of surgical and medical skill found in a culture which did not permit dissection and was, therefore, anatomically ignorant. *Susruta-Samhita* contains a description of how to soak a cadaver so that the outer tissues may be brushed or peeled away to facilitate observation, but this was hardly a substitute for dissection as a method for effective postmortem examination.

Training for the ayurvedic physician involved a long period of apprenticeship, during which the neophytes learned the Vedas, thus perpetuating orally the whole of the tradition. Training also involved practice with surgical instruments. The state played an important role in health matters. There is one inscription from the third century B.C. according to which a certain king, Asoka, provided facilities for the ease of his people. Some have read the inscription to refer to establishing hospitals; others believe that it meant that remedies were offered to those who needed them. Finally, in addition to medicine for humans, there was a large veterinary practice which has left a literature.

Ayurvedic medicine was carried by Buddhist missionaries into China in the fourth century B.C., and it may have made its way westward to touch medical development in Greece. It flourished in India through the first millennium A.D. As it was codified, however, it lost vitality, became increasingly ritualized and formal, and was finally overwhelmed by Arab practices. In the eighteenth century, European medicine entered India with the British and the French, but in the twentieth century western-trained Hindu physicians seeking their own cultural roots have again discovered the ayurvedic heritage. It is an important chapter in the history of medicine and world culture.

ADDITIONAL READINGS: Bhegvan Dash and Lalitesh Kashyap, *Basic Principles of Ayurveda Based on Ayurveda Saukhyam of Todarananada*. New Delhi, 1981; K. L. Bishagratna (trans.), *Sushruta-Samhita*, 3 vols., Varanesi, India, 1907–1911, 1963; B. L. Gordon, *Medicine Throughout Antiquity*, Philadelphia, 1949; A. C. Kaviratna (trans.), *Charaka-Samhita*, 2 vols., Calcutta, 1912; P. Kutumbiah, *Ancient Indian Medicine*, Bombay, 1962; Guido Majno, *The Healing Hand: Man and Wound in the Ancient World*, Cambridge, Mass., 1975, chap. 7; P. Ray and H. N. Gupta, *Caraka Samhita: A Scientific Synopsis*, New Delhi, 1965; L. Renou, *Vedic India*, P. Spratt (trans.), Calcutta, 1957; P. V. Sharma, *Indian Medicine in the Classical Age*, Varanasi, India, 1972; Jürgen Thorwald, *Science and Secrets of Early Medicine*, Richard and Clara Winston (trans.), London, 1962; W. D. Whitney (trans. and commentary), *Atharva-Veda Samhitā*, 2 vols., Delhi, Patna, and Varanesi, 1962; H. R. Zimmer, *Hindu Medicine*, Baltimore, 1948.

Medicine in Mesopotamia

A series of civilizations which included the Sumerian and Akkadian, the Assyrian, Babylonian, and Chaldean appeared in the region drained by the Tigris and Euphrates rivers between the fourth millennium B.C. and the first. These cultures have left extensive archaeological remains but only occasional evidence concerning their medical practices. Written sources are in the form of cuneiform clay tablets, and the largest number available, including about 1000 on medicine which have been deciphered, was found in the library of King Ashurbanipal near Nineveh. The collection dates from the seventh century B.C., but the materials are much older, with some tablets being from the middle of the second millennium.

The medical tradition to which the Ashurbanipal tablets belong was founded by the Sumerians, who also developed cuneiform writing. The tradition and the language were accepted and transmitted by each succeeding culture. The tablets, which contain lists of remedies, ingredients, diagnoses, and prognostications, suggest the existence of a complementary oral tradition. There are no medical texts as such, though some collections have titles. The largest, which was probably set down after 1000 B.C., is called "The Treatise of Medical Diagnosis and Prognoses" and comprises 3000 entries on 40 tablets. It is a list of diseases, some described circumstantially enough for modern medicine to identify them, with conditions noted which are the basis for prognosis. These prognostic signs are often of no modern medical significance at all, and the treatise has been called a sorcerer's handbook.

Medicine in Mesopotamia, as in Egypt, combined religious ritual with empirical treatment. Three types of healers are mentioned in the texts: a seer (*bârû*), specializing in divination and prognosis; a priest (*âshipu*), for exorcisms and incantations; and a priest-physician (*âsû*), who employed the rich *materia medica* and performed surgery in addition to using chants and incantations. There was a hierarchy of priest-physicians under a physician–in–chief, and during the Assyrian period the court physicians were requried to take an oath of office. The Code of Hammurabi (ca. 1700 B.C.) has a table of surgical fees and penalties for failure to pay. Both varied according to the patient's social class. Each physician was assisted by a "barber" (*gallabu*), who seems to have been responsible for such minor operations as branding slaves and drawing teeth.

Disease theory in Mesopotamia began with the Sumerians and involved the entry of evil spirits into a person due to carelessness, fate, sin (i.e., the breaking of taboos), or sorcery. The first was considered the most common. Conditions for which the evil spirits were responsible included migraine and tics, neck pain, intestinal ailments, insomnia, anorexia, impotence, anxiety, and speech impediments. Treatment followed identifying the demons responsible and meant expelling them by spells or incantations, while physical symptoms were treated empirically. Some pathological conditions were ascribed to natural causes including cold weather, dryness and dust, putrescence, malnutrition, and venereal infection. Diagnosis involved a detailed description of symptoms, which were classified according to such body parts as eye, tongue, and face. The descriptions included fluctuations in the condition, the time of day when symptoms occurred, and what symptoms were terminal.

The *materia medica* was extensive and varied. Active ingredients which have been identified include pine turpentine, oleander, mustard, opoponax, hellebore, and a favored mixture of *Artemisia judaica*, balm of Gilead, and Persian fennel. Other treatments included the "three gestures" recorded on a Sumerian tablet of about 2100 B.C. These were washing, making plasters, and bandaging. Wound dressings were made with dried wine dregs, juniper, beer, salt, oil and mud, resin or fat with alkali, and a mixture of herbs which were pounded, cooked, and strained.

While the evidence is scanty, it seems clear that an extensive religio-medical tradition existed in Mesopotamia which lasted from the Sumerian fourth millennium until the Persian invasions in the middle of the first. That this tradition was developed institutionally may be inferred from the chain of medical information, the association of medical and religious practice, the identification of a religio-medical hierarchy, and documented efforts at regulation. The parallels with Egyptian medicine are close, though not exact; and elements from Mesopotamia, especially pharmacological ones, appear among the Hebrews. Thanks to the transcription and translation of Sumerian medical tablets beginning with the work of Campbell-Thompson at Oxford, far more is now known about the medicine of Mesopotamia than at any time in history; but while it is no longer necessary to epitomize that tradition with Herodotus's report that in Babylon the sick were put on public view to elicit opinions on their illness from the passersby, much that is important remains obscure.

ADDITIONAL READINGS: R. Biggs, "Medicine in Ancient Mesopotamia," in A. C. Crombie and M. A. Hoskins (eds.), *History of Science*, Cambridge, 1969, III, 94–105; M. Levey, "Some Objective Factors of Babylonian Medicine in the Light of New Evidence," *Bulletin of the History of Medicine* 35 (January–February 1961): 61–70; S. S. Levin, *Adam's Rib: Essays on Biblical Medicine*, Los Altos, 1970; Guido Majno, *The Healing Hand: Man and Wound in the Ancient World*, Cambridge, Mass., 1975, chap. 2; A. L. Oppenheim, *Ancient Mesopotamia: Portrait of a Dead Civilization*, Chicago and London, 1964, 1965; A. L. Oppenheim, "Mesopotamian Medicine," *Bulletin of the History of Medicine* 36 (March–April 1962): 97–108.

Medieval Medicine

The medieval world lay in time between the collapse of the Roman empire in the west around A.D. 500 and the birth of the modern period roughly 1000 years later. The Middle Ages encompassed the development of several closely related cultural formations: the later Roman, or Byzantine, empire, Islam, the Latin-German west, the Greco-Slavic east, and the Hebrew Diaspora. Each of these formations in turn comprised several cultural entities, employed a variety of languages, and showed a remarkable disposition to disintegrate into multiple political components. Medically, however, there was a common heritage rooted in the Greco-Roman world. At the extremities of the system, in northern or northwestern Europe and along the Russian river system, the Greco-Roman medical inheritance was thin. In southern Europe and throughout the Moslem-Byzantine world, that heritage was dense and rich.

Until the end of the twelfth century, medicine was most developed in the wealthy commercial centers stretching from India through Mesopotamia, and Egypt to Spain and along the eastern Mediterranean coast through Anatolia to Constantinople. With the thirteenth century, however, this world declined, new centers of learning developed in the west, and medical leadership shifted to Italy and France, later England and Germany. By the time the Middle Ages ended, it was no longer Baghdad, Gondishapur, Alexandria, or Constantinople which led the way. The new centers were Bologna and Padua, Montpellier, Paris, Oxford, and Prague.

The Classical Heritage and Its Preservation The primary contribution of medical scholarship in the early Middle Ages was to preserve the Greco-Roman tradition. Galen's already elaborate system was further embellished, and observations on diseases multiplied and were made more discriminating. The major emphases in medical scholarship were codifying what was known in encyclopedias, handbooks, or texts and translating material either from Greek into Aramaic (Syriac) and Arabic or from Arabic into Latin. As a result, the medicine taught in European universities in the thirteenth, fourteenth, and fifteenth centuries was largely the same medicine taught in Byzantium and the Islamic world from the fourth through the thirteenth centuries.

The books which preserved the classic tradition were written as summaries of current knowledge and as a guide to practice. Among the most influential were the fourth-century compilations made by Oribasius, a friend as well as physician to Julian the Apostate; the *Tetrabiblion* of Aëtius of Armida, physician to Emperor Justinian I; and, from the seventh century, the collections made by Paul of Aegina.

The classical tradition moved outward from its Mediterranean base in the fifth century, when the Council of Ephesus (431) condemned the doctrines of the patriarch Nestorius and declared his followers heretics. The Nestorians fled to Egypt, where Nestorius probably died in 451, and to Abyssinia, Persia, India, and China. A substantial number settled at Gondishapur on the Persian Gulf, where a hospital and medical school were established. This center became a meeting place for all the major medical traditions: Persian, Alexandrian, Greek, Jewish, Hindu, and Chinese.

In the seventh century, when the Arab followers of Mohammed conquered Persia, they took over the medical center at Gondishapur and began translating the medical works from Syriac into Arabic. The conquerors established the seat of their government, the caliphate, at Baghdad in the eighth century, and during the ninth and tenth centuries, Baghdad became one of the world's important medical centers. In the early stages of Baghdad's medical development, primary emphasis fell on collecting and translating the available Greek classics. Among the leaders in this process were Johannes Mesuë the Elder, also known as Janus Damascenus, a Christian who in the early ninth century became a hospital director at Baghdad, and the Nestorian, Honain ben Isaac (Johannitus).

By the tenth century, when the Baghdad medical system was fully established, a group of medical writers of astonishing powers and versatility appeared, led by the famed clinician and physician Al Rhazes. Al Rhazes followed Galen's system, though his style of presentation and his clinical approach were Hippocratic. Other important Moslem scholars included the tenth-century Persian magus Haly ben Abbas; Ibn al Haitham, also called Alhazan, who worked on ocular refraction and magnification in the eleventh century; and his contemporary, Ibn Sina, or Avicenna. Ibn Sina was the most famous of the group. A flamboyant and extraordinarily successful physician, politician, and medical administrator, Ibn Sina was also a sophisticated medical philosopher who followed and expanded on Galen. His *Canon of Medicine* was an attempt to order all medical knowledge according to Aristotelian and Galenic principles. Ibn Sina was a leading source for Europe's understanding of Galen's system. Paracelsus consigned Galen's work to the flames at Basel in 1527 in the form of Ibn Sina's *Canon*.

Spain under the Ummayad caliphate was also an important medical center, producing a leading clinician in Avenzoar, an important surgeon in Albucasis, and the medical systemizers Averroës and Maimonides. Albucasis was particularly notable. His major work, a medical-chirurgical compilation known as *Altasrif (Collection)*, was the leading textbook for surgery in the Middle Ages. Based on the work of Paul of Aegina, it described various instruments and procedures, including setting fractures, manipulating dislocations, cutting for stones (lithotomies), amputating, and treating wounds. Rabbi Moshe ben Maimon, or Moses Maimonides came from Cordova to become the medical adviser to Saladin (Salah-ah-din), founder of the Egyptian Ayyab dynasty and victor over the Third Crusade. Maimonides was one of the major intellectual figures of the Middle Ages. An early exponent of psychosomatic medicine, Maimonides wrote on a wide variety of medical subjects, though his most popular work was on *materia medica*. He also stressed the importance of hygiene in therapy, an important lesson for surgery, and he was, in fact, widely quoted by such leading European authorities as Guy de

Chauliac, Arnold of Villanova, and Henri de Mondeville.

Other Jewish scholars played a leading role in medieval medicine. Their own medical traditions drew heavily on Egyptian, Babylonian, Greek, and Alexandrian sources, and they had a highly developed body of medical and hygienic rules codified in the Talmud (see Hebrew Medicine). Assaph ha-Yehudi, for example, compiled an important *materia medica* in the seventh century which used both talmudic and Greco-Roman sources; his *Medicine pauperum* was a work specifically designed to help the poor to care for themselves without a physician. One of the best known and most influential Jewish physicians was Isaac ben Solomon Israeli (Isaac, Isaacus, Judaeus), who lived from the mid-ninth to the mid-tenth century. Personal physician to Caliph Ziyudat Allah t'Agh and the Fatimite 'Ubaidallàh al Mahdī, Isaac ben Solomon wrote *On Fevers, On Urine,* and *On Diets,* which were collected and translated as *Opera omnia Isaaci* to become a standard medical text in the Middle Ages and the Renaissance. The Jews in Spain and Portugal produced authors and court physicians, though the tide of persecution which accompanied the Christian campaigns for liberation drove many away. Nevertheless, Joseph Vecinho, court physician and astronomer for King John II of Portugal, and Bernal and Marco, the naval physician and the surgeon who accompanied Christopher Columbus to the new world, were Jews. Rabbi Zemah Duran, a noted authority on obstetrics and gynecology, was forced to flee to Algiers. Some Jewish physicians served princely courts in Germany, but the number was small, and their situation was often hazardous. On the other hand, it was the German city of Würzburg in 1490 that licensed the first Jewish woman, Dr. Sarah, for medical practice. There was relatively few Jewish physicians in Austria, Bohemia, Rumania, and Switzerland, though Stephen the Great of Moldavia had a Spanish Jew as court physician.

Medicine in Western Europe Western and northern Europe stagnated medically through the early Middle Ages as the barbarian invasions destroyed Roman political control, and neither the "imperial" dynasties nor native princes were successful in maintaining order. The wealthy urban centers that characterized the Moslem-Byzantine world were absent in the west; high culture collapsed, and with it the underpinnings for medical, scientific, artistic, and philosophical development. Shelters and hospices built late in the days of the Roman empire were available for the use of pilgrims, merchants, or other needy travelers, but primary responsibility for medical services devolved upon the church. Abbeys and monasteries offered refuge to the sick or weary, while in the larger towns, hospital-like institutions took shape. Very little medicine was practiced, however, and what medical writings survived were practical care manuals or brief summaries of everyday remedies.

Educated physicians were rare. At the beginning of the ninth century, when Charlemagne needed a physician to establish medical studies, he asked for help from the caliph Harun al-Rashid, who sent Rabbi Mahir to teach the Talmud, veterinary science, and medicine in France. Jews had settled in Gaul in the Roman era, and there were still talmudic schools at Narbonne and Troyes where some medicine was taught. There is a tradition that a student of Rabbi Abban of Narbonne was called to teach medicine in the town of Montpellier, leading to the suggestion that at least one founder of the medical school there in around 1021 was an anonymous talmudic scholar.

The medical school at Salerno, founded in the ninth century, marked a new beginning. Tradition says that the school was organized by four scholars, a Greek, a Jew, a Latin, and a Moslem. Whether true or not, the story reflects the Salerno medical tradition, which was a distillation of the Greco-Roman and Arab methods and which made its primary contributions by translating materials from Greek, Arabic, and Hebrew into Latin. The Jewish scholar Donnolo and the mysterious Constantine the African were among the translators who made the Greco-Arab medical writings available to Europe. Salerno also trained physicians in the classical heritage. Galen's influence was strong, but there were independent minds as well, and Salerno's influence was likened to a fresh sea breeze in the stagnant medieval world. The anatomy and physiology were Galenic, and in diagnosis pulse and urine lore dominated. But diseases were studied first-hand, treatments were rational, the surgery was new and original, and the dietetics were effective. The school at Salerno became the fountainhead for medical development in Italy and France, and it remained vital until the twelfth century.

Between about A.D. 1000 and 1300, the European medieval world showed signs of gathering economic strength. Populations expanded, cities quickened, and a new cultural vitality appeared. The Crusades, which began at the end of the eleventh century, were evidence of the new energy, and the contacts they created hastened both cultural and economic growth.

The availability of Arabic works stimulated medicine's development, and new medical schools were founded as part of a growing university movement. Bologna, Montpellier, Avignon, Padua, and Paris extended the achievements of Salerno, and medicine became one of the major disciplines offered, while physicians took on a new dignity. In fact, university medicine was heavily theoretical and bookish—anatomy (q.v.) was not taught through dissection until the fourteenth century. Physicians held themselves apart from surgeons while a motley crew of barbers, midwives, lithotomists, cataract couchers, herb and drug sellers, gelders, and bonesetters carried on with treating ordinary people. Guild regulations systematized the trade in drugs in Italy, France, and Germany, while governments, university faculties, and guild corporations attempted to define and control the various specialties. Men of particular skills were able to make their influence felt. Though physicians were the elite of European medicine, surgeons were more active and advanced because general medicine was dominated by the Greco-Arab view, and especially by Galen. Surgery, however, advanced in the hands of the late Salernitans Ruggerio Frugardi (Roger) of Palermo and his student Rolando Capelluti (Roland) of Parma. Other important figures included Hugh of Lucca, William Saliceto, who worked at Bologna, Lanfranchi (Lanfranc), and Henri de Mondeville. The last, a contentious and difficult man, argued for avoiding suppuration by following Hippocratic hygiene, and his handbook on surgery, a collection of materials presented in lecture at Montpellier, showed rare common sense and a shrewd practicality. Guy de Chauliac, who spanned the first 60 years of the fourteenth century, was particularly erudite, having studied at Toulouse, Montpellier, and Paris and then having pursued special studies of anatomy at Bologna. A clever and innovative surgeon, the most erudite of his time, he nevertheless rejected the idea that wounds should be permitted to heal as nature willed and stressed the surgeon's interference.

By the fourteenth century, Europe had created a new medical culture. Built firmly on the universities and employing the vast body of thought and practice accumulated in the classical and postclassical worlds, medieval Europe was an extension of the medical systems which had flourished around the Mediterranean. At the same time, the non-European medical world stopped developing. Both the character and the quality of medicine practiced in the medieval west were comparable to those of medicine in Byzantium and Islam. Eastern Europe as far as Vienna, Prague, and Lithuania-Poland followed the course marked out in the west and north. The Russian lands farther east, which inherited Byzantine-Greek medicine, did little with it. Three centuries of brutal civil war punctuated by the thirteenth-century Tatar conquest left learned tradition, medicine included, moribund. When Ivan III of Moscow sent the first Russian students to Padua in the fifteenth century to take medical training, there was virtually no sign of classic medicine in Russia. Though the ancient manuscripts reposing in Russian monasteries represented at least as rich a source as the west had available, there were no means to give it life. Thus Muscovites had to go to Italy, and later to Holland, to acquire entrée to the ideas they had inherited and lost.

In the west, the medical system received from late antiquity began to crack in the sixteenth century. Direct study of anatomy, culminating in the work of Andreas Vesalius and in William Harvey's discovery of the circulation of the blood (q.v.), opened a major fissure. The medieval synthesis then began to disintegrate, though aspects of humoral theory remained vital until the eighteenth century. Seventeenth- and eighteenth-century theorizing over physiology seemed to substitute one kind of scholasticism for another. The development of clinical medicine and disease classifications based on observation were actually more fruitful. In the Islamic world, however, the synthesis reached in the medieval period remained essentially unchallenged until the eighteenth century, when questioning of medical orthodoxies began in Egypt. The most violent challenge, however, came with the establishment of European influence in north Africa and Egypt, the Middle East and India in the eighteenth and nineteenth centuries. Just as the establishment of the classical tradition in western Europe lagged centuries behind the Moslem-Byzantine world, the world of Islam has been centuries slow in transforming its medical culture. In a world perspective, medieval medicine has remained a living force into the twentieth century.

ADDITIONAL READINGS: Arturo Castiglioni, *A History of Medicine*, E. B. Krumbhaar (trans.), 2d rev. and enl. ed., New York, 1947; Fielding A. Garrison, *An Introduction to the History of Medicine*, 4th ed., Philadelphia and London, 1929; Benjamin Lee Gordon, *Mediaeval and Renaissance Medicine*, New York and London, 1956, 1960; Institute of the History of Medicine and Medical Research, *Theories and Philosophies of Medicine*, 2d ed., New Delhi, 1973; Leon MacKinney, *Early Medieval Medicine*, Baltimore, 1937; Andrew W. Russell (ed.), *The Town and State Physicial In Europe from the Middle Ages to the Enlightenment*, Wolfenbüttel, German Federal Republic, 1984; H. M. Said (ed.), "Traditional Greco-Arabic and Modern Western Medicine: Conflict or Symbiosis?" *Hamdard* 17 (January–June 1975); Charles Singer and E. Ashworth Underwood, *A Short History of Medicine*, 2d ed., Oxford, 1962; X. Soffstosch, "The Two Faces of Medicine in Old Russia," CIBA Symposium 15(2), 1976; Charles Talbot, "Medicine," in David Lindberg (ed.), *Science in the Middle Ages*, Chicago, 1978; Charles Talbot, "Medicine in Medieval England," London, 1967; René Taton, *History of Science: Ancient and Medieval Science from the Beginning to 1450*, A. J. Pomerans (trans.), New York, 1963; Oswei Temkin, *Galenism, The Rise and Decline of a Medical Philosophy*, Ithaca, N.Y., 1973; Manfred Ullman, *Islamic Medicine*, Edinburgh, 1978.

See also HOSPITAL; MEDICAL PROFESSION.

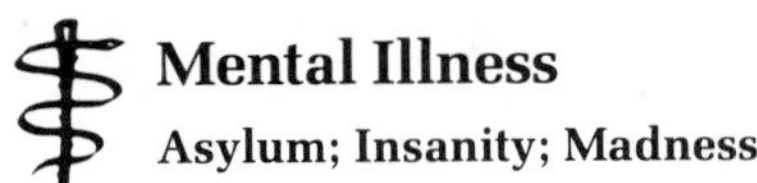

Mental Illness

Asylum; Insanity; Madness

"Madness" and "insanity" are words describing a condition of mind which produces behavior inconsistent with accepted norms. The words them selves have cultural rather than scientific meaning because concepts of mental illness are socially determined. On the other hand, the physiological or psychological causes which produce such behavior are objective evidence that an illness exists. Until the nineteenth century, the emphasis fell on behavior, and both the definition for what constituted insanity and the steps taken to deal with it were primarily social. In the nineteenth and early twentieth centuries, as mental illness came to be considered a disease, the emphasis fell on classification, causes, and treatment. More recently, medical and social approaches have drawn together. Drug therapies have eased treatment problems and permitted the release of previously hospitalized patients. This last development has begun to reduce the populations in mental hospitals for the first time in nearly 300 years while requiring, though not necessarily eliciting, a fundamental change in public attitudes toward the mentally ill.

Madness in Ancient Life Though madness is a relative concept, it is clear that certain behavior patterns have consistently signaled insanity. When Homer portrayed Odysseus as feigning madness, he had him yoke a bull and a horse to plow sand which he then sowed with salt. In the Old Testament story, when David pretended madness while seeking asylum from Saul among the Philistines, he disarranged his clothes, dribbled in his beard, and babbled; Achist, the Philistine king, recognized the symptoms immediately. Madness was also believed to disturb perceptions of reality. Ajax slaughtered sheep in the belief that they were enemy soldiers, a scene reminiscent of Don Quixote attacking sheep and windmills 2500 years later. Lycurgus, king of the Edonians, whom Dionysus sent mad, killed his own son with an ax under the impression that he was trimming a vine.

Sudden, explosive acts of violence, uncontrolled grief, joy, or rage, blood lust, and cannibalism have all been taken to indicate insanity. Herodotus, the earliest of the Greek historians and the founder of the craft, described two mad kings, Cambyses of Persia and Cleomenes of Sparta. In Herodotus's opinion, what marked Cambyses as mad were his acts of uncontrolled violence and his mocking holy rites and long-established traditions. Herodotus stressed the latter, asserting that only a mad person would make sport of the gods. Cleomenes, a brilliant if erratic ruler, showed a pattern of increasingly irrational behavior which began when he struck citizens in the face with his scepter for no apparent reason and eventually led to his family's locking him into the stocks. There he bullied and threatened his keeper, demanded a knife, and, when he was finally given it, slashed his own legs, loins, hips, and thighs with such ferocity that he died of his wounds.

Irrational behavior ran the gamut from convulsions, cries, and screams to murderous assaults. In the Bible, some mad people were compared with prophets, since the prophetic tradition involved ecstasies and trance like states. The Jews, however, considered madness not a badge of divinity but one of Jehovah's most powerful and feared weapons. Greek gods were believed to use madness to punish those who resisted or mocked them. The Hippocratic writings, which rejected divine possession as the cause for epileptic seizures and provided a naturalistic explanation for other mental disorders, also listed Pan, Hecate, Cybele, or the Mountain Mother, and the Corybantes as those gods that were believed to make people mad, while Dionysus was thought to be particularly quick to use madness against his opponents.

Greek custom offered legal means to protect the families of the mad from them and to prevent them from destroying or dissipating their property. Roman law contained the same principle and included provision for appointing guardians to protect the holdings of the mad. Neither Greece nor Rome took social responsibility for the insane, though it appears that Roman military hospitals (*valetudinaria*) accepted mental cases from among the troops. The Asclepian sanctuaries also admitted mental cases, and the methods of treatment which involved religious rituals and a mystic experience in which the god Asclepius visited patients in their dreams, fitted the needs of some neurotic conditions. Aristides, a sophist and rhetorician of the second century A.D., spent 10 years under the god's care and regained his mental health. Such opportunities, however, were for the few, as was employing a physician to care for a mental case. At base, insanity was a family problem. The seriously disturbed were kept under restraint at home. The less serious roamed abroad, though if not guarded, they were likely to be mistreated. The evil spirits (*keres*) who were thought responsible for all disasters not only could enter people to make them mad but also could fly out to enter others. As a result, the disturbed, whether merely eccentric or wildly psychotic, were feared and shunned. Spitting was thought to ward off the spirit, and clods or stones would be thrown at the insane to drive them away. So long as the insane kept to themselves, they were left alone, but when their presence became threatening, and they could not be driven away, they were tied up or imprisoned.

The Medieval View The acceptance of Christianity as the official faith of the Roman empire in the fourth century A.D. had little effect on attitudes toward the mentally ill, though a marginal benefit derived from the Christian emphasis on caring for the sick or destitute. Possession by devils, the spiritual etiology for insanity, was entirely consistent with Christian doctrines and provided attitudinal foundations for the later witch hysteria. It also contributed the more benign idea of the holy innocent, in Russia the pure fool, or fool in Christ, which equated a simple or lacking mind with God's special favor. Fools so blessed spoke freely and without restraint, and because they were holy, they were also protected and nurtured.

The position regarding the insane was markedly different in Islam. In the *Koran*, the principle was laid down that society was responsible for the kindly and humane care of the insane, and the first institutions created primarily for mental cases appeared in Moslem lands. Called *maurastans*, these centers for care of the insane were reputed to be vastly luxurious, and one thirteenth-century account portrayed the violent cases restrained with golden chains. Exaggerated though such descriptions were, Moslems were far more ready to treat the mentally disturbed with consideration than their Christian neighbors were, and as late as the nineteenth century, European travelers marveled at the tolerance and humaneness shown the insane in Moslem countries.

The Islamic tradition had some effect on late medieval European mental institutions. The first European mental hospitals were built in Spain before the expulsion of the Moslems, beginning in Granada (1365–1367). Others were built at Valencia (1407), Zaregoza (1425), Seville (1436), Barcelona (1481), and Toledo (1483). In the early sixteenth century, a pious and eccentric merchant named Juan Ciudad Duarte, who had suffered an acute psychotic experience during which he was flogged, founded and endowed a special hospital for humane care of the insane and an order to serve it. His Order of the Hospitaler, later the Order of St. John of God, became one of the most important hospital orders of the time, founding hospitals in Spain, Italy, and France, including the famed Santé de Senlis, which became a model for eighteenth-century reformers.

Elsewhere in Europe, attitudes toward the insane were little different from what they had been in the ancient past. Town records in Germany show that municipalities periodically expelled mentally deficient or insane persons, thought it is uncertain whether those expelled were natives or transients who drifted in claiming shelter and protection. Some towns turned their mental cases over to sailors or even hired a ship to carry them away. Thus the ship of fools (*Narrenschiff*) became a persistent image in literature and art, a symbol of humanity's follies and restlessness. More prosaically, it was common practice to whip those who were expelled to remind them that they were not to return. Those who ignored the warning were given a more severe beating the second time. Since whipping was a common form of punishment for sacrilege and outrageous behavior, it was a treatment to which the insane were particularly liable.

Not all the insane were sent away. Most European towns had madmen's towers (*Narrtürmer*) or cells, and the insane were also gathered into medieval hospitals. In Paris, special cubicles were set aside at the Hôtel-Dieu and the Châtelet de Melun for mental cases. The Teutonic Knights' hospital at Elbing had a madhouse (*Tollhaus*), while the Grosse Hospital at Erfurt (1385) was furnished with a mad hut (*Tollkoben*). St. Mary of Bethlem in London, built in 1247, had six men "deprived of reason" on the rolls in 1403. This hospital gave English a new word. Better known as Bedlam, a corruption of its proper name, it became famous for its population of insane folk and the ear-splitting din they made.

In popular culture, madness and demonology were never far apart. Pilgrimages to healing shrines and rituals of exorcism were common methods for driving out the devil, and possession remained a recognized explanation for insane behavior. In the fifteenth century, the church itself promoted fear of the devil and his powers by opening a formal campaign to cleanse society of those the foul fiend had corrupted. Women were considered particularly susceptible to the devil's influence. Waves of witch hysteria rolled across Europe during the next 300 years. Literally thousands of people, largely women, were tested, tried, tortured, and executed. The weak-minded, the hysterical, the neurotic, and the senescent were particularly vulnerable to the hunters, though in at least one case, recognition that a woman was insane led a panel of judges to free her.

The Age of Incarceration During the sixteenth and seventeenth centuries, demographic, economic, and cultural changes were accompanied by ferocious civil, dynastic, and class wars, devastating plagues, and a terrifying incidence of butchery and brutalization. The solution was to put a premium on peace and order and to legitimate the absolute power which promised it. By the late sixteenth century, attitudes toward all socially disruptive elements hardened, and this reaction heralded a far harsher attitude toward the mentally disturbed than any held before. Guaranteeing public order meant locking away all who might disturb it. Increasingly rational and effective political systems hastened the process, and by the middle of the seventeenth century the insane, together with beggars and the indigent poor, prostitutes, minor criminals, unemployed youths, the chronically ill, and the aged, were swept up into a new type of institution where they could be held indefinitely.

The attempt to establish social order by incarcerating the disorderly was general in Europe, but it was carried out most systematically in France. In 1656, a royal edict created a new institution for Paris called the General Hospital (l'Hôpital Général). This was an administrative system with responsibility for several institutions, including the Bicêtre, which provided facilities for insane males, and Salpêtrière, which served female mental cases. The General Hospital was an institution over which neither the courts nor the police had jurisdiction. It was created to deal with people who burdened society, but it was not subject to society's sanctions. Collectively, those from whom society was to be protected were called "the poor," and the directors of the hospital were granted "all power of authority, of direction, of administration, of commerce, of police, of jurisdiction, of correction and punishment over all the poor of Paris." The authority delegated to the directors was virtually absolute. There was no recourse against their decisions. This "strange power," this "third order of repression," locked up the mental cases. They did not emerge until the end of the next century.

Paris's General Hospital became the model for public and private institutions in France. On the eve of the revolution, general hospitals existed in 32 provincial cities, while many church-administered institutions reorganized as general hospitals. In Germany, these institutions were called houses of correction (*Zuchthäusern*). The first was founded at Hamburg in 1620, but the largest number was organized between 1650 and 1800. The "bridewell" was the early private equivalent in England, and the first public workhouse was founded in 1697. In both England and Germany, local authorities carried the heaviest responsibility. The French precedent for centralizing functions was not repeated.

General hospitals were not intended to treat the sick, and medical staffing was minimal. In the Paris General Hospital, there was just one physician to minister to 6000 inmates. The essential purpose of the general hospital was to remove indigents from the streets and turn them into sober and industrious citizens. Only people able to meet their obligations in society could be returned to society. This meant that the insane, because they were unteachable, could never be released. There was, therefore, a heavy emphasis on security. Yet some believed that because it was reason that defined humans, the reason in them could never be alienated, though consciousness of it could be clouded. It was also thought that some people played insane roles for reasons of their own. Therefore harsh treatment, including physical punishment, was justified to bring the insane to their senses, to force them to renounce their irrationality.

A contrary view held that the human being deprived of reason was less than human and lacked normal human sensibilities. This approach held that the insane were immune to physical discomfort, that they were impervious to heat or cold, that clothing was superfluous, and that they had no consciousness of pride, shame, or any of the feelings expressed by normal human beings. Like animals, the insane could be dangerous and should be kept under close restraint. Also like animals, the insane understood physical punishment, could be beaten into submission, and, when safely sequestered, were interesting to watch. Keepers displayed their wards for a fee—in some cases the inmates themselves organized the show—and people flocked to see the animal humans. At Bedlam, for example, the charge in the early eighteenth century was a penny a head, and the receipts in one 12-month period amounted to 400 pounds. This meant at least 96,000 spectators for the lunatic show.

Such attitudes toward the insane produced cruel treatment. The conditions under which they existed were unspeakable. The mad cells were usually dark, dank, cold, and rat-infested. Sanitation was virtually nonexistent, clothing was minimal in even the coldest weather, and it was not uncommon for both men and women to be seen lying entirely naked on beds of rotten straw or on the slats which covered the floor of the confinement cages. Incorrigibles were chained to the walls or to their beds, and some were locked up in cages. The only consideration was to make escape impossible. Health or comfort meant nothing.

None of the attitudes which produced "the great confinement" were new. But the determination to protect society against the unfortunates in it and the willingness to make their misfortunes the basis for punitive treatment were new. Insanity by itself was not actionable. Where there was wealth and the willingness to care for a deranged relative, the situation could be entirely different. There were also institutions which not only provided a decent physical environment for mental cases but actually tried to improve their condition. The Charité de Senlis, which was administered by the brothers of the Order of St. John of God, was a model of rational organization and humane treatment. Mental defectives, psychotics, and dangerous psychopaths were segregated from one another and from the group called "libertins," patients believed to have "amendable behavior disorders." Each case was treated individually. There were no whips, chains, detention cells, or stocks. The inmates wore a common dress modeled after a religious habit, and all were given pseudonyms. They were invited to attend religious services and were treated humanely and with dignity. Nothing more different from Bedlam or Salpêtrière could be imagined. It was also the exception.

The Era of Reform Although concern over conditions among the insane appeared earlier, action on the worst abuses began in the last decades of the eighteenth century. The movement was spontaneous, a product of Enlightenment humanitarianism, and it appeared in several places at once. It was also a movement in which dedicated individuals made major contributions, while the societies involved remained uninterested or even hostile.

In its simplest form, reform meant physically freeing the insane from their chains. Vincenzio Chiarugi, a physician at Bonifazio Asylum in Florence, was one of the first to attempt the experiment. The results were promising and led to further reforms in Italy. Philippe Pinel, who was to become a leading authority on mental illness and one of the most distinguished physicians in France, was given responsibility for the insane at Bicêtre in 1793 when the Reign of Terror was at its height. Pinel argued that the reason the insane behaved like wild animals was that, like animals, they were chained, and once they were freed, their behavior would improve. Georges Couthon, a member of the ruling triumvirate who was responsible for prisons and hospitals, reluctantly agreed to the experiment, though he threatened Pinel's life if the experiment failed, and he appears to have suspected a political intrigue. Pinel was careful to select inmates he believed could and would act responsibly, and the experiment proved a dramatic success. Ultimately, most of Pinel's mental patients were freed. Some were found to have been innocent victims of the dragnet approach favored by the French authorities. Others, who were ill, improved sufficiently when unchained to permit release. Some were retained but were given the freedom of the institution. It was still necessary to keep the most severe cases under restraint, but Pinel labored to make the controls as humane as possible.

Philippe Pinel's successes at Bicêtre brought him responsibility for Salpêtrière as well, and he introduced his new regimen at once. He also collected and published data on the patients under his care while taking students whom he instructed in his methods. The most distinguished of his pupils was Jean-Étienne Dominique Esquirol, who became one of the leaders in the asylum movement and the author of the main body of regulations governing care for the insane in France. Other influential reformers included Benjamin Rush in Philadelphia, Christian Reil in Berlin, and the Tuke family in England. In 1792, William Tuke, a Quaker and a tea merchant, founded an asylum known as the Retreat in Yorkshire, which became famous for its enlightened treatment of the insane. Though none of the Tuke family were physicians until Daniel Hack Tuke qualified in 1853, the Tukes and their asylum exerted a powerful influence on the asylum movement.

The asylum movement regarded the insane as victims of a special illness which could be cured. The treatments implemented were anything but humane and reflected the common conception that the victims were suffering some stoppage or insufficiency which robbed them of their senses. Asylum inmates were subjected to unexpected dousing with icy water, cold baths, isolation, electric shocks, and the dizzying whirl of centrifugal treatments aimed at increasing the blood supply to the head. They might also be purged and "bled to depletion," while various punishments, including beatings, were still meted out as part of the so-called moral therapies. Benjamin Rush was particularly notable for treatments as ferocious as his views on incarceration were enlightened.

In the United States, asylum directors competed with each other in making claims for the successes of their various institutions. The resulting hucksterism obscured whatever real advances were made. On the other hand, the asylum movement, which began by isolating the mentally ill, also began to accumulate information about them. This led to major advances in describing and classifying mental illnesses. Esquirol established a new system of psychopathological concepts based on direct observation, compiled statistical descriptions of mental diseases, and began to study the environment for treating mental illness. Esquirol believed that the asylum itself was a "therapeutic instrument," that all activities within the asylum, together with the building and grounds, should serve the purpose of treating mental illness. While moving toward group therapy, Esquirol also became the world's leading authority on asylum construction. He planned the National Asylum of Charenton, of which he became director, and he published a major treatise on asylum construction after visiting every place in France where mental patients were kept.

Aftermath of Reform The asylum movement established a pattern of care which has continued into the twentieth century. Special facilities of many different kinds evolved to permit treatment in environments sheltered from society. Communities modeled after the Belgian village of Gheel provided a controlled social setting in which the mentally disturbed could live and receive treatment. There, individual families, in return for a fee, would take in mental cases, particularly children. In the second half of the nineteenth century, hospital renovation and remodeling of large homes or public buildings multiplied the facilities available to care for the insane. Increase in facilities permitted special wards for different degrees of mental illness and the use of various therapies, while new hospital construction in the twentieth century created major centers for research as well as care. In Germany, France, and England, a rich variety of mental institutions appeared which ranged from polyclinics to the traditional asylum and mental wards in general hospitals. Public financing added to private funds to support European facilities. After 1850, governmental licensing and regular inspections enforced minimum standards.

In the United States, care for the mentally ill lagged. Hospital facilities were underdeveloped, public funding and control over health institutions were not common, and the institutions which existed were unregulated, often little better than prisons. In the years before the Civil War, Dorothea Dix, a Boston teacher with a strong commitment to public service, began a personal campaign for publicly supported mental institutions, and she lobbied strongly in state legislatures for her cause. Miss Dix was amazingly successful, bringing a number of state-supported mental institutions into existence, including the New Jersey State Hospital in Trenton, and in 1854 carrying both houses of Congress with a bill for federal support of the indigent insane. The bill was vetoed by President Franklin Pierce on the grounds that it would establish a precedent for transferring the burden of the indigent poor from the states to the national government. Dorothea Dix also campaigned in Europe where she was well-received.

Despite the Dix campaign and the publicity it won, treatment of the insane in the United States revealed a persistently negative attitude, and even in state institutions, patients were handled as if they were prisoners or criminals to be punished. These conditions were again publicized in the twentieth century. Clifford W. Beers, a young college graduate and businessman, suffered a severe mental breakdown which caused him to be institutionalized, first at a private hospital, later in a public institution. As he wrote in the introduction to his autobiographical *A Mind That Found Itself* (1908), "I left the state hospital in September, 1903, firmly determined to write a book about my experiences and to organize a movement that would help to do away with existing evils in the care of the mentally ill, and whenever possible to prevent mental illness itself." Encouraged by the philosopher-psychologist William James, and by Adolph Meyer, the country's leading psychiatrist, Beers established a Mental Hygiene Society which became the National Committee for Mental Hygiene in 1909. The committee became a moving force for mental health, first in the United States and later abroad. With a grant of $50,000 from Henry Phipps, a partner of Andrew Carnegie and a supporter of psychiatric causes, the committee began an active campaign. Under Dr. Thomas W. Salmon, the committee gained such prestige that during World War I it took over the government's neurology and psychiatry division. From that point on, the committee's influence expanded as it became the center for a variety of mental health interests.

The Modern Era In the course of the nineteenth century, insanity became a disease to be treated by medical means, as modern society accepted responsibility for providing treatment and care. On the medical side, the treatments which evolved, whether directed to physical or to emotional causes, proved able at most to ameliorate some conditions; and because the means to integrate many mental cases into society did not exist, institutions providing for their segregation, in part or altogether, became essential. One exception was Great Britain, where there was a strong move in the direction of permitting the mentally disturbed to move freely in society. In the United States, the hospital approach was the most common one, and mental cases comprised from one-third to one-half of hospitalized patients. The development of drug therapies since the 1960s has made the release of thousands of previously institutionalized patients possible, though public skepticism and resistance remain high. Community mental health facilities, which are substantially developed in most European countries, are lacking in the United States, and therefore the support systems, including follow-up, are far from adequate. The immediate result has been a profound disillusion with the release program which has left large numbers of people who are at best marginally competent to live in society without protection or even the means to request assistance.

Modern society has modified its attitudes since the insane were unchained and the asylum movement was founded; neurology and psychology have revealed many aspects of mental function and have contributed significantly to understanding the pathology of dysfunction; psychiatric medicine has developed sophisticated methods for dealing with both symptoms and causes; and preventive mental health plans provide some hope of controlling the development of mental problems. What has been achieved, however, is only a beginning, and the problems of mental health stand out as requiring the most serious attention.

ADDITIONAL READINGS: Silvano Arieté (ed.), *American Handbook of Psychiatry, Volume I: The Foundations of Psychiatry*, 2d rev. and enl. ed., New York, 1974; Simon Bennett, *Mind and Madness in Ancient Greece: The Classical Roots of Modern Psychiatry*, Ithaca, N.Y., 1980; Jan Ehrenwald, *The History of Psychotherapy*, New York, 1976; Michael Foucault, *Madness and Civilization: A History of Insanity in the Age of Reason*, Richard Howard (trans.), New York, 1965; Alan Krohn, *Hysteria: The Elusive Neurosis*, New York, 1978; H. C. Midelfort, "Madness and Civilization in Early Modern Europe: A Reappraisal of Michel Foucault," in B. C. Malament (ed.), *After the Reformation: Essays in Honor of J. H. Hexter*, Philadelphia, 1980, 247–265; George Rosen, *Madness in Society: Chapters in the Historical Sociology of Mental Illness*, London, 1968; Andrew Scull (ed.) *Madhouses, Mad-Doctors, and Madmen: The Social History of Psychiatry in the Victorian Era*, Philadelphia, 1981.

See also EPILEPSY; NEUROLOGY; PSYCHIATRY.

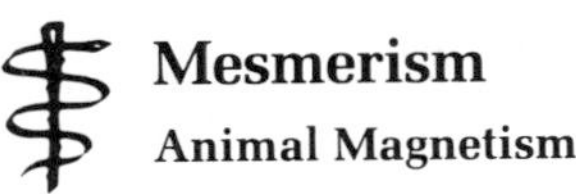

Mesmerism

Animal Magnetism

Mesmerism was a procedure and a movement which developed from the cosmological, physiological, and therapeutic ideas of an eighteenth-century Vienna-trained physician, Dr. Franz Anton Mesmer. Between 1773 and 1787, Mesmer became a controversial, even notorious, figure in Vienna and Paris. His fame and the movement he founded spread throughout prerevolutionary France and reached the American colonies, where mesmerism took firm root in the early nineteenth century. Mesmerism also reached England, but it enjoyed no success there until the second quarter of the nineteenth century.

Mesmer's Society of Harmony, founded in 1783, attracted cultists and mystics as well as scientific amateurs and respectable physicians. Mesmer's society, though not Mesmer himself, also played a role in French revolutionary politics, identifying with the moderate Girondist faction and suffering a purge at the hands of the radical Jacobins. In medical terms, mesmerism led directly into hypnotism (q.v.) and has been identified as an early stage of abnormal psychosomatic medicine, while its techniques contain early prefigurings of group therapy and psychoanalysis. Mesmer himself was not a conscious prophet of these future wonders, but his followers, even at the cost of breaking relations with him, turned the movement in that direction.

Mesmer's cosmology and physiology were in the mainstream of traditional European scientific thought. His dissertation (1766), which won plaudits from the Vienna medical faculty, treated the effect of the planets on the functioning of the human system and postulated a "universal fluid" which permeated the body, moving the vital organs to act as it ebbed and flowed throughout the cosmos. Mesmer was a physiological mechanist. Like John Brown of Edinburgh, Mesmer found neither will nor overt purpose in his cosmic tidal wash, and the therapy he evolved was a purely mechanical one which assumed that the flow had been inhibited and that a powerful shock (the mesmeric crisis) was necessary to get the organs functioning properly again.

During Mesmer's six years of training and first seven years of practice, his approach to medicine was entirely orthodox, he stood well in Vienna's social and cultural community, and he prospered. He developed the therapies which made him famous almost by accident. His inspiration was a semipermanent houseguest, Francisca (Franzl) Oesterlin, who suffered crippling periodic seizures which produced vomiting, convulsions, intestinal inflammation, urinary failure, toothache, earache, despondency, fainting fits, temporary blindness, hallucinations, and occasionally paralysis. Mesmer recorded the symptoms regularly, observed their pattern, and by a leap of imagination connected them with the cosmic rhythms of his universal fluid. Because he believed that magnetic attraction accounted for the universal tidal flow, he placed three magnets in what he thought were critical positions on Franzl Oesterlin's body. How he prepared her psychologically for treatment is not known. That she was highly suggestible and dependent on Mesmer is clear. His magnetic applications produced convulsive physical responses and a temporary remission of symptoms. When she reacted repeatedly in the same way, Mesmer was sure that his theory was correct and that he had unlocked one of nature's fundamental secrets.

Mesmer's initial success brought the first of an endless train of controversies and a basic refinement of conception. His colleague who had prepared the magnets claimed that they were responsible for the cure, but Mesmer hotly denied it. Mineral magnets, he argued, could not possibly effect animal magnetism. The magnets were simply conductors for the animal magnetism which he possessed and which he had learned to direct. The therapy, then, depended on a physician who understood how to manipulate the animal magnetism. Any person, he was to claim later, could become a magnetizer, but the power was so great that only the best, most committed, and most trustworthy persons could be admitted to its secrets. He also, quite illogically, regarded his discovery as a boon accessible to anyone which would free humanity from functional disorders. The problem was to activate animal magnetism, and it was to this end that he developed the hypnotic techniques which have become synonymous with his name.

There is no doubt that the Oesterlin woman suffered the symptoms described, nor that she was eventually relieved from them. She changed from a reclusive semi-invalid into a fat, jolly hausfrau, the wife of Mesmer's stepson and the mother of several children. Mozart, who was a familiar of the household, declared himself astonished at the change and delighted with it. Other cases followed, and Mesmer became a phenomenon whose reputation as a healer spread through central Europe. His colleagues on the Vienna medical faculty refused to accept the cures he offered as proofs for his therapeutic system, but they also sent him incorrigible cases involving organ failure or malfunction. The most famous of these was a blind girl, Maria Theresa Paradies, who eventually became a renowned concert pianist. Mesmer had partially restored her sight when a bitter controversy, first with her parents and then with the medical authorities, left his reputation in tatters and forced him to immigrate to Paris.

Mesmer's techniques were well-established by the time of the Paradies scandal. They became famous during his fabulous decade in Paris. Mesmer definitely thought he manipulated the universal fluid by using animal magnetism. It is equally unquestionable that he achieved real influence over his patients and some effect on psychosomatic conditions by a variety of psychological techniques which, however, were wholly predicated on the concept of animal magnetism. The crux of Mesmer's therapy was the crisis—everything he did aimed at achieving it. The crisis might be gentle or violent, and it could involve symptoms ranging from fever, delirium, and convulsions to catalepsy, uncontrolled weeping, and nervous twitches. These were healthy symptoms, for they meant the magnetism was working to build up the fluid pressure necessary to stimulate organs while clearing away the detritus left by nonfunctioning organs. In a patient who had been properly prepared, a gesture by the magnetizer or a touch with a magnetized artifact could produce a convulsive twitch. Gentle stroking of the area of blockage was another method, as was rhythmic massage of the "polar areas" to generate magnetic action. Mesmer was known to bend patients into a backward arc and then tip them backward and forward to start the fluid movement necessary for a crisis.

Any object could be magnetized and used to start the necessary motion, and the famous instrument for group treatments was called the "baquet." The classic version was a large tub packed with bottles of "magnetized" water lying on their sides, necks outward, submerged in water containing magnetized wooden and metal chips. Iron rods were thrust through the sides of the tub, and each patient held a rod with one hand while clasping his or her neighbor's hand with the other. As the magnetic force in the tub poured through their bodies, they would pass into crisis, falling down and writhing in apparent agony. Mesmer walked among them, dressed in a flowing gray overgarment and carrying an iron wand. His assistants, dressed in lilac suits, gave help as needed to the patients. When a particularly violent crisis occurred, the patient would be helped away to a padded "crisis room," and Mesmer or his helpers would stay with him or her until the crisis passed.

Suggestibility and dominance were at work to produce these effects, but the best tool for his purpose was the trance state, which Mesmer discovered during his sessions with Franzl Oesterlin. His French followers, Charles Deslon and the Marquis de Puységur, worked on the trance state intensively, coming finally to the realization that it provided an effective means for mobilizing the patient's will to aid his or her own cure. This line of thinking had scientific and medical implications of the first importance which were finally realized in the next century. The trance was also dangerously titillating. Young women were reported to experience erotic fantasies which gave them the appearance of being in the grip of passion and which ended with orgasmic spasms. This phenomenon was cited to prove that only the most dedicated and responsible workers should be trusted with Mesmer's powerful secret.

Mesmer took Paris by storm. He was inundated with patients, and his techniques were pilloried and praised on the stage, in pamphlets and broadsides, and in the press. He accepted rich and poor alike, as he had always done, and a penumbra of benevolence, social concern, and humanitarianism surrounded his clinics. In time his movement attracted those with grievances against authority, for, despite its success and popularity, no medical or scientific institution in Paris would accept his system. One effort was made to provide him with a building and a royal pension on the understanding that the government could name the students. Mesmer rejected the offer claiming to see in it an attempt to supervise his activities and to acquire his "secrets" at minimal cost. In 1784, a royal commission was appointed to investigate his medical claims. The verdict was that there were undoubtedly effects from Mesmer's procedures but that they did not demonstrate his scientific claims.

Disenchanted with royal authority and the academies, Mesmer agreed to form a private organization whose members would learn his techniques and whose membership fees would pay him for his knowledge. The prime movers in this project were a Lyons lawyer, Nicolas Bergasse, and Guillaume Kornmann, an Alsatian financier. The society began as a secret organization which would become public when Mesmer had been paid. It would then spread Mesmerian technique throughout the world for the benefit of all humanity. The Society of Harmony, as it was called, was a great success, founding chapters throughout France, while members carried the message abroad. Marquis de Lafayette, a charter member, informed George Washington of his intention to propagate mesmerism in America, encouraged a correspondence between Mesmer and the general, and lectured the American Philosophical Society on the subject, showing more enthusiasm than knowledge.

The Society of Harmony, which began so well, ended ill. Mesmer, despite a covenant with the organizers and 240,000 livres in membership fees, insisted on control over the organization and secrecy for his ideas. This stand, combined with bitter factional disputes, destroyed the society within two years of its founding. By 1787, Mesmer himself had dropped out of the picture. Though he lived for 30 more years, Mesmer had nothing further to contribute, and through he continued to seek scientific acceptance, his creative period had ended.

Mesmer believed himself to be a scientist and physician who had learned a great natural secret which he employed to benefit humanity. He thought animal magnetism was as real as any other natural phenomenon, but his only proofs were the methods of treatment he employed and the successes they achieved. This was no proof by any standards, and the real effects which mesmeric techniques produced were simply puzzling. Mesmer himself never questioned his doctrine, never analyzed or tested his techniques, but rather worked to perfect them. The psychological mechanisms which made mesmerism work were found by institution and accident. Mesmer was a natural psychologist of great power, and he achieved remarkable results. But he lacked the intellectual and emotional resources which would allow him to turn his intuitions into scientific realities. His followers were the ones who began to study mesmerism critically, and they were only able to do so by qualifying and ultimately eliminating animal magnetism.

Mesmerism's political side was destroyed in the French Revolution, but its association with popular science and the occult flourished. Animal magnetism was finally co-opted by the founder of theosophy, Helena Petrovna Blavatsky, to explain magic, miracles, and reincarnation. On the other hand, Mary Baker Eddy, who founded the Church of Christ, Scientist, though initially impressed with mesmerism, came to regard animal magnetism with a profound loathing. Scientifically, it was the mesmeric trance which was most significant. Redefined as hypnotism by James Braid, this aspect of mesmerism led toward abnormal psychology, psychiatry, and psychosomatic medicine. These fields developed in the second half of the nineteenth century and have been particularly important in the twentieth. Their development reveals Franz Anton Mesmer as a true blind prophet: He pointed out roads he could not see which led to destinations whose existence he never suspected.

ADDITIONAL READINGS: Vincent Beranelli, *The Wizard from Vienna: Franz Anton Mesmer*, New York, 1975; Robert Darnton, *Mesmerism and the End of the Enlightenment in France*, Cambridge, Mass., 1968; R. de Saussure, "The Magnetic Cure," *British Journal of Medical Psychology* 42 (June 1969): 141–168; Henri F. Ellenberger, *The Discovery of the Unconscious*, New York, 1970; Fred Kaplan, "The Mesmeric Mania: Early Victorians and Animal Magnetism," *Journal of the History of Ideas* 35 (October–December 1974): 691–702; Jonathan Miller, "Mesmerism," *The Listener* 90 (November 1973): 685–688; J. D. Schneck, "History of Electrotherapy and Its Correlation with Mesmer's Animal Magnetism," *American Journal of Psychiatry* 116 (November 1969): 463–464.

See also HYPNOTISM; PSYCHIATRY.

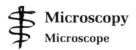

Microscopy

Microscope

Microscopy is a discipline which concerns observation of phenomena too small to be seen with the unaided human eye. Microscopy has been essential to the modern evolution of physiology and pathology. Such special fields as bacteriology, virology, histology, and cytology could not exist without it, and it has contributed as well to metallurgy, crystallography, and the development of precision tools. Today, light microscopes are the workhorses of both clinical and research laboratories as well as being the first scientific instruments which schoolchildren learn to use, while advanced electron and acoustic microscopes promise significant new advances in biological science.

Microscopy began in the sixteenth century and reached its first plateau of development in the second half of the seventeenth century. Though interested in optics, neither ancient nor medieval scientists paid attention to magnifying tiny objects. When magnification did become important, it was to bring distant objects near, and as a result microscopy has always lagged behind telescopy. Greek and Arab achievements in the science of optics were synthesized for western Europe during the thirteenth century by the Polish scholar and scientist Witelo (Vitellius; Vitellio; Vitelo) and by John Peckham, an English theologian, mathematician, and physicist who wrote a textbook on optics which remained standard for the next 300 years. Optics and perspective engaged European minds into the seventeenth century, but though mathematicians worked on the properties of lenses, glassmakers developed proficiency at making them. Preparing lenses was a practical matter which in the early stages of microscopy owed very little to theory. It now seems certain that the compound microscope was invented between 1590 and 1610 in the Dutch town of Middleberg by three spectacle makers, Hans Jansen (Janssen), his son Zacharias, and Hans Lipperskey. Lipperskey's claim to priority is less certain than the Jansens' though he was responsible for a binocular telescope. Jansen instruments were known in Austria, Italy, and England during the early seventeenth century and stimulated a popular curiosity about very small objects.

In 1646, Athanasius Kircher, a learned monk who served as professor of mathematics at Würzburg, published a book on light, and in 1671 he issued a second edition which included a description of his *smiscropium parastaticum*. This was a circular box whose upper lid was on a rotary axis. A mirror and the objects to be observed were placed opposite each other inside; there was an aperture for light, and a tube in the top was fitted with a good-quality lens. The effect was "to present to the observer a series of magnified views of the objects in the field." This instrument enabled Kircher to see "little worms" in the blood of a plague victim, a report which aroused an early though short-lived interest in the germ theory of disease. What Kircher saw was almost certainly not *Yersina pestis,* nor was his instrument either the first or the most developed microscope for its time. Many people made both instruments and observations, but the work of Robert Hooke, Antonj van Leeuwenhoek, and Marcello Malpighi was especially important, for it was these men who established microscopy as a discipline.

Robert Hooke was a distinguished English scientist of the Stuart Restoration. He served as Robert Boyle's assistant, and as a result of his microscopic demonstrations, he became curator of experiments for the newly founded Royal Society. One of his responsibilities in this capacity was to provide weekly scientific demonstrations. These usually involved some experiment in microscopic observation. Hooke's most important published work, which summarized his observations and described his techniques, appeared in 1665 under the title *Micrographia.* Published in English rather than Latin, this handsome volume contained the first descriptions of cells and used the world "cell" for the first time to describe the compartments which characterized the structure of cork.

Antonj van Leeuwenhoek, of Delft, who elevated the skills of lens preparation to high art, visited London in 1668. Though there is no direct evidence of contact, there is a close similarity between the simple microscope in Hooke's *Micrographia* and what came to be called the Leeuwenhoek microscope. Whether he knew the *Micrographia* or not, Leeuwenhoek was a brilliantly meticulous observer and artisan with an insatiable curiosity. He was trained neither as a physician nor as a scientist, yet he became one of the greatest of the early microscopists. Leeuwenhoek tailored his instruments to the observations he was making, and when he died in 1723, he was supposed to have had over 300 (some say 500) microscopes, some of which had gold or silver fittings. Most, however, were a simple body to hold the specimen and lens. As Leeuwenhoek ground each lens for a particular observation, many were left with the specimen in place. The Royal Society published his work, and he had a wide following of devoted admirers throughout Europe. Among his myriad observations, the most notable were the illustrations of red corpuscles, his work on capillaries and the circulatory system in frogs and eels, his descriptions, the first ever, of spermatozoa and protozoans, and his illustrations of bacteria.

The third and most important of the seventeenth-century microscopists was Marcello Malpighi, a professor at Bologna and Pisa. Malpighi was less interested in curiosities than in basic physiological analysis. He worked with lower animals and plants as well as human tissue, and in 1661 he supplied the missing link between arteries and veins in William Harvey's classic explanation of circulation. Malpighi identified capillary vessels in a frog lung, which proved the existence of a channel between the smallest arteries and the smallest veins. Harvey knew the channel had to exist, but he was never able to show it without a microcope. Malpighi's command of microscopy led him to other important observations, including studies in embryology which became the foundation for the field. His effectiveness as a microscopist and physiologist is reflected in the fact that his name has been attached to such organ microstructures as the Malpighian layer in the kidneys, and he is widely considered to be the founder of scientific microscopy.

Hooke, Leeuwenhoek, and Malpighi were the leading practitioners in what was potentially an extremely important art, one which attracted a host of fascinated followers. But microscopy's popularity was actually greatest among scientific amateurs, and in general the discipline was not applied systematically to solving scientific problems. Several factors accounted for this failure. Most of the questions which scientists were studying could be answered by observations with the naked eye. And where this was not true, the microscope was of little use because lenses could not give accurate readings of high magnification. The diffusion of light rays through the lenses fuzzed images or put a distorting halo around objects, while spherical aberrations changed the shape and outline of what was observed. Major errors were commonplace, Marie François Xavier Bichat, whose observations and classifications of tissues were major steps in the development of histology, never used the microscope because of the distortions it produced, and historians now believe that lens distortion was responsible for the eighteenth-century controversy over whether body tissues were "fibullar" or "globular." The myth of the homunculus, the fully formed human in each drop of sperm, was another example of creative interpretation which derived from microscopical aberration.

High standards of manufacture and some improvement in detail characterized eighteenth-century microscopes, but design retrogressed, and the main hindrances to accuracy of observation remained unresolved. The problem of chromatic distortion was solved in telescopes before the middle of the eighteenth century, but the achromatic lens was much slower to appear in microscopes, and when it did, there was still substantial distortion, even at relatively low magnifications. Though many worked on this problem, it was J. J. Lister who solved it; he published his solution in 1830. Previous lens preparations, whether chromatic or achromatic, compound or simple, were done by trial and error. The achromatic lens required the grinding and fitting together of two lenses of different materials, but there was no routine way to position the lenses. Lister worked out a formula to determine in advance the optimum distance between the lenses to eliminate both chromatic and spherical aberration. Lister's paper has justifiably been called "the most important ever published on microscopy," for it literally opened the way to modern applications of the microscope.

The influence of interested amateurs remained strong in nineteenth-century English microscopy, and the instruments produced by London makers reflected the market. Large, beautifully tooled, and magnificently finished, the English microscopes of the Victorian age were works of art dedicated to the genteel pursuit of science. They were highly effective, but both size and cost made them inappropriate for working laboratories or research institutes. Parisian workshops were the center for nineteenth-century microscopes. The French makers produced small, strong, reliable instruments which were entirely satisfactory and relatively cheap. Ironically, French research scientists were slow to accept microscopic techniques. In Germany, on the other hand, microscopy was welcomed and carried to a very high level of development. Rudolf Virchow's pioneering work on cells and cellular pathology built squarely on microscopic observations; Robert Koch, the most eminent German bacteriologist of the era, a man whose reputation was matched only by that of Louis Pasteur, was a laboratory worker of genius and an outstanding microscopist. Yet, German lens making was well in arrears of that in France. In 1846, however, Carl Zeiss established a mechanical workshop in Jena to serve university scientists. Matthias Jacob Schleiden, a botanist famous for his studies on plant cells, persuaded Zeiss to concentrate on microscopes, and Ernst Abbe, who joined the firm as a consultant in 1866 at the age of 23, made Zeiss lenses the world's leader. Abbe had been appointed as lecturer in mathematical astronomy at the University of Jena, but he was soon working full-time at optics. He designed the first successful series of immersion lenses in the history of the microscope, developed the concept of numerical aperture which established a universal standard by which to compare lenses, and improved achromatic design by shifting to lithium glass and eventually fluorite for making lenses. By the end of the nineteenth century, Abbe had moved the Zeiss Company, of which he became head, to a position of leadership in the optical industry, and Germany became famous for both microscopy and the production of instruments.

The history of microscopy to the end of the nineteenth century concerned optical microscopes whose basic operating principle involved the behavior of light waves, thus establishing an outer limit on what could be achieved in magnification, resolution, and purity of image. Improvement in body design could make instruments more convenient; refinements in the preparation and mounting of lenses or in the materials used led to more accurate observations; while improved techniques for preparing specimens made many new studies possible. Yet all these improvements ran against the limit on effective magnification imposed by the wave length of light. The first significant change from light microscopy came in the twentieth century, when electrons were found to have a wave motion and the length of the wave proved to be a function of both the mass of the particle to be observed and the speed of the electrons. Wave length decreased as electron speed accelerated, and it was relatively easy under laboratory conditions to achieve speeds which gave wave lengths shorter than those of light. Electrons as charged particles can be refracted by an electrostatic, or magnetic, field which, if of a suitable size and intensity, serves a purpose comparable to that of a glass lens and offers the opportunity to observe much smaller entities than the light microscope. Unfortunately, the electron microscope requires elaborate apparatus, is very bulky and costly, and tends to damage biological material.

While an x-ray microscope appears to be in view, the most recent development in microscopy is the acoustic microscope, which uses vibrational waves comparable in length to the electromagnetic waves in visible light. This focusing element is actually simpler than the lens of an optical microscope. The potential for resolution is limited only by the characteristics of the operating wave length, and there is relatively little aberration. The idea of using acoustics for microscopy was originated by the Soviet scientist S. Y. Sokolov more than 40 years ago, but the technology necessary to implement the idea was not available until the 1960s. Progress on the instrument has been made over the past 10 years at the Bell Laboratories and at the University of California, Los Angeles. During the past five years, work has continued at Stanford University. The acoustic microscope offers many advantages, some inherent in its basic design. In biological studies, for example, sharply defined high-contrast images can be obtained without staining beforehand, and as a result it is possible to do live tissue studies. The potential for development is immense, but while the acoustic microscope offers new opportunities in many areas, it is particularly promising as a means to further understanding of cell composition and structure, an area of the first importance for cancer studies as well as physiology in general.

ADDITIONAL READINGS: S. Bradbury, *The Microscope, Past and Present*, Oxford, 1968; S. Bradbury and G. L. E. Turner, *Historical Aspects of Microscopy*, Cambridge, 1967; Reginald Clay and Thomas Court, *The History of the Microscope Compiled from Original Instruments and Documents*, London, 1932; Alfred N. Disney, Cyril F. Hill, and Wilfred E. Watson Baker, *Origin and Development of the Microscope*, London, 1928; Brian J. Ford, *The Optical Microscope Manual: Past and Present Uses and Techniques*, Newton Abbot, U.K., and New York, 1973; P. W. Hawkes, *Electron Optics and Electron Microscopy*, London, 1972; Calvin F. Quate, "The Acoustic Microscope," *Scientific American* 241 (October 1979): 58–66.

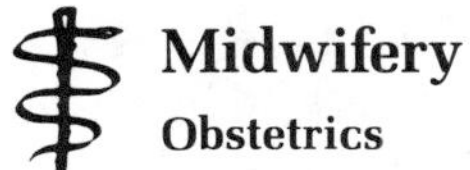

Midwifery

Obstetrics

Midwifery deals with problems of pregnancy, childbirth, and the period immediately after birth. The midwife's function is to aid the woman to deliver her child. Midwives also advise women on sexual matters, the effects of pregnancy, and life after the confinement. Midwifery is as old as birth itself and is mentioned in ancient medical texts from Egypt, Mesopotamia, China, India, and Japan. It is also discussed at length in the Hippocratic writings, as well as by Galen, Celsus, and Soranus of Ephesus. Though male physicians were interested in obstetrical and gynecological problems, midwives in premodern cultures were generally women. The movement of men into this field, the rearrangement of disciplinary boundaries which resulted, and in some countries the displacement of women from a lucrative and respectable calling have all occurred in the modern period. The issues involved in these complex processes include economic competition, sexual rivalry, the advancing demands of scientific medicine, the growth of social regulation over basic health questions, and the development of professionalism.

Under the Roman empire and throughout the European Middle Ages, midwives held a position of particular importance. All matters pertaining to generation fell within their competence. This gave them heavy responsibilities on matters of inheritance and citizenship, the maintenance of private morals, and the preservation of public health. The *Corpus jures civilis* (A.D. 533) of Justinian the Great, which codified centuries of Roman legal practice, devoted an entire section to the responsibilities of midwives and their role in the courts. Physicians, by comparison, received only a few lines. The tradition continued in the Middle Ages, though then it was ecclesiastical authority which required the midwives' testimony. In divorce proceedings, for example, it was necessary to prove that the wife was still a virgin, since impotence was the legal ground for dissolving a marriage. In 1220, Pope Gregory IX codified the common practice when he ordered that women in divorce proceedings were to be examined by midwives. The common proof of virginity and the symbol of the midwives' legal status was the intact hymen. Many contemporary medical authorities, however, denied the hymen's existence, a fact which has been interpreted by historians to indicate the antagonism and jealousy generated by the midwives' monopoly and their favored position in the ecclesiastical courts. Secular legislation followed the same course as that of the church. Midwives' testimony was important in paternity cases, in cases dealing with performance or nonperformance of marital functions, and on identity of children. The midwives continued to be called for such purposes into the nineteenth century.

Both custom and statutory regulations established the responsibilities which the midwives bore. Midwives could be held accountable for anything which happened in the course of the confinement. They were required to call for medical assistance if the birth went wrong, since they were not permitted to go beyond "natural" measures in assisting the birth. They were required to report the results to the authorities. There were severe penalties for concealing a stillbirth or in any way perverting the record. They were given the power to baptize a newborn infant that might not live, and they were absolutely forbidden to interfere with the course of pregnancy and delivery. Abortion was not only a sin but a capital crime.

Such obligations, backed by law and the authority of the Church, gave the midwife status. There were other traditions, however, of more sinister significance. Birth and everything connected with it have a ritual dimension going beyond organized religion to the roots of folk culture. The midwife, whose business was birth, was set apart and made mysterious by the special knowledge she possessed and the powers she was thought to wield. Moreover, since the practice of witchcraft gave a high value to the detritus of birth—cauls, umbilical cords, placentas, and the fetus itself—the midwife, who handled and disposed of these things, was easily implicated in their use for occult purposes. When the witchcraft hysteria washed over early modern Europe, midwives were a natural target. *The Hammer of the Witches,* for example, a classic work on witchcraft published between 1484 and 1486 by two German members of the Inquisition, charged that no one had done more harm to the Catholic faith than midwives who would kill infants in the womb or at birth, having pledged their souls to the Devil. In the sixteenth century, Germany was particularly afflicted with the mania of witchcraft, and midwives were charged, condemned, and executed for diabolical trafficking.

It is difficult to generalize about who the midwives were. Most were women, though occasional male midwives do appear, and in Germany it was found necessary to legislate against shepherds' or cowherds' performance of the midwives' functions. In medieval and early modern Europe, the midwives tended to be married women who had borne children, who were approaching middle age, and who were often widows. Their preparation to assist at births was their own experience in bearing children combined with what they could learn from established midwives and older female relatives. In general, midwives learned and passed on folk wisdom, since by far the largest part of them lacked education or were illiterate. In this respect, they exactly mirrored the society they served. There were, of course, exceptional cases. Nuns, for example, would act as midwives as part of a healing mission, and the lady of a manor house would assist at births as part of her obligation to the people on her husband's lands. There was also an elite. Educated, town-dwelling women, often of middle-class status, found midwifery a respectable way to support themselves or even to develop a career. One of the most famous of the sixteenth-century French midwives, Louise Bourgeois, fell into this category. A woman of middle-class background, she married a surgeon and with his assistance acquired a large fund of information and a huge practice. She served Marie de Medici, wife to Henry IV of France, through six confinements, and she published a number of books detailing her secrets and relating her experiences. She lost the royal favor when a tribunal of physicians suggested she was negligent and therefore culpable when the Duchesse d'Orleans contracted sepsis after delivery and died in 1627. Even so, Louise Bourgeois was eminently successful and influential, and her career showed the sort of opportunities which midwifery held out to women of talent, ambition, and schooling.

The introduction of municipal regulations and the first licensing rules in the fifteenth century added status to the midwives' vocation. In 1452, the city of Regensburg laid down the first comprehensive municipal code governing midwifery.

The code required proofs of competence and character. It also provided municipal funds to aid aged or disabled midwives. By the sixteenth century, municipal codes were common, and in England, the Tudors moved toward establishing a centralized system of licensing for midwives as part of their general policy of royal control over social and economic functions. In addition, the economic growth which marked the sixteenth and seventeenth centuries added to urban wealth and expanded the population capable of paying well for medical services. Urban midwives benefited accordingly, and it became worthwhile to pursue a degree of training beyond what was necessary to meet municipal requirements.

By the seventeenth century, midwifery had developed a distinct social hierarchy, with a few outstanding women serving royal, noble, or wealthy commercial households. Others made satisfying careers among the urban middle classes and even contributed to the literature on midwifery and obstetrics. Prominent among these was the legendary Jane Sharp, whose *Complete Midwife's Companion* (1671) provided a systematic and comprehensive survey of the art. In the eighteenth century, Louise Dargès Lachapelle and Marie Anne Victoria Boivin were notable as administrators, teachers, and writers on midwifery. Away from the affluent court and urban classes, however, midwives tended to be what they had always been. When the British government began registering practicing midwives in the last quarter of the nineteenth century, they discovered that while midwives attended some two-thirds of the births in the kingdom, most were marginally educated, and many were illiterate.

The changes occurring in the fifteenth and sixteenth centuries which regularized the practice of midwifery also redefined its status, and by the nineteenth century women in the most lucrative practices had been replaced with trained physicians and surgeons. Advances in anatomical knowledge and the expansion of formal training in medicine at the university level led to hostility against people who claimed expertise but lacked scientific knowledge. The midwives became the target for attacks based on their ignorance and dangerous incompetence. In 1575, for example, the most influential surgeon of the age, Ambroise Paré, launched a wicked sally against the midwives; his attack was preceded by Eucharius Roesslin's broadside of 1513 and followed by Witkowsky's parody on the "expert opinion" of a midwife published in 1616. Because the women who served as midwives had no access or limited access to formal education even if they had been prepared to take it, there was little that they could do to respond. In this climate, the licensing regulations which improved the status of midwifery could also be used to block midwives from a desirable practice. In the eighteenth century, fear of this abuse prompted the Paris guild of midwives, like the spokeswomen for unregistered midwives in England in the nineteenth century, to resist recognition and registration.

The criticism of midwives for having inferior training masked a conflict among disciplines seeking to provide health services and a bitter competition for the richest kinds of practice. While surgeons wished to expand the functions they could perform and acquire status closer to that of physicians, both physicians and surgeons saw the opportunity to expand their practices at the midwives' expense. Men trained as physicians or surgeons began to perform the midwives' actual functions. Only custom stood in their way, and once men came to be accepted in that role, there was little that the midwives themselves could do. They lacked both social influence and political organization.

Though there were preliminary forays, the male invasion of the midwife's domain occurred in the seventeenth century. Traditionally, a midwife was not permitted to use surgical instruments (a monopoly of the barber-surgeons' guilds) and was required to call in a surgeon if the baby had to be dismembered and extracted or if a cesarean section was required. Physicians provided medical advice on all conditions preceding and following birth. It was the female midwife, however, who actually delivered the baby. In the seventeenth century, male physicians and surgeons began to do that too. Working entirely by feel—with the woman's genitals hidden under a great cloth drape tied at her waist and on the seated physician's neck—he performed the delivery. One factor which aided the male physician was the invention of the obstetrical forceps (q.v.), the first successful tool for easing birth. The female midwife was not permitted to use the forceps.

The change toward surgeons and physicians acting as midwives was notable first in the royal courts. As early as 1628, Peter Chamberlen, a member of the family of Huguenot émigrés who first developed the forceps in secret, attended Queen Henrietta of England when she miscarried. In France, in 1671, Jules Clément attended Mme. de Montespan at the birth of the Duc de Bourgogne, the first child of the dauphin and dauphine. Clément won the title of "accoucheur" for his work.

Courtly women became convinced that a male surgeon-accoucheur was superior to the traditional female midwife, and the conviction spread through aristocratic circles into the wealthy mercantile and professional classes. Surgeons and physicians who specialized in lyings-in found lucrative practices which they supplemented further by offering lessons in obstetrics and midwifery. Some of the most eminent contemporary medical men carried on such practices and in the process popularized the growing body of scientific information available concerning parturition. Among these, the Scot William Smellie was one of the most notable. Trained in Paris, the eighteenth-century capital of medical midwifery, Smellie settled in London in 1739, where he taught his craft in his home. He made a number of improvements in forceps design in 1744 and from 1751 to 1753, and he published an important book, *Midwifery*, in 1752. It was an eminently practical work which contained the first systematic treatise on the safe employment of forceps. Other men who contributed to medical midwifery and obstetrics included William Hunter, Charles White of Manchester, Johann Roederer of Göttingen, and Peter Camper of Amsterdam. White's work was particularly important, for he emphasized asepsis in midwifery a full half century before Ignaz Semmelweis carried out his famous campaign against puerperal fever (q.v.) in Vienna at the end of the 1840s.

By the middle of the nineteenth century, the professional status of physicians and surgeons had been established, together with the idea of the general practitioner. Obstetrics was a recognized discipline, and gynecology was becoming organized. Medicine oversaw the whole spectrum of generative and female problems. On the continent of Europe, particularly in France and Germany, licensing regulations, medical curricula, and medical practice provided specifically for midwives as paramedical professionals who practiced in hospitals and who, though subordinate to licensed physicians and surgeons, claimed a status clearly in advance of nurses. Indeed, German midwives in the later nineteenth century received more and better training in obstetrics than most American doctors. In England, the situation was different. The midwife had no special status, and with medical education largely closed to women, there was little opportunity to acquire the training necessary to qualify for obstetrics. Midwives had not disappeared, however. They represented the main assistance available to the working classes, the urban poor, and the rural population. Though the affluent purchased the help of the medical profession, the majority of English people consulted the traditional midwife.

Social reformers urged professional recognition, registration, and licensing for midwives on the grounds of improving health care and opening a career opportunity for educated middle-class girls and women. Opposition to the proposal came from medical men worried over competition in the valuable obstetrical practices, from established social opinion which considered marriage and a family the only acceptable occupation for a woman, and from women practicing midwifery, who feared that licensing would be used to drive them out of the market. Nevertheless, progress was made, much of it due to the work of Louisa Hubbard. A Midwives' Institute was founded in 1881, and after a hard political fight, Parliament passed the Midwives' Act of 1902, which established educational standards and defined the relationship between midwives and the medical profession. Jealousy and competition continued until public responsibility was established for fees for physicians called in for consultation by midwives. The Midwives' Institute was transformed into the College of Midwives, becoming the Royal College of Midwives in 1947. In the United Kingdom today it is estimated that graduates of the Royal College of Midwives attend some 80 percent of deliveries. In the twentieth century, midwifery in England attained the status it had won earlier on the Continent and in Japan.

Midwifery in the United States followed a course of development similar to that in England, though the modern outcome has been quite different. Midwives played an active part from the colonial period into the early nineteenth century, and some achieved a considerable standing. Notable among these were Anne Hutchinson and Mrs. Fuller, Ruth Barnaby, Margaret Jones, and Elizabeth Phillips. Medical midwifery appeared in the second half of the eighteenth century. The initiator and strong early influence was William Shippen, Jr., who received his college training at the College of New Jersey (now Princeton University) and then studied with his father, Dr. William Shippen. He went to England in 1757, where he worked on anatomy, surgery, and midwifery with John and William Hunter in London. He then moved on to Edinburgh to study under William Cullen and the second Alexander Monro before returning to the colonies. He settled in Philadelphia, where he announced a course of lectures on anatomy, surgery, and some aspects of midwifery in 1763, and he followed this with a private course in midwifery. Shippen became professor of anatomy and surgery at the College of Philadelphia, but he continued to offer private tuition in midwifery. He established a tradition for extramural instruction which continued even after the University of Pennsylvania included midwifery in its regular curriculum.

During the nineteenth century, American medical schools expanded, and, as in England, stress fell on professional development and medical specialties. No attention was paid to midwifery, as obstetricians struggled to obtain recognition for their specialty within medicine. The general level of medical education in the United States after 1865 was very low compared with that in France, Germany, or England, and training in obstetrics was abysmally poor. There was neither licensing, training, nor regulation for midwives, yet the first statistics on attended births showed that in 1910, 50 percent of all births in the United States were attended by midwives. The percentage in urban areas was undoubtedly much higher.

The waves of immigration to the United States from central, southern, and eastern Europe brought the midwife tradition with it, and midwives were the normal resort for birth assistance among the large black minority. Unfortunately, the skilled and educated European midwife usually did not emigrate, and the immigrants who arrived, especially in the later nineteenth century, often came from backward rural areas. The kinds of birth care available to southern blacks and to European immigrants offered little to choose between. Since obstetrics and medicine in general lagged as well, the choices available to American women facing childbirth were not palatable, a fact borne out by the U.S. maternal mortality incidence, which was the third highest among countries which kept such statistics. There was also a very high incidence of neonatal ophthalmia. Maternal mortality owed primarily to puerperal fever, a condition which could be controlled by rigid rules governing cleanliness of attending physicians, nurses, or midwives; neonatal ophthalmia was controllable with silver nitrate applied to the newborn infant's eyes. That both conditions were rampant implicated both midwives and doctors.

The solution which emerged between 1900 and 1930 vastly improved medical and particularly obstetrical training, reformed hospital procedures, produced a significant expansion in hospital facilities, substantially reduced puerperal sepsis and neonatal ophthalmia, and equated proper birth care with medical supervision and hospitalization. The process was aided by the end of mass immigration with World War I, the decline of birthrates in the 1920s, and a progressive consciousness among women who demanded the "best" care for their confinements. This was identified with hospitalization and the doctor. Midwife practice declined sharply. New York City had 1700 midwives who were responsible for 40,000 births in 1919. In 1929, 1200 midwives were attendant on 12,000 births. In that same period, the total number of births also declined by 25 percent. The practice of midwifery was prohibited in some states, while in others the practice continued under close supervision. The midwife disappeared from the most visible areas of American life, and American medicine dealt with birth as a medical problem to be "cured" rather than a natural process to be realized.

During the 1960s and 1970s, there was a revolution in attitudes toward women, sex, and childbearing. This has been particularly notable among the educated urban middle class in the United States. It was evolved with the general concern for women's rights, the women's liberation movement, and the much broader concern for reaffirming nature against manipulative science and exploitive economics. The influence of the movement has been felt in most advanced societies, and it has become an issue for westernized groups in traditional and former colonial societies. When childbearing is the question, the new outlook has reaffirmed a natural approach to birth in which the mother performs a normal function as the central figure in a united family. Both parents participate in prenatal sessions, and birth itself takes place, so far as possible, without medically manipulative techniques, preferably with the father present and helping. Hospitalization is still considered desirable, but there is a growing demand for birth at home as the most natural place for birth to happen. In turn, this has led to a new interest in midwifery and agitation against the laws prohibiting or restricting its practice. Most advanced nations integrated midwifery into the practice of modern medicine by establishing training programs and licensing rules and providing a defined area of practice. The United States did not follow that course but gave precedence to a clearly professional medical approach. Under a variety of pressures, it now appears not only that there is a call for the reestablishment of the midwife but also that there is a reaction against established medical practice as it applies to childbirth and the women's role.

ADDITIONAL READINGS: E. H. Ackerknecht, "Midwives as Experts in Court," *Bulletin of the New York Academy of Medicine* 52 (1976): 1224–1228; Thomas G. Benedik, "The Changing Relationship Between Midwives and Physicians During the Renaissance," *Bulletin of the History of Medicine* 51 (Winter 1977): 550–564; Irving S. Cutter and Henry R. Viets, *A Short History of Midwifery*, Philadelphia and London, 1964; Jane B. Donegan, *Women and Men Midwives: Medicine, Morality, and Misogyny in Early America*, Westport, Conn., 1978; Jean Donnison, *Midwives and Medical Men: A History of Inter-Professional Rivalry and Women's Rights*, London, 1977; Thomas R. Forbes, *The Midwife and the Witch*, New Haven, 1966; Harvey Graham, *Eternal Eve*, London, 1950; Frances E. Kobrin, "The American Midwife Controversy: A Crisis of Professionalism," *Bulletin of the History of Medicine* 40 (July–August 1966): 350–363; Judy B. Litoff, *American Midwives: 1860 to the Present*, Westport, Conn., 1978; Walter Radcliffe, *The Secret Instrument: Birth of the Midwifery Forceps*, London, 1947; Richard W. Wertz and Dorothy C. Wertz, *Lying-in: A History of Child-Birth in America*, New York, 1979.

See also GYNECOLOGY; OBSTETRICAL FORCEPS.

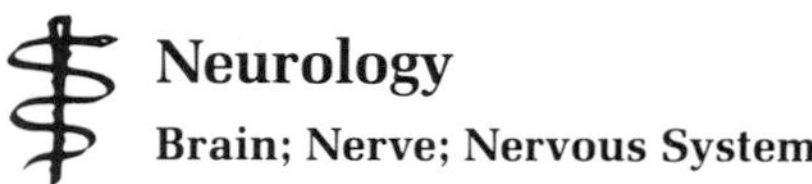

Neurology

Brain; Nerve; Nervous System

Neurology is a modern medical discipline dealing with the organization and functioning of the brain and nervous system. It includes the physiological bases for perception, rational thought, speech, and the control mechanisms which keep the body functioning. To the degree that consciousness, motivation, and emotional disturbances have physiological roots, neurology contributes to such varied disciplines as psychology, psychiatry, language studies, communications theory, and philosophy. The basis for its integrity as a field of knowledge, however, lies in the systematic study of the brain and nervous system.

Historical Background Neurology has developed during the last two centuries, with its most important growth occurring since 1880. Evidence that the brain and nervous system attracted medical attention is, of course, much older. Prehistoric remains show that craniotomies were one of the earliest successful surgical procedures performed, and though archaeologists have searched in vain for trephined skulls among Egyptian remains, other evidence including the Edwin Smith papyrus (ca. 1700 B.C.) shows recognition of brain disorders and the performance of skull repairs. In fact, however, most ancient medical systems gave less attention to the brain than to the heart or viscera. This was true in Egypt, Mesopotamia, and among the Jews, but in Greece there was a division of opinion. The main line of Greek philosophy and science considered the heart the seat of life, but an influential minority, which included such leading medical figures as Alcmaeon of Croton, Hippocrates of Cos, and the Alexandrian anatomists Herophilus and Erasistratus, emphasized the brain. Five hundred years later, when Galen of Pergamum systematized the Greco-Roman medical heritage, he followed the Hippocratic and Alexandrian view on the brain's importance, and it is this tradition which has reached across the Middle Ages to the modern period.

Ancient medicine was religion and philosophy rather than empirical science, and even the Hippocratic writings, which were strong on clinical detail, revealed only a rudimentary understanding of anatomy and physiology. What was known about the brain's anatomy and the nerves resulted from dissections at the Alexandrian school, compounded with Galen's much-later work. Modern authorities have come to appreciate Galen as a comparative anatomist as well as a medical philosopher. His dissections of ox brains, for example, have been replicated following the original texts, and his descriptions have proved to be generally accurate. Since no one approached Galen's command of his subject, and since the postclassical Mediterranean and European worlds were oriented to tradition and authority, Galen's errors and misinterpretations went unchallenged for over 1500 years. One doctrine which Galen promoted which was particularly important for the early history of neurology was that the brain generated a "vital spirit" which was then carried through the hollow nerves to the muscles which it activated. This idea, one of the longest-lived in the classical heritage, was still respectable at the end of the eighteenth century. It has been suggested recently that electrochemical nerve impulses and brain waves provide modern analogues for Galen's vital spirit, though it is also generally believed that Galen's doctrine inhibited the early growth of knowledge on the functioning of the brain and nervous system.

The New Era: 1600 to 1800 Later Roman, Byzantine, and Moslem authorities preserved the Galenist tradition but added nothing to it. In Europe, it was not until the sixteenth century that new material on brain and nerve structures appeared as part of the general reform of scientific studies. The anatomical work of Andreas Vesalius and his school at Padua was particularly notable, though neither the Vesalians nor their seventeenth- and eighteenth-century successors approached the problems of brain and nerve function. Seventeenth- and eighteenth-century workers corrected and improved Vesalius while producing more detailed, specialized works. The well-known English physician and anatomist Thomas Willis published an anatomy of the brain in 1664 which established an improved system for classifying cranial nerves. In 1685 Raymond Vieussens brought out his detailed description of the central and peripheral nervous systems. In the eighteenth century, Jacob Winslow's comprehensive anatomy (1733) and Samuel von Soemmering's description of the brain and classification of the cranial nerves (1778) were the most important of many contemporary works. Winslow's book remained a standard reference for nearly a century, while Soemmering's system supplanted that of Thomas Willis.

The seventeenth and eighteenth centuries also produced an extended and sometimes clamorous philosophical debate over the human soul, mind, and consciousness, the nature of perception, the influence of environment, and the basis for a scientific study of human beings. These problems raised issues which were fundamentally neurological, but there was no methodology appropriate for studying them empirically. Much of the controversy, therefore, was carried out through abstract, a priori reasoning. The French philosopher René Descartes, who formulated an intellectually sophisticated interpretation of the human beings as a "machine," was the most important contributor to the argument, and the late Charles Singer called Descartes's *Treatise of Man* (1662) "the first modern book entirely devoted to the subject of physiology." In his *Treatise,* Descartes speculated on the reception of external stimuli, their processing, and the development of reactions. His general thesis, that external stimuli are received and transformed into various actions, and his approach, which combined an integrative concept with functional discrimination, have proved surprisingly durable. Unfortunately, how those functions were performed or whether they actually were performed could not be demonstrated.

Medical theorists entered the debate as iatromechanists (see Physiology) or vitalists who sought techniques to prove or disprove their hypotheses. They concentrated on actions which they could measure, and they began to make both structural and functional distinctions among nerve, muscle, and connective tissue. They were not prepared to study the brain or nerves as such, but they collected evidence and promoted theories relevant to brain and nerve functions.

There was also a beginning effort to study nerve function directly. The Reverend Stephen Hales, a talented amateur and indefatigable experimenter in the first half of the eighteenth century, became curious about the location of reflex actions. He decapitated a frog and then stimulated its reflexes by pricking the skin. Only destruction of the spinal cord ended response. Anyone who had butchered a chicken knew about convulsive reflexes, but Hales pursued a further point systematically. He did not, however, publish his results, but Robert Whytt, the Edinburgh physician and physiologist, learned of them and repeated the experiments. He published his findings in *An Essay on the Vital and Other Involuntary Motions of Animals* (1751), which identified reflex as "an unconscious sentient principle . . . residing in the brain and spinal cord" and noted that reflexes persisted when only a segment of the spinal cord remained.

The experimental work which Hales and Whytt did pointed the direction which the most fruitful early studies on brain and nerve functions would take. Animal experiments using frogs, fowl, dogs, cats, and later rats and monkeys permitted controlled studies which could be reproduced. One of the earliest and most effective methods was surgical extirpation, in which a segment of cord or brain was removed from a living animal and the results recorded. In 1809, Luigi Rolando used this method to demonstrate that the cerebellum, which controlled involuntary motion, augmented and reinforced the voluntary movements initiated in the cerebrum. Marie Jean Pierre Flourens carried out more extensive experiments which showed what portions of the brain controlled which functions. Working with pigeons, Flourens was able to prove, for example, that removing the entire cerebral hemisphere brought blindness while removal of one hemisphere only blinded the opposite eye. He concluded that "vision depends on the integrity of the cerebral cortex."

While animal experiments were responsible for neurology's early progress, improvements in technology were also important. Luigi Galvani raised the question of nerve impulse as electricity in the second half of the eighteenth century, and Alexander von Humboldt rationalized and confirmed the basic idea in 1811. Studying the behavior of electrical impulses in the nerves, however, required new instrumentation. Though a galvanometer was developed by 1821, it was unable to register the electrical charge in nerve impulses, and it remained to Emil Du Bois-Reymond, a student of Johannes Mueller, to develop an effective instrument. Once the nerve impulses were recorded, Hermann von Helmholtz, another Mueller student best known for the doctrine of conservation of energy, undertook to measure their speed. Surprisingly, the nerve impulse was found to move at a slow 35 to 40 meters per second, raising the further and more important question of how nerve impulses and muscular responses were triggered. These questions required a level of knowledge which did not become available until the twentieth century.

Nineteenth-Century Foundations Experimental physiology played a vital role in mapping areas of brain function in the early nineteenth century. Franz Josef Gall, a brain anatomist and dissector of great skill who founded phrenology (q.v.), began to lecture in 1796 at the University of Vienna on the "faculties" of the brain, how they controlled a person's behavior and character, and their location in specific areas. Gall's approach to functional specialization had no anatomical or physiological foundation, but it was consistent with other, more scientifically rooted thinking. In 1811, for example, Sir Charles Bell rejected the idea of the brain as "a common sensorium," arguing that its anatomical complexity demanded a high degree of functional specialization. In 1822, the French experimental physiologist François Magendie supported and completed Bell's arguments. He reported that the nerves connecting the brain to the body found separate incoming and outgoing pathways, and he refined Bell's location of motor and sensory function. Finally, Flourens's experiments on the cerebellum performed in 1824 showed a progressive deterioration in response the deeper he cut. This reinforced the notion of a specialized topography in the brain.

During the next four decades, studies on functional specialization shifted toward clinical questions, followed by the development of new electrical techniques. John Hughlings Jackson, working with brain-damaged patients at the Hospital at Queen's Square, London, reported evidence in 1864 and again in 1870 showing that the brain had specific motor areas which governed individual movements. Paul Broca, a French surgeon, made postmortem examinations of aphasia cases. He connected the loss of capacity to speak or comprehend speech with damage to specific areas of the cortex, especially on the left side, and he began to map those areas of the brain. Carl Wernicke, a young Breslau professor, continued and refined this work during the 1870s. It was also at this time that Gustav Fritsch and Edward Hitzig of Berlin developed an electrical method for brain mapping. Hitzig worked with war-wounded who had portions of skull destroyed and the brain exposed. He gave mild galvanic shocks to the exposed brain and noted which muscles reponded. The two men expanded their work, using experimental animals to locate those areas of the brain which controlled muscle movement. This technique, which became known as electrical stimulation of the brain (ESB), proved invaluable and was used with especially good effect by the English neurologist Sir David Ferrier, who began systematic mapping work in 1873, and by Charles Beevor and Victor Horsley. The latter provided a detailed guide to brain function in monkeys which was plotted on numbered squares. Ferrier was credited with a nearly final definition for the motor cortex.

Electrical stimulation worked well on impulses going from the brain to the muscles, but sensations received through the nerves and transmitted to the brain proved more difficult to study. Nevertheless, a Liverpool physician, Richard Caton, using an improved reflecting galvanometer, was able to show alterations in brain electricity when external stimuli were received. He also may have identified the electroencephalogram, or brain waves. However, his work, which he reported between 1875 and 1887, was not widely known, and portions of it were rediscovered and published by Adolph Beck, a Polish scientist, who was inspired by the work of Ivan Sechenov, a Russian student of the Mueller school. Sechenov studied electricity in the brain and spinal column and summarized his results in 1890. A tangled controversy over priority in discovering the electroencephalogram ensued, involving Caton, Beck, Fleischl von Marxow (Vienna), and V. Y. Danilevskii (Kharkov). Danilevskii's dissertation (1877) placed him second after Caton and ahead of both Marxow (1883) and Beck (1890).

Interest in the brain and nerve function was becoming intense, and by the end of the nineteenth century, a great deal was known about the nature and direction of nerve impulses, the role of electricity, and functional specialization of the brain and nervous system. The question of what was happening, however, raised the further problem of how it happened. Scientists were becoming interested in the composition of the nervous system and how it was linked together. Progress in these areas depended on developments in microscopy as well as surgical experimental techniques, and it also involved the problem of learned behavior.

Cells and Communication The development of cellular theory in the first half of the nineteenth century owed to improved microscopy and particularly the achromatic lens. Jan Evangelista Purkinje, a Czech working at Breslau, gave the first detailed account of nerve cells in 1837, demonstrating that they had a protoplasm-filled main body which enclosed a central body and a fibrous "tail" extending from the main body. The nature of the tail, or "process," was not clear, though von Helmholtz thought that in many cases nerve fibers were composed of nerve cell processes, a view supported by more detailed work on nerve fibers by the Danish student A. H. Hannover. But the basic problem of the nerve cells' role in electrical action and the related problem of whether or how the nerve cells were connected remained unanswered.

Progress on understanding nerve cell function began to be made when methods for fixing and sectioning tissue for microscopic study improved in the 1850s and 1860s, while Joseph von Gerlach's carmine stain (1854) greatly improved contrast. It was still very difficult to observe nerve connections through the microscope, however, though it had become clear that nerve cells had each one main process and that "nerves" were bundles of these processes. But there agreement stopped. One school of thought adhered to a theory set out by von Gerlach that the nerve cells were connected by a network of fibers. The network served to conduct impulses from cell to cell. This was known as the reticularist theory. Their opponents criticized the argument without having any clear alternative, though in 1887, Wilhelm His, a noted histologist, and Auguste Forel suggested that nerve cells not only were not connected but also had "free endings" in the central nervous system's gray matter. Available microscopy neither confirmed nor denied their views, and the reticular theory gained new support from findings by Camillo Golgi, who had discovered a new stain for central nervous system tissue. The Golgi stain, which required a week to prepare, revealed the nerve cell clearly, showed its process, and for the first time revealed smaller processes (dendrites). But the junctions remained unclear. Golgi, nevertheless, supported a reticularist position which was challenged by an obscure Spanish histologist, Santiago Ramon y Cajal. Cajal became a master microscopist whose ambition was to unravel the problem of the brain cell, what he called "the aristocrat among the structures of the body" containing the promise of "knowing the material course of thought and will." Cajal, who shared a Nobel prize with Golgi in 1906, became the Italian's critic and competitor. He improved the Golgi stain and, working systematically with embryonic tissues of birds and small mammals, began to develop new images and descriptions which he published at his own expense. In 1889, he went to the Berlin conference of the German Anatomical Society, where his demonstrations, delivered in halting, clumsy French, astounded and converted some of Europe's leading biological scientists, including Rudolf von Koelliker.

Cajal's theory became the basis for what Wilhelm Waldeyer named the neuron doctrine. It held that each nerve cell is a self-contained unit with an axon reaching toward but not connected with another cell. Nerve fibers are composed of these processes, but it is the cell which forms the communicating links in nerve tissues. The processes are insulated against each other except for the axon end, which makes contact with the next cell.

Cajal's 1889 presentations supported the views outlined by His and Forel and swung the weight of evidence against the reticularist theory. Cajal continued to build on this early work, improving his stains and contributing to a fuller understanding of nerve pathways and the flow of electrical impulse. But his primary contribution, as Sir Charles Sherrington pointed out, was that he "solved at a stroke the great question of the direction of nerve currents" and swept away the reticularist theory. Cajal held that nerve circuits were valved, and he located the valves "where one nerve cell meets the next one." It was Sherrington who named that valvular connection, later found to be a gap, the synapse.

Reflexes Experimental animal studies continued to be important at the end of the nineteenth and in the early twentieth centuries, especially in the field of reflexes. Here, Sherrington developed surgical techniques of extraordinary delicacy to isolate particular connections in animals' spinal columns. Ultimately he was able to decerebrate dogs and monkeys, creating animals which were virtually machines which functioned reflexively. Sherrington's research showed the integrative function of the nervous system. He demonstrated "spinal shock," the loss of reflex after the spinal cord is cut, following which the reflexive action returns. He showed that the common flexion reflex was intended to remove the limb concerned from danger, while the reflex itself was not limited to those segments of the spine through which pain passes. A sensory stimulus going to one segment of the spinal cord would carry motor stimuli to be discharged from all segments which activate the limb's flexor muscles. The reflex arc, as Sherrington envisioned it, had to involve at least two neurons with a transverse barrier between one cell and the next which permitted the impulse to pass with varying degrees of ease. This connection was what Sherrington named the synapse. Clear pathways would channel responses, and there was a distinct pattern of priority. Like reflexes arriving simultaneously reinforce one another; unlike reflexes pass through successively rather than simultaneously. From the various segments of spinal cord through the brain, coordination is carried out in successively broader and more complex patterns. The end result is singleness of action despite conflicting sensory impulses.

Sherrington's work, which carried from the last decade of the nineteenth century through World War II, provided a broad base of fact and interpretation for spinal reflex. It was among the most important work done in modern neurology. At the same time, in Russia, Ivan Petrovich Pavlov was working on another aspect of the problem, the conditioned reflex. Pavlov was deeply influenced by Ivan Sechenov's work, *Reflexes of the Brain* (1866), which summarized the author's understanding of doctrines he had learned from Du Bois-Reymond, Helmholtz, and Claude Bernard. Sechenov's thesis was that reflexes controlled both conscious and unconscious action, while physical life was shaped by the environment, and particularly by the nervous system's perception of that environment. The environment influences action through the nervous system, which receives and interprets stimuli, and as a result all actions from the most simple and mundane to the most exalted "are mere results of a greater or lesser contraction of definite groups of muscles." With so radical a view, Sechenov ran afoul of the czarist authorities, and he finally resigned from the Academy of Sciences over "a matter of principle." He was denounced, the police claimed he had been fired, students rioted, and Sechenov became a symbol. More important, his experimental and laboratory work contributed directly to the growth of physiology and neurology in Russia.

Pavlov admired Sechenov immensely, and while his own fame grew, he always credited Sechenov with shaping and directing his thought. Pavlov's work on conditioned or learned reflexes brought neurology and psychology firmly together while focusing attention on reflexive function in glandular secretions. Its materialist orientation placed him among the progressive prerevolutionary intelligentsia in Russia and after 1917 made his research ideologically acceptable to the Bolshevik leadership. This point became significant after the middle 1920s, when party political control and Stalinist ideas began seriously to limit intellectual, cultural, and scientific development.

Pavlov's early work dealt with digestion and demonstrated that "reflexes ... automatically controlled the chemistry and motility of the digestive system." This research won him the Nobel prize in 1904, provided him a method for studying reflexes, and set him on the road to his exhaustive exploration of the conditioned reflex. He continued in the course for 25 years, until his death in 1936 at the age of 87. Pavlov distinguished two types of reflex: innate, or inborn, and learned. The former, studied by Sir Charles Sherrington, was located in the spinal cord and brain stem, functioned even when the brain was removed, and was stable. The conditioned reflex had to be learned, was highly unstable—it could be lost through inaction, inhibited by stronger reflexes, or even transformed—and was located in the cerebral cortex. Pavlov concluded that the study of a specific reflex would reveal the way the brain dealt with stimuli and would provide information leading to a general theory of human function.

The particular phenomenon on which Pavlov began was "psychic secretion," the process which produced salivation at the sight, smell, or even thought of food. His digestive studies had established that salivation was reflexive, so it was possible to test reflexive reactions and ultimately to chart and compare them by combining other stimuli with food. In his experiments, the appearance of food would start salivation by the subject; then a bell would ring when food was presented. Ultimately the ringing bell alone would start the salivary flow. The problems of carrying out the research were immense, since all events surrounding a particular stimulus became part of the stimulus and had to be reproduced to get an accurate replication. Pavlov first developed a research cubicle with one compartment for the dog to be tested and a second for the researcher. Outside noises continued to intrude, so in 1910 he designed a special research tower which almost entirely eliminated exterior stimuli. The building was constructed in Leningrad after the revolution.

Pavlov's study of conditioned reflex exemplified an approach to research in which a single operation was repeated over and over again with infinite variations. The results became the basis for a theory of human behavior. To the extent that the work involved physiological analysis, the basic discoveries were made in the digestive studies. His work on conditioned reflexes multiplied stimuli and refined the methods for recording the results. Among his conclusions, two central ones concerned "irradiation and concentration of excitation" and inhibition. In the first, he found that when a stimulus was introduced, not only that stimulus, for example, a ticking metronome, would produce reflexive action, but all stimuli similar to it would have a similar effect, and even dissimilar stimuli received in the early stage could produce the reflex. As the experiment progressed, however, the stimuli which produced the effect grew fewer and more concentrated, until, for example, only ticking in a particular range would release the reflexive action. Similarly, one stimulus could override another. The smell of meat would trigger salivation, while the crack of a whip—which was associated with pain—would stop the salivating. Pain was the stronger stimulus and inhibited the salivary reflex. Ultimately, Pavlov concluded that the process of concentration of stimulus was, in fact, the result of inhibition which blocked all but the strongest stimulus to a particular reflex. By combining these ideas he projected a theory in which the brain, composed of millions of active cells, was every moment receiving countless stimuli from outside and within, to each of which there was a conditioned response. All these stimuli and responses, as he put it, "meet, come together, interact, and they must, finally, become systematized, equilibrated, and form so to speak, a dynamic stereotype." It was in the brain that these countless actions were ordered, and Pavlov envisioned the results in terms of a constantly shifting center of action within the cerebral cortex. "If we could see through the cranium," he wrote, "and if the zone of optimum excitability was luminous, we should see, in a man who was thinking, the supposedly luminous point of optimum excitability perpetually moving about. We would watch it continuously changing in shape and size. It would be surrounded by a zone of more or less dense shadow occupying the remainder of the hemisphere."

Pavlov's contribution to understanding the results of reflex action was enormous. That contribution, however, rested on propositions concerning transfer of information from cell to cell which could not be demonstrated. His general theories proposed patterns of action similar to brain waves, though the electroencephalogram was not discovered until 1924, and it played no part in Pavlov's thinking. His most important contribution ultimately was in the direction of behavioral psychology, and the behavioral school, founded by John D. Watson, has used his approach. Freudian psychologists, however, have been critical, and neurologists quite correctly argue that Pavlov's research went far beyond what could be shown physiologically. Nevertheless, his concept of the conditioned reflex and his myriad experiments place him among the leaders of twentieth-century science.

Institutes and Interdisciplinary Studies Work on the anatomy and physiology of the brain and nervous system advanced steadily through the twentieth century in response to a succession of technological advances and the maturation of interdisciplinary method. The latter produced a growing number of research institutes bringing specialists from many fields together to work on neurological problems. The earliest of these institutes were at Vienna (1882) under Heinrich Obersteiner; Leipzig (1882) under Paul Flechzig; and Zurich (1886) under Constantin von Monakow. Other institutes were founded before World War I in Madrid, Frankfurt-am-Main, St. Petersburg, Philadephia, and Amsterdam. The international Institute for Brain Research was established in 1901 to encourage government support for research and the interdisciplinary method. After 1918, a number of new institutes were created in Berlin, Moscow (where Lenin's brain was subjected to a searching analysis), Montreal, and Bristol. Interdisciplinary research in neurology was slow to develop in the United States. The first institute was founded in 1928 at Northwestern University, in Illinois, and it closed in 1942 when its founder, Stephen Ranson, died. In that year, however, the Chicago Neuropsychiatric Institute of the University of Illinois Medical School was founded. In the postwar period, the U.S. Public Health Service organized neurological studies under the National Institutes of Health and the National Institute of Neurological Diseases and Blindness. The Brain Research Institute of the University of California, Los Angeles, was established in 1961 and exemplifies the interdisciplinary approach. At its opening, 14 university departments and divisions were represented, and the staff comprised 67 leading scientists.

The growth of interdisciplinary studies and research centers for neurology reflected the growing commitment by industrialized societies, even those which had suffered most from the devastations of World War I and its revolutionary aftermath, to basic research in the medical sciences and its economic potential. An interdisciplinary methodology, advanced research technology, and broad financial support for the increasing cost of the necessary instrumentation have combined in the twentieth century to bring the study of the anatomy and physiology of the brain and nervous system to unprecedented heights. In this process, technology played a particularly important role, making possible major achievements in the study of nerve impulses, chemical factors in nerve and brain function, brain mapping, and the discovery and use of electroencephalograms.

Electricity and Chemistry Research on electrical impulse in nerve function stood still after the middle of the nineteenth century until more effective measuring devices were available in the first decade of the twentieth century. In 1909, the Dutch physiologist Willem Einthoven, who had invented the electrocardiagram, brought out a string galvanometer which responded to and recorded electrical activity in the heart. This instrument was, as one authority stated, "the culmination of electro-mechanical measuring instruments in nerve physiology," and Einthoven used it to study electrical activity in the retina and the role of electricity in muscle tonus.

The string galvanometer was limited in range, but developments in electronics leading to John Ambrose Fleming's radio tube (the thermionic vacuum diode) and Lee De Forrest's thermionic vacuum triode made amplification of nerve currents and voltages possible. The amplified currents could be recorded without difficulty by the galvanometer or other device. An instrument using amplification was devised by Alexander Forbes at Harvard in 1920 for "amplifying such action currents in the nervous system as are too small to be recorded satisfactorily with the string galvanometer alone." So rapid was development in this area that in 1931 Edgar D. Adrian remarked: "The amount of amplification which can be obtained nowadays is far greater than we are ever likely to need in physiological work." He also thought that while amplification and recording had brought in direct evidence of a kind which was lacking before, "the field now open is so large that it will be a long time before the method has exhausted its usefulness." Cathode rays, which were discovered in 1858, led to a cathode-ray tube and the invention in the mid-1920s of a cathode-ray oscillograph which gave a graphlike picture of electrical waves. It was this type of instrument which Herbert S. Gasser and Joseph Erlanger of Washington University (St. Louis) developed to study frog and rabbit nerves. The instrument could detect and record minute voltages and currents while measuring quantities and frequencies and reproducing intricate wave forms at high frequencies.

In 1931, electronics gave the neurologists a far more effective microscope than the light microscope, whose potential was exhausted. The electron microscope opened a new world of observation, revealing for the first time many aspects of cell structure previously unseen, including a new perspective on the synapses. Radio Corporation of America (RCA) developed the first commercial electron microscope in 1939 and began selling them in 1940. By the 1960s, over 9000 were in use. In 1965, a three-dimensional scanning electron microscope was used at the University of California to photograph synaptic junctions in three dimensions with a magnification of 20,000 times.

New technology carried neurology to new levels of sophistication and at the same time advanced new problems. Amplifiers gave detailed evidence on nerve impulses as message carriers, but there was also evidence that a chemical as well as an electrical process was at work. Claude Bernard raised the question around 1850, when he discovered that curare blocked certain nerve impulses at the nerve end juncture. It was also noted that nicotine stimulated contraction when applied to a nerve-muscle preparation, but curare stopped it. These facts raised questions about the electrical nature of nerve impulses, but little more was done until 1921, when Otto Loewi, a German physiologist, took up the problem and proved that the heart, when stimulated, secreted a substance directly responsible for certain muscular actions. The identity of the substance was unknown to Loewi, though he believed that the sympathetic nerve secreted adrenaline. His other substance he called *Vagusstoff* after the nerve origin for it. An English physiologist, Henry Dale, had found a substance in 1914 in ergot which was called acetylcholine. Acetylcholine affected muscle response at certain nerve junctions, and when Dale heard of *Vagusstoff*, he thought it might be acetylcholine. In 1929, Dale and H. W. Dudley isolated acetylcholine from the spleens of freshly killed horses, and in 1936 they proved that it was secreted at nerve endings after electric stimulation of motor nerve fibers. Acetylcholine was the chemical agent with which the nerves worked on the muscles. Loewi showed that it was a chemical inhibitor, the enzyme cholinesterase, which interrupted the acetylcholine stimulator and produced the nerve impulse pattern. Dale and Loewi shared a Nobel prize for physiology or medicine in 1936 for their work on the chemical activator.

Chemicals and Brain Waves Other chemical agents were found at work in the nervous system. Walter Bradford Cannon identified the stimulative role of adrenaline (epinephrine), and this led to a classification of nerves according to their transmitter substances. Cholinergic nerves secreted acetylcholine, and adrenergic nerves secreted adrenaline. But this work applied only to the peripheral nervous system. There was indirect evidence of chemical action in the central nervous system, but experimentation was difficult. Research at Oxford by Edith Bülbring and J. H. Burn in 1941 indicated the presence of acetylcholine, and this was confirmed by J. H. Mitchell of Cambridge in 1960. There was also evidence of monamines in the central system, including noradrenaline, dopamine, and serotonin (5-hydroxytryptamine). Other transmitters have been suspected though not definitively placed.

The presence of chemical agents in the brain raised the possibility of using drugs to combat mental conditions and to alter behavior. In 1943, a Swiss biochemist, Albert Hoffmann, accidentally ingested lysergic acid diethylamide (LSD). He suffered severe hallucinations and loss of emotional control and had to be tranquilized. He repeated the accident purposely and suffered the same symptoms. LSD was found to inhibit the action of serotonin, but subsequent work showed that it also blocked noradrenaline and adrenaline. By 1967, it was believed that LSD could block any of six mechanisms and that its action was both unpredictable and dangerous. Similar studies were done on reserpine, benzedrine (amphetamine), and tranquilizers such as chlorpromazine. All acted to inhibit functioning of transmitters.

It was possible to do relatively little with central nervous system failures unless they were susceptible to surgery before the discovery of the chemical aspect of brain function. Once the transmitter-inhibitor pattern was known, however, work on correcting or controlling basic problems in brain function developed. The action of botulism and tetanus on the nervous system was explained. In the former, the action of botulism toxin prevented the release of acetylcholine, which meant the muscles went flaccid and the victim was unable to move. Tetanus toxin affects an unknown transmitter necessary to inhibit contraction, and the muscles lock into spastic paralysis. Nothing can be done with these conditions except to use antitoxins. Parkinson's disease, a degenerative nervous condition identified in the nineteenth century, was considered incurable until it was associated with chemical transmission in the nerve system. It is now thought that normal movement depends on the balance between two pathways of motor control nerves, one cholinergic, the other adrenergic. The disease occurs when there is a reduction on the adrenergic side, and some relief is given by reducing the cholinergic activity by drugs or surgery. In the late 1960s, however, it was found that the adrenergic side could be stimulated with a drug called L-dopa (levodihydroxyphenylalanine), which raises the dopamine level in the central nervous system and acts on the precursor of noradrenaline, presumed to be the transmitter substance. L-dopa was reported to be highly effective in 1969 with postencephalitic patients at Beth Abraham Hospital in the Bronx, New York. Ninety percent of those afflicted with Parkinson's disease responded to the treatment. Thirty percent had a spectacular recovery, and 30 percent made a modest improvement. The remainder either were refractory or were affected adversely. Chemical substances have been similarly effective in controlling or managing epilepsy (q.v.)

Understanding chemical action in the brain and nervous system has created a useful tool for further research, particularly in understanding the neurophysiological bases of behavior. Chemical exploration of the brain, which began systematically in 1953 with studies in Sweden by Bengt Andersson, has clearly established that specific chemicals will selectively stimulate certain brain cells; therefore "drive-oriented behavior," as a recent scientist wrote, "can be triggered and sustained by chemical means." This fact, important as it is for research and therapy, has also led to developing chemical nerve gases of extraordinary toxicity which inhibit the enzyme cholinesterase and whose action is very swift. Such compounds pose profound dangers in peace as well as war since storage is a problem. Sarin, for example, the nerve gas which created controversy at the opening of the 1970s, can eat through most metals and is contained only by silver.

The electroencephalogram (EEG), or brain wave, offers another important technique for research, diagnosis, and treatment of neural problems. Discovered by Johannes Berger in 1924, though not publicized until 1929, brain waves are traceable impulses emanating from the cerebral cortex which reflect states of consciousness, external stimuli, and mental operations. The first waves identified were called alpha and beta, and subsequent discoveries have received other Greek alphabetical designations. Initially, Berger's discovery was ignored, but in 1934 Edgar Adrian and B. H. C. Matthews of the physiological laboratory of Cambridge University affirmed the importance of the waves, though differing in interpreting alpha waves. Subsequently the waves were used for diagnosis in epilepsy cases, and during World War II, they were found to be valuable in working with a variety of brain injuries. As instrumentation improved, the waves could be used to distinguish between severely retarded and normal subjects, establishing a basis for further diagnostic work. It was found that newborn infants developed no EEG for 6 to 13 days, indicating that at birth the brain is still incomplete. Work with brain waves has led into the study of brain function, research on sleep, diagnosis of psychiatric disorders, and different approaches to tension problems, persistent or migraine headache, and high blood pressure. The potential in brain wave research is very large.

Conclusion Modern neurology faces many unanswered questions, including a definitive appreciation of memory. Its accomplishments in just over a century, however, are enormous. Though not all the particulars are in place, there is now a well-defined image of how the brain and nervous system work, and this has led in turn to more effective measures for identifying and managing or treating dysfunction. Whether neurology holds the final answer to emotional disturbance and neurosis is still a matter for debate. But the results of chemical blockage on behavior, the dispersal of functions throughout the system, the definition of consciousness in terms of brain waves, and the complex integrative processes which coordinate the system's functioning all underscore the contemporary importance of neurology for understanding and treating a wide range of mental, emotional, and nervous problems.

ADDITIONAL READINGS: Edwin Clarke and C. D. O'Malley, *The Human Brain and Spinal Cord*, Berkeley and Los Angeles, 1968; Alfred Meyer, *Historical Aspects of Cerebral Anatomy*, London, New York, and Toronto, 1971; F. N. L. Poynter (ed.), *The History and Philosophy of Knowledge of the Brain and Its Functions*, Oxford, 1958; Leonard A. Stevens, *Explorers of the Brain*, London and Sydney, 1973; J. Z. Young, *Programs of the Brain*, Oxford, 1978.

See also ANATOMY; EPILEPSY; PHYSIOLOGY; PSYCHIATRY.

New World Medicine

Pre-Columbian civilization in North and South America ranged from seminomadic tribes in the northern forests and plains to settled cliff dwellers with an established agriculture in the North American southwest to the Mayans, Aztecs, and Incas in Mexico and Peru and their vast urban complexes. Created by migrations of a considerable antiquity, these cultures flourished between 1000 B.C. and A.D. 1500. Even the most developed of them, however, have left only scattered written sources, and most of what is known comes from archaeological and anthropological studies combined with observations made by Europeans in the sixteenth and early seventeenth centuries. Where medicine is concerned, these data are very rich, and while it is difficult to identify such supporting structures as hospitals or training institutes, a great deal is known about disease and therapeutic practices.

Beliefs and Practices In common with all other known ancient cultures, American Indian civilizations combined medicine and religion. Depending on the particular culture, priests, shamans, medicine men, or sorcerers were entrusted with the rituals which served as the basis for diagnosis and cure. Supernatural agencies were believed to cause illness, often as a punishment for human error or misbehavior, and Indian cultures in Mexico, the Yucatán, and Peru identified specific diseases with particular deities. North American Indians endowed all nature with spirits, some highly malevolent, and also connected disease with witchcraft and enchantment, the restless and vengeful spirits of dead animals, wandering souls, demons, and deities. The wind was considered particularly dangerous, a phenomenon which was virtually universal in ancient cultures, as was the importance attached to breath or "internal" air.

Health practices in pre-Columbian cultures stressed hygiene, and the societies were free from many Eurasian diseases such as plague, cholera, smallpox, chicken pox, measles, scarlet fever, diphtheria, malaria, and typhoid. The absence of such diseases also meant the absence of immunities, and when European infectious diseases arrived they devastated the Indian cultures. Cancer and skin diseases were rare, but there is strong evidence of syphilis (q.v.) and a probability that yellow fever (q.v.) was also indigenous. Paleopathologists have identified deficiency diseases, arthritis, and endemic goiter, while North American Indians, particularly in the Great Lakes region, were especially susceptible to pneumonia and pleurisy. However, the perpetual problem of maintaining an adequate food supply was probably the most important single factor which affected Indian health before the European invasions.

Elements of rational medical treatment showed through the religious rituals. Amerindian medicine was naturalistic, emphasizing herbals, diet, emetics, diuretics, and bathing, especially steam baths. The *materia medica* was extensive. Some 1200 medicinal herbs have been identified as available to Aztec and other Mexican practitioners, and a modern physician, Dr. Nicolas Monardes, experimented with several hundred Mexican herbals to demonstrate effect. He concluded that the pharmacopeia was rich in remedies which contained active elements. Hallucinogens such as peyote and mescaline served ritual functions, and sarsaparilla was used as a diuretic. There were curatives for skin eruptions and chlorines for sexual stimulation, and tobacco was used as a specific against headache or stupor. Rubber was used in various ways, but especially for a kind of syringe and to act as a blistering agent for treating rheumatism and pleurisy. Cacao (cocoa) was the Aztecs' most important tonic and medicinal beverage. It was powdered and boiled in water with honey, vanilla, and pepper. This product went to Europe with Cortés in 1529, where it became a favorite drink, a specific for "wasting diseases," and a stimulant, and it eventually appeared in cocoa butter suppositories.

The Incas of Peru similarly used a wide range of natural products, including mineral substances, and they were famed among the Spanish for the quality of their medicine. Two products among hundreds attracted European attention: cinchona, the so-called Peruvian bark, which was effective against fevers, won an enormous reputation in Europe, and as quinine (q.v.) it became a staple for the treatment of tropical fevers. Similarly, coca leaves, which grew only in the Peruvian valleys, reached Europe in the nineteenth century as cocaine, serving as an anesthetic and narcotic. Peruvian Indians chewed coca leaves to improve circulation, stimulate breathing, increase muscular energy, speed the metabolism, and deaden hunger. The coca leaf helped to make physical labor at high altitudes possible, though the Indians probably consumed no more than a leaf a day. Since the leaf was known to be addictive, intoxicating, and deadly when misused, it was strictly rationed, and only priests had unrestricted access to the supply.

The highly developed Inca state appointed herb collectors, and itinerant apothecaries went throughout the country with their stocks of mineral medicines and dried herbs. Among these, there was a wide variety of purges, abortifacients, and diarrhea remedies including the bark of *raluntici*, which contained tannic acid, and argillaceous earth, which had silicon, aluminum, and magnesium in it. Other substances included unripe maize tassels for a diuretic, for bladder ailments, and for dropsy; petter tree resin for intestinal parasites; martella leaves, which had an antiseptic effect, for inflamed eyes; papaya juice for eczema; and a salve of lard and sulfur to apply to scabies, a remedy still considered effective. As in Egypt, copper sulfate was used for eye infections, while sulfide of arsenic, which the Incas called *hampiyoe hampei*, or death medicine, was used in restricted doses for verrucae and leishmaniasis. On balance, though information is less accessible, Peruvian Inca culture appears to have been the most highly developed medicinally of the Amerindian civilizations.

North American Indian tribes had a similar though less extensive *materia medica*. They used sassafras, holly, sunflower seeds, and infusions of flaxseed or inhaled the smoke from burning twigs when treating chest conditions. Steam houses were the primary means for treating rheumatism, arthritis, and neuritis, while the Dakotas and Ponchas used pasqueflowers to form a blister as a counterirritant treatment. Other treatments for rheumatism and arthritis included hot sheep dung or ground cactus (balm of Gilead) poultices, while hallucinogens included decoctions of foxbain, mushrooms, peyote beans, and jimsonweed.

Mayan records indicate anatomical knowledge comparable to that of Europe before Vesalius, but none of the Amerindian cultures developed surgery to any degree. There are Mochias (west Mexican pre-Aztec) pottery figures which suggest amputated legs and feet, and mummies have been found with amputated feet and wooden cylinders fitted over the stump as prosthetic devices. There are no written records, however, nor is there any direct evidence on how they handled bleeding, pain, shock, or sepsis. North American Indians showed skill in wound management, using healing herbs and cobwebs in wounds and closing open wounds with the jaws of leaf-cutter ants. They also splinted fractures, though often without attempting to set the break, and it has been asserted that North American Indians used a version of the tourniquet to control bleeding.

Skull trephining was common among the Indians of Peru and Mexico. The purpose is not clear, but so many trephined skulls have been found that it has been estimated that 2.5 percent of the Peruvian population underwent the operation. On the other hand, there is no evidence of trephining north of Mexico. The success rate was very high, judging from the amount of bone growth on the edges of the wounds, and the instruments used were made from flint, quartz, obsidian, bronze, and copper. Aztec wound healers splinted broken bones and inserted stone-pine splinters into bones which did not heal. Tonsillectomies were performed with obsidian knives, and pulverized obsidian seems to have been used to counteract suppuration. Boils or other eruptions were opened to drain. Even so, surgery among the Amerindians remained a means to repair damage and appears to have developed very little beyond that point.

Though wound healers, fracture specialists, and herb gatherers appear in the record, it seems that the clear separation between priests and physicians was only beginning to take place at the time of the Spanish conquest. Spanish accounts praised Inca physicians and the quality of their cures, and there was a class of "possessors of medicines" and surgeons recognized as separate from the priest class. There are also hints that some Inca medical functions were under state control. Though available evidence on the culture of Inca, Aztec, and Mayan medicine is scattered and incomplete, what exists suggests a level of development comparable with that of Eurasian cultures before the modern period, with the closest parallels being Egypt and Mesopotamia. The North American Indians, on the other hand, compare most closely in medical culture with the Eurasian steppe peoples.

ADDITIONAL READINGS: A. W. Crosby, *The Columbian Exchange: Biological and Culture Consequences of 1492*, Westport, Conn., 1972; Benjamin Lee Gordon, *Medicine Throughout Antiquity*, Philadelphia, 1949; Francisco Guerra, "Maya Medicine," *Medical History* 8 (January 1964): 31–43; Jürgen Thorwald, *Science and Secrets of Early Medicine*, Richard and Clara Winston (trans.) London, 1962; V. J. Vogel, *American Indian Medicine*, Norman, Okla., 1970; Abner I. Weisman, *Medicine Before Columbus as Told in Pre-Columbian Medical Art*, New York, 1979; Abner I. Weisman and Celia Behrman, *These Were Their Gods: The 'Graven Images' of the New World as Medical Therapy Before Columbus*, New York, 1979.

Nursing

Professional nursing, one of the most critical support functions in modern medicine, developed in response to complex diagnostic and therapeutic techniques, the exponential growth of health facilities, the constantly enlarging pool of persons claiming medical care, and the multiplication of health services through schools, industry, and governmental institutions. The modern nurse is also the product of major developments in society. Nursing has been basically (though not exclusively) a woman's vocation, and its establishment as a recognized profession was an important victory in women's drive for independence. More broadly, the emergence of the professional nurse was part of the modernizing process which created increasingly specialized social structures to perform specifically defined tasks. One distinguishing feature of this process was the establishment of objective criteria for determining qualifications. In the case of nursing, these criteria were defined in terms of educational standards and were institutionalized in registry or licensing regulations.

Historically, attendance on the sick was a household chore normally performed by women or slaves, but there is some evidence that trained personnel were used when developed medical traditions existed. The Indian *Samhitas*, which were compiled early in the first millennium A.D. from a much older tradition, spoke of attendants (nurses) who had the ability to prepare medicines and administer them, to care for the patients' physical needs, and to carry out a physician's instructions without question. The ideal attendant was cool, competent, loyal, and knowledgeable. Similarly, the Hippocratic writings from the fifth and fourth centuries B.C. noted the importance of trained attendants in difficult cases. These attendants were most likely students preparing to be physicians. The Roman *valetudinaria* for soldiers, slaves, and gladiators probably had trained slaves for attendants. Evidence concerning attendants in the older Egyptian and Mesopotamian cultures is obscure or nonexistent.

During the first millennium A.D., trained attendants were used in the hospitals of the eastern Roman (Byzantine) empire and throughout Islam. That tradition was largely lost, however, in the Latin west. Both Christianity and Islam recognized a moral obligation to care for the sick, but in the Christian world that responsibility was given special force by the emphasis on love, humble service, and the abnegation of self. Caring for the sick was a Christian duty, "a sacred vocation based upon Christ's actual command," and a major component in the Christian ideology of service. The wealthy Roman matron Fabiola, who turned her home into a hospital in which she personally nursed the needy sick, exemplified the Christian commitment to selfless service that remains a fundamental element in nursing ideology. Nor was Fabiola an isolated case. There was a group of such wealthy women in early-fifth-century Rome known as the Circle of St. Jerome which nursed the needy; in the east, this role fell to the deaconesses (from the Greek *diakonein,* "to minister"), a group formally recognized in the church hierarchy. Deaconesses also appeared briefly in the west after the eighth century.

Religious orders of one kind or another accepted responsibility for those who needed help. They provided nursing in the general sense of caring for physical needs, but there was little preparation or medical content in their work. This remained true until the nineteenth century. Advances in science, education, and medicine accomplished over the period from the thirteenth to the nineteenth century had no discernible effect on nursing. To the extent that the sick, the poor, the injured, or the insane had care, it was provided by religious orders as acts of Christian charity. There were many such organizations. All monastic orders were charged with caring for God's poor, which included the sick, and each monastery or convent had an *infirmarius* or *infirmaria* who oversaw the infirmary and, with the help of assistants from the religious community, ministered to the sick. During the Crusades (1096–1204), the Knights of St. John of Jerusalem (later called the Knights of Malta), the Teutonic Knights, the Knights Templar, and the Knights of St. Lazarus were active in nursing as well as hospital building and administration. The last-named was organized to care for lepers. In the thirteenth century, orders began to appear which were predominantly or exclusively for the care of the sick. The most important of these included the Order of the Holy Ghost, organized by Guy de Montpellier; the Augustinian Sisters, the oldest of the purely nursing orders; the Order of St. John of God, founded in the sixteenth century; and the Sisters of Charity, founded in the seventeenth century by St. Vincent de Paul.

In England, the Protestant Reformation destroyed monastic medicine and the nursing orders in the sixteenth century, leaving a large gap in care facilities which was not effectively repaired until the middle of the nineteenth century. Hospitals became places to deposit social problems of all kinds, the sick poor included. They were desperately overcrowded and a social scandal. Even nursing in the medieval sense was hardly possible, and what was done fell into the hands of illiterate, often dissolute women from the indigent classes. The English voluntary hospitals founded early in the eighteenth century offered some improvement, though not in nursing. The situation in European hospitals was marginally better, thanks to the continued presence of the nursing orders. Their numbers, however, were inadequate, given the rate of hospital growth. The authorities supplemented their efforts by encouraging the healthiest patients to aid the sick, by recruiting from the prisons, and by hiring the cheapest possible hand laborers.

Early interest in nursing reform in the second half of the eighteenth century was part of the hospital and prison reform movement, which dealt primarily with the conditions in which patients and prisoners were kept. In nursing, reform meant supplying humane services where none existed before while improving the quality of the service offered. The form these efforts took was to organize new nursing orders. It was still believed that holy orders were necessary to discipline as well as to protect women working in hospitals and to consecrate work which otherwise would be debasing. Among the new orders organized between 1800 and 1850, the Sisters of Mercy and the Irish Sisters of Charity, founded by Catherine McAuley in the period 1827–1831 and Mary Aikenhead (Sister Mary Augustin) between 1812 and 1833, were particularly influential. There were several Church of England nursing orders as well, and the most important for reform of hospital nursing, St. John's House, founded in 1848, was also the first.

The Deaconess Institute, established in 1836 by Theodore Fliedner, the pastor of Kaiserswerth near Düsseldorf, marked a significant advance. Pastor Fliedner was interested in prison reform and social welfare, and his institute was intended to train women who could "ameliorate the condition of the sick poor." Nursing was only one aspect of his program. Nevertheless, in 1838 the institute took over the Elberfeld city hospital, and by 1842 it had a 200-bed facility in operation at Kaiserswerth. The deaconesses were required to be able to read, write, and do arithmetic. They were also expected to pass the state's pharmacy examination.

The first clear break with the order, or "motherhouse," concept came in 1859, when the countess Agénor de Gasparin founded La Source, a special nursing school, near Lausanne in Switzerland. This school, which still exists, emphasized training for a vocation. The countess considered the organized discipline of religious orders incompatible with the confronting and solving of problems by a free individual on the basis of knowledge and a trained mind. She also believed that women who did nursing had been educated for a particular job and should be salaried. Religious vows were an unnecessary encumbrance.

In England, the Crimean War (1854–1856) awoke public opinion to the need for a new approach to nursing and produced an authentic heroine in Florence Nightingale. Miss Nightingale, who came from a prosperous, cultured, middle-class background, found a focus in nursing for her great need to serve. Educated well beyond the level of her class and sex, she studied nursing abroad, staying briefly at Kaiserswerth (1851), and again in Paris with the Sisters of Mercy (1853). Her strong convictions about nursing were well-known among the influential people who formed her social circle, and when W. H. Russell's shocking dispatches from the Crimea revealed that Britain's sick and wounded "lacked the commonest appliances of a workhouse sickward," it was natural for the secretary of state at war, Sidney Herbert, to ask his friend Florence Nightingale to put matters right. Miss Nightingale's offer to do just that crossed the secretary's request.

Florence Nightingale's extraordinary success during the Crimean War led to a successful public subscription to establish a nurses' training program. Arrangements for ward experience and medical lectures were made with St. Thomas' Hospital in London, and the first of thousands of Nightingale nurses began the course in 1860. The Nightingale system stressed firm discipline, a corporate identity, and dedication to nursing as a vocation. Florence Nightingale recruited her "probationers" from girls of good character with lower-middle-class artisan or rural background. Well-to-do middle-class women were accepted as paying lady-pupils. The probationers received a stipend during training and generally stayed one year. Lady-pupils, who were usually better-educated and were prepared to take administrative or teaching duties, stayed in training for two years. The Nightingale schools became a source for teachers and administrators who carried the system throughout Britain and the empire, particularly Canada, Australia, and New Zealand. The Nightingale school was also influential in the United States, though in modified form.

Nightingale schools were the culmination of the first period of nursing reform and the beginning of nursing's modern development. During the next 40 years, nurses' training institutes sprang up throughout Europe and North America and began to develop in Europe's colonies as well. The Red Cross contributed to this growth. In 1859, a Swiss banker, Jean Henri Dunant, witnessed the battle of Solferino (June 24, 1859) between Austria and the Franco-Italian forces of Emperor Napoleon III. Dunant's horror at the absence of medical support and the terrible condition of the wounded led him to found the International Red Cross in 1864. This organization became a powerful influence in developing nurses' training, especially in the less-advanced areas of Europe and in the nonwestern world.

In Germany, religious orders dominated nursing, and the professional element developed slowly. In 1907, there were 26,000 Roman Catholic sisters and 12,000 deaconesses in a total nurse population of about 75,000. Only 3000 were members of the professional German Nurses' Association. Twenty-five years later the situation was virtually unchanged. For every lay nurse, Red Cross included, there were three Protestant nursing sisters and five Roman Catholic sisters. France was more secular. After the Franco-Prussian War (1870–1871), programs to improve nursing were introduced. Courses began at the Salpêtrière and Bicêtre hospitals in 1878, and by 1906 there were several private nursing schools with attached paying hospitals. The Nightingale system was introduced at Bordeaux in 1901, and a two-year program was established at Salpêtrière. Following World War I, the government created a state nursing diploma (1922), and 10 years later lay nurses outnumbered the nursing sisters by nearly two to one (16,500 to 8500). There were 80 recognized nursing schools, of which just 25 were in the hands of nursing orders. Of the 55 secular schools, 30 belonged to the Red Cross.

Nursing in the United States developed after the Civil War (1861–1865). When the war broke out, women in both the north and the south formed committees to provide relief and support for the medical services. A New York City group led by Dr. Elizabeth Blackwell, a former associate of Florence Nightingale, and Louisa Lee Schuyler met in Cooper Union on April 26, 1861, to form a Ladies' (later Women's) Central Relief Committee. Louisa Lee Schuyler was elected president. The purposes of the organization were to identify the army's nursing needs, establish relations with the military medical staff and serve as its auxiliary, establish a central stores depot, and create "a bureau for the examination and registration of nurses." The association joined with other groups to petition President Lincoln for a central commission to oversee medical support for the army. On June 9, 1861, their appeal was answered by the creation of the National Sanitary Commission. Louisa Lee Schuyler served with the commission, and the Women's Central Association became an adjunct to the commission with responsibility for coordinating the work of similar relief organizations throughout the country. One important function was to provide nursing care. Some of the societies were able to offer training, though most of the nursing done by the more than 2000 volunteers who served was admittedly amateur.

The Women's Central Relief Association comprised a nucleus of dedicated women whose influence on nursing continued into the postwar period and helped promote hospital and nursing reform. The first schools of nursing in the United States were founded at New York's Bellevue Hospital (1872) and in New Haven and Boston (1873). These schools followed the Nightingale system in most particulars. By 1900, there were 433 schools of nursing in the United States, and 137 of them offered a three-year training program. In 1899, Teachers College, Columbia University, began to offer college-level courses for nurses, and in 1910, the University of Minnesota set up a five-year program leading to a bachelor's degree in nursing as well as a nursing diploma. By 1916, there were 5 such university programs in existence, a number which increased to 175 fifty years later. By then, 1125 American programs were graduating some 32,000 nurses per year. Though it began slowly, nursing in the United States matured and expanded very rapidly.

The development of nursing in Russia differed in important respects from that in other European countries and the United States. Before the middle of the nineteenth century, religious orders such as the Sisters of Mercy provided some nursing, but many medical functions, nursing included, were performed by paraprofessionals called feldshers who in many rural areas served also as physicians. In 1864, the creation of the zemstvo, or county council system, enlarged local responsibility for medicine and public health, and in 1867, the Red Cross was organized in Russia. Women from the educated classes became volunteer Red Cross nurses, a two-year (later three-year) training program was begun, and the government permitted military hospitals to be used for that purpose. By 1897, four hospitals were training nurses, and nearly 3000 had completed the course. When the revolution came in 1917, there were 64 training hospitals and 17,000 nurses in training.

In the years immediately after the revolution, nursing had a low priority, but as other health institutions expanded, nurses became essential. There was substantial resistance to their introduction from both physicians and the public. In 1927, a program was outlined, and a curriculum was introduced in 1928. Within 10 years, there were 95,000 students in the program. In 1965, the Soviet Union counted 684,100 nurses actively employed. In the Russian case, nursing emerged as part of a consciously created health program sponsored by the government which took shape between 1928 and 1938 and was fully in place by the outbreak of World War II.

Professional standing for nurses was slow to come, though professional organizations began to appear in the later nineteenth century. The British Nurses' Association, founded in 1887 by the former matron of St. Bartholomew's, Mrs. Bedford Fenwick, was the first. It gained 1000 members in its first year, and in 1892 it was chartered as the Royal British Nurses' Association. By 1930, similar bodies existed in 35 countries. The first national nurses' association in the United States, the Nurses' Associated Alumnae of the United States and Canada, was organized in 1896. It became the American Nurses' Association in 1901. In many countries, the Red Cross served as the national nurses' society, and in the United States the Red Cross acted as the registry for nurses for the Army and Navy.

A professional identity led to further efforts by nurses to define and protect their status through high entrance requirements, prescribed curricula, and licensing regulations. Physicians' opposition and rivalries within the nursing profession drove the early proponents of educational requirements and licensing to take extreme positions. Nursing in the second half of the nineteenth century was still more domestic than medical science, but women who attended the early nursing schools had a vested interest in preserving their positions by setting entry and educational requirements as high as possible. When successful, their efforts created nursing shortages and tended to cut off recruitment among lower-class women who lacked educational advantages.

The licensing battle in England went on for nearly 40 years. A Royal College of Nursing was established in 1916 to provide statutory recognition for trained nurses. Its authority, however, was limited, and a General Nursing Council was formed in 1919 with powers to approve hospital schools, formulate a recommended syllabus, and conduct examinations. A nurses' registry was finally established in 1922 and 1923 which guaranteed a minimum level of training for all nurses. In the United States, national nursing organizations and the state governments worked jointly toward defining standards and educational requirements. New York State passed the first registry law in 1938, and it was put into effect on July 1, 1940. This law established the difference between the registered nurse, who had fulfilled state requirements for a licensed professional nurse, and the practical nurse, who met less stringent training requirements.

For many modern women, nursing has fulfilled the promise of an independent professional career. Great Britain by 1965 had nearly 100,000 nurses in service, while in the United States there were 500,000 professional nurses active, with the same number on the inactive lists. There were 250,000 practical nurses and 400,000 nurses' aides, raising the total nursing contingent above 1.5 million. Yet the need for nurses grows inexorably, and the World Health Organization has made the provision of adequate nursing in all countries one of its goals. Despite the economic development of the field, the realization of this goal remains remote. Nursing has achieved its fullest development in the most advanced, affluent societies. In this respect, as in its professionalization and specialization, nursing shows its integral connection with modern scientific medicine and the societies it serves.

ADDITIONAL READINGS: Brian Abel-Smith, *A History of the Nursing Profession*, New York, 1960; Vern Bullough and Bonnie Bullogh, *The Care of the Sick: The Emergence of Modern Nursing*, New York, 1978; Celia Davies, *Re-Writing Nursing History*, London, 1980; M. A. Nutting and L. L. Dock, *A History of Nursing*, 4 vols., New York, 1907, 1912; M. M. Roberts, *American Nursing: A History and Interpretation*, New York, 1954; L. R. Seymer, *A General History of Nursing*, London, 1932; F. B. Smith, *Florence Nightingale: Reputation and Power*, London, 1982; C. Woodham-Smith, *Florence Nightingale*, New York, 1951.

See also HOSPITAL; MEDICAL PROFESSION.

Nutrition

The science of nutrition is a twentieth-century discipline treating the composition of foods, the elements required by living bodies to remain healthy, to grow, and to reproduce, the processes by which food products are transformed into useful elements within an organism, and the pathological conditions which result from dietary deficiencies. The chemistry and physiology essential to nutritional science evolved during the eighteenth and nineteenth centuries. "Nutrition" did not appear as an English word until the mid-fifteenth century and was used infrequently until the second half of the nineteenth century. Before 1850, the word "diet" was more commonly used. The interest in foods, diet, and health, however, is very old, and early attempts to regularize dietary concepts belong as much to the history of religion and law as they do to medicine and science.

Diet and Tradition Human beings have lived most of their existence on earth without any codified nutritional system. Omnivorous creatures, humans apparently have eaten what appealed to them, leaving it to experience to show which foods were safe, nutritive, and satisfying. The evidence of expanding population growth throughout history and the development of increasingly complex and sophisticated civilizations show that human food selection has maintained the minima necessary for reproduction and growth. Since it also appears that no new food crops or animals have been domesticated in the historic period, it follows that the means to meet food requirements have been present from the earliest times.

Though human foods have not changed, the means for producing them have undergone radical alterations. Originally hunters and gatherers, humans began to domesticate necessary plants and animals over 10,000 years ago, thus establishing more regular and predictable food sources. At the same time, as more settled creatures, they codified rules governing planting, harvesting, and food preparation. These rules entered into religion, law, and mythology. The intimate connection among religious rituals, agricultural practices, and food taboos demonstrates the antiquity of humanity's efforts to demarcate acceptable forms of sustenance, though the rationale for specific ritual practices, as, for example, those summarized for the people of Israel in the biblical Book of Leviticus, is now virtually impossible to reconstruct. Nevertheless, the persistence of ritual rules and prohibitions in the folk heritage of most peoples attests to the importance of foods and shows one method for bringing the provision, preparation, and choice of foods under rational control.

Food and Health The association between food and health implicit in religious prescriptions has been made explicit throughout the history of civilized socieities. Egyptians, according to Herodotus, Greek historian of the fifth century B.C., believed that food was the root of all disease and that good health therefore required regular purging. More precisely, the quantities of food consumed were connected with the preservation of health. Socrates, who instructed late-fifth-century Athens on morality and the nature of the good, urged moderation in eating and drinking, warned against satiety, and believed that a person should eat only when hungry and drink only when thirsty.

The contemporary Hippocratic writings warned against both overindulgence and too great abstemiousness, giving the opinion that too slender a diet was more dangerous than too generous a one.

Popular fads affected dietary prescriptions. At the beginning of the third century A.D., Athenaeus, an Egyptian-born Greek writing in Rome, reported a variety of unusual diets which supposedly supported life and promoted creative effort. His book, *The Sophists at Dinner,* told of men who lived on milk alone, or on water and figs, or on meals with no liquids. This modish asceticism reflected ideas among well-to-do Romans which may be thought of as compensation for the gluttony which passed for good living among them. Galen, the most influential of the late classical medical writers, considered correct dietary choice fundamental to a long and healthful life. This conviction, drawn from the Hippocratics, was also a central theme in late medieval and early modern medical, dietary, and scientific writing.

Beginning with Roger Bacon in the thirteenth century and continuing to the foundation of modern geriatrics with Sir John Floyer at the opening of the eighteenth century, the conviction that diet was the fundamental element in health and long life provoked a variety of studies. Echoing the classics, Sir Francis Bacon argued in the sixteenth century that while medicine could cure disease, only sound diet could prolong life, a doctrine which received its fullest development in Luigi Cornaro's influential book *The Sure and Certain Method of Attaining a Long and Healthful Life* (1558).

Luigi Cornaro was an early victim of gross overindulgence who, faced with the collapse of his health and probable death, resorted to a drastic experiment. He followed a daily diet of 12 ounces of solid food which included vegetables, bread and egg, and 14 ounces of wine. He observed and recorded his reactions to this diet and, as it proved successful, to its subsequent variations. Eventually Cornaro reduced his food intake to just one egg. He lived to the age of 99, living proof of the idea that abstemiousness was healthy.

Abstemiousness was only part of the picture. The distinction between food and medicines was never clear in premodern writings on diet. Many foods were believed to have curative powers, and it was common to associate particular foods with particular physical conditions. The Hippocratic writers, for example, warned that garlic, pulses, and vetch brought on flatulence, as did cheese, and they prescribed dry, sour, or bitter foods for dropsy and cold decoctions of wheat, lentils, and bread for intestinal distress where there was no fever. The Hippocratic authorities considered linseed, wheat flour, beans, millet, eggs, milk, and barley mush valuable for treating dysentery. But they warned against beef, especially for those of a melancholic disposition, and they noted that goat's meat and young pork were likely to be difficult to digest. Though particulars varied, the Hippocratic approach was typical. The Egyptians prescribed liver for night blindness; the Chinese asserted the curative powers of rhubarb, particularly as a purgative; cinchona bark was a new world specific for malaria; and in the sixteenth century, North American Indians showed the French explorer Jacques Cartier how to cure scurvy (q.v.) with an infusion of what seems to have been pine bark and needles. Finally, a diet of rich foods was considered an essential counter to the wasting effects of tuberculosis in the nineteenth century. Herbalist traditions in every society mixed common foods with botanical exotica to provide remedies for all manner of conditions, and until modern chemistry revolutionized the pharmaceutical industry, the lines separating herbalism, dietary prescriptions, and everyday food preparation were hopelessly blurred.

Scientific Nutrition While tradition stressed the importance of food for health throughout human history, the techniques necessary to analyze foods and their effects within living systems only gradually became available. It was not until the last decade of the nineteenth century that the essential elements which healthful diets had to provide began to be understood. In the twentieth century, those elements have been identified, and their roles have been explained, and nutritional science has begun to consider the more subtle consequences of dietary practices.

Broadly speaking, the prerequisites for the evolution of modern nutrition took shape with the appearance of scientific method. Its progenitors included the great scientific innovators from Roger Bacon in the thirteenth century through such sixteenth-century giants as Vesalius and Paracelsus to the modern men of the seventeenth century, William Harvey, Robert Boyle, and Isaac Newton. Many of these men wrote on nutritional problems as well as in the fields on which their fame rests. Paracelsus, for example, outlined a self-regulating chemical physiology which contained the germ of a metabolic theory; and Robert Boyle studied the effects of food on the composition of bodies, worked on the chemical analysis of blood and urine, and moved toward the definition of life as a "slow-burning process."

Nutrition owed a special debt to chemistry, which provided the tools to analyze the composition of foods and the concepts necessary to understand digestion, the nutritive process itself, and metabolism. The main steps included Joseph Black's rediscovery (after van Helmont) of carbon dioxide (1757), Henry Cavendish's discovery of hydrogen in 1766, and Daniel Rutherford's identification of nitrogen six years later. The most important development, however, was the discovery of oxygen by the Swedish apothecary Carl Wilhelm Scheele (1774). Robert Boyle had already shown that a candle could not burn nor an animal live in an airless environment, thus suggesting that breathing and burning were similar. Oxygen was the element common to both processes. The great French chemist Antoine Lavoisier subsequently proved that respiration was a process of combustion in which oxygen was burned in the body to produce carbon dioxide and water. Lavoisier further established (1780) the ratio of oxygen to carbon dioxide (inhaled and expelled) through experiments with guinea pigs, and in 1789 he showed that the amounts of oxygen used varied according to whether the organism studied was at rest or working, whether the food intake was raised or lowered, and whether the body cooled. This work led directly to the concept of a self-regulating system (metabolism) for the transformation of food values into energy. On the basis of this work, Lavoisier has been called the father of modern nutritional science.

The discovery and definition of the metabolic process opened further fields for study. Chemical analysis offered the means to identify the composition of food substances, to classify those substances, and to study how they performed their life-supporting role. In the early nineteenth century, René Réamur, who is best known for his thermometer, used birds to show that digestion was a chemical process, not a mechanical one, and that once stomach acids were obtained, digestion could be carried on outside the stomach. In 1823, the English physician and chemist William Prout proved that the acid contents of the stomach contained hydrochloric acid which was separable by distillation, while the actual digestive process was observed by Dr. William Beaumont at Fort Mackinac on the U.S.-Canadian border. Dr. Beaumont successfully treated a man who had suffered a severe gunshot wound. The grateful patient permitted him to leave a "window" into his abdomen through which the workings of his digestive system could be overseen and samples withdrawn. Beaumont carried out these observations over a 10-year period and published them in 1832.

By the middle of the nineteenth century, most of the basic components in diet were known, as were the composition of bones and teeth and some of the roles of proteins, carbohydrates, fats and minerals. Statements concerning dietary requirements began to be made, the proportions of necessary food elements in diet were under study, and in 1862 the British government went so far as to ask Dr. Edward Smith, an English physician who specialized in nutrition, to formulate a diet for workers which would maximize nutritional values at the lowest possible cost. Such projects were entirely premature. Nutritional science had developed greatly between 1750 and 1850, but the major barrier to its ultimate achievement was only beginning to be understood. It was becomming clear that proteins, carbohydrates, fats, and minerals did not in themselves constitute a life-supporting nutriment, but why that was true was obscure.

The evidence that there were nutritional elements which were present only in natural foods and which were essential for life was scattered and largely misunderstood. Though scurvy, for example, was known to result when a limited diet was fed and to disappear when certain foods were introduced, the reasons for the illness or the cure were not apparent. William Stark, an eighteenth-century physician interested in nutrition, was an early victim of the ignorance concerning necessary dietary elements. Determined to observe the effect of certain diet changes on his own condition, Stark began a diet of bread and water on July 12, 1769. Over the next several months he gradually added olive oil, milk, roast goose, boiled beef, fat, and veal. He fell ill on February 18, 1770, and died five days later. An autopsy was performed, but it failed to reveal a specific cause of death, though it now seems clear that he succumbed to dietary deficiencies.

In 1816, François Magendie, the eminent French physiologist, used dogs to show that nitrogen had to be available in the animals' food in order for them to survive. There was no other source. Studies in this area advanced rapidly, especially under the impact of work done by Justus von Liebig, the famous German chemist and physiologist who by mid-century claimed to have established a rational theory of nutrition including a metabolic concept. Liebig's conclusions were sharply questioned during the 1860s however. During the Prussian seige of Paris (1871), J. B. H. Dumas, a physician in charge of a nursery, proved conclusively that the dietary constituents defined by the Liebig school could not sustain life when synthesized artificially. With no natural food available, Dumas had to feed a large number of infants and young children. He compounded a formula by emulsifying fat in a sweetened albuminous solution. The resulting mixture contained proteins, carbohydrates, and fats, but it utterly failed to nourish the children. Dumas described his experiences in an article on "The Constitution of Milk and Blood" (1871), and within two years laboratory tests on mice completely confirmed his conclusions. Though the control mice thrived on milk, they could not survive on artificial compounds of fats, proteins, and carbohydrates. These results also corresponded with studies on animal nutrition carried out by the retired French mineralogist J. B. Boussingault, who had noted as early as 1822 that there was a connection between iodized salt and the prevention of goiter, and whose studies on his own herds showed the importance of calcium for animal growth.

In 1883, Max Rubner, a student of Carl Ludwig and Carl von Voit, was able to show that metabolism was proportional to the body's surface area and, in 1902, that the dynamic action of foods was greatest for proteins and least for carbohydrates. By 1906, it was possible for Sir Frederick G. Hopkins, one of the most distinguished nutritional scientists of the early twentieth century, to conclude that it was impossible for any animal to live on an artificial mixture of proteins, carbohydrates, and fats, even when necessary inorganic matter was supplied. Hopkins believed that the animal body was adjusted to live on plant tissues or other animals which contained countless substances other than the standard nutritional components. In support of this view, he pointed to the etiology of rickets and scurvy, which indicated that there was some mysterious dietary element critical to nutrition. When it was missing, deficiency diseases developed. At the time Hopkins wrote, nutritionists working on the deficiency diseases were close to identifying the dietary missing link. In 1907, the existence of such a link was asserted, and five years later the Polish-American biochemist Casimir Funk named it the "vitamine." Subsequent progress was rapid. By 1915, new criteria for scientific nutrition had been established, deficiency syndromes had been isolated and evaluated, and the basis for understanding the nutritional roles of various foods, from the parts of plants (leaves, stems, seeds) to milk, egg yolk, and meat, had been established. Moreover, the initial steps toward synthesizing vitamins in the laboratory had been taken. The physiology of metabolic process was in place, and the development of a fully scientific basis for nutritional standards had been established.

In 1943, the U.S. National Research Council published the first of its *Recommended Dietary Allowances* series, which, in successive editions, has become a standard guide for nutritional requirements. Subsequent nutritional research has begun to explore the more subtle emotional, cultural, and physiological consequences of diet, and particularly of dietary deprivation. The Keys study on the biology of human starvation, published at the University of Minnesota in 1950, began the systematic evaluation of behavioral changes arising from diets producing weight loss of up to 25 percent. Other studies on the consequences of anemia and protein-energy malnutrition suggest substantial effects on energy levels, intellectual capacity, and disease resistance. This work is also connected with the effort to find adequate food sources to maintain the health of the world's population.

The period from 1890 to 1950 saw the establishment of a definitive, medically sound nutrition; the period since 1950 has raised the much larger problem of nutritional needs and the world's health in the twentieth century.

ADDITIONAL READINGS: Adelia M. Beeuwkes, E. Neige Todhunter, and Emma Seifrit Weigley (compilers), *Essays on History of Nutrition and Dietetics*, Chicago, 1967; L. S. P. Davidson and R. Passmore, *Human Nutrition and Dietetics*, 4th ed., Edinburgh and London, 1969; Karl Y. Guggenhein and Ira Wolinsky, *Nutrition and Nutritional Diseases: The Evolution of Concepts*, Lexington, Mass. 1981; Charles B. Heiser, Jr., *Seed to Civilization: The Story of Man's Food*, San Francisco, 1973; Clive M. McCay, *Notes on the History of Nutrition Research*, F. Verzan and Hans Huber (eds.), Bern, Stuttgart, and Vienna, 1973; E. V. McCollum, *A History of Nutrition*, Boston, 1957.

See also DEFICIENCY DISEASES; PELLAGRA; SCURVY.

Obstetrical Forceps

Forceps are a two-bladed instrument made of metal which act as pincers or pliers to seize, hold, and manipulate various objects. They are used in watchmaking, industry, and surgery, and they played a particularly important role in midwifery and obstetrics. Prior to the invention of the midwife forceps in the seventeenth century, there was no tool available to aid in difficult births. Cesarean sections were performed when there seemed a chance to rescue a live baby from a dead or dying mother. When a mother was unable to give birth, the baby was destroyed to save her life. Hooks known as crotchets were sometimes used to dismember and remove the child from the birth canal, or a crainiotomy could be performed, in which the head was perforated to provide a purchase and then the baby was dragged out. These operations were performed by surgeons, and it was commonly accepted that when the surgeon was called, mother or child and probably both were doomed.

Men entered the practice of midwifery in the seventeenth century, and it was a family of male midwives, the Chamberlens, who invented and used the obstetrical forceps. The Chamberlens were French Huguenots who went to England in 1569 to escape persecution in France. Dr. William

Chamberlen, the father of the family, settled first in Southhampton and then moved to London. His children included two sons, both named Peter, who are known as the Elder and the Younger. Both men were enrolled in the barber-surgeons' company and became known for their obstetrical skills, their individualism, and their contentiousness. They served at court, and Peter the Elder became physician to King James I. Independent, even unruly, the Chamberlens ignored the rules of both the barber-surgeons and the Royal College of Physicians. The latter prosecuted Peter the Elder for the illegal practice of medicine in 1612 and his brother for the same offense in 1620.

Peter the Younger had a son who was also called Peter, who started medical training at age 14 at Emmanuel College, Cambridge. He also studied at Heidelberg and Padua, where he received a doctorate in 1619, and he was enrolled in the Royal College of Physicians in 1628. Dr. Peter Chamberlen became the successor to his uncle as the royal midwife, attending in his uncle's stead at the birth of Charles II in 1630. He continued to flourish under Oliver Cromwell's commonwealth, and when the Stuarts were restored, he was reappointed physician-in-ordinary to Charles II in 1660.

The Chamberlens built reputation and wealth on their powers as midwives. The key to their success was the obstetrical forceps, which Peter the Elder probably invented, though Dr. Peter, the son of Peter the Younger, has also been credited. The forceps permitted them to deliver more women more successfully than any previous practitioners. They kept their instrument a close secret, however, and they went to extraordinary lengths to mislead observers. When they arrived to assist at a birth, they brought a large, apparently very heavy box with them which was decorated with gilded carvings and which required two men to carry. The woman to be delivered was kept blindfolded and was never permitted to see what instruments were used. The lying-in room was kept locked, but persons listening outside the door heard strange noises, including ringing bells. The Chamberlens not only kept their secret but endowed it with an unquestionable aura of mystery. This proved very effective advertising.

In 1670, Hugh Chamberlen, the son of Dr. Peter Chamberlen, took the family secret to France. He was apparently prepared to sell it for 10,000 livres to Jules Clément, the royal accoucheur, and François Mauriceau, a leading young French authority on midwifery. Mauriceau set Chamberlen a test: Under his care was a dwarf, deformed by rickets, who was already in labor. If Chamberlen could deliver this woman using his secret appliance, he could deliver anyone, and the French would pay Hugh the price. The experiment failed. After three hours of struggle, Chamberlen was unable to budge the baby, and the mother died undelivered. The baby died as well when it was taken by cesarean section. The French rejected the Chamberlen secret instrument.

Hugh Chamberlen returned to England, where he became involved in a number of schemes, the last of which was fraudulent, and he was forced to flee the country. He went to Holland, where he was still reported to be living in 1720. When and where he died is not known. To raise money, he is alleged to have sold the Chamberlen secret to a Dutch physician, Rogier van Roonhuyze. What he actually sold van Roonhuyze is not known, but it was apparently not the obstetrical forceps. Nevertheless, several individuals, beginning with van Roonhuyze, his colleagues, and his students, claimed to know the secret, and van Roonhuyze appears to have sold information to several others. In 1747, John Peter Rathlauw, a Dutchman who had studied surgery in London, published a book in which described what he claimed was the Chamberlen secret possessed by van Roonhuyze. Rathlauw alleged that van Roonhuyze and the Amsterdam Medico-Pharmaceutical College had refused him a license to practice midwifery because he would not purchase information on the secret. What he published was a description of some tools which a disaffected apprentice had seen in van Roonhuyze's medical bag. These tools included two curved levers which could be connected by a hinged joint. Whatever this may have been, it was not the Chamberlen forceps, though it was a workable tool which Rathlauw improved.

The Chamberlen secret was never freely and fully divulged to the medical world. But the last of the Chamberlens, Dr. Hugh Chamberlen, Jr., who died in 1728, permitted the secret to escape during the last years of his life. In 1733, Edmund Chapman, a surgeon and male midwife, published the first detailed account of the forceps, which he called " a noble instrument to which many now living owe their lives," and gave instructions for their use. An example of the Chamberlen forceps was discovered in 1813, hidden in the floor of the former family home at Woodlawn Mortimer Hall in Essex. The cache contained instruments that belonged to Dr. Peter Chamberlen. By the time it was found, the contents were of purely antiquarian interest. Forceps were in use before 1733, and while contemporaries recognized that the Chamberlens invented them, the originals had already been modified.

In the course of the eighteenth century, it seemed that every person who had to do with forceps tried to improve the design, but the basic tool remained essentially what the Chamberlens had invented. The Chamberlen forceps had two wide, flat blades curved to fit the child's head. The blades were put in place separately and then locked together to provide a firm hold on the head. By gentle pulling, the head was then extracted. Since the head was larger than the shoulders, trunk, or hips, the rest of the body followed easily once the head was freed. It was some time, however, before the doctor-midwives realized that if the pelvic ring was too small, no amount of effort with the forceps could bring the head through, and cesarean section was the only answer. Anesthesia and aseptic surgery in the nineteenth century finally made the cesarean section an acceptable alternative.

Inevitably, the obstetrical forceps were abused, used to aid births when they were not needed or where they could not be effective. William Smellie, one of the great teachers and practitioners of midwifery in eighteenth-century London, took the lead in establishing a conservative approach to the use of forceps and laid down specific cautionary rules for practitioners to follow. Smellie's influence was immense. He taught 1000 or more students, and his methods were nearly universally approved.

The forceps did reduce birth mortalities. It is recorded at the Rotunda in Dublin, for example, that when the long, curved forceps were introduced around 1855, the number of craniotomies was halved. Before their introduction, the rate was 7 craniotomies in every 1000 births. One recent authority notes that probably no other instrument did so much toward saving mothers and babies.

The question of whether the Chamberlens were justified in withholding their invention has been widely discussed. The consensus is that they were not. However, a somewhat different historical judgment is indicated. The Chamberlens behaved like the highly skilled artisans they were, with a valuable service to sell. Their behavior was consistent with seventeenth-century social and economic principles. It was consistent as well with the emerging efforts to restrict competition by defining standards for physicians. The Chamberlens were prosecuted for breaking just those rules. The modern medical professional combines a humanitarian and altruistic ethic with materialistic self-interest. The social aspect to the history of medicine involves the evolution of rules and organizations designed to protect the interests of trained practitioners selling invaluable services. Such organization and regulations have social utility as well. The Chamberlens' defense of their monopoly underscores the element of economic interest which inheres to the practice of medicine in modern society. The fact that such behavior is roundly criticized points up the fundamental tension between interest and ideals which is a continuing issue when questions of medicine's social role arise.

ADDITIONAL READINGS: Harvey Graham, *Eternal Eve*, London, 1950, Chap. VIII; Edwin M. Jameson, *Gynecology and Obstetrics*, New York, 1936, Chap. V; Walter Radcliffe, *The Secret Instrument: Birth of the Midwifery Forceps*, London, 1947.

See also MIDWIFERY.

Ophthalmology

Ophthalmology, a medical specialty dealing with diagnosis and treatment of eye conditions, originated in the later Middle Ages and acquired its current form in the course of the nineteenth century. In classic and medieval times, little was known in Europe about the eye's anatomy or how it functioned. The most important optical contributions of the premodern era belonged to Arab science and most notably to Ibn al Haitham (Alhazan), whose eleventh-century *Treasury of Optics* included such concepts as refraction and magnification through a glass sphere. It was the latter principle which Roger Bacon employed in the thirteenth century when he proposed a reading glass for the elderly and for other people whose eyes were weak.

By the sixteenth century, however, reliable information on the eye and its functions had begun to appear. Clear and accurate descriptions of the eye's structure began with Andreas Vesalius; Franciscus Maurolycus demonstrated the retina's role; and in 1604 Johann Kepler described the cornea and lens as refracting media. Spectacles to correct visual defect were introduced in the sixteenth century—Raphael painted Pope Leo X holding concave lenses. Hieronymus Fabricius correctly placed the lens behind the iris, though it appears he failed to understand the significance of his discovery. Georg Bartisch of Königsbrück, a barber-surgeon who became court oculist for the elector of Saxony, wrote on eye diseases in the vernacular and employed anatomy, physiology, and optics in his work. His writings published in 1583 showed wide experience with cataracts, and he discussed diseases of the conjunctiva, tumors on lids, trachoma, and ptosis, as well as a variety of other conditions. Bartisch is sometimes credited with founding modern ophthalmology.

Specialization in the treatment of eye diseases began very early. Medieval medicine differentiated physicians, surgeons, and barber-surgeons from irregular healers, or quacks (see Quackery). Among the irregulars, eye specialists called oculists and cataract couchers were particularly important. Cataracts were a common affliction which required surgery, and the methods for treating them were described in Indian as well as Greco-Roman texts. In fact, though cataract couching had been carried on for centuries, very little was known about the condition or about the lens of the eye. Galen believed that cataract was caused by a humor from the brain which solidified behind the lens. Cataract couching involved breaking up the solid matter and pushing it away, actually displacing the lens, a fact that was not accepted until late in the eighteenth century. Irregular oculists and couchers were often highly skilled, and, unlike regular physicians and surgeons, they had acquired a wide experience with eye operations. Regular practitioners were reluctant to operate on cataract. Lazare Rivière, a professor of medicine at Montpellier, commented in 1640 that when surgery for cataract became necessary, "it should be left to the itinerant quacksalvers who practice it," especially as the outcome of such operations was so uncertain.

This abdication of responsibility created a recognized need which only irregulars were meeting, and this led regulatory bodies to give a measure of approval to the irregulars' work. The Rhineland city of Worms, for example, wrote an apothecary code in 1582 permitting experienced lithotomists, oculists, and teeth pullers to practice provided they gave no medicines internally. London's barber-surgeons' company also granted irregulars licenses, while in Florence the guild code enrolled irregular healers including oculists with doctors and apothecaries. Inevitably there were frauds among the irregulars, and cataract couchers had a bad reputation for exaggerated claims and surgical incompetence. Many, however, were effective operators, and as a group they remained active well into the first half of the nineteenth century in Europe and even longer in the United States.

Science supported regular medicine on optical matters. After Kepler, René Descartes explained the process of accommodation in his *Dioptrics* (1637), and in 1664 Robert Hook discovered the principle of measuring for minimum visual angle. He also explained the correct position of the lens, what cataracts really are, and how to extract them. His views were ignored, however, until the early eighteenth century, when Pierre Brisseau (1705) and Antoine Maître-Jan (1707) showed that cataract was a condition in the lens. The French academy approved the argument in 1708, but more than 50 years passed before the opinion was generally accepted. Nevertheless, lens removals occurred. Charles de Saint-Yves, for example, undertook to couch a cataract in 1722 and displaced the lens into the interior chamber of the eye. His success was the first recorded instance of removal of a lens from a living body. It was another eighteenth-century French surgeon, Jacques Daviel, who described cataract correctly as a senile degeneration of the lens and published an account in 1748 of his operation for lens removal. Even Daviel vacillated between couching and lens excision before finally settling on the latter. Once he had determined his course, however, his lens extractions proved largely (89 percent) successful.

Other surgical procedures were important in the early history of ophthalmology. Bartisch described complete excision of the eyeball in 1583, an operation which continued to be performed regularly, first for a protuberant eye, and more commonly in the nineteenth century when injury to one eye threatened the onset of sympathetic blindness in the other. Squint, or strabismus, also came to be corrected surgically. The traditional treatment for this condition, the result of overreaction of the extrinsic ocular muscles which produces a permanent deviation in the eyeball from its normal axis, was a mask with holes over the eyes. The theory was that the squinted eye would straighten itself when its vision was impaired. This procedure appeared in the later Greek texts and was still recommended in the sixteenth century. It is possible that the first operation in which the affected muscle was cut was performed by the famous oculist and charlatan Chevalier John Taylor in 1738, and it is also possible that he performed the operation more than once. (Though deemed a quack, Taylor had both surgical and medical training and had studied with William Cheselden at St. Thomas' Hospital, London; he is also supposed to have had training on the Continent, and he held an appointment as oculist to King George II.) Taylor did not, however, establish a tradition or an accepted procedure, and while Johann F. Dieffenbach successfully cut an eye muscle for squint in 1839, others failed, and it remained to Albrecht von Graefe to develop the basic method for the modern operation in 1853.

By the opening of the nineteenth century, there was a nucleus of physicians and surgeons committed to specialized studies on the eye who organized eye hospitals and clinics and gave formal courses in ophthalmology. In 1803, the University of Göttingen introduced ophthalmology as a special course, and Vienna established the first clinic in 1812. The London Eye Infirmary, which was destined to become one of the leading schools of ophthalmology, was established by John Saunders in 1805. It was the model for the New York Eye and Ear Infirmary (1820), the first such institution in the United States, and for the Boston Eye Infirmary (1824). France, a leader in eye studies in the early eighteenth century, failed to keep pace, and the first private eye clinic established in Paris (1832) belonged to a German immigrant, Dr. Julius Sichel, who had studied under Georg Joseph Beer, the first professor of ophthalmology at Vienna. The clinic was a huge success. C. J. F. Carron du Villards set up the first eye dispensary in Paris (1835), while L. A. Desmarres, who became Sichel's assistant, consolidated what became the modern French school of ophthalmology. The new ophthalmology also reached the United States, where George Frick of Baltimore, another of Beer's students, published the first book on the subject in 1823. Frick's work was essentially a summary of Beer's lectures.

Advances in the science of optics very early made correction of defects in vision possible. Spectacles, or reading lenses, were commonplace by the eighteenth century, though they were selected rather than prescribed. There was no systematic way to estimate the degree of visual error in a person's eyes, and people needing glasses simply rummaged through collections of different lenses until they found what seemed to fit. The corrections were mainly for old vision, nearsightedness and farsightedness. Astigmatism was not known until Thomas Young identified it at the opening of the nineteenth century. Lenses to correct the condition came later still. There is a tradition that Benjamin Franklin originated bifocals, while the first contact lens appeared in 1877. Frans Donders, a Dutch ophthalmologist, led the way to a modern system for prescribing and fitting glasses. He was able to separate errors of refraction from those of accommodation, and his book on the subject, *Anomalies of Refraction and Accommodation* (1864), is an acknowledged classic. His countryman and contemporary, Hermann Snellen, contributed to rational prescription by developing a set of "test types," standard letters of different sizes which test visual acuity. Others contributed as well, but Snellen's types proved exceptionally effective and are still in use.

Ophthalmology's status as a medical field owed less to optics than to operations and ultimately to the development of the means to study the eye's anatomy, physiology, and pathology. The first major work on the eye's pathology did not appear until 1808, when James Wardrop of Edinburgh published his *Essays on the Morbid Anatomy of the Human Eye,* which dealt with eye conditions anatomically. By 1830 eye pathology had advanced to the point that the blindness owing to glaucoma could be distinguished from that produced by cataracts. The investigation of the eye, however, was external and superficial, with only a magnifying glass to assist the examiner's own vision. Relating eye conditions to general health was virtually impossible, and ophthalmology was therefore largely surgical. A most dramatic change came when Berlin's Hermann von Helmholtz invented the ophthalmoscope (1851) and the ophthalmometer (1852), instruments which permitted a physician to investigate the interior of the eye and which revealed conditions significant for other areas of the body, especially the brain. The ophthalmoscope also permitted accurate measuring of refraction, a function which it still performs. Albrecht von Graefe, also of Berlin, who developed the modern operation for strabismus, expanded these clinical applications of the ophthalmoscope and has been credited with initiating the modern era of ophthalmic surgery. Among his most important contributions was introducing iridectomy (1857), the removal of a portion of the iris, in glaucoma cases. This marked a major step toward a satisfactory treatment of the condition.

Ophthalmic diagnosis and surgery place particular emphasis on specialized applications in microscopy. The first attempts to use the microscope on the eye of a living patient were made in 1823, but it was not until 66 years later that a microscope appropriate to this purpose was successfully developed. It was the contribution of Louis de Wecker. The slit lamp, an instrument essential for illuminating the areas to be observed, was invented by Sweden's Allvar Gullstrand, who won a Nobel prize in 1911 for his studies on the refractory system, the shape of the cornea, and the changes which occur in lens accommodation. Theories on color vision were offered first by Thomas Young in the eighteenth century and were refined by Hermann von Helmholtz in the mid-nineteenth. The theory postulated that the retina contains elements in the nerve endings which react to the primary colors, red, yellow, and violet (Helmholtz said blue). These theories have stood up well and have served as the basis for studying color blindness.

Replacements for the natural eye involved technology of another sort. Artificial eyes have been used from early days and are mentioned in early Egyptian medical records. Various materials were employed, including gold and silver with enameling to counterfeit the appearance of the human eye. Ambroise Paré described such an eye in the sixteenth century. Glass eyes appeared in the seventeenth century, manufactured first in Venice and later in Bohemia and France. Glass eyes of German manufacture led the field from 1835 to 1933, when their export was prohibited. Deprived of German glass eyes, the importing countries developed their own versions, including plastic ones.

Despite important work in France, Britain, and Italy, Germany led the way in developing modern ophthalmology. The United States benefited from this achievement when German specialists emigrated from central Europe in the two decades following the revolutions of 1848 and 1849. Many came to New York, and in 1862, Dr. Julius Homberger, a man who had studied with both Graefe and Sichel, founded the *American Journal of Ophthalmology,* the first ophthalmological journal in the United States. Seven years later, another German émigré, Dr. Herman Knapp from Heidelberg, established the *Archives of Ophthalmology.* Fittingly enough, the American Ophthalmological Society was organized in New York in 1864.

New York's leading role in American ophthalmology underscored the importance of large cities for the growth of medical specialization. In urban environments, there was a concentration of wealth and population which created a market able to afford specialist care as well as a large pool of potential subjects for clinical investigation. Cities concentrated public health problems. Hospitals, dispensaries, and clinics were essential to cope with the disease consequences of poverty, overcrowding, and inadequate nutrition, but they also provided unique opportunities for study. Using the techniques of clinical pathology, specialist knowledge flourished. At the same time, cities in the industrializing era were centers for a radically expanding middle class which learned to value the professionally trained medical doctor and then demanded the further services of specialists. Ophthalmology as a specialized practice followed the course of European and American urbanization, with the heaviest concentration of training facilities, research centers, and practitioners in New York, London, Paris, and Berlin. In the twentieth century, with a multiplicity of significant urban centers, and with an urbanized culture spreading to smaller cities and towns, a wider dispersion of specialists, ophthalmologists included, has occurred. But even today, a more general medicine is practiced in predominantly rural areas, and the association between urbanization and specialization continues to hold.

Modern ophthalmology is closely tied to general medicine, and most medical curricula provide an introduction to the subject for all medical students. As a specialty, however, ophthalmology requires a prescribed course of training in addition to the regular medical curriculum and involves special licensing requirements. Ophthalmologists most commonly work on patient referrals from general practitioners, and surgery, particularly for cataract, is an important part of their practice. The basic conceptions and many of the procedures of ophthalmology were established by the end of the nineteenth century. Technological refinements in diagnostic instruments, aids to vision, and surgical procedures have since made the specialty more effective, but its most important advances (especially since World War II) have concerned the prevention of eye problems through the application of specialized knowledge in society. Some of the most prominent of these include regular school inspections of children's eyes leading to early diagnosis, isolation, and treatment of infectious conjunctivitis; maternal and infant care directed at preventing ophthalmia in newborn babies; and regulations governing light levels in schools and factories. Recognition that granular conjunctivitis, or trachoma, is both chronic and infectious has produced effective isolation and quarantine for treatment of immigrants, though the problem remains serious and endemic among the poor of both developed and undeveloped countries. Testing for vision impairment in schoolchildren and the availability of glasses to correct those problems have improved eye health in general. Ophthalmology's medical-scientific foundation was established by the opening of the twentieth century; its growth since then has elaborated on those achievements.

ADDITIONAL READINGS: Fielding H. Garrison, *An Introduction to the History of Medicine*, 4th ed., Philadelphia, 1929; Benjamin Lee Gordon, *Medieval and Renaissance Medicine*, New York, 1959; David C. Lindberg, *Theories of Vision from Al Kindi to Kepler*, Chicago, 1976; George Rosen, *The Specialization of Medicine with Particular Reference to Ophthalmology*, New York, 1944, 1972; Charles Singer and E. Ashworth Underwood, *A Short History of Medicine*, 2d ed., Oxford, 1962; Owen H. and Sarah D. Wangensteen, *The Rise of Surgery: From Empiric Craft to Scientific Discipline*, Minneapolis, 1978.

See also MEDICAL PROFESSION; QUACKERY; SURGERY.

Orthopedics

Orthopedics is a medical specialty concerned with deformities, diseases, and injuries of the bones, joints, ligaments, tendons, and muscles. The term originated with Nicholas Andry in 1741 in a treatise on preventing diseases in children, and the field has remained closely associated with pediatrics (q.v.). It is also integral to the history of surgery (q.v.). The subject matter of orthopedics makes it one of the oldest fields of medical treatment. Accidents resulting in sprains, fractures, or dislocations are as old as human life, and, not surprisingly, these matters appear in the earliest medical records. Because such injuries were common, communities had to deal with them whether there were physicians available or not, and a rich heritage of folk treatment developed.

In medieval and early modern Europe, bonesetters were among the most ubiquitous of the irregular practitioners, though unlike lithotomists or cataract couchers, they tended to be sendentary. Bonesetters were more like midwives in that they provided a service needed in every community, though the bonesetting function does not appear to have been sufficiently lucrative to become a full-fledged trade. Artisans and craftsmen, most notably carpenters and blacksmiths, often supplemented their income by acting as bonesetters, while retired sailors were prominent as well. No ship's captain could be comfortable without some person aboard who was responsible for treating injuries, and when there was no surgeon available, a member of the crew had to be deputized. The ship's carpenter was often the choice. England's preeminent maritime status was probably an important factor in the rise in the number of bonesetters available, though this phenomenon alone cannot account for the leadership in orthopedic matters England achieved in the late nineteenth and early twentieth centuries.

Bonesetters gained what knowledge they possessed from more experienced practitioners. In this they were similar to other popular medical specialists who performed particular functions. And, as it was with the midwives or lithotomists, some individuals attracted considerable attention. Certain English families, for example, were famed (later notorious) as bonesetters. Among the best-known names were Hulton, Thomas,

Crowther, and Taylor. A descendant of one of these families, Hugh Owen Thomas, of Liverpool, should probably be called the founder of modern orthopedics in England. His father was a bonesetter, and while Hugh Thomas was fully educated for the medical profession, he never entirely escaped the stigma of his father's vocation.

It was inevitable that the quality of individual bonesetters would vary enormously, but while the competing interests of the medical brotherhood gave its members every reason to denigrate bonesetters' skills and impute their honesty, many bonesetting irregulars were capable and competent. Their primary function was to set fractures and treat sprains and dislocations. Some, however, went further, attempting to correct deformities by manipulations, splints, iron braces, or stiffened bandages. They were not surgeons and made no attempt at surgical corrections. As they were uneducated in medical matters in general, they avoided the obvious signs of illness, particularly inflammations. As trained medical men, especially surgeons, made inroads on their practice, the bonesetters shifted their emphasis toward exercise, manipulation, and massage, and by the middle of the nineteenth century they had lost much of their standing. Their role was gradually taken over by hospitals, clinics, and accident services though there is also a hint of the bonesetters' previous function in modern chiropractic.

From the middle of the eighteenth century through the end of World War I, orthopedics was one branch among many in medicine, more particularly surgery; and while various achievements were recorded by individuals, an orthopedic specialty was, at most, in process of formation. The first orthopedic institution may have been J. C. Lettsom's special hospital established at Margate in the later eighteenth century for victims of scrofula. This disease, later recognized to be a tubercular condition, was a common affliction which produced crippling effects when it attacked the joints. Lettsom believed that treating this disease required a much longer period than would be possible in existing hospitals, and he favored fresh air and sunshine for their therapeutic effect. His open-air hospital at the seaside was the first of many established in western European countries.

Surgical orthopedics also began in the eighteenth century, when Jean-André Venel set up an orthopedic institute at Orb in the canton of Vaud in Switzerland in 1780. His particular interest was in correcting lateral curvatures and spinal torsion, and he published a study on the subject in 1788. Several medical men introduced the use of spinal braces in the eighteenth century, and in 1779 Jean-Pierre David published a detailed account of spinal deformation from caries which included pathological data from autopsies. Percivall Pott, a surgeon at St. Bartholomew's Hospital in London, published a pamphlet on palsy arising from spinal caries in the same year. Spinal caries came to be known as Pott's disease, though his essay was less comprehensive in scope than David's and in fact described the consequences of the disease rather than the disease itself. It remained to Montpellier's Jacques M. Delpech to point to the tubercular character of spinal caries in 1816.

Delpech was, in fact, a ground breaker in the field of orthopedic surgery, and he appears to have been the first surgeon to attempt to correct clubfoot by sectioning the Achilles tendon by working the knife under the skin. The operation was performed on May 9, 1816, but Delpech did not return to it. The man who did, and who not only established orthopedic surgery on solid ground in Germany but contributed as well to its development in England, was Georg F. L. Stromeyer of Hanover. Fifteen years after Delpech, Stromeyer carried out a tenotomy on a 14-year-old clubfooted boy which was successful. In eight weeks, the patient was pronounced cured. Stromeyer became an advocate of subcutaneous tenotomy for all deformities which arose from muscular defects, thereby practically creating modern surgery of the locomotor system.

Stromeyer's hospital, founded in 1830, became a center for the study of deformities, and in 1831 it attracted, among other students, a young Englishman named William John Little who had already qualified as a member of the Royal College of Surgeons and was studying for a doctorate at Berlin. Little, who was himself clubfooted, was specializing in that condition and more generally in the anatomy of the foot. Convinced that clubfoot resulted from disordered muscle action, Little found Stromeyer's thinking entirely to his taste. He submitted to a subcutaneous tenotomy which was successful, learned the Stromeyer method, and returned to Berlin, where he defended his thesis, entitled "The Nature and Treatment of Club-Foot" and received his degree. Little then returned to London to perform his first subcutaneous tenotomy of February 20, 1837, and in 1838 he established the Orthopedic Institution, which taught the Stromeyer method and his own doctrines. His institution became the Royal Orthopedic Hospital in 1843, and in 1909 it merged with the National Orthopedic and the City Orthopedic to form the Royal National Orthopedic Hospital.

The improvement in orthopedic bandages made possible by Anthonius Mathijsen's quick-setting plaster of Paris in 1854 was a particular boon to surgeons attempting to correct deformities. Another advance, the so-called Thomas splint, an iron leg or army support with a ring at one end which facilitated extension of the injured member, was devised by Hugh Owen Thomas and still remains in use. Thomas was not only a gifted orthopedist but also a man whose ideas affected the development of orthopedics in both England and the United States, though to achieve their full effect they required an intermediary. Thomas himself was difficult, contentious, and sensitive to slights. He attacked bonesetters and surgeons alike, and he ended by alienating himself from both. On the other hand, he served the working classes of his district with sympathy and devotion. At one point in his career, Thomas was the medical officer for no less than 28 trade union and friendly societies, and he still had time to serve as consultant to a newly formed hospital for deformed children. Hugh Thomas resisted surgery. He would avoid excising a joint at almost any cost. He did his most important work on fractures and deformities, and he wrote extensively on both. Characteristically, he had his books printed privately and made no attempt to circulate them, and when he died in 1891, they were found stacked to the ceiling in a special room in his house.

Hugh Thomas was noted for the brute force and violence with which he attacked manipulations, but once the hard part was done, he insisted on absolute rest for the injured limb, and he tailored his own splints, casts, and bandages to guarantee it. Apart from the Thomas splint, he was probably best known for the method called passive congestion, or "damming the circulation," which he recommended for delayed union in fractures; he also promoted what was to become known as "carry-through" treatment. Once a fracture was joined, Thomas believed that a skilled orthopedist was needed to oversee the recovery or else an unsatisfactory union might result. His argument received dramatic confirmation in a British Medical Association investigation of fracture healing carried out in 1912. Follow-up studies on 3000 fracture cases produced results as startling as they were unwelcome. In 40 percent of the cases studied, there was malunion of the fracture, and in 60 percent of those cases where the union was deemed good, functional results were poor. Fracture treatment by (relatively) inexperienced doctors was unsatisfactory; orthopedic specialists were necessary to achieve reasonable results, and specialist oversight was essential if a satisfactory end even to an acceptable joining was to be achieved.

Though Hugh Thomas was a seminal influence in orthopedics, his effect on the field would probably have been negligible had it not been for his nephew, Robert Jones. Jones accepted his uncle's ideas and carried them into every new project in which he became involved. An effective orthopedic practitioner, Robert Jones was not an original medical thinker, but he was as social as his uncle was misanthropic, and he had a genius for institutional development.

Robert Jones began the most fruitful period of his life in 1881, when he was elected surgeon at the Stanley Hospital, Liverpool, and to the Manchester Ship Canal. In both institutions he introduced his uncle's techniques, and at the canal he pioneered an association to provide injury treatment and first aid, thus taking a step on the road which led eventually to the modern accident or emergency service. He was also interested in institutions for aiding crippled children, and he allied with Agnes Hunt, herself a cripple who was also a nurse, who organized a hospital at Baschurch in 1904. Jones began by treating her, ended by joining her, and helped to create an institution now recognized to have been the model for nearly all the crippled children's hospitals and homes in England.

World War I produced opportunity for him of another sort. It became apparent, with the casualties during the fighting of 1914 and 1915, that there was going to be a massive rehabilitation problem which no one was prepared to meet. In 1915, Jones opened an orthopedic center for war wounded at Alder Hey in Liverpool. It was run according to his uncle's therapeutic principles, and it was received with great enthusiasm. Jones became the man responsible for organizing the rehabilitation of England's wounded. Several new centers reflecting the Thomas-Jones approach were opened, including a giant 800 bed military hospital in Shepherd's Bush. Before the war was over, there were 15 such institutions, with a total of 30,000 beds. But each of those centers required personnel, and in the end, the rehabilitation hospitals themselves became major instructional institutions, providing training in orthopedics and especially orthopedic surgery. When the American expeditionary forces arrived in Europe in 1917, the English hospitals were in full force. They provided both experience and examples for the United States, contributing thereby to orthopedic advance and the development of rehabilitation facilities for American wounded.

Robert Jones, who was knighted for his wartime efforts, came to be recognized, in Fielding H. Garrison's words, as the "guiding spirit of the British and American orthopedic services during the war," and his contributions to the application of orthopedic medicine to social problems continued in the postwar world. The establishment of fracture clinics in Liverpool and London followed the example of the Manchester canal accident society and the wartime rehabilitation centers, and the subsequent creation of the accident service of the Carnegie (Illinois) Steel Trust and the Vienna (Austria) Accident Insurance Company Hospital for injured workers followed Robert Jones's example. When the British Orthopedic Association announced in 1943 that it supported creating accident centers to provide organized treatment for all accident victims, they were extending what had become a fundamental principle in the Thomas-Jones position.

Although orthopedics had its most significant modern development in England, the specialty had a long-standing tradition on the Continent, and it appeared relatively early in the United States. Orthopedic hospitals arrived early in the nineteenth century, and by the end of the century, American orthopedic surgeons were well-established and had done some original work. Initially, New York and Boston were the most important centers and were visited regularly at the turn of the century by Europeans observing American techniques. One of the most important achievements was Fred H. Albee's work on bone transplantation and the use of bone grafts in treating Pott's disease, fractures, and deformities. This work was done between 1911 and 1915 in New York. A circle of New England contemporaries also attracted attention. These included Edward H. Bradford, Robert W. Lavell, and James W. Sever, who promoted the treatment of scoliosis by plaster jackets applied in suspension, and E. G. Abbott, of Portland, Maine, who treated lateral curvature of the spine by applying jackets in flexion.

Subsequent to World War I, orthopedics grew rapidly as a specialty, taking over a wide range of conditions from general practitioners and surgeons. The specialty acquired academic foundations as medical schools developed orthopedic departments or specialized programs within surgical curricula. The establishment of the Nuffield chair of orthopedics at Oxford in 1937 was a landmark in the development of the discipline. By the middle of the century, orthopedics had become a firmly established specialty with an expanding practice and an important role in the maintenance of public health. Individuals, particularly surgeons from Europe and America, all contributed techniques and procedures to the field, but the institutionalization of the discipline and its advance as a specialty with social applications owed most to its English leadership.

ADDITIONAL READINGS: E. M. Bick, *A Source Book of Orthopedics*, 2d ed., Philadelphia, 1948; Frederick F. Cartwright, *The Development of Modern Surgery*, London, 1967; R. Ted Steinbock, *Paleopathological Diagnosis and Interpretation: Bone Diseases in Ancient Human Populations*, Springfield, Ill., 1976; F. Watson, *The Life of Sir Robert Jones*, New York, 1934, 1980.

See also SURGERY.

Pathology

Pathology is the systematic study of abnormal conditions arising in the body. It seeks to identify such conditions with specific causes and to explain why and how the cause identified has produced the results it has. Pathology combines anatomy, physiology, and theories of disease. It is directly relevant to therapy, epidemiology, preventive medicine, and immunology, and there is hardly a field in medicine to which it does not contribute in some fashion. Similarly, its methods of investigation draw on many medical specialties. They begin with surgical dissection and anatomical observation but proceed through microscopy in all its refinements to biophysics and especially biochemistry. In sum, pathology is the point of critical convergence for medicine and the biological sciences. The history of pathology treats the evolution of the concept and the development of methods appropriate to it. Consequently the history of pathology reflects the major stages in the history of western medicine and, in a broader sense, western culture.

The early history of pathology follows in the track of the history of gross anatomy, and the history of physiology provides clues to the way early students answered questions concerning the physical effects and symptoms of disease. In the Greco-Roman tradition, humoral theory (see Humors) accounted for the consequences of disease without reference to morbid anatomy. The reasoning was a priori, philosophical, and abstract. Necropsies, postmortem examinations, and cadaver dissection for scientific purpose were not commonly practiced in the Greco-Roman world. The sole significant exception was the medical center at Alexandria in Ptolemaic Egypt, where the religious prohibitions on desecrating dead bodies were relaxed to permit dissection. Vivisection on condemned criminals appears to have been practiced as well. The Alexandrian tradition, lost when the library was destroyed in 48 B.C., had very little effect on physiological thinking or the pathology it produced. Humoral doctrine dominated and continued to do so among the Christian and Islamic cultures of Europe, western Asia, and north Africa.

The first phase in the history of scientific pathology began in late medieval Europe and culminated in the eighteenth century in the work of Giovanni Battista Morgagni. During this period, the church relaxed its rules against dissection and agreed to necropsies to determine cause of death. The first documented necropsy was held in 1341. Others were authorized following the onset of the black death. Dissections for teaching purposes were permitted through the fourteenth and fifteenth centuries. In 1507, the first book on morbid anatomy appeared. This was a posthumous publication by Antonio Benivieni, a surgeon in Florence. The book, entitled *On the Hidden Causes of Disease,* gave clinical descriptions of over 100 cases with the results of 20 postmortem examinations, 10 of which Benivieni conducted personally. Benivieni is known as the founder of morbid anatomy. In Paris, Jean Fernel devoted one-third of his textbook on medical practice, published in 1554, to pathology, but his information came largely from classical sources, and Fernel himself was a humoralist. Nevertheless, he sought to correlate clinical observations with postmortem appearance while developing a method for classifying postmortem results.

Neither dissections nor postmortems were sufficient to overthrow humoralist doctrine. The new morbid anatomy was actually no more than scattered observations; the meaning of the physical changes described was entirely uncertain; and even the association of particular clinical manifestations with pathological conditions was at best tentative. Humoral theory was not just traditional. It provided explanations which adequately covered the facts as they were known. Moreover, factual results from early medical empiricism were inconclusive, a condition which even the first generation of microscopes was unable to alter. Consequently, development in pathology was glacial. There were, however, some achievements. Among these, Marcello Malpighi, the seventeenth-century anatomist, histologist, and pathologist, deserves special mention for his use of microscopic examination; Johann Wepfer continued and refined the correlation of case histories with postmortem findings; and Théophile Bonet compiled a major retrospective collection of necropsies from the preceding two centuries.

During the eighteenth century, the pace quickened, and more work on pathological subjects accumulated. The methods employed were the simple ones of describing diseased conditions in detail and correlating the descriptions with clinical evidence. It was this method which reached its most complete expression in Morgagni's massive *On the Seats and Causes of Disease,* which appeared in 1761. Morgagni was an empiricist and a quantifier who argued that the number of observations yielding the same results gave an index to the reliability of the results. Moreover, he recognized the importance of background information. His reports on cases routinely included such data as age, sex, marital status, and occupation. He also probed for previous illness, family history (to identify possible hereditary factors), and environmental conditions affecting the patient. His ultimate purpose, to which he was fanatically committed, was a comprehensive catalog of disease phenomena, cross-referenced and indexed. Though the subject was pathology, the approach was structural, static, and, at base, definitional. The concept of disease development was missing, and the vital organs provided the basis for classification.

Morgagni's contribution was to present morbid anatomy systematically as a discipline in its own right. He was a brilliant and dynamic teacher, and students flocked to him. His book was translated into English in 1769 and German in 1774; other collections appeared in subsequent years which were modeled on his. Morgagni summarized a tradition which had begun nearly 500 years before, and his work was the most comprehensive and authoritative that tradition had produced.

Rapid changes in scientific thought and cultural development overtook Morgagni's approach to morbid anatomy before the century was out. As the Morgagni method spread across Europe, the information accumulated from countless cases threw up anomalies which simple correlations between clinical observation and postmortem description could not resolve. The characteristic intestinal lesions in putrid or typhoid fevers, for example, correlated with the initial symptoms which pointed to an intestinal affection. But there were other symptoms, especially cerebral, and in 1829, Pierre Bretonneau argued that dothienenteritis (typhoid) was accompanied by an intestinal eruption but was not caused by it. Morgagni's system rested on too simple a view of cause and effect to explain these phenomena. Further observations on intestinal lesions in typhoid cases suggested a biological response in which the lesions were actually the product of a morbid process. This concept was different from the linear cause and effect implied in empirical pathology. With its introduction, the second phase of pathology's modern development began.

Dynamism and process are ideas belonging generally to the nineteenth century, though their roots are in the eighteenth. The concept of purposeful growth went back to Aristotle, but it reappeared in the early eighteenth century in Leibniz's monadology and after 1765 in Johann Gottfried von Herder's idea of "spirit of the people" (*Volksgeist*), a kind of cultural seed which controls a people's historical development. In medicine, John Hunter's lectures on surgery showed an appreciation of the developmental idea, as did his views on blood and the generation of tissues, and his nephew, Matthew Baillie, grasped fully the implications for pathology of the developmental concept when he referred to "changes of structure arising from morbid actions" and regretted that knowledge about structure was still inadequate to lead certainly "to the knowledge of morbid actions, although the one (structural change) is the effect of the other." Part of the resolution lay in reconsidering what structures were important. Traditional pathology dealt with organs. Marie François Xavier Bichat stated his belief at the opening of the nineteenth century that "the more one will observe diseases and open cadavers, the more one will be convinced of the necessity of considering local diseases not from the aspect of the complex organs but from that of the individual tissues." Bichat did not think that physics or chemistry—"the law of dead bodies"—explained the "phenomenon of living." Only "sensibility and contractability" were relevant to living tissue.

Though the classical approach to pathology retained a strong following, the idea of growth, or process, gained force to create a crisis around 1830. The Parisian pathologist Jean G. C. F. Lobstein proposed to resolve the problem by a further application of Morgagni's method which would take vital, or developmental, factors into account and would attempt to determine to what degree specific disease phenomena were attributable to structural alteration. Lobstein's ideas inspired Karl von Rokitansky in Vienna. Rokitansky was one of the best-known morbid anatomists of the day, and he built his basic studies on some 30,000 postmortems which he had performed himself together with the results of 60,000 others he had available. But Rokitansky also accepted the idea that symptoms which pertain to disease effects on vital forces could not be expected to have a local seat but would belong to some more pervasive element, probably the blood. This led him to explore altered conditions in the blood, and it was this enterprise which lay behind the foundation of the Institute of Pathologic Anatomy and Pathologic Chemistry at Vienna in 1862.

Johannes Mueller took a different and more fruitful approach. He argued in 1834 that it was necessary to go beyond autopsy to investigate the structure of altered tissues, and he took up the problem in his *On the Finer Structure and Form of Morbid Tumors* (1838). This approach reached back to Bichat's basic point, but it looked forward as well to the concept of cellular pathology, which Mueller's student, Rudolf Virchow, formulated in 1858. The idea of tissue, which had evolved from Albrecht von Haller's fibers, was revised by Theodor Schwann, who established the cell as the basic unit of normal tissues. It was further established that cells multiplied by division and that both normal and diseased cells were themselves the product of other cells. Karl Remak applied the principle of successive generation to neoplasms. Virchow synthesized these concepts, including the idea that all cells are the product of preceding cells, into a system of cellular pathology. This involved a new approach to understanding the nature of disease through microscopic analysis of cell anatomy and the changes which take place. Though the genetic, or developmental, principle had led there, Virchow's method was at base a traditional morphological one which defined and correlated pathological cell transformation with clinical symptoms. Causal relationships were implied, but while cellular pathology was brilliantly effective in describing the development of cancers, it was inadequate as a general theory of disease.

Rudolf Virchow's cellular pathology concluded the second phase of pathology's evolution. The third phase began in the fourth quarter of the nineteenth century and continues to the present. In 1877, at a meeting of the Society of German Naturalists and Physicians, the inadequacy of Virchow's cellular pathology as a general theory of disease was set against the new discoveries in bacteriology. The problem, as Edwin Klebs argued, was that cellular pathology was "a theory which does not provide clarification of the causal conditions of diseases." and (more harshly) that it was "an extreme doctrine which regards all morbid processes as purely internal events and completely neglects the importance of external factors which provoke diseases." Virchow had doubts concerning microbial disease theory which, in fact, were amply confirmed in such conditions as deficiency diseases, while the actual effects of microbial infection were found to be far more complex than the early bacteriologists thought. On the other hand, Virchow himself remained committed to a morphological approach to pathology, correlating the symptoms of disease with the observed cellular effects. His fear was that a germ theory would reawaken the concept of disease as a "living entity" which the romantic German nature philosophy had postulated at the opening of the nineteenth century, which was embodied in such popular enthusiasms as Brownianism (see Brownian System). Nevertheless, bacteriology provided the first concept of disease causation which could be demonstrated empirically. Yet the pathology of infective diseases, as of disease in general, was not automatically explained when causation had been determined. The issue of how diseases produced the deviations from normal structures and functions remained to be answered. It was necessary better to understand normal physiological function in order to grasp the body's potential for defending itself. The tools for these purposes were at hand in biochemical analysis and experimental medicine.

At the same time that the intellectual foundations for cellular pathology were developing, biochemistry and experimental medicine were coming to the fore. Animal experiments had played a part in medical research from the earliest days and were central to Galen's physiological studies. In the seventeenth century, Richard Lower carried Harvey's conclusions on circulation into a systematically developed interpretation of the effects of stagnation in the venous circulation, publishing his conclusions in 1669. Early in the eighteenth century, Johann Conrad Brunner made several discoveries pertinent to the digestive tract. After removing the pancreases from a number of dogs, for example, Brunner found them hungrier than before, perpetually thirsty, and frequently voiding urine. His dogs were, in fact, diabetic, though he lacked the chemical means even to approach that conclusion.

Experimental pathology worked best with animals, though some early experimenters used themselves as subjects. This was the case, for example, with John Hunter. Indeed, Hunter was so active an experimenter that Rudolf Virchow later credited him with founding experimental pathology; and Virchow himself, in addition to his brilliant microscopic forays, used experiments extensively to simulate disease conditions. In his study of embolisms, Virchow injected experimental animals with a variety of substances ranging from bits of real thrombi and tissue to air, starch, and even fat. This experimentation was as important for his final conclusions on embolism as was his dissection of cadavers. Other German scholars, most notably Ludwig Traube, relied heavily on experimental work, and even Vienna's Rokitansky, with tens of thousands of autopsy reports at hand, was able to assert: "Pathological anatomy applying its methods of observation and investigation to the living body, requires an experimental pathology to establish the conditions surrounding the origin, existence, and involution of the anatomical disturbances it discovers." In the twentieth century, experimental pathology has outstripped morbid anatomy and autopsy as a means for understanding the consequences of disease, a fact which indicates the importance of physiological function as opposed to static structures as pathology's primary point of attack.

Claude Bernard in France and Julius Cohnheim in Germany became the leading experimentalists of the middle nineteenth century, and their influence came to rival that of Virchow. Julius Cohnheim provided one of the critical elements in understanding inflammation, demonstrating by irritating the cornea of a frog that the corpuscles responding to the injury came from the blood, and he was able to show their actual passage through the capillary walls to the eye. This demonstration appeared to overset Virchow's conviction that local cell changes produced the reaction. As it happened, what Cohnheim demonstrated was only one part of a complex physiological process which Salomon Stricker—who was able to demonstrate cellular change before any cells could pass through the capillaries—and Elie Metchnikoff further explained. The latter's exposition of small and large phagocytes eventually gave support to both the Cohnheim and the Stricker-Virchow view. Claude Bernard studied the role of the liver in regulating sugar metabolism and laid the groundwork for understanding the so-called organs of secretion. His work on the pancreas and the vasometer mechanisms, both fundamental to physiology, also had important pathological applications.

Animal experimentation was the primary source for information on internal secretion and particularly those glands important for metabolic function: the thyroid, parathyroids, pituitary gland, pancreas, adrenals, and sex glands. Moritz Schiff created symptoms of thyroid insufficency in dogs by surgically removing the thyroid gland, and Theodor Kocher, a surgeon from Bern, reported in 1883 that humans showed the same symptoms when the thyroid was removed surgically to counter other diseases. Apart from glands, organ pathology was studied intensively in Germany, where Friedrich Theodor von Frerichs, working in Kiel, Breslau, and finally Berlin, led the way. Best known for his studies on the liver, Frerichs did his most important experimental investigations on jaundice, and he relied to such a degree on chemical analysis that he stands as one of the leaders in chemical as well as experimental pathology. His students, who included Bernhard Naunyn and Paul Ehrlich, have become synonymous with the emphasis on chemistry in understanding disease process.

Interest in the chemical composition of the body and its fluids as diagnostic indicators was integral to the early development of clinical medicine (q.v.), while the evolution of chemical analysis as a basic diagnostic tool took place in the nineteenth century. It was in this guise that chemistry supported physiology. To be more than random observation, however, chemical pathology required an institutional foundation, and it found that base in the German laboratories which developed in the second quarter of the nineteenth century. The primary influence here was Justus von Liebig and his circle of chemical physiologists. As early as 1828, Friedrich Wöhler was able to convert organic ammonium cyanate into urea, the chief end product of nitrogen metabolism in the human system. And this achievement was followed in short order by the work of Felix Hoppe-Seyler, who forwarded physiological chemistry, and Emil Fischer, the acknowledged leader in the field. Fischer, who was at Berlin, worked across the spectrum of biological chemistry, trained a number of talented students, and contributed much to the critical field of the chemistry of proteins and carbohydrates. Fischer's work helped open new avenues for understanding disease effects in the human body, most particularly the processes involved in what can be called the degenerative lesions, including necrosis, gangrene, and suppuration. Biochemistry also held the keys to immune reaction and chemotherapy (areas where Paul Ehrlich was a leading figure), calcification, and the effects of vitamin deficiencies and nutritional requirements in general, and blood chemistry radically expanded the understanding of a host of functional disorders, including uremia and diabetes. Finally, biochemistry was centrally important to the other major components in the late-nineteenth-century medical revolution, bacteriology and cell theory.

Twentieth-century pathology has shifted its geographical base from Europe to the United States and has infinitely elaborated and refined the basic areas of development created in the nineteenth century. The strong tendency to ever greater degrees of specialization in particular organ complexes characteristic of modern medicine has produced an enormous quantity of new pathological data as each specialty has developed further understanding of the disease processes peculiar to it. Generalizing concepts from studies of nutrition, immune response, or environmental factors in disease continue to reflect the enormous importance of biological chemistry for understanding relationships within the body and the disease processes which result from breakdowns in those relationships. It is in this area that pathology shows its greatest potential for achieving an advance in understanding comparable in significance to that which was won in the second half of the nineteenth century. Beyond that, modern pathology remains that branch of medicine concerned with understanding the changes disease brings about in the physiological and biochemical makeup of the human system and the structural alterations which follow. Its potential for advancing its goals has been infinitely enlarged by refinements in research technology and the multiplication of data for analysis and classification. Within the limits of the scientific approach to disease, pathology's most important unsolved problem concerns the processes involved in generating cancerous growth; and resolving that question holds a potential for reformulating the understanding of biological process itself and forcing a reconsideration of what disease as a whole may entail. Here, pathology stands in a central position among the medical disciplines, with the possibility of a major contribution to the biological sciences on which its present standing rests.

ADDITIONAL READINGS: Sir Howard Florey (ed.), *General Pathology, Based on Lectures Delivered at Sir William Dunn School of Pathology, Oxford University*, London, 1962; Jack Kevorkian, *The Story of Dissection*, New York, 1959; P. Klemperer, "Morbid Anatomy Before and After Morgagni," *Bulletin of the New York Academy of Medicine* 37 (1961): 741–760; Esmond R. Long, *History of American Pathology*, Springfield, Ill. 1962; Esmond R. Long, *History of Pathology*, London, 1928; Rudolf Virchow, *Cellular Pathology as Based upon Physiological and Pathological Histology*, Frank Chance (trans.), L. J. Rather (intro.), New York, 1971; Rudolf Virchow, *Disease, Life, and Man: Selected Essays*, L. J. Rather (trans. and intro.), Stanford, 1959.

See also: ANATOMY; BACTERIOLOGY; CANCER; CELLS; CLINICAL MEDICINE; IMMUNOLOGY; PHYSIOLOGY.

Pediatrics

Pediatrics is a modern medical specialty dealing with the care and treatment of children. Until the middle of the nineteenth century, its subject matter was intertwined with general medicine, obstetrics and midwifery, orthopedics, physical culture, and education. More recently, under the impress of disciplinary specialization and professionalization, pediatrics has focused on the care and treatment of childhood diseases outside of orthopedics while maintaining limited and necessary ties to obstetrics. The history of pediatrics is also closely associated with public health. In the eighteenth and nineteenth centuries, physicians concerned over high infant and child mortalities promoted various programs for medically sound child rearing. These efforts produced a network of institutions which had the effect of socializing basic medical knowledge.

References to child rearing and children's diseases are scattered through medical fragments remaining from the ancient world. The earliest known pediatric work is an Egyptian papyrus of the second millennium B.C. containing ritual incantations for use when a child or its mother was ill. Among later sources, the Hippocratic writers of the fourth and early third centuries in Greece provided clinical detail and therapeutic recommendations for such common children's problems as fever, diarrhea, convulsions, mouth ulcers, vomiting, and cough. Soranus of Ephesus, who wrote on obstetrics in the first half of the second century A.D., covered children's diseases and child care. Aulus Cornelius Celsus in the first century A.D. and Oribasius in the fourth included material on children in their compilations.

The most important medieval treatise on children's care was an anonymous twelfth-century Latin manuscript entitled *The Children's Practice,* whose recommendations appeared in various guises over the next 400 years. At base it was a practical guide which mixed common sense and everyday usages with bits of classical erudition.

With the advent of printing, popular works on the care and treatment of children multiplied. Paulus Bagellardus published Europe's first printed book on children's diseases at Padua in 1472, and it was followed in 1513 by Eucharius Roesslin's *Rosengarten,* a widely respected and highly influential treatise on birth and child rearing which went through more than 100 editions. Different versions were published in English, French, and Dutch, and the book was still in use in 1730. Thomas Raynalde published *Rosengarten* in England in 1540 as *The Byrth of Mankinde,* a literary and medical landmark, but Thomas Phare's *Boke of Children* (1545), the translation of an earlier French work, was the first English book to deal exclusively with children's diseases. In the same period, Ambroise Paré, France's leading surgeon, devoted whole chapters of his writings on obstetrics to the handling, care, and feeding of the newborn, and he also discussed the coughs, rashes, and diarrheas to which older children were subject.

During the seventeenth century, clinical medicine (q.v.) gave the available literature on pediatrics a new tone. Disease descriptions became more precise and discriminating, specialized works appeared, and medical statistics called attention to the high death rates among mothers, infants, and children. England's Thomas Sydenham led the way. He identified measles as a separate condition rather than a phase of smallpox, recognized and described scarlet fever as a special disease entity, and provided the first circumstantial account of chorea minor, or St. Vitus' dance. His contemporaries, Donald Whistler and Francis Glisson, established the clinical characteristics of rickets (q.v.). Whistler published first, but Glisson gave the more complete account. The most popular text on children's diseases for the late seventeenth and early eighteenth centuries was Walter Harris's *Concerning Acute Diseases in Infants* (1689), which gave detailed and useful summaries on many different conditions. Harris followed Franciscus Sylvius's system, which taught that disease resulted from a concentration of acids in the body, and he recommended an alkaline compound of his own creation which contained chalk, cuttlefish, eggshells, oyster shells, pearls, and coral. The popularity of his book was such that it was translated into several languages, and its influence was strong through the middle of the eighteenth century.

During the eighteenth and early nineteenth centuries, medical interest in pediatrics continued to expand while social institutions specifically designed for children began to appear. Enlightened spirits had been deeply shocked by the staggering infant mortality rates recorded routinely in Europe's major cities. One mid-century estimate for London claimed that mortality among children ages 1 to 10 exceeded 80 percent, while the death rates before the age of 1 were undoubtedly higher. One answer was to provide care for children whose parents could not or would not care for them; another was to publicize the best methods for child rearing to assist concerned parents and to inform ignorant ones. Chartered by Thomas Coram in 1739, the London Foundling Hospital opened in 1745, and a hospital physician, William Cadogan published *An Essay upon Nursing and the Management of Children from Their Birth Through Three Years of Age* in 1750. Cadogan argued that infants were human beings with a right to life and liberty, that parents and society were obligated to protect that right, and that proper attention to the infant's health was a necessary first step. Cadogan criticized close-swaddling, strongly supported breast-feeding, and filled his treatise with practical advice on diet, clothing, cleanliness, and exercise.

Twenty-four years after the foundling hospital opened, George Armstrong founded his Dispensary for the Infant Poor, where in the course of 12 years he distributed advice and medicines to over 35,000 children. Public subscriptions failed to support the dispensary, and Armstrong carried the financial burden himself until 1783, when he was finally unable to meet his expenses, and the institution closed. Its example, however, inspired John Bunnell Davis, who initiated the modern approach to child hygiene and public health nursing. Davis opened a new children's dispensary in 1816, and in 1817 he published his *Cursory Inquiry into Some of the Principal Causes of Mortality Among Children,* in which he laid down his conviction that infant mortality owed in great part to mothers' ignorance of sound health practices. He used the dispensary as a command post from which trained volunteers went out to counsel and assist new mothers. Young physicians studied with him, and at the middle of the century the dispensary became the Royal Waterloo Hospital for Children and Women, the main center for British pediatric training.

Other developments important for pediatrics occurred contemporaneously. Nicholas Andry, a French physician interested in the causes of deformity in children, concluded that mishandling and improper care were responsible in many cases, and he wrote a treatise entitled *Orthopedics or the Art of Preventing and Correcting Deformities of the Body in Children* (1741). His countryman Jean Charles des Essartz took the broader view in a study published in 1760 that correct physical training in childhood was essential for healthy adults. He wrote just two years before the appearance of Jean Jacques Rousseau's *Émile,* which presented a new theory of child development and education, combining prescriptions for physical, moral, and intellectual training. Rousseau marked the culmination of a major change in attitudes toward childhood which had been in process for at least a century and which emphasized preserving and developing the individual child as a unique and important being.

Clinical studies on children's diseases continued to multiply. In Sweden, Dr. Nils Rosen von Rosenstein published a pediatric handbook in 1765; in 1784 England's Michael Underwood published his *Treatise on the Diseases of Children.* This was destined to be the most influential English work in the field of pediatrics until the middle of the nineteenth century. Underwood was a London physician specializing in children's diseases, obstetrics, and gynecology. Entirely clinical in his approach, he produced the first published descriptions of scleremia and malignant familial jaundice in the newborn, while the 1799 edition included a section on congenital heart disease in children. The same edition also discussed the chemistry of milk. In the early nineteenth century, French physicians contributed new disease classifications and important single disease discoveries. Of the latter, one of the most important came in 1826 when Pierre Bretonneau definitively separated diphtheria (q.v.) from scarlet fever, named the disease, and performed the first successful tracheotomy for a diphtheria patient. In 1828, Charles Michel Billard introduced autopsies correlated with clinical findings to found a new classification of children's diseases, while Frédéric Rilliet and Antoine Charles Barthez published their authoritative *Clinical and Practical Treatise on Children's Diseases* (1838–1843). Poliomyelitis (q.v.) was beginning to attract attention as a disease syndrome, and in 1840 Jacob von Heine and Oscar Medin separated its effects from those of other diseases and described them. Polio was known for some years as Heine-Medin disease.

In the later nineteenth century, pediatrics advanced with the general growth of professional and scientific medicine. The germ theory of disease, immunization, and a better understanding of nutritional balance and the pathological consequences of vitamin deficiencies, together with the definitive identification of causal organisms in a host of children's diseases, provided unprecedentedly powerful tools for promoting children's health. Modern hospitals offered improved facilities for children's care, while a growing band of specialists in children's diseases was available to treat them. At the same time, a complex institutional structure was coming into existence to serve pediatrics and to socialize the results of its scientific work.

During the French Revolution, when good health was portrayed as the citizens' right and children were considered the basis for the republic's future, a national health program was drafted which provided both maternal and child care. Only fragments of the plan were implemented. In the German states, Johann Peter Frank, the leading authority on public health and sanitary police, promoted statistical studies on birthrates and infant mortality as well as health education, and B. C. Faust, a German physician, compiled a handbook for school use in 1794 called *The Catechism of Health,* which was widely distributed through state agencies. Nevertheless, centralized health programs on a national level remained for the future, and local initiatives dominated social action on children's health. In France, for example, in 1854, the mayor of the village of Villiers-le-Duc offered a bounty to every mother who kept her child alive through his or her first birthday. Advice on winning the bounty stressed cleanliness and correct diet, and though the villagers had little beyond intuition to assist them, they worked to such good effect that infant mortality declined by one-third, from 300 per 1000 live births to 200. The program was renewed in a far more ambitious form in 1893. As soon as pregnancy was established, the expectant mother was placed under a physician's care, regular examinations and consultations followed, and when the baby was born, it was examined and weighed every two weeks. The baby was breastfed for its first year, and the village maintained a herd of cows to provide clean milk for mothers and children. Infant mortality from 1893 to 1903 in Villiers-le-Duc was recorded at zero.

Other communities stopped short of this example, but there was widespread interest in milk stations and consultation centers. In 1859 the New York Infirmary for Women and Children began to recruit "sanitary visitors" to instruct poor women on the most recent methods of caring for infants and children. In 1874, the New York Health Department prepared an instructional pamphlet for distribution to mothers, and two years later it organized teams to identify and treat cases of summer diarrhea. A milk station was set up in 1878. Pierre Budin, professor of obstetrics at the University of Paris, laid down a plan for a national system of consulting centers in 1892. By 1907 there were 497 such centers throughout France. In the same period, two Parisian pediatricians, J. Cornby and Gaston Variot, organized the systematic development of clean milk stations, and in 1893, Nathan Strauss brought the system to New York. By 1902 it provided a monthly total of 250,000 bottles of milk. The milk station idea spread through Europe from Germany to Spain, and it was enthusiastically received in England in 1899. The first German consultation center was organized in Berlin in 1905; 73 more consultation centers and 17 milk stations appeared over the next two years; by 1910 there were over 300 infant welfare centers, staffed by volunteers from the Society for Infant Welfare.

The formal organization of child hygiene and welfare work began in 1908 when New York City set up a division of child hygiene under the city health department. This division, the work of S. Josephine Baker, a physician and child health inspector, was the first of its kind in the world. It became a much-imitated model for other cities in the United States and abroad. The Baker approach was not unlike that of the early dispensaries in England. Prevention was considered the key to reducing infant mortality. New mothers were identified from the municipal birth registers, and a public health nurse was dispatched to visit and, if necessary, to educate the mother on how to keep her baby well. The results were astounding. Twelve hundred fewer deaths were recorded in the visited districts than in the previous summer, with control over summer diarrhea being a major factor. Nutrition also improved as the division's milk station sold milk prepared for babies at a lower price than store milk. The milk station was also used for on-the-spot consultations.

The New York experience inspired other cities and states, but it had resonance on the national level as well. In 1912, the federal government established the U. S. Children's Bureau to collect information on conditions among children and to make that information generally available. Two health activists, Florence Kelley and Lillian Wald, conceived the idea of the bureau and sponsored its development. The bureau specialized in prenatal and maternal care. In France, Adolph Pinard organized a "maternal dispensary" in 1890, and a similar institution appeared in London the following year. By 1942 nearly 75 percent of British mothers had received prenatal care, and the number rose further after 1945. The U. S. Children's Bureau published a pamphlet on prenatal care in 1913 which became one of the government's most popular publications, and the bureau initiated a strong publicity campaign to remove births from the home to the hospitals. As late as 1935, two-thirds of the babies born in the United States were born outside hospitals, but the picture then changed radically, and in 1956 95 percent were born in hospitals, with physicians attending in 97 percent of the cases. In the last two decades, mounting hospital costs and a growing conviction that "interventionist medicine" adversely affects family cohesion have somewhat eroded the belief that hospital medicine is necessary for a baby's healthy start in life, and natural childbirth and birth at home have come to be highly prized.

As education became public, schools took on an increasing role in children's health. General legislation in the first half of the nineteenth century attempted to make the French schools responsible for health and hygiene, but the effort failed. Physical inspections were established in 1842, however, and school medical inspectors were provided in 1879. In Germany, Hermann Cohn of Breslau gave eye examinations to schoolchildren beginning in 1866. He tested the sight of 7568 children and opened the way to further studies on the health of school-age children. School medical services were organized in New York starting in 1871. Similar institutions appeared in Europe in the next two decades, and the National Educational Act set up a medical department for the board of education in Great Britain in 1907. The national school lunch program began in the United States in 1938, and the National School Lunch Act, passed in 1946, provided grants-in-aid for state-administered school lunch programs. Similar plans were put into effect in other nations.

Until the end of the nineteenth century, there was relatively little medicine could do to cure children's diseases. The same, of course, was true for adult diseases. Interest in physical training and nutrition preceded the knowledge of physiology and biochemistry necessary to make it effective. The sanitary movement and social medicine undoubtedly bettered conditions in hospitals and asylums while promoting improvements in city living, but their systematic development required the germ theory of disease, bacteriology, and immunology. Though pediatrics began to be taught as a special discipline in the middle of the nineteenth century, it was not until the end of the century that pediatricians were able to deal effectively with childhood diseases. The rate of advance after 1900, however, was relatively rapid, and by 1950 nutritional research, hospital medicine, antibiotics and penicillin, effective antisepsis, immunization, and a battery of supporting diagnostic, therapeutic, and surgical techniques made bearing and raising children safer than at any time in history.

As the elevated child mortalities of preceding generations have declined, recent debates have centered on the high costs of keeping premature or deformed babies alive. The medical technology for child care has reached an extraordinary level of sophistication. Supporting institutions on municipal, regional, and national levels have developed concomitantly. The main issues for the present and future of child care concern maintaining public health and health delivery systems already in place in the world's advanced societies while creating the institutions necessary to channel modern knowledge to the families needing it in less affluent and advanced societies. Pediatrics, like modern medicine in general, finds its strongest contemporary challenges on the social rather than the medico-scientific side. There is little evidence from the 1980s that the intensity of those challenges will abate.

ADDITIONAL READINGS: A. F. Abt, *Abt-Garrison History of Pediatrics*, Philadelphia, 1965; Joan Bel Geddes, *Small World: A History of Baby Care from the Stone Age to the Spock Age*, New York, 1964; Thomas E. Cone, *A History of American Pediatrics*, Boston, 1979; George Rosen, *A History of Public Health*, New York, 1957; George Frederick Still, *The History of Pediatrics: The Progress of the Study of Diseases of Children up to the End of the Eighteenth Century*, London, 1931, 1965.

See also: GYNECOLOGY; MIDWIFERY; specific disease articles.

Pellagra

Pellagra is a niacin deficiency disease whose symptoms include severe symmetrical dermatitis, diarrhea, and mental changes. It affects only people whose staple grain is maize (American corn), and it has had a serious incidence through southern, central, and eastern Europe, in Egypt, in the southern United States, and in central and south Africa. Pellagra does not appear in the medical classics, and its first detailed description dates to 1763 when a Spanish physician, Julian F. N. Casal, not only portrayed pellagra accurately but associated it with the maize-based diets of poverty-ridden Asturian peasants. Since maize was brought to the old world from the new, pellagra is a relatively recent disease problem.

Pellagra has been closely identified with Italy, and the word itself is Italian for "sour skin." But pellagra was also known in Europe as "the maize disease," and it was thought that under certain circumstances maize produced a toxin which poisoned those consuming it. A minority held the view that pellagra was a product of poverty and that an improved and balanced diet, together with better living conditions, was needed to counteract its effects. The toxin theory was the more popular, and in France it led to a successful governmental campaign against maize. Pellagra simply disappeared by the end of the nineteenth century. In Italy, pellagra seemed to be associated with spoiled maize, and it was declared illegal to sell the grain in a wet or moldy state. This created hardship for the peasants, however, and the government established public maize driers, or dessicators, throughout the countryside to remove excess moisture. In addition, the government subsidized rural bakeries to provide inexpensive wheat bread for the public. These efforts, though based on misperceptions, effectively reduced pellagra's incidence in Italy, and by 1928, the disease was largely under control.

A particularly serious pellagra epidemic occurred in the southern United States in 1907. The peak was reached between 1928, when 6969 deaths were recorded, and 1930, when it was estimated that there were 20,000 cases in the state of Georgia alone. After 1930, the case incidence fell dramatically, and by the end of the decade, pellagra was no longer a problem. The outbreak resulted from a nearly exclusive concentration on cash crops, most notably cotton, and the parallel decline of food crops for personal consumption. Cornmeal (from maize) was the diet staple for poor whites and blacks alike, and it was supported by salt pork, lard, and molasses. This diet was hardly adequate, but it had been made worse at the turn of the century when coarse-ground cornmeal gave way to a fine, machine-ground variety from which the available niacin was removed in the milling process. In 1912, Joseph Goldberger of the U.S. Public Health Service proved that pellagra was a deficiency disease caused by the absence of a "pellagra-preventive," or P-P. In 1927, the U.S. Agricultural Extension Service opened a campaign to convince farmers that they had to begin raising food crops for their own use and diversify their diets. This campaign was aided by the collapse of the cotton market and the onset of the depression. Cotton acreage declined sharply; food production for home consumption rose; diets improved; and as the extension service program heightened public awareness of diet and proper food preparation, pellagra disappeared. The pellagra-preventive was finally identified in 1937 as nicotinic acid, or niacin, but by then the pellagra battle had already been won. After 1937, it became possible to add further protection by enriching cornmeal with niacin, while economic growth in the period since World War II has changed the socioeconomic character of the south and has made the possibility of another pellagra outbreak remote.

Pellagra also declined in eastern Europe through the era of World War II. Rumania recorded 55,013 cases with 1654 deaths in 1932, but the disease almost entirely disappeared over the next three decades. A similar pattern appeared in Yugoslavia, and in Egypt as well. The causes for this development appear to have been an improvement in living standards, and especially the diversification of diet. Food enrichment was not a factor. Pellagra remains a problem, however, among the maize-eating peoples of sub-Saharan Africa and in parts of India where *Sorghum vulgare* is eaten. There are some maize eaters for whom pellagra is not a problem. The Indians of the Yucatán, for example, eat a maize-based diet, yet they are free of pellagra. The reason may be that they soak the grain in a solution of water and lime which liberates the "bound" niacin; it may also owe to the beans they eat with the cornmeal. It is now believed that as living standards rise and as diversified diets become more widely available, pellagra will cease to be a significant public health problem anywhere.

ADDITIONAL READINGS: W. R. Aykroyd, *Conquest of Deficiency Diseases: Achievements and Prospects*, Geneva, 1970; Kenneth J. Carpenter (ed.), *Pellagra, Benchmark Papers in Biochemistry*, vol. 2, Stroudsburg, Pa., 1981; H. F. Harris, *Pellagra*, New York, 1919; Daphne A. Roe, *A Social History of Pellagra*, Ithaca, N.Y., 1973.

See also DEFICIENCY DISEASES; VITAMINS.

Penicillin

Penicillin was the first of the modern antibiotics to be discovered, and it remains the most important single remedy available for a long list of diseases caused by bacteria. Penicillins are natural by-products from molds of the genus *Penicillium* in the process of growth. They are also produced by *Aspergillus*- and *Cephalosporium*-type molds. There are hundreds of species of molds that are classified *Penicillium,* and each species produces several strains. Hence there are literally thousands of "penicillins" in the world. Both ancient medical texts and folk traditions recommend the use of molds, especially in wound dressings, but there is no known connection between these folk practices and the modern discovery of penicillin, which was strictly a twentieth-century achievement.

The history of penicillin is marked throughout by coincidence and luck, but there was hard, systematic research as well. Sir Alexander Fleming, a Scottish bacteriologist working in the Inoculation Division of St. Mary's Hospital, London, is the man credited with identifying penicillin. Fleming did important work on wounds and natural resistance to infection during World War I, demonstrating that the harsh antiseptics used to cleanse wounds damaged natural defenses against infection while failing to destroy the bacterial causes for infection. In 1922, he identified the enzyme lysozyme, a component in tears and most of the mucous fluids in animal and human bodies and a substantial element in egg albumin. This substance was not effective against pathogenic bacteria. It is, however, part of the body's defense system, coming in to play before immune reactions are triggered and functioning in exposed areas where there is no blood supply. Fleming was opposed in general to chemotherapy, holding to the view that once infection had entered the body, it was the body which would have to contain it. He was not, however, dogmatic on the point. One of his earliest assignments at St. Mary's was to administer Paul Ehrlich's Salvarsan treatment, introduced by the director, Almroth Wright, in consequence of his personal friendship with Ehrlich. Lysozyme was a different matter, belonging to that class of substances which bodies produced in their reactions against outside intrusions.

The identification of penicillin came at the end of August or the beginning of September 1928, just six years after the lysozyme discovery. The exact date remains stubbornly obscure. After a brief holiday, Fleming was inspecting various cultures left in petri dishes in his St. Mary's workroom. A mold had appeared on one which seemed to have destroyed staphylococcus colonies on the same dish. The reaction caught Fleming's eye. He took scrapings of the mold and, after some preliminary investigation, published a paper in 1929 describing the event and identifying the mold (incorrectly, as it happened) as *Penicillium rubrum.* His authority here was the mycologist C. J. La Touche, who was also working in the inoculation department. The fact that the mold was actually *Penicillium notatum* made no real difference in subsequent developments.

Fleming's paper, which appeared in the *British Journal of Experimental Pathology,* contained two important points. First, it was clear that not all forms of penicillium molds produced bacteria-inhibiting penicillin. Fleming had noted a fact of real significance. Second, he pointed out that while the penicillin strongly affected such gram-positive bacteria as staphylococci, streptococci, gonococci, meningococci, diptheria bacillus, and pneumococci, it had no toxic effect at all on regular tissues and did not interfere with leukocytic, or white cell, defense functions. This point was doubly important in the light of Fleming's general views on chemotherapy and wound treatment. Penicillin appeared to be strong and safe. On the less desirable side, penicillin had no effect on gram-negative bacteria, including those responsible for cholera and bubonic plague. Worse, penicillin was difficult to produce, it was very unstable, it required special care, and while it appeared to be useful for wound dressings or laboratory functions, it was altogether too difficult to use to be practical clinically.

Although the point was not publicized until 40 years later, Fleming was never able to recreate the reactions he observed under the circumstances he described, nor was anyone else able to do so, though many tried. Moreover, among the many ironies and coincidences in the penicillin story, not the least was that whatever Fleming may have seen, his belief that the penicillin was directly attacking the staphylococcus colonies was incorrect. The discovery, in fact, included a misinterpretation of the event described.

Alexander Fleming did relatively little with penicillin in succeeding years, and the scientific community in general paid little heed to what had been reported. In 1938, however, a team of young scientists at Oxford, led by the pathologist Howard W. Florey and the emigré biochemist Ernst B. Chain, began to organize a long-term research project which included a major section on microbial antagonisms. Florey, who had studied in the United States and had contacts there, was encouraged by the Rockefeller Foundation to apply for a research grant. The application was filed on November 20, 1939, and the proposal was funded early the following year. Penicillin was one substance among many the group intended to study, and the first work done on it was under the false assumption that penicillin, like lysozyme, was an enzyme. The Oxford group used molds from the original Fleming *Penicillium,* and while early tests produced unimpressive results, progress was made toward a reliable method for assaying the level of penicillin present and assigning a stable measure. By 1940, the technique for extracting, purifying, and stabilizing penicillin for laboratory work had been achieved. This was a major step, because the difficulties of working with the substance had been one reason for Alexander Fleming's pessimism about its clinical value.

The first laboratory tests for effectiveness followed, but on a very small scale. Four laboratory mice were injected with penicillin after being infected with a strong streptococcus strain. Four other mice were infected as controls. Two of the penicillin-treated mice survived, and two died though they resisted the infection. The four control animals were dead in less than 24 hours. Though the test was a limited one, it appeared then, as Florey put it, that "penicillin was a chemotherapeutic drug of great power" which not only did not damage the host's cells in its successful attack on bacteria but would "stop the growth of bacteria in all parts of the body." It was, in fact, a systemic agent.

Penicillin was first injected into a human patient on January 27, 1941. The woman who received the initial 100 milligrams had no infection. She reacted to the injection with a rising temperature followed by symptoms of rigor. A second trial produced the same result, which was then traced to a pyrogen in the substance which was not, however, associated with the therapeutic agent and which could be separated by chromotography. Testing in rabbits identified the pyrogen's presence, and subsequently such testing became mandatory for all clinical penicillin.

The first penicillin treatment began on February 1, 1941, when a policeman with an advanced staphylococcus infection complicated by streptococcus was given penicillin for five days. Though his condition was desperate, with terrible abscesses and deep bone damage, one eye destroyed and his lungs becoming affected, the treatment momentarily arrested the progress of the infection, and the patient began to recover. Unfortunately, the supply of penicillin available was limited, and when it was gone, there was no way to replenish it quickly. The patient began to lose ground, fell into a relapse, and died. It was clear that when penicillin was given in massive doses, it could deal with the most difficult infection, but that its administration had to continue until the disease was eliminated.

Treating adults with the limited quantities available would invite another tragedy, so the group turned to children on the assumption that the smaller body mass would require less of the precious substance. Between February and June, five children were treated. All were at a stage where normal therapies had failed, yet only one failed to recover, and the child who died was proved on postmortem examination to be free of the infective bacteria. He died from an arterial rupture in the head. These cases showed that huge doses of penicillin were not toxic, that recovery began almost immediately, and that the most difficult infection could be treated successfully. They also showed that treatment had to be continued until the disease was extirpated, and that for general use, far larger stocks of penicillin were needed than could be produced with known laboratory methods.

Although World War II had begun in September 1939, a period of quiet set in following the German-Soviet partition of Poland. Then, in April 1940, the German assault on western Europe began, which resulted in the occupation of Norway, Denmark, the Netherlands, and Belgium, the fall of France, and the evacuation of the British expeditionary force from Dunkirk. A German cross-channel invasion of Britain was feared. Against this backdrop, the work of the Oxford group seemed of small significance, and neither the British government nor the British pharmaceutical industry responded to requests for help in developing the technology for mass production of penicillin. There was some interest in the substance in the United States, however. Florey's initial reports led to requests for penicillin cultures, and Martin Dawson, working at Columbia Presbyterian Medical Center in New York, had produced penicillin and tried it on patients even before the Oxford group carried out their clinical applications. The Rockefeller grant also meant American connections for the British scientists.

During the summer of 1941, Florey and Norman C. H. Heatley, an expert on microtechnique, visited the United States to work on developing methods for producing penicillin in quantity. Their reception was mixed, but the U.S. Department of Agriculture was interested and referred them to their Northern Regional Research Laboratory in Peoria, Illinois, where work was going forward on fermentation processes. Heatley worked for several weeks with the Peoria group, and three major developments emerged. First, it was discovered that penicillin yield could be increased 10 times by adding corn steep liquor, a by-product of cornstarch manufacture, to the culture medium. Second, a systematic search for variants on Fleming's *Penicillium* uncovered far more productive strains. Finally, a beginning was made on a new process for growing penicillin mold in deep tanks rather than on the surface of media in shallow dishes. These developments from the corn-producing American middle west opened the way to mass production of penicillin.

The American pharmaceutical industry, under prodding from Alfred N. Richards, chairman of the Committee on Medical Research of the Office of Scientific Research and Development, began to take an interest in penicillin. Richards, who knew and was impressed by Florey's work, convinced three major houses, Merck and Company, E. R. Squibb and Sons, and the Charles Pfizer Company, that they should cooperate in developing penicillin. Richards appears to have been influenced by penicillin's potential as a military medicine at a time when war was threatening. By December 1941, when Japanese attacks on Hawaii and the Philippines brought the United States into the war, the groundwork had been laid for mass production of penicillin. Nearly three more years were necessary, however, before the quantities needed were actually made. In early 1943, penicillin production in the United States was barely sufficient to treat 100 persons, but by 1944, production had escalated to 300 billion units per month. When the Allies invaded Europe in June 1944, there was sufficient penicillin on hand to treat all severe casualties among the American and British invading forces. By the time the war ended in Europe in May 1945, all military needs could be met, and penicillin was coming onto the civilian market.

While production expanded, the evidence was mounting that penicillin was uniquely effective. The testing begun in 1942 repeatedly demonstrated penicillin's powers, especially when injected and used systemically. So, for example, in one group of 91 patients suffering from staphylococcal infections with bacteremia present, penicillin treatment held the mortality to 40 percent. Normally, all of those patients would have been expected to die. Forty-eight of 55 patients with osteomyelitis either recovered or improved, and good results on streptococcal and gonococcal infections resistant to sulfonamides were reported. In 1943, John F. Mahoney of the U.S. Public Health Service found penicillin highly effective in treating syphilis, and in the last year of the war, penicillin contributed to a radical rise in the rate of recovery from battle wounds, which approached an unheard-of 95 percent.

The development of penicillin gave rise to controversies and, in one case, charges of sharp practice and unprofessional behavior. One member of the Peoria Department of Agriculture research team, Andrew J. Moyer, who worked closely with Norman Heatley in the early stages of the Peoria project, later used his special knowledge to acquire United Kingdom patents on corn steep liquor and other elements in the media used to cultivate penicillin. The Oxford group had taken no patents on the grounds that public funds had led to the development of penicillin and the public should have the benefit. This stand provided no protection for British rights, however, and when Moyer was able to use his patent claims to divert what was alleged to be millions from the British economy, the Oxford scientists were criticized for not protecting British interests. Though Moyer would have been in violation of the law had he sought American patents for processes on which he worked while an employee of the U.S. government, he was within his rights in acquiring British patents. For many, however, the millions in royalties which he gained were tainted by what was widely interpreted as an action of doubtful morality.

A longer-lived controversy developed over the question of priority in discovery of penicillin.

Though Fleming, Florey, and Chain were given a joint Nobel prize, there has been a considerable argument over the public image of Fleming's role. The historical records now clear, and the different contributions made by the leading figures are hardly in doubt. Alexander Fleming identified penicillin, preserved the mold, and called attention to its properties. Florey and the Oxford circle developed penicillin, first as one of a group of substances with antibiotic potential and later as a positive chemotherapeutic agent of power and importance. Though the contributions differed, and the exaggerated reverence for Sir Alexander Fleming as the sole or primary contributor to penicillin's development is not justified, it is clear that he can no more be written out of the story or reduced to a peripheral role than can his Oxford colleagues. There is credit enough for all to share while appreciating the special character of each contribution.

With widespread use, and early abuse, penicillin itself has been brought into medical perspective. Early in 1942 it was observed that some staphylococcus strains resisted penicillin, excreting a substance called penicillinase, an enzyme which deactivated the penicillin action. In subsequent years, it was noted that resistant staphylococcus survived, multiplied, and passed the characteristic on, and that people working in hospitals were likely to harbor resistant varieties. By the early 1950s, this led to rigid aseptic procedures in hospitals to reduce the chance of communicating resistant staphylococcus, and with the help of newer antibiotics, an equilibrium was reached.

Resistance also began to appear in 1946 among gonococcal strains. The gonococcus had been one of the most susceptible to penicillin action, but by 1960 British physicians were using 50 times the dosage which had earlier sufficed to cure gonorrhea, and in 1976, strains of gonococci were identified which could only be affected by concentrations of penicillin too high to be obtained through blood and tissue. Syphilis has shown a similar resistance, and the two phenomena together added to the difficulty of resisting the burgeoning venereal disease problem of the 1970s.

Finally, though penicillin is not toxic for most people under most conditions, the enormous dosages required for some diseases can damage the liver and the brain. This problem has been eased by combining penicillin with other antibiotics. In 1949, however, it was shown that penicillin also set off violent allergic reactions which could be fatal. This fact, together with the resistance factor, has led to practicing greater discretion in prescribing penicillin, limiting its use to those conditions which positively require it, using smaller doses, and attempting to identify penicillin allergies in individuals before treatment is needed.

The development of other antibiotic drugs has removed some of the pressure from penicillin, and there are many conditions for which it is useless. Even so, penicillin is the best cure for a considerable number of diseases, and the only cure for some. Together with the sulfonamides and other antibiotics, penicillin fulfills the hope for effective cures of bacterial diseases which was first voiced when bacteriologists proved the germ theory of disease in the last quarter of the nineteenth century. In societies where such remedies are available, as well as the people and the institutions needed to produce and administer them, it is possible to speak of curing disease and to mean it. This development is one of the most radical changes to have occurred in human history, and penicillin has contributed significantly to it.

ADDITIONAL READINGS: Helmuth M. Boettcher, *Miracle Drugs: A History of Antibiotics*, Einhart Krawer (trans.), London, 1963; H. F. Dowling, *Fighting Infection: Conquests of the Twentieth Century*, Cambridge, Mass., 1977; Sir Alexander Fleming, *Penicillin: Its Practical Application*, London, 1946; H. W. Florey, E. Chain, et al., *Antibiotics: A Survey of Penicillin, Streptomycin, and Other Antimicrobial Substances from Fungi, Actinomycetes, Bacteria, and Plants*, 2 vols., London, New York, and Toronto, 1949; Robert G. MacFarlane, *Howard Florey: The Making of a Great Scientist*, Oxford, 1979; André Maurois, *The Life of Sir Alexander Fleming, Discoverer of Penicillin*, Gerard Hopkins (trans.), London, 1959; John C. Sheehan, *The Enchanted Ring; The Untold Story of Penicillin*, Cambridge, Mass., 1982; Gordon T. Stewart, *The Penicillin Group of Drugs*, Amsterdam, London, and New York, 1965; David Wilson, *Penicillin in Perspective*, London, 1976.

See also ANTIBIOTICS; CHEMOTHERAPY; SULFONAMIDES.

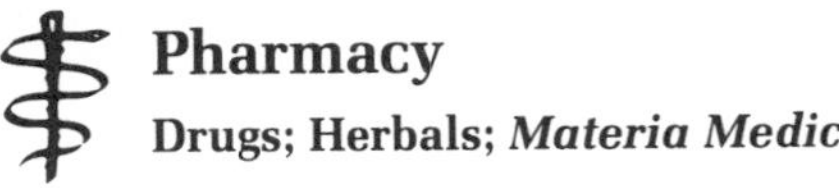

Pharmacy

Drugs; Herbals; *Materia Medica*

The Ancient Heritage Pharmacy is a modern profession with an ancient tradition whose history begins with the human being's first efforts to find materials in nature to control or relieve the effects of disease. How that search began can only be surmised, since the oldest surviving written sources are from the beginning of the third millennium B.C. Those sources, however, reveal a fully developed tradition in which natural products are used for specific medical purposes.

The oldest source for pharmacy may be the original of the great Chinese herbal compilation, or *Ben cao,* which has been attributed to the semilegendary emperor Shennong (ca. 2700 B.C.) and contains both a classification of medicinal plants and a guide to medical compounds. Cuneiform clay tablets found in the library of King Ashurbanipal near Nineveh record the *materia medica* used in the Mesopotamian cultures of Sumer, Akkad, Babylon, and Assyria between the fourth and first millennia B.C. Of 30,000 tablets found, 800 deal with drugs or drug preparations. The collection dates from about 500 B.C., but the information is of indeterminate age. The tablets refer to vegetable drugs, 150 mineral drugs, and a variety of substances with medical uses, including alcoholic drinks, fats and oils, animal parts and milk, and honey and wax. Instructions for compounding and administering drugs show familiarity with some chemical principles and complex refining procedures.

The Egyptian medical papyri, particularly the Ebers papyrus (ca. 1550 B.C.), provide further insight into ancient pharmacy. About 700 drugs and 800 compounds are mentioned, with botanicals far outnumbering animal or mineral substances. Most of the methods used today for administering drugs appear, while compounds and doses are given in stated units, commonly a measure rather than a weight. Drug preparations were probably made by specialists who oversaw the work of technical assistants. Hindu medical texts are also rich in pharmaceutical data. In the *Susruta-Samhita* (ca. A.D. 450), a major Brahmanic medical text, there are references to more than 700 drugs. Some have been identified with China, others with Iran. India was a pharmaceutical crossroads, receiving materials and ideas from both east and west Asia. It is less clear to what degree Indian pharmacy and medicine may have influenced Mediterranean culture in the classical period.

The Greco-Roman Era The Greek tradition was the beginning point for European pharmacy. Greek culture had a strong drug orientation, especially in religious practices. The Dionysian revelers combined hallucinogens with alcohol, and hypnotics, or somnifacients, were probably used in the Asclepian temple practice. It is believed that Greek pharmacy drew on Egyptian and west Asian sources, since they recommend similar medications. The Hippocratic writings, compiled in the fifth and fourth centuries B.C., contain a variety of recommended drugs and other substances. Even though Hippocratic medicine stressed diet rather than drug intervention, there are more than 200 specific preparations mentioned as well as pharmaceutical processes including the preparation of fomentations, gargles, pessaries, pills, ointments, and oils.

A class of pharmaceutical botanists called *rizotomoi* (Greek for "root mass") collected indigenous roots and plants and sold them for medications as well as food. They also classified herbs and herbal cures. Among the most important of these naturalists were Diocles of Carystos, who lived in the fourth century B.C., and Crataeus, who produced the first-known illustrated herbal. His drawings of medicinal plants were used in Dioscorides's *materia medica* (A.D. 60). Dioscorides was the most influential and respected of the pharmaco-botanists. His *Materia Medica in Five Books* has been called "an intellectual milestone in the development of pharmacy and botany." It was translated into English in 1665 and is still in print.

The Greek tradition in pharmacy, as in medicine generally, was synthesized in the writings of Galen of Pergamum in the second century A.D. Galen followed a humoral physiology in which balance among the body's constituent elements was critical for health. He was interested in the humoral effects of different drugs, and he developed a classification system based on those effects which presented 473 different drugs and a number of formulas. Galen prepared his own materials. Many Roman physicians went to compounding specialists called *pigmentarii,* but Galen criticized the practice. In fact, preparing and selling drug preparations was an important business in both Greece and Rome. There are more than a dozen terms to identify these entrepreneurs, and it appears that they sold directly to the public as well as to physicians.

Roman encyclopedic writers preserved substantial parts of the classic tradition. Among these, Aulus Cornelius Celsus and Paul of Aegina were particularly important. Celsus, who wrote in the first century B.C., was rediscovered and his *De medicina* republished under the sponsorship of Pope Nicholas V (1478) at a time when no other classic book on medicines was in print. Paul of Aegina, who lived in Alexandria in the seventh century A.D., gave a comprehensive review of Greco-Roman medications in his *Seven Books on Medicine*. His sources included Dioscorides, Galen, and Oribasius of Pergamum. His work became widely known in the late medieval and early modern period. These works, together with Galen, Pliny's natural history, and the dispensatory of Scribonius Largus, compiled in A.D. 43, were among the most important sources from which Europe drew its later knowledge of classical pharmacy.

The Medieval World Between the fifth and eleventh centuries, the classical pharmaceutical tradition virtually disappeared in western Europe. Monastic medicine produced a practical literature which included some prescriptions, while the so-called leech-books, that is, handbooks for a basic medical practice which appeared in vernacular languages, gave lists of indigenous botanical drugs with instructions for their preparation and use. In the eleventh century, Odo of Meune, the abbot of Beauprai, used Latin sources and possibly translations of Arab works to produce a poem on the properties of drugs which has been termed the first independent herbal written in the medieval west. The abbess Hildegard of Bingen (1098–1179) also produced two treatises on health and medications entitled *Physica* and *Causes and Cures*. These works were actually the first tentative beginnings of a new pharmaceutical literature.

The most important influence on medieval pharmacy came from the Arab world, where the classic Greek tradition was synthesized with west Asian influences. Eighth- and ninth-century Arabic works treating drugs and their uses showed a high degree of specialization and greatly expanded the quantity of recommended drugs and their classification. General works on medicine compiled in the tenth and eleventh centuries contained pharmaceutical sections which included this new material. The most important general works were those of al-Ràzi (Rhazes), Ali Ibn 'Abbas (Haly Abbas), Abu-l-Qasim al-Zahrawi (Albucasis), and Ibn Sìnà (Avicenna).

The Arab works reached western Europe through Spain, southern Italy and Sicily, and the Byzantine empire. The Salerno school of medicine, founded in the eighth century, was particularly important. It was there that works based on Arab sources first appeared when the Jewish scholar Donnolo published his *antidotarium* in the tenth century. In the eleventh century, a man known as Constantine the African appeared at Salerno to begin translating Arab manuscripts into Latin. He translated whole treatises, not just fragments, making entire works available to western scholars. Salerno also produced the most popular health and cure book of the Middle Ages. Entitled *Regimen sanitatis,* this book was a collection of dietary and pharmaceutical rules written in verse. The original version contained 364 lines. It was annotated and edited by Arnold of Villanova, a leading physician with strong chemical interests, and the book attained a tremendous popularity. After the invention of the printing press, it was published in all major European languages, and it ran through more than 300 editions.

Pharmacists, Physicians, and Apothecaries Medieval monasteries maintained herb gardens and compounded specifics which they sold to the public. Until the Reformation, monastic pharmacies were common, and in Catholic countries they continued to be important until the nineteenth century. In the towns, drugs were available from grocers and spice merchants as well as apothecaries and physicians. The organization of trade in therapeutic drugs and compounds and regulations governing those who dealt in drugs began to appear in guild rules, municipal statutes, and, in the thirteenth century, by decree of German emperor Frederick II. His proposals for regulating pharmacy in the Kingdom of the Two Sicilies were set down between 1231 and 1240. They separated the physician from the pharmacist, recognized pharmacy as a special field of knowledge, laid the groundwork for governmental supervision of pharmaceutical practice, and attempted to establish a code of ethics for the craft. The emperor also ruled that the number of pharmacies should be limited and that prices should be fixed. This decree was of negligible effect in its own time, but it foreshadowed future developments.

On the European continent, guilds provided the institutional structure within which pharmacy developed. In Florence, physicians and pharmacists were organized into a single guild which was classified in 1236 as one of the seven major arts in the city. Italy was the center of the European trade in drugs and spices before the sixteenth century. Guild lists covering the years 1297 to 1444 contained 70 different callings, but the pharmacists and drug wholesalers outnumbered all the rest. The guilds were responsible for sick and poor members, the examination of candidates, the location of pharmacists who passed the exams, the regulation of the distance between pharmacies, drug prices, the collection of government taxes, and supervision over the production and sale of food, liquors, pastries, and medicinal herbs.

Pharmacy guilds in France and Germany were similar to those in Italy, but the development in England was different. No pharmacists' guilds appeared to establish standards for the craft, and when the apothecaries were organized (ca. 1300), it was as part of the grocers' guild. There was no distinction among physicians, apothecaries, and surgeons. The term "leech" covered them all, and the drug trade emerged as part of the commerce in spices and followed French usage. Initially, a trader in drugs and spices was a *mercier,* or trader in small goods. In time, these traders were separated into pepperers, or wholesalers, and spicers, or retailers. "Spicer" and "apothecary" eventually came to be used interchangeably. However, there was a difference, because the apothecaries considered themselves prescribers as well as purveyors of drugs and wanted the same status as physicians. In 1540, when Henry VIII empowered the College of Physicians to "search, view and see the apothecary wares, drugs, and stuffs," the apothecaries responded with a demand to be examined for medical practice and not just as apothecaries. In fact, the apothecaries practiced medicine, including surgery, as well as dispensing drugs.

In 1607 James I recognized the apothecaries as a special body in the grocers' company, and 10 years later they gained their independence, organizing the Masters, Wardens, and Society of the Art and Mystery of the Apothecaries of the City of London. The grocers, from whom the apothecaries divided, were forbidden "to make, compound, or apply medicines or medicineable compositions." The grocers were to be traders; the apothecaries were to be the skilled artificers.

The apothecaries' society became rich and powerful. It founded a cooperative for producing pharmaceutical products which became a commercial company in 1682, winning a monopoly on the right to supply drugs to the navy. In the eighteenth century, it became the main drug supplier for the East India Company. Further, in 1703, the House of Lords confirmed the apothecaries' right to sell drugs without a physician's prescription. On the other side, the apothecaries faced a challenge from druggists, the former middlemen between the drug wholesalers and the apothecaries, and the chemists, that is, preparers of chemical substances who were skilled in distillation and processes requiring fire. Both the druggists and chemists compounded medicines for sale.

Education, Regulation, and Monopoly Rights As a result of its peculiar history, pharmacy in England developed with a minimum of regulation. One result was that scientific achievement played a much smaller part in pharmacy's early history in England than it did in France, Germany, or Italy, while professionalization came more slowly. The French guilds and their German counterparts emphasized long apprenticeships, stiff examinations, and formal education. Beginning in 1484, apothecary candidates in Paris were required to concoct a "masterpiece," that is, a compound of galenicals requiring special skills acquired during an apprenticeship which could last up to 10 years. In 1536, formal academic work was added. Apprentices were required to attend two university lectures per week on the art of the apothecary. Pharmacy was introduced into university curricula, a chair of surgery and pharmacy was established at Montpellier in 1601, and in 1675, Louis XIV founded a chair of pharmaceutical chemistry in Paris.

Academic requirements were added to apprentice training in Germany in the eighteenth century. Prussia had the most advanced system of qualification. The second-class certificate, which served country and small-town practitioners, required five years of apprenticeship, six years as a clerk, and a practical examination. The first-class certificate for city apothecaries also required five years of apprenticeship but stipulated seven years as a clerk combined with study at the Collegium Medicum in Berlin. There the candidate was expected to take courses in chemistry, botany, the characteristics of drugs and compounds, and practical pharmacy. This system was maintained until 1854. The emphasis on a long apprenticeship and academic work established a high standard for French and German pharmacists which led them into advanced research and gave them professional standing equal to that of most physicians and academic scientists.

The German pharmacy guilds regulated the number of apprentices to be accepted, the number of pharmacies to be established, the prices to be charged, and the standards to be maintained. This last required a degree of standardization of drug preparation, and in 1541 Valerius Cordus published his Dispensatorium, a pharmacopeia which became the official standard for practice in Nuremberg. Similar pharmacopeias were completed for Basel (1561) and Augsburg (1564). The London pharmacopeia (1618) was the first to establish a national standard, and the Prussian *Pharmacopeia Borussica* (1799) was the first to incorporate the new chemistry.

In Germany, opening a pharmacy was a privilege conferred by a political unit, most commonly a municipality. A privilege, or *privilegium*, was a feudal writ which spelled out in precise detail what rights were granted and what responsibilities were entailed. No pharmacy could be set up without a writ, and the terms of the writ determined whether the right was hereditary, whether it established a monopoly, what such a monopoly would cover, and even what real estate might be acquired or used for shop premises. A later version of the *privilegium* was called a concession. These were normally awarded in an open competition among qualified pharmacists and provided for the right to operate a pharmacy during the lifetime of the holder. Since pharmacists could nominate their successors, and since the granting authorities tended to respect the nominations, concessions could, in effect, be inherited or sold. These rights were highly prized. Sheltered against competition, and with monopoly rights over cosmetics, liquors, and similar products, a pharmacy owner was guaranteed a substantial living. Governments, following the guild tradition, restricted the number of pharmacies, and it was not until the occupation of Germany after World War II that free establishment of pharmacies was permitted, and then only in the U.S. zone. In 1959, the German Federal Republic accepted the principle of free location, thereby oversetting nearly 1000 years of precedent.

Pharmacy in Early America Pharmacy in the United States followed the English rather than the continental pattern. The regulatory tradition, so strong in continental Europe, was weak in England before the nineteenth century and virtually nonexistent in America. Even the late-developing apothecaries' society had no American counterpart. There was no serious interest in establishing rules to govern the training of pharmacists, and the trade in drugs and natural products was virtually unrestricted.

In the eighteenth century, American drugs were sold by importing wholesalers, by physicians who dispensed their own prescriptions, by apothecary shops, and in the general store. There was no distinction among apothecaries, physicians, merchants, and wholesale druggists. All sold drugs and other items, and many practiced medicine. Some thought that drug dispensing should be a special vocation. Benjamin Franklin recommended that the apothecary at the new Pennsylvania General Hospital (1751) be restricted to dispensing drugs since there was so much work to do, and John Morgan, the second person to hold the apothecary's post, argued for the separation of pharmacy and medicine. Morgan had studied in France and Italy, but when he returned to Philadelphia, he found that it was impossible to maintain European standards of pharmaceutical practice, and he kept a shop where he sold "anything to anyone." He was also the first teacher of pharmacy, pharmaceutical chemistry, and *materia medica* at the medical school of the College of Philadelphia, later the University of Pennsylvania.

During the Revolutionary War, a pharmaceutical division separate from but equal to the medical section was organized for the Continental Army, drugs were manufactured on a large scale, and the first practical formulary was introduced. In the years following the war, however, American pharmacy reverted to its customary entrepreneurial anarchy. The traffic in therapeutic compounds and substances flourished. Patent medicines of English as well as American manufacture became the staple of "drugstores" and, promising relief for virtually all of man's ills, cut deeply into the trade of the more staid and respectable physician-apothecary drug shops.

"Druggists" separated from dispensing physicians. In 1750, there were only 6 drugstores in Philadelphia which were not owned by physicians. By the end of the revolution, that number had tripled, and by 1821, Philadelphia and its environs had 130 stores with no medical connection which sold drugs. The same pattern appeared in Boston and New York.

Pressure for licensing, standardization of drug products, and quality control came from physicians who had the support of some drug dealers and compounders. The movement centered in Philadelphia. In 1820, J. Richard Coxe, with 16 prominent druggists and the backing of the University of Pennsylvania, proposed a plan for licensing pharmacists which envisioned a supervised apprenticeship of three years in an apothecary shop and two courses of university lectures on chemistry, *materia medica,* and pharmacy. This proposal failed of its purpose, and the following year the Philadelphia druggists and apothecaries organized a College of Apothecaries, which became the College of Pharmacy in 1822. The college took responsibility for establishing standards and policing its members, and in 1825 it began to publish the *Journal of the Philadelphia College of Pharmacy,* the first pharmacy journal in America. The Philadelphia College became the model for the Massachusetts College of Pharmacy (1823) and for societies for the city and county of New York (1829) and for the state of Maryland (1840). Later St. Louis (1854) and Chicago (1859) followed Philadelphia's lead. Pressure for standardization produced the first *United States Pharmacopeia* in 1820, and the Massachusetts College of Pharmacy experimented with fixing drug prices.

Congressional failure to legislate workable controls on imported pharmaceutical products and the chaotic condition of the domestic drug trade were national issues which local organizations were unable to influence. In 1851 the recently founded American Medical Association supported demands by physician-pharmacists for controls over drug imports, but its leaders pointed out that pharmacy in the United States had no identity and no recognized spokesperson. Representatives of the various colleges of pharmacy met on this issue in September 1851. Urged on by William Procter, Jr., then editor of the *American Journal of Pharmacy* and a leader of the Philadelphia group, they broadened the issue from imported drugs to all aspects of pharmacy. Procter called for a national association. In October 1852, at a meeting of 20 pharmacists at the Philadelphia College of Pharmacy, the American Pharmacy Association was organized to deal with educational standards and professional qualifications, drug standards, and professional ethics. This organization became the institutional core for pharmacy's modern development in the United States.

Curricula, Licensing, and Regulation in the United States At the midpoint of the nineteenth century, occasional university courses on chemistry, *materia medica,* and pharmical chemistry were all that was available, and what existed was directed toward future physicians rather than pharmacists. Edward Parrish, a member of the Philadelphia College of Pharmacy, believed that the solution was to have pharmacists rather than physicians teach the material, and, further, that practical rather than scientific training would meet the largest need. In 1842, he established a School of Practical Pharmacy in a drugstore near the University of Pennsylvania. His success with it was purely local, but it showed the direction which future educational training might take.

Following the Civil War, educational institutions of all kinds expanded, and many new programs, schools, and institutes for pharmacy were established. The most important were the state university programs introduced at the University of South Carolina (1867), the University of Michigan (1868), and the University of Wisconsin (1883). The Michigan program was strong academically and innovative in teaching methods, but it did not include apprentice training and thus lost the approval of the American Pharmacy Association. The Wisconsin program, which was organized at the request of Wisconsin pharmacists and carried out through a department of the university created by a legislative act, balanced practical and academic education while preparing students for the licensing examination. The Wisconsin plan was eminently successful and served as a model for other departments and schools of pharmacy. In 1905, a survey of 80 pharmacy schools showed that 32 were associated with a college or university. By 1975, when 73 schools were surveyed, 69 were college- or university-related, and there was at least 1 accredited school of pharmacy in 43 of the 50 states.

While state licensing of pharmacists began early, the practice did not become general until the end of the nineteenth century. The pharmacists' association was opposed to both federal and state regulatory legislation, but as the demand for regulation increased, the American Pharmacy Association began to consider what would be acceptable regulatory practices. The result was a model legislative proposal for the guidance of state legislators. The model was first constructed in 1870 and then revised in 1900 when regulation had come to be accepted as desirable. It provided that the pharmacist was not a merchant or storekeeper and that pharmacy was a distinct profession working for the public's good. The favored regulatory institution was a state board composed of practicing as well as academic pharmacists. The board would be responsible for examining, for registration procedures, and for enforcement of a pharmacy code. This approach became standard through the United States in the twentieth century.

Although the United States lagged in developing local and intraprofessional systems for regulating pharmacy, in the twentieth century the federal government has been the most active of any government in defining and enforcing rules for the sale and use of therapeutic drugs. This emphasis was part of a shift in American political ideology which occurred in the post-Reconstruction period. It involved a reinterpretation of the principle that government exists to provide the greatest good for the greatest number to introduce the idea that government must protect society against exploitation by those on whom they rely for life's necessities. Under the constitutional umbrella of the interstate commerce clause, a federal Food and Drug Act was passed in 1906 which defined the government's responsibility for maintaining minimum safe standards. The regulations applied directly to drugs. The 1906 act, however, was inadequate. A succession of tragic incidents in the 1930s, including the premature release of live antipolio vaccine and the deaths of 73 people who took the so-called Elixir of Sulfanilamide in 1937, produced a much stronger Food, Drug, and Cosmetics Act in 1938. Further amendments to the act were legislated in 1962, largely in response to the thalidomide scandal which rocked Europe when thousands of mothers gave birth to deformed babies after taking thalidomide early in their pregnancies. The 1962 act mandated a review of all drugs admitted to use between 1938 and 1962 to determine efficacy and effect.

Strong drug regulation has forced a more cautious approach to new pharmaceutical products. Critics have pointed to a blighting effect on the development of new substances, while the testing program has been blamed for escalating drug costs. Such criticism has had little effect as the federal government has remained firmly committed to extensive testing in the interests of consumer protection. Attempts to combat the use of addictive drugs have been less successful (see Drug Abuse). With no clear idea of what should be controlled, or how to control it, and with substantial popular resistance, all levels of government have sunk into an enforcement quagmire, and the illicit production and sale of forbidden drugs have become a multi-billion-dollar business. The problem is international, and no effective solution to it is in sight.

The Pharmaceutical Industry In the nineteenth century, scientific advances in chemistry, bacteriology, microbiology, and biochemistry revolutionized the pharmacopeia. The active therapeutic agents in natural drugs began to be identified and refined. Narcotine was isolated from opium in 1803, morphine was identified in 1806, emetine and strychnine in 1817, quinine in 1820, nicotine in 1828, atropine in 1833, and cocaine in 1860. Such discoveries made it possible to standardize quality, eliminate impurities, make dosages more accurate, and achieve a more discriminating understanding of drugs' effects. And this led in turn to attempts to create the natural product synthetically. One result was improved versions of natural agents and whole families of new products. Another result was the feasibility of mass production, thus moving another step forward in pharmacy's transformation.

The industrialization of drug production began in workshops which developed techniques for manufacturing a specific product or process. A tablet compression machine, for example, was introduced in England by William Brockedon in 1843 and in the United States by Jacob Denton in 1864. In 1838, Robert Shoemaker of Philadelphia began manufacturing sticking plaster, and in France, a method for mass-producing sugar-coated pills appeared in the 1830s. The process was refined by William R. Warner, another Philadelphia pharmaceutical manufacturer, in 1866. Warner also began production of small pills (parvules) on a large scale. In France, a national pharmaceutical cooperative began large-scale manufacturing in the 1850s, though most drug production was carried on in laboratories at the back of apothecary shops or in drugstores.

In the United States, the Civil War stimulated large-scale drug production. E. R. Squibb, for example, was a Brooklyn physician and pharmacist who served in the U.S. Navy from 1847 to 1857. In 1858, he opened a laboratory to supply medicines to the U.S. Army. The demand was small, however, and despite support from a number of physicians, the Squibb laboratory had difficult times until war broke out in 1861. Then Squibb expanded rapidly, completing a new laboratory in 1862 as well as enlarging and refurbishing his old quarters. He moved into factory-style production, using steam power to turn the mills for powdering drugs, and his work force expanded to 40 people. Squibb's earliest and most valuable contribution was to discover methods for producing chemically pure ether and chloroform, a major step toward safety in anesthetics.

Squibb was already a large-scale producer in 1865, but other major firms were moving into production. In 1841, George R. Smith founded the Philadelphia concern which became Smith, Kline, and French. They expanded rapidly during the war period. Sharpe and Dohme were established in Baltimore in 1860 to produce natural drug products. They entered chemical manufacturing in 1886. The Eli Lilly Company was founded in Indianapolis in 1876 and opened a branch, the first of its kind, in Kansas City, Missouri, in 1882. Parke-Davis and Company, which was founded in 1867, established one of the earliest research institutes in the industry in 1902. Finally, Merck and Company, a branch of one of the leading German chemical firms, came to the United States in 1891.

Drug production in the United States, France, and England was subordinate to the chemical industry in Germany, which established and maintained leadership amounting to a monopoly on the synthesis of drug products beginning with salycilic acid (1874) and antipyrine (1863). German leadership continued into World War I, and the chemical and drug industries remained strong until World War II. American development benefited from German achievements. Until 1917, American drug companies brought their supplies from Germany or from branches of German firms producing in the United States under German patents. When the United States entered the war in 1917, German chemical patents were seized and distributed to various American companies. Abbott Laboratories, for example, claimed several German discoveries for their own under the rubric "first made in America." These included chlorazene, dichloramine-T, arsphenamine, neoarsphenamine, and sulfarsphenamine. Sterling Drug, Inc., followed a different course. Founded in 1900 to promote an analgesic called Neuralgine, Sterling bought assets of the U.S. branch of the German Bayer Company, Bayer of New York, which manufactured and sold aspirin, certain physicians' drugs, and dyestuffs. Sterling marketed aspirin under the Bayer trade name, sold the dye business, and created the Winthrop Chemical Company to make physicians' drugs. When the United States entered World War II, all "limiting agreements" on markets and products with German firms were disavowed, and Winthrop Chemical began to break down German products to identify and manufacture their active ingredients. It took less than a year, for example, to begin manufacturing Atebrin, an antimalarial preparation used extensively by U.S. forces in the Pacific theater, on a mass scale from products available in the United States. The Sterling Company's sales reflected these developments, rising from $3,801,902 in 1918 to $47,678,024 in 1944. Between 1944 and 1967, Sterling's sales jumped again to $198,703,000, and by 1970 had reached $594,412,000.

The greatest growth in pharmaceutical manufacturing occurred after World War II and owed to the discovery of sulfonamides, penicillin, and the other antibiotic drugs which could be mass-produced. The sulfonamides (q.v.) were a by-product of the German dye industry, penicillin (q.v.) was an English discovery which was then developed for mass production in the United States, and the other antibiotics (q.v.), beginning with streptomycin, were essentially American achievements. The American drug industry came to dominate large-scale drug production for the world market by exports and through overseas branches of American firms which are now found in more than 60 foreign countries. There are between 600 and 700 American firms which produce prescription drugs, with something over 1000 manufacturing laboratories. Just 20 companies control up to 75 percent of the market, but no single firm controls more than 10 to 20 percent. American firms, like the German leaders of an earlier era, invest substantially in research, putting $677 million (11.9 percent of sales) into research in 1971. In turn, between 1940 and 1971, U.S. firms originated 557 single chemical entities which are regularly available on prescription. This figure comprises two-thirds of the new medicinal substances introduced into drug therapy. The other third was divided among Germany, Switzerland, the United Kingdom, and France.

Conclusion The drug industry in the twentieth century is very big business. It covers prescription drugs, restricted nonprescription drugs, nonprescription drugs, and cosmetics. In most countries which accept the western scientific approach to medicine, compounding and sale of the first class of materials and sale of the second require licensed pharmacists whose professional status rests on a prescribed course of formal study, practical experience, and examination. Since World War II, drugstores which combine prescription service with the sale of nonprescription drugs, cosmetics, and a wide variety of other consumer products and services have appeared in Britain and western Europe. They originated in the United States. At the same time, the development of new drug therapies for bacterial and viral diseases, for various forms of cancer, and for degenerative conditions of the circulatory and cardiovascular system have revolutionized medical practice. Increasingly sophisticated anesthetic compounds and substances which resist infection systemically have greatly enlarged surgery's capacity.

There are, however, problems. Critics point out that pharmacy companies' aggressive marketing tactics have strongly influenced medical treatment as the line between scientific reports and product advertisement has become blurred and indistinct. Busy physicians are seldom in a position to compare a pharmaceutical house presentation with recent research reports and have learned to rely on what amounts to the seller's description of the product. General advertising has encouraged the public's reliance on drug preparations; news stories and public relations campaigns elevate the public's consciousness of and expectations for particular substances; and the cost of modern pharmaceuticals, especially those marketed under brand names, has skyrocketed. The availability of "generic" drugs has provided a partial response to this problem, but there is resistance on the part of physicians and consumers alike.

Government regulations and testing requirements have added significantly to the costs of modern drug development, though the history of the drug industry makes it apparent that such regulation in the interest of consumer safety is essential. However, even the testing on which regulation must rely has become problematic, as evidence multiplies that independent laboratories contracting to carry out testing procedures have ignored negative results or even failed to test at all. In sum, while pharmacy's development as a discipline and a profession has been a powerful and positive influence on the history of modern medicine, the problems associated with that growth are similarly significant as part of the modernizing process and drive home the extent to which economic, social, and political factors are fundamental to the healing vocation.

ADDITIONAL READINGS: Frank J. Anderson, *An Illustrated History of Herbals*, New York, 1977; Alfred Burger (ed.), *Medicinal Chemistry*, 3d ed., 2, New York, 1970; E. P. Claus, V. E. Taylor, and L. R. Brady, *Pharmacognosy*, 6th ed., Philadelphia, 1970; Wyndham Davies, *The Pharmaceutical Industry*, Oxford, 1967; Harry F. Dowling, *Medicines for Man: The Development, Regulation, and Use of Prescription Drugs*, New York, 1970; Chauncey D. Leake, *An Historical Account of Pharmacology to the Twentieth Century*, Springfield, Ill., 1975; Glenn Sonnedecker (ed.), *Kremer's and Urdang's History of Pharmacy*, 2d and 4th eds., Philadelphia, 1951, 1976; James Harvey Young, *American Self-Dosage Medicine: An Historical Perspective*, Lawrence, 1974; James Harvey Young, *The Toadstool Millionaires: A Social History of Patent Medicines in America Before Federal Regulations*, Princeton, 1961.

See also ANTIBIOTICS; CHEMOTHERAPY; IMMUNOLOGY; PENICILLIN; QUACKERY; QUININE; SULFONAMIDES.

Phrenology

Phrenology, a pseudoscience which developed at the end of the eighteenth century, achieved a widespread following in France, England, Scotland, and the United States in the first half of the nineteenth century and faded away after 1850 to disappear by the beginning of World War I. It was longest-lived in the United States, where the *American Phrenological Journal* continued publication until 1911. Phrenology attained its greatest scientific respectability in France between 1800 and 1830, and its most important medical applications were made in England between 1830 and 1850.

In general, phrenology belonged to popular science, though it attracted both scientists and physicians, especially in the early days. It became part of philosophical argument concerning the nature of the human being. It became involved in and contributed to campaigns for reform of penal codes and the educational system, and it was caught up in the early history of psychology. It contributed as well to forensic medicine and the development of physical anthropology. Phrenology began in anatomy and physiology, particularly the advancing understanding of the brain and nervous system, and Franz Josef Gall, the man who originated the doctrine, was widely recognized for his valuable work on brain anatomy. Gall's interests centered on the cortex. He developed his own system for dissecting the brain which enabled him to demonstrate cortical unity, he linked the nervous system with the brain by showing the presence of a gray matter in both, and he identified the fibrous character of white matter. Gall, as a recent student pointed out, was "a great anatomist" whose work helped to transform the understanding of the nervous system as a whole.

The doctrine of phrenology held that the brain was the source for thought and will, that it controlled character, and that its configurations were an unfailing guide to an individual's total personality. The brain, it was believed, contained separate "organs" which occupied specific areas. These organs controlled the qualities, or "penchants," which shaped an individual personality. The size of the organ was critical, while the ensemble of qualities each individual possessed formed the total personality. The brain was not accessible to inspection, but Gall conceived of the idea that the topography of the skull—its depressions and protuberances—provided a guide to the brain configurations which lay beneath. A trained observer could tell at a glance something of the character of any person by considering the general shape of the head. Closer examination with the fingertips and measurement with calipers would make a more discriminating reading possible. Such a reading, or "cranioscopy," would help the observer to help the individual to a better understanding of his or her personality and potentiality.

Gall identified 27 penchants. His collaborator, Johann Caspar Spurzheim, with whom Gall later broke, found 33. In time, as areas were subdivided, more were added, but this was not a serious issue. Gall had predicted that the number would vary, and that as the understanding of the brain advanced, greater discrimination in function could be anticipated. The question of how to measure the areas did give trouble. Gall used such relative terms as "quite small," "very small," and "very large." Many followers felt that more precise measurements expressed in area or volume would give greater validity to the conclusions reached.

A more serious objection was that the brain determined what personality was to be, leaving little or no freedom to the individual. Phrenologists parried this objection by arguing that their science promoted self-awareness. The individual should know his or her capacities in order to exploit them to the fullest while recognizing what penchants he or she possesses which require caution and control. In the United States, phrenology was used to determine what capacities a person possessed as a preliminary to planning his education and career. Used this way, phrenology in American pointed toward personality testing and contributed to the ground swell of opinion which produced progressive education.

The qualities phrenologists identified defined those characteristics which would be part of any individual's role in society. Since Gall was more concerned with developing a physical science for humanity, it was Spurzheim's refinement of Gall's ideas which gained the widest followings. Spurzheim divided the qualities of personality into feelings and propensities and knowing faculties. The former were located at the back of the brain, with the nobler sentiments toward the crown. Knowing was toward the front of the brain. Among the penchants in the first category were adhesiveness (community orientation), combativeness, amativeness (the penchant for physical love), destructiveness, and acquisitiveness. Also in this category were such sentiments as self-esteem, love of approbation, benevolence, hope, and conscientiousness. The knowing faculties were what permitted perception of the external world and judgment about it. Those which concerned weight, breadth, color, texture, locality, number, order, or tune involved sense perception. In this group there were also reflecting faculties, which distinguished humans from animals and included compassion, wit, causality, and imitation. No two people were exactly alike in their combination of qualities; therefore; only individual evaluations were possible. Moreover, while cranioscopy could describe what a person was and what would influence his or her behavior, it made no claim to fortune-telling or reading the past. Such refinements appeared as phrenology turned into fairgrounds entertainment.

From the beginning, though it was controversial, phrenology received a respectful hearing, and its originator was accepted into the highest scientific as well as social circles. Unlike his slightly earlier contemporary, Anton Mesmer, Gall won and then maintained a strong scientific reputation. Early in his career, he was offered a post as physician to the Austrian emperor, a position he declined in order to continue his researches. He was forced to stop teaching in Vienna in 1802 and finally to leave the city in 1805 for publicizing a materialistic and atheistic doctrine, but when he toured northern Europe from 1805 to 1807, he was warmly received by scientific societies, philosophers, and princes. Settling in Paris in 1808, he was well received by the medical and scientific fraternity. He remained in Paris until his death in 1828. Though Gall's life was complicated by shifts in the political winds, and his doctrines remained a point of dispute, his standing was always high. That reputation, however, rested on his abilities as an anatomist and skilled dissector. Gall's reputation as a scientist made phrenology more credible, though literally hundreds of brain dissections generated no evidence to support phrenology as such.

The experience in England was somewhat different. While Spurzheim gave the movement scientific respectability, it was received as a formulated doctrine to be widely applied. It attracted the attention of leading members of the medical profession, though Charles Bell, a Scot and one of Great Britain's outstanding students of the brain, rejected it, and it proved to be especially strong in Edinburgh thanks to the advocacy of the Combe brothers, George and Andrew. George Combe became the main spokesperson for phrenology in the English-speaking world. His writings were particularly effective, and it was he, following Spurzheim, who introduced the doctrine to the United States in the 1830s and was responsible for its spread there.

During the period from 1820 to 1850, phrenology was highly popular, becoming a kind of middle-class game and ending by establishing itself as a staple in workingmen's clubs and mass popular entertainments. Initially, it attracted the medical profession as well. According to one estimate, exactly one-third of the 120 members of the Edinburgh Phrenological Society in 1826 were physicians and surgeons. A decade later, of 110 members, just 19 were "medical persons." Part of the movement's early appeal undoubtedly owed to the concept of a "science of man" based on firm anatomical observation and a physiological approach. Soon, however, it became apparent that phrenology was not in step with the critical experimental work carried on by François Magendie in Paris or the new German physiology developing with Johannes Mueller. Gall's work had been done in the period from 1790 ot 1810; in the 1840s it was plainly, as John Stuart Mill pointed out in exasperation, entirely out of date. Another factor was that phrenology offered little to medicine as medicine was understood. That François Broussais, the most brutal of the heroic bleeders left in the nineteenth century, was also a supporter of phrenology in France underscored a growing gulf between modern medicine and the residue of the eighteenth century.

There were two notable attempts to bring phrenology into line with medical needs in the 1830s and 1840s. John Elliotson, a brilliant if erratic physician and heart specialist in London, became an enthusiastic phrenologist. He was also, however, a noted mesmerist, and he combined the two ideas into something called phrenomesmerism. What the mesmeric trance provided was a means to manipulate penchants and qualities. Elliotson came to dominate London phrenology, and he brought forward a manipulative aspect that aimed at attempting to change behavioral patterns. Elliotson gained renown, even notoriety, for he was a powerful advocate and an influential man. Inevitably, in his mesmeric hospital, phre-

After 1650, most physiologists used a mechanical model to frame descriptions of body function. But they differed fundamentally on how the system functioned. The great French philosopher and mathematician René Descartes gave the first comprehensive expression to the mechanistic view. Descartes was neither a physician nor an anatomist, though he had observed a number of dissections and may have performed some. In his essay *De homine* (1662) Descartes compared the body to a perfect clockwork mechanism which God set in motion and which then functioned according to mechanical laws. Descartes knew Harvey's work, but he chose to ignore it, postulating instead a "cardiac fire" which heated the blood to near the boiling point, causing it to expand and spread outward to the farthermost parts of the system. Each organ system within the body functioned separately and in response to similar stimuli. There was also a divinely created soul which dealt with voluntary actions but which had no role in bodily functions as such. Though Descartes was sharply criticized for the factual shortcomings of his doctrine, his conceptions remained.

Iatrophysics The seventeenth-century iatrophysical movement was as empirical as Descartes was philosophical. Led by Giovanni Borelli and Giorgio Baglivi, the iatrophysicists studied muscle function, gland secretions, respiration, cardiac action, and neural response. Borelli was a physician and mathematician from Pisa who worked in Rome under the sponsorship of Sweden's Queen Christina. His main contribution was a book, *De motu animalium* (*On Animal Motion*) (1680–1681), which summarized his observations on birds in flight, fish swimming, muscular contraction, the mechanics of respiration, and a host of other subjects. He believed that there was a "contractile element" in the muscles themselves whose action was triggered by a process similar to chemical fermentation. This principle operated in the heart, which Borelli thought functioned automatically because it was a muscle, and he attempted unsuccessfully to calculate the actual force exerted by the heart during contraction. He also used a thermometer to check whether body heat developed in the left cardiac ventricle and concluded that it did not. He viewed respiration as a purely mechanical process which introduced air through the lungs into the blood. Borelli knew about the experiments conducted by Otto von Giericke and Robert Boyle in which small animals died in "rarified" air, and he held that "aerated blood" contained elements necessary to life. The life-sustaining function of air was to act as a vehicle for "spiral and elastic particles" which entered the blood to impart an internal motion to it.

Borelli's contemporary, Giorgio Baglivi, who was professor of anatomy at the papal school in Rome, represented the culmination of the iatrophysical movement in Italy. His *Praxis medica* (1699) affirmed that "a human body, as to its natural actions, is truly nothing else but a complex of chymico-mechanical motions, depending upon such principles as are purely mathematical." Baglivi, like Borelli, considered the motive force for body action to be located within the body itself; and while he agreed that the heart's action stemmed from the fact that it was a muscle and therefore possessed a contractile principle, he extended that view to include the meninges and their extensions, the membranous fibers of the small muscles, which he considered to be in a state of continuous pulsation. He also noted that the automatic contractions of the heart persisted even when it was removed from an animal and cut into pieces. Significantly, Borelli saw another kind of muscular force residing in the voluntary muscle fibers, which required conscious will to be put in motion.

Iatrochemistry Parallel to and competitive with mechanistic physiology was the iatrochemical movement, which was rooted in Paracelsus' chemical system and was systematized by Johannes (Jean) Baptiste van Helmont. Van Helmont rejected Paracelsus' generalized archeus, or indwelling spirit, substituting for it the idea that each organ had its particular archeus, or *Blas* (spirit), which controlled it. He considered all vital processes to be chemical, and each owed to the action of a special ferment, or gas. These ferments were invisible spirits capable of transforming food, which was turned thereby to living flesh. This transformative process occurred throughout the body, but particularly in the stomach, duodenum, liver, and heart. Van Helmont thought that body heat was a by-product of fermentation, not a force generated in the heart to digest food, and he believed that the whole system was controlled by a soul (*anima sensitiva motivaque*) located in the pit of the stomach. One explanation for his locating it there is that a blow to the solar plexus brings unconsciousness, obliterating the reception of sensory data and closing off the motivating or directing function.

Van Helmont began his career as a Capuchin friar, and he was always comfortable with mystical and nonempirical explanations. He was also an early modern scientific observer who knew a great deal about bile, gastric juices, and stomach acids. He approached the discovery of nitrogen, which he called "gas sylvestre," and he had some insights into the processes later identified as the immune system. In these areas he was much in advance of Paracelsus, but his general physiology and the pathology it generated were traditional and abstract.

Another leader of the iatrochemical movement was Franz de la Boë, also known as Franciscus Sylvius. Sylvius taught at Leyden. He was a physician and a follower of William Harvey who understood the significance of blood circulation for general physiology. Though a iatrochemist, he was highly critical of van Helmont's mystical ideas, seeking to substitute for them a process which combined chemical analysis with circulation theory. Sylvius concentrated on digestion, arguing that this essentially fermentive process took place in the mouth, in the heart—where the digestive fire was kept burning by chemical reactions—and in the blood, moving outward to bone, tendon, and flesh. Sylvius was a synthesizer and a teacher rather than an investigator. He speculated in glands, secretions, and especially the role of saliva and pancreatic juices in digestion. Most important, however, he focused attention on chemical action as part of body function.

Eighteenth-Century Systematizers The eighteenth century systematized sixteenth- and seventeenth-century physiology, and three men, Friedrich Hoffmann, Georg E. Stahl, and Hermann Boerhaave, dominated the field. Hoffmann lectured at Halle and Boerhaave at Leyden. Both were highly successful teachers whose students carried their ideas throughout Europe. Hoffmann was a thoroughgoing Cartesian whose *Systematic Rational Medicine* (1718, 1740) was a monument to seventeenth-century work. Boerhaave, the better-known of the two, was also firmly mechanistic, but he was more empirical and less indebted to the past. He believed that body functions were controlled by placement and vessel size, and he considered the solid parts of the body to be vessels, or vascular structures, which contained, directed, modified, divided, or secreted body fluids. Other solid structures were "mechanical instruments" which supported or determined certain motions. Bodily fluids also had such mechanical properties as coherence and elasticity, and Boerhaave concluded that life or death, health or disease, lay with "the motion, obstruction and stagnation of these bodily fluids."

A reaction against mechanistic doctrines appeared in the physiology of Georg E. Stahl and spread through the work of the talented physicians of Montpellier. Stahl returned to the idea of a purposive spirit which animated the body. An excellent physician and chemist, Stahl was also a religious man who found faith and science compatible. He believed that God created both a body and a soul. The body was subject to corruption when death overtook it. The soul (*anima*) feared death and directed the body's action to avoid death by promoting wisdom and foresight. The body's functions resulted from an urge to live. The Montpellier school took up Stahl's animism and refined it. Its most important member, Théophile de Bordeu, demonstrated that Boerhaave's mechanistic explanation for gland secretions was physically impossible, but he also argued against a metaphysical explanation for bodily functions. Bordeu believed that each body organ was endowed with the capacity to respond to appropriate stimuli. Thus vital function was integral to the organs themselves.

The leading physiologist of the eighteenth century was Albrecht von Haller, a student of Boerhaave whose massive publication list included Europe's first comprehensive treatise on physiology, *Physiological Elements of the Human Body* (1757–1766). Haller approached his subject empirically, combining numerous animal experiments with scholarly erudition. He followed a conventional mechanistic approach which postulated God as the creator and first mover in a universe which, once started, ran according to mechanical laws. The body was a machine composed of passive and extended matter which was kept in motion by immaterial forces analogous to

Newton's gravity. The forces could not be known, but their effects could be. Haller offered two important ideas to the history of physiology. First, he distinguished three separate patterns for the organization of tissues in which the structure of the tissue varied with the function it performed. This marked an important stage in the early history of cell theory. Second, in 1752, he published his seminal study, *On the Irritable and Sensible Parts of the Body.* This book, based on animal experiments, has been termed an "epoch-making work in the history of physiology." In it Haller developed his idea that certain parts of the body possessed sensibility and reacted to pain, while others, which he called irritable, reacted with contractions when stimulated. Haller classified bodily structures according to the irritability-sensibility factor. The system proved overly schematic, for many structures could be both irritable and sensible, but the doctrine provided a comprehensive explanation for vital function which could be studied empirically and did not depend on an immaterial principle. Haller was now able to suggest why the heart pulsated. He argued that the heart was the most "irritable" organ in the body. Composed of various layers of muscular fibers, it was stimulated by the flowing in of blood and responded with systolic contractions. Embryologists would have to explain how the heart started in the first place.

Progress at the Dawn of the Nineteenth Century Though notable for its system building, the eighteenth century saw substantial progress in a number of specialized fields. It was this type of work rather than the more speculative philosophies which became the hallmark of nineteenth-century physiological research. Advances were recorded toward understanding digestion as a chemical rather than a mechanical process. In metabolic studies, Antoine Lavoisier, the French chemist who died on the guillotine, was able to show that respiration and combustion were the same process and that both required oxygen. Lavoisier and his collaborators, Pierre S. de la Place and Armand Sequin, also proved that increased physical exertion or food digestion required larger quantities of oxygen than the body did at rest. A further refinement, provided by Jean H. Hassenfratz and Lazaro Spallanzani, was that oxidation occurred in the blood and throughout the entire physical system. By the opening of the nineteenth century, the understanding of respiration and metabolism approached the views held today.

Information on the nervous system also expanded. Nicolas Saucerotte trephined dogs' skulls to discover which areas produced front- or back-leg paralysis, while William Cruikshank related the medulla to respiration and Georg Prochaska worked out the reflex system. In the next century, Charles Bell, François Magendie, and Johannes Mueller provided the anatomical details for Prochaska's system. Reflex and nervous response were also the subject of electrical experiments as Luigi Galvani demonstrated that electrical current stimulated nervous and muscular response. Valuable work was also done on blood physiology, especially the role of clotting lymph and white blood cells, and the anatomical basis for understanding sight and hearing was established. Théophile de Bordeu expanded the available information on gland function, and at the end of the century, Marie François Xavier Bichat offered his system for classifying cellular tissue.

Nineteenth-century physiology separated itself organizationally and methodologically from anatomy. At the same time, the organizational structure of the discipline expanded, professional societies and journals proliferated, and the number of scientists engaged in physiological research substantially increased. Systematization disappeared with the eighteenth century to be replaced by detailed studies on particular organs and organ systems, the maturation of chemical analysis, development of an experimental method, and the improvement of microscopy. Factual answers to speculative questions about vital manifestations indicated that the philosophical battles over cause which characterized the eighteenth century had shifted ground, and new attention to questions of genesis, development, and growth rendered the simple mechanistic theories of the previous 200 years out of date.

At the beginning of the century, German physiology was caught up in the controversy over F. W. C. von Schelling's Nature Philosophy, a radical unitary approach to science which denied empiricism and emphasized intuition and a priori philosophical speculation. It found a medical counterpart in the Brownian system (q.v.), a theory of disease and treatment devised by John

Brown of Edinburgh and promoted by Schelling himself in the early days of the nineteenth century. Schellingism retarded scientific development in the early nineteenth century, but it was a more positive influence on cultural history, aesthetics, and literature. It contributed little to physiology beyond a lingering fear of vitalist explanations, which were often incorrectly identified with romantic nature science.

The French School The nineteenth-century French school of physiology built on the work of François Magendie, who has been called "the true founder of modern experimental physiology and medicine," and culminated with Claude Bernard, Europe's leading physiological methodologist. Other distinguished French physiologists included Julien J. C. Legallois and Marie-Jean P. Flourens. As a whole, the group was notable for its stringent empiricism, its emphasis on the particular experiment, its extensive use of vivisection, its close attention to structural detail, and the conviction that all one needed to know was in the subject observed. Magendie, who worked at the Collège de France, exhibited these characteristics to an exaggerated degree. A thoroughgoing skeptic, Magendie avoided all theoretical statements and only generalized the cumulative results of his experiments. He particularly favored vivisection, killing literally hundreds of animals, especially dogs, in the course of his work. He refused to specialize, studied one problem after another, and therefore contributed information on a variety of subjects. His particularized, vivisectionist, experimental methodology spread throughout Europe between 1815 and 1850, though he never developed the network of disciples which followed Johannes Mueller, Carl Ludwig, or even his own colleague and successor, Claude Bernard.

Claude Bernard was the most brilliant star in the French school, an important figure in the history of physiology, and a notable influence on the European cultural scene. A prolific experimentalist and a fine writer, Bernard published over 300 titles between 1834 and 1878, and a number of publishable manuscripts were among his papers when he died. Like Magendie, Bernard was essentially an experimentalist and vivisectionist. He ranged across the whole front of physiological research, making notable contributions to digestive studies and carbohydrate metabolism, the functioning of the nervous system, and the effects of poisons. Unlike Magendie, Bernard was willing to generalize and even hypothesize. His *Introduction to the Study of Experimental Medicine* (1865) is a classic work on methodology, the first lucid and systematic explanation of theory and practice in physiological and medical experiments. Bernard accepted Newton's dictum that one may know the consequences of a natural law without knowing the primary cause behind the law itself. Bernard concentrated on secondary causes of vital manifestations, organic functions themselves, and the milieu within which functions took place. He called attention to the fact that vital functions occurred in and through structures capable of growth, and he spoke of this ability as "a vital force which cannot be denied, and is as clear as daylight." His most important proposition was that all organic functions take place in a milieu, or environment, and that stability of the environment is a precondition for the organ's ability to grow and function—for its autonomy. The environment, which includes the structures through which functions take place, determines the functions themselves. Bernard allowed for development within the system, and by emphasizing the milieu, he called for a physiologically sophisticated method which would study the whole organism in terms of its parts' relationships with each other and with the world outside itself.

German Physiology Nineteenth-century German physiology found its leading figures in Johannes Mueller and Carl Ludwig, the respective contemporaries of Magendie and Bernard. Although some German physiologists studied with Magendie, there was only minimal contact between the French and German schools, a fact which was reflected in profound differences in methodology, institutional organization, temperament, and cultural milieu. Mueller and Ludwig trained literally hundreds of students. Personal relationships between teachers and pupils were extremely important, and students tended to identify themselves throughout their careers with the men who trained them. Institutional organization strengthened this characteristic. French science was centralized in Paris, with only limited opportunity for study and research in the provinces. In Germany, however, political centralization came very late, and a multiplicity of states traditionally supported institutes and universities in which there was great local pride. The tradition continued after unification in 1871. The result was that in Germany there were a dozen or more university departments and research institutes of substantial standing which carried on varied research programs and provided a broad system of scientific facilities throughout the country. They also enlarged the opportunities for employment. German physiology developed a community spirit, its methods tended toward the institutional, and there was a greater appreciation for technological advance. The replication of experiments, quantification, the application of physical and chemical analysis, and the use of advanced microscopy were all characteristic features of German methods. The qualitative, surgical methods used in France were less common east of the Rhine.

Johannes Mueller led German physiologists in the first half of the nineteenth century. Mueller was a vitalist whose early studies dealt with the laws and relationships governing motion in various animals. His teacher at Berlin, Carl Rudolphi, had been a strict empiricist who trained under Magendie and who resisted Mueller's generalizing tendencies. Mueller showed Rudolphi's influence, though he remained convinced that it was best to establish an interpretive context in which to evaluate experimental results. Mueller was originally interested in psychology, but after a collapse brought on by overwork in 1827, he dropped that interest to concentrate on glands and their secretions, genital structures, blood and blood vessels, tissues, and the voice. His methods stressed laboratory work, comparison of specimens, and especially microscopy. With Theodor Schwann, he contributed to the basic work on the structure of cells (q.v.), and his student Rudolf Virchow established the field of cellular pathology. Mueller taught in Bonn from 1824 to 1833 and then went to Berlin, where he remained until he retired in 1858. In addition to Virchow and Lehmann, Mueller's students included Ernst Brücker, Hermann von Helmholtz, and Emil Du Bois-Reymond. These men, who were among the profession's leaders in the second half of the nineteenth century, were especially notable for developing physical and chemical factors in physiology.

Carl Ludwig led German physiology in the second half of the nineteenth century. His approach stressed chemical and physical elements and evolved toward a quantitative method which was anatomical, analytic, and nonsurgical. Ludwig studied hydromechanisms and blood pressure. He developed the first instrument for recording variations in fluid pressure (the kymograph). When he moved to the Vienna Military Academy in 1855, he concentrated on respiration, blood, and innervation of blood vessels. He moved to Leipzig in 1865 to become director of the New Physiological Institute. During his tenure there, Leipzig became the world center for physiological studies. Over 200 students came there to work with Ludwig, and when they left, they maintained close touch with the institute. Ludwig was famous for the interest he took in his students' research and for the personal contributions he would make as the work progressed. Hugo Kronecker, Ludwig's associate in the institute, was in charge of maintaining personal contact with the international community of alumni.

The British Era Germany's preeminence in physiology waned in the last decade of the nineteenth century when Brücke, Helmholtz, Carl Ludwig, and Du Bois-Reymond died, all between 1892 and 1896. Though Germany remained strong in the field, leadership passed to Great Britain, where it remained until World War II. British physiology was moribund until the second half of the nineteenth century, when William Sharpey began its revival at University College, London. Michael Foster continued the work. He established continental ties, built up a student following, helped to found the British Physiological Society (1876), wrote the first authoritative study on general physiology in English (1877), founded and edited the *Journal of Physiology* (1878), and helped to organize the physiologists' first international congress (1889). English physiology drew on both the French and German tradition, though the German was the stronger of the two. The most important centers were University College in London and Cambridge University.

British work followed the established patterns of close analysis of particular organs and organ complexes. There was also a growing tendency to restrict research to a particular area or cluster of problems. Thus Charles Scott Sherrington was essentially, even exclusively, a neurophysiologist.

His findings revolutionized the field (see Neurology). Sherrington's method was surgical and morphological, closer to the classic French style than to the German. Other British physiologists worked primarily with chemical problems. Sir Frederick G. Hopkins has been called the founder of biochemistry in Britain, and the balance of his work was concentrated in that area, with a special emphasis on nutrition. Hopkins played a critical role in developing knowledge concerning those "accessory food factors" which, with proteins, carbohydrates, fats, and minerals, are essential to growth. For his work in this area, he shared a Nobel prize for physiology and medicine in 1928 with Christiaan Eijkmann, the man who established the cause of beriberi. Sir Henry Dale was another distinguished physiologist, who became director of the Wellcome Physiological Research Laboratory. His most important contribution was to identify the action of acetylcholine on the heart. He, too, shared a Nobel prize for physiology and medicine. Though the tradition of studying many subjects within the field of physiology was represented, especially among the older generation, including Sir Edward Sharpey-Schafer, who worked on the brain, histology, and internal secretions, specialization was becoming the rule, and Britain's most important work had a biochemical foundation.

Characteristics of Contemporary Physiology
English leadership in physiology faded with World War II, and changes in conception and methodology, institutional organization, and scope which had begun 50 years earlier utterly transformed the discipline. Methodology has spread outward until the technical requirements for physiological specialties have become specialties themselves, requiring elaborate support and maintenance systems. Microscopy is one example. Specialization moved in another direction, calling for greater detail and specificity on particular organs or systems, which in their turn became complexes of specialties. Generalization has moved toward considering life so broadly that human physiology has become a source of data for studying more generalized functions, a development which has had the effect of weakening the traditional connection between medicine and physiology.

In the end, deepening the understanding of life processes can only improve knowledge on human functions and thus strengthen medicine's ability to diagnose and treat disease. Change, however, is unsettling, and the extraordinary growth of physiology and its disciplines in the modern period is both evidence of scientific development and a threat to the more settled intellectual and social systems embodied in classic physiological studies. When physiology separated from anatomy in the nineteenth century, it was essentially a European discipline of modest size. Only 124 delegates attended the first international congress held in Basel in 1889. By 1926, 33 nations could send 581 delegates to Stockholm, and in 1953, 41 countries sent 2188 participants. The 1968 meeting in Washington, D.C., attracted 51 nations and 4300 participants. Of that number, nearly half (2040) were from the United States, where all scientific and medical fields have expanded dramatically since World War II. In 1937, there were 631 physiologists registered in the United States; in 1954, the number reached 1400.

As could be expected, physiology continues to be basically a western phenomenon. Initially, the field attained its growth and independence in France and Germany while planting colonies of students all around Europe, in North America, and eventually in Japan. This situation continues to be true. In 1968, only two Asian countries, Japan and India, participated in the international meetings, and there were no delegates whatever from nonwhite Africa or the Islamic world. Large delegations from the main Latin American countries showed the degree to which those nations, as well as eastern Europe, have become integrated into the western scientific system. It also indicates how widely the growth of scientific physiology has spread. The virtual absence of Asian and African participants underlines the double cultural system which exists in the modern world.

Specialization within physiological studies and numerical as well as geographical expansion have meant a major explosion of data, evidenced in the proliferation of meetings and journals. In 1950, there were already 250 publications dealing with physiology which totaled some 68,000 pages. At that time it was estimated that simply to read this material would require three times the total amount of working time available. The amounts have not declined since 1950. Specialization generates increased quantities of data, which in turn make the discriminating judgments necessary to further specialization possible. This process was already well under way in British physiology at the opening of the twentieth century. In important respects, physiology is a discipline whose extraordinary success in identifying and understanding particular and connected phenomena has ended by destroying the discipline as it was originally conceived. William Harvey provided the starting point for that process—its end is not yet in sight.

ADDITIONAL READINGS: Theodore M. Brown, "The College of Physicians and the Acceptance of Iatromechanism in England, 1665–1695," *Bulletin of the History of Medicine* 44 (January–February 1970): 112–130; Allen C. Debus, "The Paracelsians and the Chemists: The Chemical Dilemma in Renaissance Medicine," *Clio Medica* 7 (September 1972): 185–196; G. L. Geison, *Michael Foster and the Cambridge School of Physiology: The Scientific Enterprise in Late Victorian Society*, Princeton, 1978; F. Grande and N. B. Vassilier (eds.), *Claude Bernard and Experimental Medicine*, Cambridge, Mass., 1967; A. L. Hodgkin, et al., *The Pursuit of Nature: Informal Essays on the History of Physiology*, New York and London, 1977; Lester S. King, *The Growth of Medical Thought*, Chicago, 1963; J. M. D. Olmsted and E. H. Olmsted, *Claude Bernard and the Experimental Method in Medicine*, New York, 1952; Walter Pagel, *Paracelsus: An Introduction to Philosophical Medicine in the Era of the Renaissance*, Basel and New York, 1958; Karl S. Rothschuh, *History of Physiology*, Guenter Risse (trans.), Huntington, N. Y., 1973; Wolfgang Schneider, "Chemistry and Iatrochemistry," in Walter Pagel, *Science, Medicine, and Society in the Renaissance*, 2 vols., London, 1972, 1, 141–150; Joseph Schiller, *Physiology and Classification: Historical Relations*, Paris, 1980; Sir Edward Sharpey-Schafer, *History of the Physiological Society During Its First Fifty Years, 1876–1926*, Cambridge, 1927; W. P. D. Wightman, *Science and the Renaissance: An Introduction to the Study of the Sciences in the Sixteenth Century*, 2 vols., Edinburgh, 1962, 1, chaps. 11–13.

See also ANATOMY; CLINICAL MEDICINE.

Pneumonia

Pneumonia is an inflammation of the lungs which results from several pathogenic microorganisms, from chemical agents which may be inhaled, from radiation, from allergic reactions to foreign particles which find their way into the lungs, and as a by-product of other diseases. The old and infirm, especially those with chronic heart conditions, are likely to develop pneumonia, and this group, together with infants, is the most susceptible. Winter is the time of greatest pneumonia mortality, and the largest part of pneumonia cases is caused by bacteria, with the pneumococcus (*Diplococcus pneumoniae*) the leading cause of pneumonia deaths. Modern chemotherapies applied at the onset of pneumonia symptoms have largely eliminated the long-drawn-out, costly battles with the disease, and pneumonia is far less common today than even 50 years ago.

Because of the multicausal character of pneumonia, diagnosis of the disease was very difficult before the various bacteria causing it were isolated; and even since, unless postmortem examinations are routinely done, pneumonia mortality figures must be considered to be educated estimates. A recent estimate of pneumonia deaths for the twentieth century gave the figures 202.2 per 100,000 in 1900; 103.9 in 1935; and 30.9 in 1970. Though it would be an obvious exaggeration to say that pneumonia has all but disappeared from modern life, its powers as a killer have been considerably reduced, and it hardly generates the fear it did in the past, when the onset of pneumonia was like a sentence of death.

Pneumonia has been a human problem from the earliest times. Mummified remains from the tenth century B.C. show signs of pneumonia, and early medical sources discuss disease conditions which include it. The Hippocratic writings of the fifth and early fourth centuries B.C. refer to a condition called "peripneumonia," a term which was to continue in use for 2,000 years and which covered all acute diseases of the chest with pains in the side. According to Hippocrates, when breathing was painful, when there was coughing, and "the sputa expectorated be of a blond or livid colour, or likewise thin and frothy, and florid," the physician should bleed "largely and boldly," especially if the pain were acute.

In the second century A.D., Aretaeus of Cappadocia gave a more detailed description of pneumonic disease while offering a similar though more violent course of treatment. He called peripneumonia an inflammation of the lungs with acute fever and "heaviness of the chest." There was normally no pain when the disease was limited to the lungs, for lungs are "naturally insensible, being of loose texture, like wool." Pain occurred when there was inflammation of any membranes and particularly those attaching the lungs to the chest. When respiration was hard and breath hot, the patient would struggle to get erect to ease breathing, and "there [was] thirst, dryness of the tongue, desire of cold air, aberration of mind," and a cough which, though often dry, sometimes brought up "a frothy phlegm, or slightly tinged with bile, or with a very florid tinge of blood." This last was the worst sign of all. To counteract these symptoms, Aretaeus bled furiously from both arms simultaneously, purged, gave "attenuent and diluent drinks," applied mustard to the chest, and prescribed soda in a decoction of hyssop and, when the fever retreated, wine "devoid of astringency." This treatment actually changed very little until the twentieth century. Aretaeus, like all ancient authorities, regarded pneumonia as a dangerous, high-mortality disease, but there is very little evidence to show what high mortality meant, and in the following centuries, nothing further of significance was added to the record.

New information on pneumonic diseases appeared with the revival of clinical medicine together with the interest in anatomy, physiology, and pathology in early modern Europe. In the seventeenth and eighteenth centuries, medical writers began to try to identify and classify pneumonias on the basis of clinical and eventually postmortem data. The early results were confusing. Thomas Sydenham, writing in the second half of the seventeenth century, mixed peripneumonia and pleurisy together, though he noted that peripneumonia had the greater effect on the lungs. Hermann Boerhaave in the eighteenth century saw two different kinds of peripneumonia. Boerhaave may have been attempting to describe the difference between lobar and lobular pneumonia. The most important development in this period, however, came from postmortem examinations. In the middle of the eighteenth century, Giovanni Battista Morgagni described the pneumonic lung consolidations which produced a texture like solid flesh, while Matthew Baillie, the first pathologist in Britain to relate case histories to postmortem findings, accurately described hepatization of the lungs. Leon Auenbrugger in the second half of the eighteenth century and René Laënnec early in the nineteenth century developed techniques for discovering what was happening in living patients' lungs during the course of pneumonia attacks. Auenbrugger used percussion, literally thumping on the thorax, to identify areas where fluid was accumulating. Laënnec's stethoscope (q.v.) and the auscultation method permitted him to diagnose pneumonia in its early stages and to separate pneumonia from pleurisy. Finally, in 1849, Karl von Rokitansky differentiated between lobar and lobular pneumonia.

Pneumonia was very active throughout the early modern period. It was recognized to be a disease of worldwide incidence which was most severe during cold, wet weather and was notably worse where living conditions were poor. August Hirsch, the eminent German pathologist and epidemologist, identified several waves of pneumonia epidemics which he asserted had swept over Europe and North America from the sixteenth to the nineteenth centuries. By the time his work appeared in its second edition (1881–1883), the author had accepted a bacterial cause for pneumonia, and he suggested that the different clinical symptoms the disease showed resulted from differing bacterial causes as well as varying environments.

The bacterial causes for pneumonia were actually identified in the 1880s. Louis Pasteur isolated what was later named the pneumococcus from the saliva of a pneumonia patient in 1881. Three years later, Albert Fraenkel demonstrated how the pneumonia-causing agent produced the course of the disease. Carl Friedländer had identified the bacilli in the lungs of some pneumonia patients a year earlier. In 1886, Anton Weichselbaum confirmed the work of these earlier investigators. Fraenkel's bacterium became the pneumococcus and was recognized to be the most common bacterial cause for pneumonia. Friedländer's organism was found to be different and much rarer, producing a severe pneumonia in an estimated 1 percent of known cases.

The work done by Fraenkel, Friedländer, and Weichselbaum was the beginning of an identification parade which, over the years, has identified and described dozens of pneumonia-causing bacteria. During World War I, Raymond Dochez, Oswald Avery, and a team of scientists at the Rockefeller Institute developed a typology for classifying this milling crowd. The various strains of pneumococci responsible for acute lobar pneumonia were organized into types I, II, and III. One half of all cases fell into one of these classes. A miscellaneous type IV was added and has grown steadily to include some 70 different strains. Types I and II have proved to be responsible in the classic cases of lobar pneumonia among young adults; type III is most common in old or debilitated patients; and type IV has most commonly been at the root of infant pneumonia cases.

The typing of bacterial causes was an important step in analyzing the disease, but there was no effective cure for acute cases. This point was driven home with terrible finality in the influenza (q.v.) epidemics from 1918 to 1920, in which millions perished. In the beginning, the pneumonic complication of influenza infection was almost totally irresistible. Lung cavities filled rapidly with a pink, frothy liquid, and the victim's bluish coloration announced oxygen starvation and the onset of asphyxia. Postmortems revealed marked differences between common pneumonias and those generated by the influenza attack. As the influenza epidemics continued, however, the proportion of pneumoina cases in which pneumococci could be identified increased as against the pneumonia resulting from the primary influenza infection.

Treatments for pneumonia through the early twentieth century were surprisingly traditional. Both cupping and bleeding were still used in Europe into the 1920s, as were strong emetics, though the counterirritant method of drawing threads through the skin was abandoned. Even so, pneumonia therapy in the 1920s still reflected the idea that so dangerous a disease required very strong medicine. One treatment recommended three grains of calomel to open the bowels and a gastric irritant expectorant mixture which was given every four hours to bring up sputum. Digitalis to "strengthen the heart muscle" was sometimes included, morphia was used as a hypnotic in the first two days, and chloral mixtures or bromides were employed after that. Barbiturates eventually replaced bromides, brandy and oxygen were both used as stimulants, and if further stimulation were required, physicians would turn to strychnine or coramine. Fluids to the amount of 15 pints in 24 hours were employed to flush out the toxins. The battle might persist for eight or nine days until a "crisis" was reached, when either the fever broke, the other symptoms subsided, and convalescence could begin, or the patient died.

Typing of pneumococci led to antiserums for each type. When the type of pneumococcus at work could be identified, antiserums provided effective treatment. This development was well along when Prontosil, the azo dye containing sulfanilamide, reached the market in 1935. Sulfanilamide was effective against streptococcal infections and was helpful in staving off diseases where pneumonia would follow as a secondary effect. Sulfapyridine, which affected some pneumococci, appeared soon after, and the chemotherapy of pneumonia was begun. Penicillin (q.v.), which was known to be effective against bacteria causing pneumonia, became available for emergency civilian use in 1944 and 1945, and by 1946 it was in general use. Both sulfa treatments and penicillin had their exponents. The former was more familiar and was of recognized effect. It was also easier to administer than penicillin, which required a series of injections. The sulfa treatment could be done orally. Penicillin, however, appeared to be more effective. Pneumonia mortality where penicillin was used declined to just 6.4 percent of the cases treated, while the sulfa preparations had a 14.3 percent mortality. Both, of course, were a marked improvement over the routinely anticipated 30 percent mortality without the new drugs. With understanding of both penicillin resistance and the allergic reaction penicillin could generate, caution in prescribing it took over. By this time, however, there were whole clusters of effective antibiotics available, including Chloromycetin, Aureomycin, and Terramycin, which permitted a variety and balance in treatment.

Under the barrage of new drugs, pneumonia has receded as a major disease. Indeed, with massive antibiotic assaults in the first stages, pneumonia often has no chance to develop, and when it does, complete recovery in 10 days to two weeks is common. Pneumonia remains a serious threat to the old and bedridden, and infants continue to be susceptible. But with the modern therapies available, even in those groups the incidence and even the mortality can be held low. Though a significant cause of death in earlier days, pneumonia has ceased to be a major factor where therapies are available. In common with other leading causes for death before the twentieth century, pneumonia has been brought within the circle of regularly effective treatment.

ADDITIONAL READINGS: E. M. Brockbank and William Brockbank, "Pneumonia," in Walter R. Bett (ed), *The History and Conquest of Common Diseases*, Norman, Okla., 1954, 84–98; H. F. Dowling, *Fighting Infection: Conquests of the Twentieth Century*, Cambridge, Mass., 1977; August Hirsch, *Geographical and Historical Pathology*, Charles Creighton (trans.), London, 1883, III, 116–168.

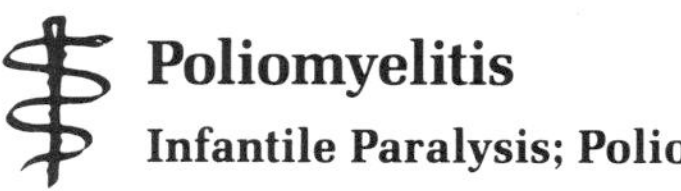

Poliomyelitis

Infantile Paralysis; Polio

Poliomyelitis is a viral infection which has had its worst effects in advanced, affluent, and hygienic societies. It is a disease, moreover, whose recent history has been marked by bitter rivalries among medical scientists, scandalous errors in judgment, and a sharp conflict of interests among foundations using advertising techniques to attract contributions, public health officials charged with making objective decisions on new drugs and treatments, and scientists pursuing research. Though no cure for polio is known, the means effectively to control the disease are readily available and have been successfully employed since 1954. Epidemiologists are cautious, however, about predicting the eradication of poliomyelitis, and they are quick to emphasize that control depends on maintaining high immunity levels.

The Disease Poliomyelitis is a viral infection of the intestinal tract which belongs to the class of picornaviruses, i.e., small (Italian: *piccolo*) viruses containing ribonucleic acid (RNA). Neutralization tests have established three antigenic types of poliovirus, called 1, 2, and 3. Type 1 has been responsible for most large outbreaks, with type 3 occasionally involved; type 2 is associated with sporadic clinical cases. Immunization must be maintained against all three, though natural infection confers such immunity. The only reservoir for poliovirus is the human being, and the virus is found worldwide. Infection is common, with the vast majority of incidents passing unnoticed. Paralytic polio is an unusual occurrence, though it was the mounting incidence of paralytic cases which aroused interest in the disease in the nineteenth century. Since infection produces immunity, poliomyelitis appeared first as a children's disease, especially for those under the age of five, and this gave the disease the name infantile paralysis. During the twentieth century, increasing numbers of adults have been attacked by paralytic polio because immunizing infection was not occurring during childhood. This was a direct consequence of improved hygiene and public health policies.

Polio virus enters the body through the mouth by ingestion or inhalation. It then lodges either in the tonsils or the surrounding lymphoid tissues of the pharynx, or in the lymphoid follicles of the ileum. The synthesis of viral RNA begins within two hours. Soon after, it is excreted into the lumen of the gut and will be found in cervical and mesenteric lymph nodes. Three days later, poliovirus can be recovered from throat secretions and from feces. It remains about a week in the throat but will be found for several weeks in the feces. There are usually no apparent symptoms when the virus does not spread beyond the lymph nodes (nonapparent infection); clinical symptoms begin to occur when the virus passes into the bloodstream and is carried to the central nervous system. This only happens in a small percentage of cases. It is estimated that from 90 to 95 percent of poliovirus infection is symptomless, limited to the gut, and can only be detected by laboratory tests. During the incubation period, an infected person may show signs of an "illness of infection," with headache, sore throat, and fever. This condition may persist for two or three days, but unless there is some viral meningitis, it may well be considered influenza or not be noted at all. In such minor infections, there are no neurological signs.

When poliovirus passes through the lymph system, enters the bloodstream, and is carried to the central nervous system, paralysis will appear, though the degree of paralysis and its permanence will depend on the quantity of poliovirus which attacks, where the attack concentrates, and whether or not extensive neuron destruction occurs. Where damage is not extensive, paralyzed muscles may regain the ability to function in from four weeks to six months; most recovery is complete by six months, however. Paralysis is asymmetrical, involving muscle groups (in order) of legs, arms, back, thorax, and diaphragm. It is possible for partial or total respiratory paralysis to occur. Though sensory loss is rare, retention of urine may follow extensive paralysis. Approximately 10 percent of paralytic cases involve paralysis of muscles controlled by cranial nerves (bulbar polio) which may be especially serious because the soft palate and pharynx are involved, and where laryngeal muscles are affected, there is danger of asphyxia. Bulbar and spinal polio may occur together. Such major paralytic attacks can produce a substantial mortality, usually from respiratory obstruction by secretions or atelectasis. Bulbar polio develops a mortality of up to 20 percent of cases; spinal paralysis has a mortality of from 5 to 10 percent, with the highest rate among infants in their first year and the elderly. Even so, paralytic polio, as one authority put it, "is not, in one sense, a disease on its own at all. It is a rare and serious complication of a common and trivial infection."

Early History Despite intense modern interest in poliomyelitis, no systematic attempt to identify it or to define its extent has ever been made for ancient times. There are indications, however, that paralytic polio, though never abundant or widespread, appeared sporadically. The oldest visual evidence is a stela from the Eighteenth Dynasty (1580–1350 B.C.) of Egypt, which portrays a crippled priest whose withered and shortened left leg is held in the *equinus* position associated with flaccid paralysis. Some of the cases of clubfoot described in the Hippocratic writings (fifth century B.C.) may include deformities caused by polio, and there is mention of a paralysis which came on in the summer or late fall. A vase of the fourth century B.C. from the Louvre collection of early Roman pottery depicts a crippled man leaning on a stick. His lower limbs appear to have been damaged by a poliolike paralysis. In the second century A.D., Galen, the classical physician whose writings dominated the medieval world, discussed clubfoot as being either congenital or acquired. Acquired clubfoot was thought to occur in infancy, an idea which could indicate the presence of polio.

References during the European Middle Ages are hardly less equivocal. There is an entry for 708 and 709 in the Ulster annals which refers to "a pestilence called *baccach* ("Lameness") which is in the right diagnostic region, but there are no supporting data. Excavators in southern Greenland, however, did find 25 fifteenth-century skeletons which show bony deformations suggestive of polio. Nothing more definite appears until the eighteenth century. Sir Walter Scott (1771–1832) suffered polio as a child and recorded his experience of a disease which left him lame but healthy. In 1789, Michael Underwood, a London physician and obstetrician, brought out the second edition of his *Treatise on Diseases of Children* which included a new section on what he considered an unusual disease. Its symptoms he could describe, but he had no knowledge about it. He remarked that this disease "seems to arise from debility, and usually attacks children previously reduced by fever" in the age group one to five years. The symptoms of this wasting paralytic condition seem clearly to signal polio. In 1808, Christopher Carlander, then chief health officer at Götborg in Sweden, wrote a letter describing several children who developed fever and paralysis in their lower limbs. Carlander did not consider this an epidemic, though he seems to have suspected contagion. During the early nineteenth century, reports of a fever and paralysis came from many places, including the United States, where George Colmer, a London-born physician, described an outbreak in Springfield, Louisiana, in 1848.

Polio Defined: 1850 to 1900 The first comprehensive and authoritative study on polio was written by Jacob von Heine and published in 1840. Heine's work began the modern medical history of polio, while the gradually increasing incidence of paralytic polio concentrated attention on it. Heine recognized that an acute attack involved "an affection of the central nervous system, specifically the spinal cord," but he and the medical profession generally were unaware of the broad extent of polio infection and the role of nonapparent, or weak-case, carriers. Heine focused on the paralysis, and this emphasis remained central even after the epidemiology of polio was more fully understood a century later.

The first recognized evidence that polio was epidemic came from Scandinavia. Fourteen cases of paralytic polio appeared in Oslo, Norway, in 1868. They were treated as spinal meningitis. Thirteen further cases were reported at Umeo in northern Sweden in 1881. These were treated by Karl Oscar Medin, an early Swedish pediatrician whose work, together with Heine's, was of sufficient importance that early in the twentieth century polio was called Heine-Medin disease. In 1886, 9 cases were reported from Mandel, Norway. The following year, Stockholm had 44 cases.

During that same period, polio outbreaks were reported in Italy (1889), France (1885), and Germany (1886). Boston, Massachusetts, had 26 cases in 1893, and in 1894, the first large reported outbreak took place in Rutland County, Vermont. There were 132 cases.

The pattern of a gradual increase in paralytic cases, the only ones that were clinically observable, was epidemiologically significant, but there was no way that the evidence could be correctly interpreted. Improved personal hygiene and public sanitation were reducing the opportunities for early exposure and immunity, while in remote areas, levels of infection and immunity were further reduced through low levels of contact with potential carriers. Two American physicians, James J. Putnam and Edward W. Taylor, noted during the Boston outbreak that urban dwellers appeared to have a greater immunity than rural or suburban populations. They also wondered whether the acute, paralytic form of the disease they treated had not become especially prevalent. Though such thinking was coming close to the truth, it was not systematic, and there was no basis in clinical observation for building a viable disease theory.

Epidemic Polio: 1900 to 1930 From 1899 to 1903, poliomyelitis reached epidemic proportions in Scandinavia, and in 1905, an outbreak in Sweden recorded 1031 cases. This outbreak proved to be particularly significant owing to the work of Ivar Wickman, who became convinced that there were probably as many "abortive," or nonparalytic, cases as paralytic ones, or more, and that they were equally infective. Wickman was the first to grasp the significance of the fact that the infection could bypass the nervous system entirely and to argue that while the paralysis was dramatic, it was epidemiologically wrong to concentrate on it, because those who escaped paralysis were nevertheless infective. But this created the further question of what then constituted a "reportable" poliomyelitis attack. It was plainly impossible to report all suspicious illnesses, and until reliable bacteriological tests became available, this problem was insoluble. Nevertheless, Wickman's clinical observations and intuition had led him to stress the contagiousness of the disease and the role of mild, nonparalytic cases as carriers. He also raised the possibility of nonapparent cases, that is, unrecognized cases, which were carriers as well. His instincts were confirmed by laboratory testing in 1907.

Wickman's emphasis on contagion fitted the scientific disposition of his time. Bacterial causes for disease were already an established fact at the opening of the twentieth century, and parallel with the bacteriological revolution there was a revolution in the study of pathology (q.v.). Thirty-five years before the Swedish epidemic, Jean-Martin Charcot and his associates had identified and confirmed the pathological effects of polio in the spinal cord, connecting the destruction of motor cells with the onset of paralysis. When the immunologist Karl Landsteiner demonstrated the polio virus in Vienna in 1908, it was an expected discovery. What was not appreciated at the time was that there was more than one viral type involved. Until this fact was understood, the epidemiological picture would be incomplete, and no effective immunization program would be possible. Lansteiner's discovery, however, meant that polio diagnosis could be made firm, that immunity levels could be tested, and that nonapparent cases could be identified.

Most of what Ivar Wickman had argued was confirmed in Landsteiner's work. Tragically, despite scientific confirmation, Wickman was passed over for a professorship at Stockholm, and in 1914 he committed suicide. Wickman's type of clinical work was out of vogue, and most of his basic contributions fell into obscurity. Research shifted focus toward the neurotropic aspects of the disease and especially toward microscopic analysis. The issues which Wickman elucidated only returned to the mainstream 30 years later.

By 1912, a sound etiological and epidemiological picture of polio was taking shape, but the discoveries of the first years of the twentieth century were matched by polio's continuing spread. It had become epidemic in the three Scandinavian countries, the United States, Canada, Switzerland, England, Wales, and Australia. Though New York reported 750 cases in 1907, 1200 would be nearer the actual total, and there were epidemics in Mason City, Iowa (1910), Cincinnati, Ohio (1911), and Buffalo and Batavia, New York (1912). In 1911, Sweden had the worst polio outbreak yet recorded—a total of 3840 cases—but the United States was displacing Scandinavia as the leader in polio cases. In 1916, New York City reported

9,000 polio cases, an incidence per 100,000 population of 185.2. The national incidence figure, which had been 7.9 per 100,000, jumped to 18.5. In 1917, a Public Health Service report summarized the position. Poliomyelitis was an exclusively human disease which transferred directly from person to person by some still-undetermined mechanism; the infection was far more prevalent even than the number of clinically recognized carriers and mild abortive cases; and paralytic cases represented a relatively minor factor in the spread of the disease. An epidemic involving from 1 to 3 recognized cases per 1,000 was thought sufficient to immunize the general population to such an extent that the epidemic would decline spontaneously for lack of susceptible cases. Moreover, a relatively low incidence rate was sufficient to limit incidence in a future epidemic. Finally, in the face of widespread inapparent infection, quarantine, sequestration, and isolation were ineffectual and disruptive.

Medicine and Polio: 1920 to 1950 Polio continued to be a significant problem in the period between the two world wars, and while its incidence grew, by 1939, a shift in age groups from children to adults was becoming statistically clear. In 1934, during an outbreak in Los Angeles, California, 5.4 percent of the doctors attending cases and 10.7 percent of the nurses contracted polio. Cases appeared in 1941 and 1942 in the British Middle East army in Egypt and the U.S. armed forces in north Africa and the Pacific. This made polio a military disease for the first time and called forth special efforts.

Polio incidence remained limited in the military, but the problem of adult infection was growing. In 1949, U.S. Public Health Service figures showed the shift: In 1916, 95 percent of the cases reported were children 9 or under; in 1947, that figure had fallen to 52 percent. In 1916, only 3 percent of the recorded cases were in the age group 10 to 19; in 1947, that figure had risen to 38 percent. And the total numbers of cases continued to grow. By the opening of the 1950s, case incidence in the United States had gone above 30,000 per year. Even in proportional terms, this was a much higher rate than that of the next highest country, the United Kingdom, which approached 4000 per annum.

Knowledge about polio almost kept step with the mounting incidence. The most important development was the reclassification of the disease from a nasal infection to an intestinal disease. Work in Dr. Max Theiler's laboratory at the Rockefeller Institute in 1934 showed that there were viruses which affected mice in precisely the way human poliovirus affected people. The mouse virus would not infect humans, but mouse polio studies provided a model for studying the human disease. In 1939 it was established that the mouse virus could be found in the intestines of healthy mice. The war interrupted this work at the Rockefeller Institute, but in Denmark, Dr. Herdis von Magnus took it up to establish that Theiler's original (TO) mouse virus was in nearly all laboratory mouse colonies; that the great majority of laboratory mice had acquired immunity; and that newborn mice raised away from exposure to the mouse colony were between 10 and 250 times more susceptible to infection.

Applied to humans, this work held the key to why polio was increasing in advanced societies. The polio virus lived in the intestine, and in societies with poor sanitary facilities, there would be early exposure to it. Better sanitation meant less exposure, lower immunity levels, and increased susceptibility. Polio virus had been found in excreta as early as 1912, but after 1915 research had concentrated on the nose and throat passages because these seemed to offer the most direct route to the nervous system. In 1937, the Yale Poliomyelitis Group began to follow up new evidence that polio was an intestinal infection. The idea was sharply contested, but once it came to be accepted, it meant that children themselves were reservoirs of infection and that polio was spread by entirely healthy carriers.

Another critical piece of the polio puzzle was identified in 1931 when F. M. Burnet and Dr. Jean Macnamara announced that they had identified two different strains of polio virus and thus raised the question of how many different strains of polio virus there might actually be. Though the Yale group confirmed the Burnet-Macnamara findings, it was not until after World War II that the problem was finally solved. In 1946, the National Foundation for Infantile Paralysis financed systematic research on the typology of poliovirus, and in 1953, the now-established types 1, 2, and 3 were announced. Since the foundation had parceled out the research to a number of university laboratories, the typing project became a prototype for cooperative interuniversity research programs in the postwar United States.

Not all the efforts in these seminal decades succeeded. There was one major failure whose repercussions were still felt 20 years later; as a cautionary tale, it should be recalled whenever new therapeutic drugs are tested. There had been high hopes after 1916 that a serum drawn from convalescent polio cases might offer a cure, or at least some immunity from the disease, but those hopes had died by 1931. Nevertheless, thinking on prevention tended in the light of other successful campaigns to focus on immunization, and as more information on the virus and how it attacked became available, there appeared to be a basis for developing a vaccine. Two men, Dr. Maurice Brodie in New York and Dr. John Kolmer in Philadelphia, had the inside track, and both announced polio vaccines in 1934. The vaccines were tried on human beings in 1935 with disastrous results. The Brodie vaccine used a formalin-inactivated virus. The principle was sound, as Dr. Jonas Salk's vaccine showed two decades later, but Dr. Brodie, apparently influenced by the competition with Dr. Kolmer, rushed his vaccine into use without adequate testing. Dr. Kolmer's preparation, a live but "attenuated" virus, was even more questionable, but the institute he headed, together with the William S. Merrell Pharmaceutical Company, put over 21,000 doses into circulation. The results, according to a report printed in the Journal of the American Medical Association, were 12 vaccine-related cases of poliomyelitis, 9 from the Kolmer treatment and 3 from the Brodie. There were 6 deaths, 1 where the Brodie vaccine was used and 5 with the Kolmer vaccine. The cases occurred where paralytic polio was not epidemic.

Both the Kolmer and the Brodie undertakings were publicly reviewed and criticized at the meeting of the Southern Branch of the American Public Health Association in November 1935. Several errors were identified. The chemistry, especially in the Kolmer preparation, was considered crude; there was a common failure to take into account what was known concerning the antigen differences in polio strains; and there was inadequate animal testing before using the vaccines on people. The Brodie and Kolmer experiments were premature. Their failure developed resistance to the vaccine approach, which was commonly acknowledged to be dangerous, and to attempts to study vaccines' effects on human subjects. This fear persisted into the 1950s inhibiting research and reinforcing demands for absolute safety.

The War on Polio: 1920 to 1950 Poliomyelitis is an expensive disease to study and to treat, and the history of polio cannot be separated from the development of institutions whose primary function was to promote public support for research, treatment, and prevention. One of the earliest appeals for public funds to aid polio-stricken children was in Australia, and though Dr. Jean Macnamara, who organized and directed the appeal, later diverted some funds to research, her primary fund-raising effort was for treatment. In Sweden, there was an annual appeal for a fund to be given to the king on his birthday. The king then determined how the fund was to be spent. In 1938, when King Gustav V was 80, he dedicated his annual fund to research on disabling diseases, especially polio, and he repeated the dedication in subsequent years. This fund became the base for the Swedish National Association Against Poliomyelitis.

The institutionalization of private philanthropy reached its most complete development in the United States. Prior to the establishment of the polio foundation, research on polio had to compete with other specialties before the Rockefeller Foundation or the National Research Council. Only the National Tuberculosis Association (now the American Lung Association), which was organized in 1904, was dedicated to a single disease, and it only began to give research grants in 1915 (see Tuberculosis). With the rise in polio incidence between 1900 and 1920, public opinion began to call for a "campaign against polio" and an institution to direct it. Undoubtedly the successful campaigns waged by the Army Medical Corps and the Public Health Service against yellow fever and malaria supported the idea of a similar assault on polio.

The antipolio campaign became a reality when Franklin Delano Roosevelt, former under secretary of the Navy and an emerging figure on the national political scene, became involved. Roosevelt had contracted paralytic polio in 1921. Though crippled by the disease, he battled back successfully to be elected governor of New York and, in 1932, President of the United States. Roosevelt's example was inspirational, but he was determined to contribute as well to organizing the struggle with polio. In 1927, he established the Georgia Warm Springs Foundation, which concentrated on care after attack and emphasized rehabilitation.

More was needed, and in 1929, Jeremiah Milbank, a New York philanthropist, proposed the formation of an international committee for the study of infantile paralysis, to comprise a panel of experts on the subject who could identify critical scientific issues and coordinate work on them. When Franklin Roosevelt was elected President, his political status and personal success in combating polio were enlisted for fund-raising purposes. The President's Birthday Ball Commission was set up to promote a gala social event on January 20, Roosevelt's birthday, and to administer the funds accumulated. The money was to be used for polio research, and the first 16 grants were made in 1935. It was this commission which became the staging for the National Foundation for Infantile Paralysis which President Roosevelt inaugurated under the direction of his former law partner Basil O'Connor.

The national foundation brought affluence to research workers who previously had only small budgets from a few granting agencies. The foundation undertook a massive public relations campaign whose focus was the March of Dimes, a symbol of the power of numberless small contributions ordinary people could make. Publicity was essential, and therefore every advance which research scientists announced was exploited to demonstrate the value of the work and to promote further giving. Polio discoveries became news, investigators were under pressure for the "breakthrough" which was always imminent, and both scientists and administrators became involved in promotion activities.

Science lost its private, personal character, and some scientists felt, as one researcher put it, that the foundation inhibited scientific advance because "Madison Avenue methods did not mix with anything but pseudo-science." Yet major accomplishments flowed from the foundation's support, including the viral typing program and the Salk vaccine. There were others who believed that the public relations approach exaggerated the polio problem at the expense of other diseases, and it was also argued that research was actually less well-funded than the popular and highly visible treatment programs or even the cost of fund-raising.

The foundation was undoubtedly successful as a fund-raiser. Its annual income between 1938 and 1962 averaged $25 million and its total receipts were $630 million. Fifty-nine percent of its budget went for medical care programs, 8 percent was spent on education, 11 percent on research, and 13 percent on administration and fund-raising. Other societies came into existence after World War II to deal with polio. In 1948, the European Association against Poliomyelitis and Allied Diseases was founded, and after 1952, the World Health Organization took on a leading role. The National Foundation for Infantile Paralysis, was, however, the largest, the most powerful, and the most influential organization in the polio campaign, and it became a significant model for fund-raising societies and for the coordination of research efforts.

Sister Kenny An Australian nurse, Sister Elizabeth Kenny, symbolized another aspect of the polio era. Standard treatments for paralytic polio victims included immobilization in a variety of braces, casts, and forms. Elizabeth Kenny, who began working with polio victims in the Australian bush in 1910, rejected the standard approach. She used several different techniques to encourage patients to move and use their paralyzed members. Claiming to have brought polio victims "back to normalcy," she campaigned for public support for her methods, engaging in debates and public confrontations with her opponents. Her message of hope came at a time when public opinion had been sensitized to polio issues, and when she visited the United States in 1940, she met with an enthusiastic reception. Minneapolis and the University of Minnesota gave her a particularly warm welcome, and while she received support from specialists all over the country, Minneapolis remained the capital of Sister Kenny's healing enterprise, and the Elizabeth Kenny Institute was founded there in 1942.

Sister Kenny's critics were legion, but their number multiplied as she became involved in a bruising battle with the medical research establishment. Elizabeth Kenny was determined not to fall under the control of the National Foundation for Infantile Paralysis, and the foundation, in its turn, refused to make a major grant to her program. Her supporters then established the Sister Kenny Foundation in 1945, which guaranteed her independence. The foundation made research grants and, in cooperation with the University of Minnesota and the Minnesota State Health Department, supported work on live oral polio vaccine.

Sister Kenny was a controversial figure who inspired a nearly fanatic devotion in some followers. Unfortunately, in fighting the political and administrative battles her program entailed, she lost touch with ward work, where she was notably skilled, especially in dealing with children. Some of the attacks on her were scurrilous, and her last years were filled with bitter conflict. Even so, Sister Kenny's work was of the first importance in reforming the techniques of aftercare in paralytic poliomyelitis.

The Salk and Sabin Vaccines: 1950 to 1970 The 1950s opened with a burgeoning polio epidemic. Incidence in the United States reached 50,000 cases annually. The accumulation of scientific knowledge, especially the results of the successful poliovirus typing campaign, made a new approach to immunization practical, though fears of a repeat of the 1935 Brodie-Kolmer debacle counseled caution. The National Foundation for Infantile Paralysis decided in 1950 to begin work on the vaccine problem, and they found a leader for their program in Dr. Jonas Salk of the University of Pittsburgh. Dr. Salk favored a killed virus vaccine. He had worked with formalin-inactivated influenza vaccine during World War II, and he was familiar as well with the administrative and logistical problems involved in vaccine testing.

On January 23, 1953, Dr. Salk reported a series of successful preliminary tests, and his results were published in the *Journal of the American Medical Association* in March. A favorable editorial appeared in April, and the Immunization Committee of the National Foundation for Infantile Paralysis decided to move ahead. The foundation was firmly committed to the Salk vaccine, though there was also support for a live oral polio vaccine. The Salk vaccine was clearly safer, however, and it was ready for immediate testing. The problem with the Salk vaccine was that it required multiple shots and a booster to achieve immunity. The live oral vaccine was not so advanced, was more chancy, but could confer full immunity for all three types of poliovirus with a single application. When the immunization committee met, however, discussion was foreclosed, and the only issues explored concerned how best to administer the killed vaccine tests.

An elaborate double-blind testing procedure was established which involved 1,829,916 first-, second-, and third-grade children in 44 states. The plan operated on two levels. The first involved between 600,000 and 700,000 children who received the vaccine. First- and third-grade schoolmates were observed as controls. All results were coded, and the codes were kept secret to the end of the tests to avoid premature revelations. The tests were done between March and June 1954. The results were announced on April 12, 1955, the tenth anniversary of Franklin Roosevelt's death.

There was a lively public interest in the tests, and the licensing committee of the National Institutes of Public Health prepared to meet to decide on licensing the vaccine as soon as the report was in. A last minute mix-up gave the press word that the tests had been entirely successful before the explanation could be made, but the report was unequivocal: There was "no evidence that cases of poliomyelitis attributable to the inoculation of vaccine occurred during the 1954 Field Trial." The vaccine was safe—and, as Dr. Salk said when pressed to define the term, "What is safer than safe?" With a 50 percent protection rate established, licensing followed at once.

But the tests were not to finish without one more paroxysm of tragedy. Just 15 days later, children vaccinated with polio vaccine began to sicken with the disease. The public was outraged, and the entire program faced cancellation. The basic question was whether this was an accident or whether the vaccine itself was dangerous. The evidence said accident. The Public Health Service's Communicable Disease Center responded quickly and was able to trace the outbreak to seven lots of vaccine manufactured by Cutter Laboratories in California which contained some live virus. The vaccine itself was sound, but better control measures by commercial houses manufacturing the vaccine were essential. In this outbreak, 204 cases of polio resulted, three-fourths of which were paralytic, and 11 of the victims died. Subsequently, the program was continued, and 4 million doses of the vaccine were administered between April 22 and May 7 with no further incidents.

Though the Salk vaccine was safe, it was less efficient or effective than the live attenuated virus vaccine, and the multiple shots required created serious logistical problems, especially in less-developed countries. There was, therefore, continued pressure to move ahead with the oral vaccine. At the time the national foundation took over the Salk vaccine, Dr. A. B. Sabin reported excellent progress with his oral vaccine. When the Salk program succeeded, the foundation showed little interest in the Sabin product, but in July 1957, the World Health Organization began to organize testing for it. Twenty field trials of three oral vaccines, the Sabin included, were carried out in 20 countries during 1958 and 1959, and critically important evaluative conferences were held in 1959 and 1960 under sponsorship of the Pan-American Health Organization, with funding from The Sister Kenny Foundation.

Though tests showed that an attenuated oral vaccine was safe, the World Health Organization insisted on higher standards than any which the current series met. Since all three vaccines had been developed in the United States, all would need to meet stringent U.S. Public Health Service licensing standards administered under an ad hoc committee. The vaccines developed by Dr. Hilary Koprowski, the Lederle Laboratories, and Dr. Sabin went through intensive testing over a period of four years. In 1964, all three types were licensed for manufacture. The carnival atmosphere which had attended the announcement of the Salk vaccine was entirely absent from the introduction of Sabin-type oral polio vaccine.

Oral vaccine has gradually supplanted the Salk-type vaccine as the vaccine of choice, except in Sweden, and the movement toward worldwide immunization against polio which these two vaccine types have made possible has radically reduced polio incidence in precisely those countries where it had been most threatening. The most dramatic improvement came in the United States, where an average annual incidence of 37,864 in the years 1951 to 1955 fell away to 570 for 1961 to 1965. Most of the improvement came with the Salk vaccine, though the oral vaccines introduced in 1964 have continued and reinforced the pattern.

Polio has been brought under effective control, though there are aspects to the disease which are still not understood, and the maintenance of control in developing countries still poses significant problems. Stable social, political, and economic conditions are essential for effective public health programs in general, and the principle applies as well to maintaining high immunity levels against poliomyelitis. The absence of such stability in major areas of the world is a public health problem of considerable consequence in which a recrudescence of poliomyelitis is only one of the dangers to be faced.

ADDITIONAL READINGS: William Beatty and Geoffrey Marks, *Epidemics*, New York, 1976; Harry F. Dowling, *Fighting Infection: Conquests of the Twentieth Century*, Cambridge, Mass. 1977; P. J. Fisher, *The Polio Story*, London, 1967; Aaron E. Klein, *Trial by Fury: The Poliovaccine Controversy*, New York, 1972; J. H. Parish, *A History of Immunization*, London, 1965; chap. 29; John R. Paul, *A History of Poliomyelitis*, New York and London, 1971; John R. Wilson, *Margin of Safety: The Fight Against Polio*, London, 1962.

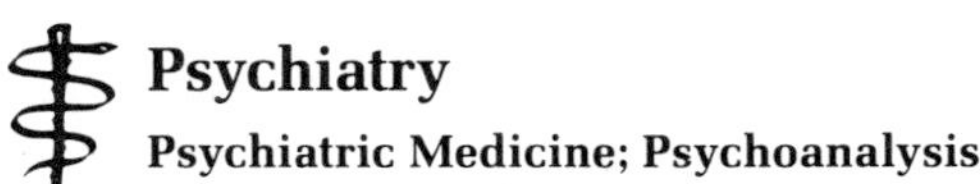

Psychiatry

Psychiatric Medicine; Psychoanalysis

Psychiatric medicine is a modern specialty dealing with the causes for and treatment of mental dysfunction and emotional disorders and their effects on general health. Until the end of the nineteenth century, medical explanations for mental illness stressed physiological causes. The conviction that the mind was a major source for hysterical or neurotic behavior developed late in the nineteenth century and found its most radical expression in Freudian psychoanalysis. During the twentieth century, psychiatry has become increasingly eclectic, recognizing the interplay between psychological and physiological causes. Modern psychiatrists receive both medical and psychiatric training, and those who wish to be licensed as psychoanalysts take work in that specialty as well. Preparation for Freudian psychoanalysis traditionally includes analysis of the candidate himself or herself.

Origins Psychiatric medicine began with the Hippocratic writings, which portrayed mental illness as the result of natural causes. In the treatise *On the Sacred Disease*, the Hippocratic writer asserted that epilepsy was caused by an accumulation of phlegm in the brain, not by divine act.

In other treatises, a similarly naturalistic explanation was given for phobias, melancholies, puerperal insanity, and hysteria. Melancholia resulted from an accumulation of black bile, and hysteria, considered to be exclusively a woman's disease, was caused by displacement of the uterus. Treatment for these conditions meant correcting their physical causes by bleeding, purging, diet, or prescribed specifics.

Most subsequent classical medical writers included some information on mental diseases, and a few made notable suggestions. In the first century A.D., Soranus of Ephesus advocated nurturing and nonviolent treatment for the insane, an idea which contrasted sharply with conventional wisdom. His near contemporary, Aretaeus, studied the effect of emotional disturbances on personality. His observations enabled him to identify and describe the successions of manic and depressive states separated by periods of lucidity in what was known as the "circular disease." In the preceding century, the Roman philosopher and orator Cicero argued that mental illness was a special disease category. Turning against humoral explanations, he suggested that melancholia came from emotional causes rather than an accumulation of black bile. He also believed that mental disorders could generate physical illness.

The classical tradition which the Middle Ages inherited remained firmly humoral in its explanations for disease, but in the sixteenth century, the brilliantly eccentric Paracelsus seemed to propose that chemical substances were involved in mental disorders and that what was thought might affect the state of mental health. Other works on mental disease remained closer to the humoral tradition. In 1586, Timothy Bright published his *Treatise on Melancholy,* which prepared the way for Robert Burton's more famous *Anatomy of Melancholy* (1621). Burton's melancholic was moody, cold, bitterly ironic, eccentric, misanthropic, and suicidal. Europeans suggested that the melancholic was a peculiarly English phenomenon, possibly a by-product of the climate. Thomas Sydenham, the most distinguished English physician in the seventeenth century, published an extraordinary description of hysteria and its effects in his *Epistolary Dissertation on the Hysterical Affections* (1682). It was Sydenham's conviction that hysteria was the chronic disease physicians were most likely to encounter. It affected men as well as women and could simulate any form of organic disorder including paralysis, vomiting, headache, heart palpitations, and even kidney stones. Sydenham's close observations on those he treated brought him very close to a modern conception of hysteria, though without a method for explaining what he observed.

Physiology and Psychology: 1700 to 1900 The eighteenth-century physiological systematizers and anatomists continued the tradition of physical explanations for mental conditions but added little to psychiatric understanding. A materialist psychology emerged in the debates over learning and perception, but important as this was for the intellectual history of the Enlightenment, it only reinforced the idea that insanity was a departure from the human being's inherent reason brought about by damage to the brain, bad education, or perverse intent. Whatever cause applied, incarceration and firm discipline were the required treatment. At the end of the century, Anton Mesmer manipulated the subconscious mind, but his doctrine rested on traditional theories of universal spirit force and flow. His followers until the time of Bernheim and Charcot were more interested in the techniques they used than in explaining the mind's nature or the psychological dynamics which affected mental health.

Although physiological explanations remained dominant, there was some interest in the early nineteenth century in appraising psychological factors as causes for mental disorders. In 1818, Johann C. A. Heinroth published a history of the diagnosis and treatment of mental diseases. Though fuzzy and unsystematic, his etiological explanations went beyond physical causes, and he proposed a gentle therapy according to which severe methods (shock, physical restraint, and punishments) should be reserved for the most intractable conditions. Heinroth was also an exponent of individual treatment. Each case required diagnosis and prescription, and detailed case histories were essential.

Heinroth's ideas ran against the materialist tide and were submerged in the masses of experimental and clinical data which the physiologists on one hand and the asylum managers on the other were collecting. The asylum movement had begun in the late eighteenth century as part of a pervasive effort to reform prisons and hospitals.

Led by Phillipe Pinel and Jean-Étienne Dominique Esquirol in France, Christian Reil in Prussia, William and Samuel Tuke in England, and Benjamin Rush in the United States, the reformers had begun to unchain the insane and create institutions designed for their care. Once they were segregated, it became possible to observe mental patients' behavior systematically, to compile clinical records and case histories, and to begin a new and more accurate classification of emotional disorders. Esquirol's work was particularly important. He outlined a new system of psychopathological concepts and gave what became modern definitions for illusion, hallucination, remission, intermission, dementia, and idiocy based on observations of thousands of cases. By the middle of the nineteenth century, the asylums provided a broad base in observed facts for classifying mental diseases. Using this material, Karl Kahlbaum, an asylum doctor, developed a basic method for studying mental disorders, which Emil Kraepelin, often considered the founder of modern psychiatry, described as "the careful pursuit of the course and culmination of mental diseases in individual cases, including autopsy." He noted that as a result of this method, modern physicians "can distinguish a set of clearly defined somatic pictures of diseases, which we are able to recognize symptomatically."

After the middle of the nineteenth century, the emphasis in psychiatric research shifted to university centers where scientific teams worked on specific problems. The models for these centers were the institutes for physiological and pathological research which grew up between 1800 and 1850. The university research institute freed the physician-scientist from ward work, provided the most advanced research technology, perpetuated the physiological interpretation of mental illness, and fostered an interdisciplinary methodology. The etiological assumptions for this work were laid down in 1830 in J. B. Friedreich's *Attempts at a History of the Literature of the Pathology and Therapy of Psychic Illnesses,* which was the first work of its kind. Friedreich stressed physical causes, refuted the psychological arguments offered by Heinroth and his followers, and became the standard authority on the subject for the next half century. Included in the tradition which developed was Wilhelm Griesinger, the founder of university psychiatry, who asserted that "mental illnesses are brain diseases" and organized research on brain pathology to locate mental disorders. Theodore Meynert and Carl Wernicke also played leading parts. Meynert theorized that mental disturbances arose from functional opposition in brain cortex and brain stem, while Wernicke's research on aphasia advanced the understanding of brain specialization and localization. Wernicke, however, combined physiology with associationist psychology, while Meynert exempted sexual deviations from his physiological explanations, considering homosexuality, for example, as psychological in origin. Though not a dominant theme, the recognition of psychological factors in analyzing mental conditions was significant.

The period between 1880 and 1920 brought a revolution in psychiatric understanding. The physiological approach yielded new information on brain and nerve dysfunction, bacteriology opened the possibility for identifying specific brain diseases with infective agents, and a start was made on synthesizing physical and psychological explanations. Psychosurgery and drug therapies followed. More attention was given to identifying and manipulating psychological dynamics. Jean-Martin Charcot and Hippolyte Bernheim worked with hypnotism (q.v.) as a method for diagnosing and treating hysterics. Emil Kraepelin combined anatomical studies, experimental psychology, and the case history method to revise the classification of mental diseases. In 1899, he defined the two major psychoses whose causes appeared to be within the mind itself: manic-depressive psychosis and dementia praecox. He further subdivided the latter into hebephrenia, catatonia, and paranoia. Eugen Bleuler refined the concept of dementia praecox into schizophrenia.

On the neurological side, John Hughlings Jackson was developing his thesis that nervous or mental disorders were actually a dissolution of, or regression from, higher functions which were the product of evolution. The clinical symptoms resulted from activating more primitive functions. Such theories formed the background for the work of Adolph Meyer, the leading non-Freudian psychiatric theorist in the United States. In Meyer's psychobiological approach to mental disorder, the disease was seen as a faulty response to situations which the patient faced. His prescriptions for diagnosis included both medical examinations and extensive life histories. Pierre Janet worked exclusively with psychological factors to create an early version of "dynamic psychiatry." He proposed a general theory which accounted for nearly all the phenomena of the mind, and he correlated hysteria with what he called "subconscious fixed ideas." He proposed to treat the conditions hysteria produced with "psychological analysis." He also developed interpretations of neurosis and "mental energy" as well as postulating an underlying psychic structure for the mind's operations. Though Janet remained within the medical psychological tradition, there were many similarities between his work and that of the early psychoanalytic school.

Psychoanalysis Psychiatry followed the models of scientific medicine in the late nineteenth and early twentieth centuries, but the results were less impressive. There was no organizing principle, no doctrine comparable in power to the germ theory of disease, no consistent approach to treatment. Even the classifications of mental illness were inadequate, while the boundaries between psychological and physiological phenomena were blurred and indistinct. Freudian psychoanalysis, the most radical psychiatric method to develop in this period, offered solutions to many of these problems. Psychoanalysis offered a theory which accounted for neuroses and proposed a therapy consistent with the theory. Moreover, the theory was flexible, possessed considerable explanatory power, and in its broadest application was both an explanation for the dynamics of personality and a theory of civilization. It was particularly significant for the history of art, culture, and morality. Psychoanalysis had an extraordinary impact on high culture in the west, especially in the fevered decades between the world wars, and, despite a decline in medical significance over the last quarter century, it remains one of the twentieth century's most important intellectual determinants.

Psychoanalysis and the psychoanalytic movement were the creations of Dr. Sigmund Freud. Alfred Adler and Carl Gustav Jung developed variations on Freud's basic themes, and subsequent generations of Freudian interpreters, including Karen Horney and Erich Fromm, broadened the application of Freud's ideas. Freud was trained at the University of Vienna in traditional anatomy and physiology, with special emphasis on neurology. Though his interests were in research, he had no prospects to advance in physiology and was forced to prepare for medical practice. He received his M.D. with a specialization in clinical neurology in 1881. Freud had developed an interest in hysteria, which he shared with his friend and older colleague Dr. Joseph Breuer. Breuer's reports on his work under hypnosis with a certain Anna O., a classic hysteric, inspired the line of thinking which led Freud toward psychoanalysis. Both men saw the succession of hysterical affections which Anna O. suffered as arising from unresolved conflicts buried beneath the level of consciousness. Some of these problem areas emerged under hypnosis, and the patient gained some relief by talking about them.

In 1885, Freud visited Charcot's Paris clinic and studied his methods; but after a period of enthusiastic acceptance, Freud turned away from hypnotism to develop free association, the conviction that sexual problems lay at the root of mental disorders, and his classification of the component areas of the mind (ego, id, superego) and the functions they perform. A rigorous course of self-analysis led Freud to his seminal *Interpretation of Dreams* (1900), and his ideas began to acquire a European following. In 1908, 42 psychiatrists and psychologists attended the first international congress on psychoanalysis, and by 1910 the psychoanalytic movement was firmly established.

Freud's study of mental disorder carried him far away from the established medical approach. He was primarily concerned with problems which were not the result of injury or physiological malfunction. He separated treatment of the mind from that of the body, and he concentrated on explaining psychological dynamics without reference to neurology. Among the most important ideas Freud developed were the dynamic unconscious and the means to understand it through free association and the analytic interview, the explanation of symptoms in terms of dynamic functions, and the interpretation of dreams. Other important concepts included repression and defense mechanisms, child sexuality and its stages of development, the Oedipus complex, the sexual foundations of neurosis, and the therapeutic power generated by developing and resolving a transference neurosis.

Psychiatric Medicine Since 1920 The psychoanalytic method was both an explanation for disease and a means to cure it. On the other hand, analysis commonly took years, it was a highly individual method unsuited to hospital or clinical work, and, as both experimental psychologists and medical psychiatrists charged, its methods lay beyond the scope of ordinary tests for scientific reliabililty. Freud's insights appeared to be intuitive, an interpretive structure reared on a surprisingly narrow base in data, and it was virtually impossible to establish whether it actually helped people or not. Nevertheless, Freudian psychoanalysis became firmly established, and, by concentrating exclusively on emotional questions, it successfully moderated the exclusively physiological attack on psychological problems.

The phenomenal growth of psychoanalysis in the twentieth century overshadowed important achievements in the medical treatment of mental problems. The consequences of bacterial infections for brain function were identified, beginning with syphilis, and the discovery that counterinfection with malaria (the Wagner-Jauregg procedure) was effective against syphilis was hailed as "a model of organic mental illness and treatment." The cause for viral encephalitis was identified in the 1917 influenza epidemics; more recently, dietary deficiencies have been implicated in mental diseases, together with chromosomal aberrations which affect metabolism and produce failures in the endocrine system.

Medicine developed a variety of manipulative techniques for treating neurosis symptoms or even deep-seated psychoses. Some had a measure of success. Others proved to be frightening failures. Insulin, which was found to control diabetes mellitus (q.v.), was employed in short treatments for schizophrenia. Manfred Sakel stumbled on the method while using insulin to treat morphine addicts. Insulin shock, though difficult to administer and dangerous to use, brought some positive results. Ladislaus Joseph von Meduna, while working with epileptics, developed a shock treatment in which camphor was the convulsive agent. The camphor treatment, though considered superior to insulin, was also dangerous, producing convulsions so violent that patients could suffer broken bones, and the time gap between administration and reaction was unpredictable. Finally, in 1938, Ugo Cerletti, working at a neuropsychiatric clinic in Genoa, began to use electric shocks. This treatment, whose antecedents were in eighteenth-century galvanism, proved to be less dangerous, more controlled, and less expensive than chemical shock therapies. It has proved to be especially useful for alleviating symptoms in severe depression, though it does not affect the causes producing the condition.

Psychosurgery to alter behavior enjoyed a brief popularity in the 1930s and 1940s. It has returned to favor in recent years for particularly recalcitrant cases. Egas Monis, working at Portugal's University of Lisbon, claimed that certain "obsessive" and "melancholic" cases could be improved by excising the frontal lobe. He performed the first lobotomy in 1935, and the procedure won acceptance as a treatment for psychotics resistant to shock therapy. Public opinion reacted against the treatment on the grounds that the cure was as bad as the disease. Intractable patients were made easier to handle and less contentious, but they were reduced to the status of unrecognizable automatons. Once done, the operation was irreversible.

The stimulants, tranquilizers, and vitamin preparations which have become available in the last three decades have revolutionized custodial care, permitting treatment of the mentally disturbed on an outpatient basis and, for the first time since the eighteenth century, substantially reducing the numbers of mental patients in institutions. Drug therapy has become a standard method for dealing with psychiatric problems of all kinds and is the most successful common treatment currently available. The most explosive growth, however, has been in psychotherapy itself, where techniques involving group sessions, family therapy, sensitivity training, consciousness-raising, game- and role-playing, and behavior modification through stimulus and reinforcement have revolutionized the treatment of mental problems. The ideology of psychiatric care has shifted from emphasizing cure to helping people live with their problems and avoid destructive behavior. The potential for treating mental problems is unlimited, and the demand for such treatment continues to grow. Psychiatric medicine has developed strongly eclectic tendencies while synthesizing the physiological and psychological approaches to the treatment of mental disorders.

ADDITIONAL READINGS: Erwin H. Ackerknecht, *A Short History of Psychiatry*, Sulammith Wolff (trans.), New York, 1935; Frank G. Alexander and Sheldon T. Selesnick, *The History of Psychiatry: An Evaluation of Psychiatric Thought and Practice from Prehistoric Times to the Present*, London, 1967; Silvano Arieti (ed.), *The American Handbook of Psychiatry, Volume 1: The Foundations of Psychiatry*, 2d rev. and enl. ed., New York, 1974; J. A. Brown, *Freud and the Post-Freudians*, Baltimore, 1961; Jan Ehrenwald (ed.), *The History of Psychotherapy*, New York, 1976; Henri F. Ellenberger, *The Discovery of the Unconscious: The History and Evolution of Dynamic Psychiatry*, New York, 1970; Reuben Fine, *A History of Psychoanalysis*, New York, 1979; Ernest Harms, *Origins of Modern Psychiatry*, Springfield, Ill., 1967; J. G. Howells (ed.), *The World History of Psychiatry*, New York, 1975; Ernest Jones, *The Life and Work of Sigmund Freud*, 3 vols., New York, 1953–1957; Donald S. Napoli, *Architects of Adjustment: The History of the Psychological Profession in the United States*, Port Washington, N.Y., and London, 1981; Teizo Ogawa (ed.), *History of Psychiatry: Mental Illness and Its Treatment*, Tokyo, 1982; Jacques M. Quen and E. T. Carlson (eds.), *American Psychoanalysis: Origins and Development*, New York, 1978; Duane Schultz, *A History of Modern Psychology*, New York, San Francisco, and London, 1975; Bennett Simon, *Mind and Madness in Ancient Greece: The Classical Roots of Modern Psychiatry*, Ithaca, 1980; Russell G. Vasile, *James Jackson Putnam: From Neurology to Psychoanalysis: A Study of the Reception and Promulgation of Freudian Psychoanalytic Theory in America, 1895–1918*, Oceanside, N.Y., 1978; Dieter Wyss, *Psychoanalytic Schools from the Beginning to the Present*, New York, 1973.

See also EPILEPSY; MENTAL ILLNESS; NEUROLOGY.

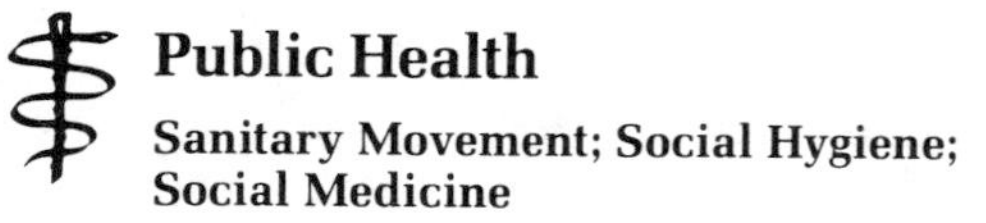

Public Health

Sanitary Movement; Social Hygiene; Social Medicine

Introduction Public health is an interdisciplinary field which uses scientific medicine, engineering specialties, and the social sciences to study the effect of various environments on human health and to mobilize the technologies necessary to protect and promote community well-being. Public health means social action and is best performed through government. The most consistent pattern in the modern history of public health has been from less governmental regulation to more and from smaller governmental units to larger. By the third quarter of the present century, most advanced societies had well-developed national public health authorities. The functions those authorities control vary, reflecting different national traditions, but the general tendency has been toward centralization of responsibility and rationalization of function.

Technological expertise and scientific knowledge determine the effectiveness of public health programs, but social needs and cultural values influence their extent and character. Historically, modern public health developed its institutional base between the sixteenth and the nineteenth centuries. The scientific discoveries which made public health effective came later and generated a further expansion of investigatory, regulatory, educational, and therapeutic institutions. This growth also created significant problems leading to charges of overregulation, excessive costs for the social benefits derived, and retardation of economic growth.

While advanced societies weigh the costs of their achievements, the major problems in underdeveloped societies have been to find the economic means to implement and sustain basic projects in disease control, nutrition, and waste disposal and to create the administrative structures necessary to apply established technology. This serves to emphasize the fact that in both backward and advanced societies, the future of public health is closely tied to social and economic issues. The miracles promised by the medical revolution of the last 100 years will require a further miracle of productivity and planning in order further to improve standards of life in the underdeveloped world while maintaining existing standards in advanced societies.

The Ancient and Medieval Worlds Organized community action to deal with social needs appears in the earliest records of ancient civilizations. Archaeologists investigating the lost urban cultures of northern India (ca. 2500–1500 B.C.) at Mohenjo-Daro and Harappa have uncovered large-scale planned cities with sophisticated water and waste disposal systems. Urban sites in Middle Kingdom Egypt (ca. 2300–1800 B.C.) show comparable facilities, including toilets. The arrangements at Cretan Knossos are the most elaborate of all, with baths, running water, and flush toilets as well as sewers. Similar though less sumptuous facilities have been found at Troy and throughout Asia Minor. Pre-Columbian America was similarly served. The Incas were quite advanced in public health engineering, and they showed an understanding of environmental influences on health by using a rotation system for highland military units which had to serve in lowland valleys.

Among more recent and accessible civilizations, Rome provides the best example of well-developed public health facilities. Though less advanced medically than Greece or the eastern Hellenistic principalities, Rome applied its engineering, administrative, and legal skills to the construction of an integrated public health system which included aqueducts for bringing fresh water to the capital, an extensive administration for overseeing the water and sewage systems, hospices and retreats for travelers along major commercial routes, a system of military medicine with hospital facilities in the provinces, and state-subsidized medical care for the population of the capital. The level of technology was advanced, though hardly more so than in other ancient Mediterranean cultures, and the Romans extended it into the European hinterlands as well as across north Africa.

From the fifth through the ninth centuries A.D., the traditions of Mediterranean civilization were largely obliterated in the west. Urban civilization disappeared and with it the need for maintaining complex health facilities and rules. Some fragments, however, remained. Monastic orders used simplified versions of Roman facilities such as baths, toilets, and piped water, though even the most elaborate, such as the ninth-century abbey of St. Gall in Switzerland, were primitive by comparison with the Roman original. With political authority in recession, the church took responsibility for the poor and indigent while ministering to its own servants, and the medieval world's primary contribution to public health lay in developing the concepts and institutions which formed the underpinnings for the modern hospital (see Hospital).

The medieval world itself began to change in the twelfth and thirteenth centuries, and by the fifteenth century a new social order had taken shape. Trade expanded, towns grew, and the public's health again became a pressing matter. The most serious problems involved keeping water supplies clean, disposing of waste, and protecting food supplies. In the thirteenth century, water began to be piped into towns, and by the opening of the fourteenth century, Bruges in modern Belgium had built an entire water system for the municipality. Towns tried to control river pollution. Tanners, for example, were not allowed to wash their skins or dyers to dump their surplus dyes in waters the public had to use. In some places, even washing clothes in the rivers was forbidden.

Within the growing towns, waste of all kinds had become a major problem. The style of life was still rural. Houses were similar to those in villages, and it was common to keep domestic animals and fowl. Litter collected in the public ways, and because most streets were unpaved, the mud in rainy periods made them virtually impassable. Various regulations were invoked. Some German cities prohibited pigpens which faced the street. Municipal slaughterhouses were established, and many towns undertook to pave their main thoroughfares. Waste canals were dug which drained to covered waste pits. Every large house in Paris was required to have a room for waste disposal which drained into the waste canal, and Milan wrote municipal ordinances to determine the placement of cesspools and sewers while requiring that they be buried deeply enough so that there was no smell. London used the Thames for waste, and in 1309 the first in a long catalog of futile regulations governing dumping in the river was enacted.

Cities also tried to control conditions in their food markets. Regulations mandated daily sweeping and the disposal of waste and refuse. Foods were inspected for spoilage or adulteration, and there were firm rules against selling old or spoiled meat and fish to local residents. In Basel, leftover fish were displayed at a special "inferior food" stall and sold only to strangers; Zurich required dead fish not sold in one day to be destroyed; while in Florence, meat which was not sold on Saturday could not be held over for the following Monday.

Disease control was another vital public health function in the medieval world. War and expanding trade brought waves of epidemic disease into Europe from the eleventh through the sixteenth centuries. The two most significant were leprosy (q.v.), which peaked in the early thirteenth century, and the bubonic plague (q.v.), which arrived in the fourteenth century. Elaborate methods were invoked to seclude lepers, and leprosaria were constructed in abundance. By the year 1200, there were thought to be 2000 in France alone, and a figure of 19,000 has been given for the whole of Europe. Leprosy also provided a model for dealing with bubonic plague, which was treated as both epidemic and contagious. To protect communities against infection, people entering the area were isolated and watched for signs of the disease. The period of observation varied from 14 to 40 days. This approach to communicable diseases remained the mainstay in epidemic control until the twentieth century.

The Early Modern Era: 1600 to 1800 In the medieval world, public health issues were met in a haphazard, ad hoc fashion. The emergence of the centralized monarchies in the sixteenth and seventeenth centuries brought a new political culture into existence, although tradition and primitive administrative methods dictated that public health functions would continue to be local matters. Nevertheless, the political philosophies supporting royal absolutism stressed the monarchs' moral responsibility for the welfare of their subjects while developing economic doctrines which equated public welfare with prosperity. Mercantilism, Colbertism, and cameralism all emphasized these goals, thus drawing attention to the need for better health regulations and facilities.

The continental monarchies took a particular interest in medical and public health issues, generating early systems of state licensure for medical specialties, codes for epidemic control, and policies directed at improving the physical well-being of the people. Theorists explained the role of medical police, and these doctrines, introduced in 1655 by Veit Ludwig von Sackendorff, received their most thorough exposition in works published by Johann Peter Frank between 1779 and 1817. The social philosophies of the eighteenth-century Enlightenment reinforced these doctrines. Beginning from humanitarian assumptions, the *philosophes* emphasized the importance of the state's acting to protect and promote the health and physical welfare of society. Denis Diderot's *Grande encyclopédie* (1751–1772) was particularly influential, and Diderot himself proposed an extensive scheme for public assistance which included medical care and old-age insurance. The Enlightenment tradition carried into the nineteenth century with Benthamite utilitarianism and utopian socialism.

Two further developments in this period were important for the future of public health. These were the use of statistics for analyzing social issues and the move toward a comprehensive social approach to health problems. In the seventeenth century, England's John Graunt had begun to study mortality statistics systematically, thus founding a discipline of crucial importance for epidemiology (q.v.) and for public health generally. And in the eighteenth century, states began systematically to collect population data. Russia's czar Peter the Great (1682–1725) initiated a nationwide census numeration (revision) for tax and other public purposes, and the exercise was repeated at regular intervals through the eighteenth and nineteenth centuries. In 1748, Sweden established a centralized system for collecting statistics, and in 1766 Per Wargentin published the first mortality table for an entire country. France began to collect detailed social statistics during the revolution and went on to evolve the most effective and accurate of the European systems available before 1850. Such French physicians and mathematicians as the Marquis de Laplace, Daniel Bernoulli, the Marquis de Condorcet, and Philippe Pinel developed the analytic techniques for applying statistics to public health questions.

Statistics were valuable for identifying problems in public health. Proposals for national public health plans and the foundation of the social medicine, or social hygiene, movement provided a beginning point for solutions. The eighteenth-century approach through medical police found a parallel in the comprehensive programs proposed between 1790 and 1794 in the French revolutionary assemblies. The constituent assembly failed to act on proposals for a central health commission, but in 1791 the legislative assembly combined health and public assistance into a single commission under Rochefoucauld-Liaincourt, who presented a plan covering health inspectorates, child care, a national inoculation campaign, and medical services for the indigent and for children. Foreign war and mounting domestic violence effectively foreclosed action on this proposal until 1794, when some provision for medical services was introduced, and in 1802 an advisory health council was set up in Paris. Subsequently similar councils were organized in other cities, and the national public health administration originally proposed in 1790 was finally legislated in 1848. By then other factors had become important in shaping public health policies, but the proposals of the revolutionary era formed a critical precedent.

The Emergence of Public Health Systems: 1800 to 1900 The establishment of national public health administrations and the introduction of legislation concerning broad areas of community health resulted from the impact of industrialization. Medicine's contribution to public health policies came through its support for an environmental approach to disease causation. The sanitary movement in England and the social hygiene movement on the Continent shared the conviction that health and disease were functions of social conditions. In its most radical form, the social hygiene (or social medicine) movement called for the transformation of society to create a truly healthful environment. Contagionist doctrines lost ground to miasmal explanations for epidemic diseases, and even the dramatic discoveries that typhoid and cholera were waterborne did not turn the tide. Later demonstrations proving the germ theory of disease failed to convince the most dedicated supporters of the environmental hygiene movement that their approach required modification. Ironically, once the weight of the bacteriological argument had broken the back of the environmentalists' resistance, decades were lost in the search for bacterial causes for conditions stemming from nutritional deficiencies and other systemic and environmental causes. The balance has only been redressed in the twentieth century.

The sanitary, or social hygiene, movement peaked between 1840 and 1880. This was also a period of serious epidemic infection, most notably from cholera and typhoid, while tuberculosis remained an insidious and dangerous threat. Modern public health administration took shape within this context. England led the way in 1842 with what George Rosen has called "the fundamental document of modern public health," the famous *Report on an Inquiry into the Sanitary Condition of the Labouring Population of Great Britain.* Edwin Chadwick, supported by two Benthamite physicians, Southwood Smith and Neil Arnolt, wrote the report, which described a condition of life characterized by massive overcrowding, inadequate waste disposal, polluted water, bad diet, and high rates of disease and mortality. The report argued that the economic costs of such conditions were insupportable, that society would gain immeasurably by taking the steps necessary to create a healthy social environment, and that the problems which needed to be solved were essentially engineering problems requiring an administrative organization to mobilize and apply the funds and technological skills. A second report in 1843 reinforced these conclusions, and in 1844 and 1845 a royal commission recommended establishing a national authority to oversee public health with a local health board in each community to deal with water supply, drainage, and cleansing. In 1846, Parliament began to implement these recommendations by passing the Liverpool Sanitary Act, the first comprehensive sanitary measure in English history, which empowered the Liverpool town council to appoint a medical officer of health, a borough engineer, and an inspector of nuisances. Other legislation dealing with waste disposal and disease prevention was enacted in 1846 and 1847, while the promised National Health Act was passed on August 31, 1848.

The National Health Act initiated a series of steps which ended just 98 years later with the National Health Service and the modern British system of socialized medicine. It created a general board of health with provision for local health boards on petition of not less than 10 percent of local taxpayers, or on a rise in mortality above 23 per 1000 of population. The backbone of the system was the local boards, which dealt with water supplies, sewers, waste disposal, "offensive trades" (slaughtering, tanning, dyeing, etc.), the placing and maintenance of cemeteries, and other matters connected with environmental cleanliness. The local boards included a health officer formally qualified in medicine, an inspector of nuisances, a surveyor, a treasurer, and a clerk. The central board coordinated local efforts and had the power to initiate surveys and investigations. The act was allowed to lapse in 1854, in part as a result of resentment at the reformers' messianic zeal and abrasive manner, but other health legislation was introduced, and in 1875 the health act itself was restored.

Other countries were moving in the same direction. In Germany, where the social hygiene movement attained its fullest theoretical development, public health administration could build on the strong cameralist tradition and was firmly established even before political unification in 1871. The hygienists, led by Rudolf Virchow, Solomon Neumann, and Ralph Leubuscher, developed a broad environmental theory of disease based on group studies which correlated health and conditions of life and claimed to identify the particular causes in the environment responsible for disease and mortality. The social hygienists' action program was first presented to the Berlin Society of Physicians and Surgeons on March 30, 1849. The proposal argued that citizens who, for whatever reason, were unable to cope with environmental problems, that is, conditions arising from the nature of the soil, industry, the food supply, or housing, should be able to call on the state for assistance and that the state had the right, indeed, the obligation, to take whatever steps were necessary to resolve the problem. Where such questions as epidemic disease or mental illness were concerned, neither personal nor property rights should be permitted to inhibit state action. The hygienists also contended that it was the state's responsibility to supply trained medical personnel to meet these obligations, while Virchow argued that political democracy and the right to work were essential to society's health and welfare. Other less extreme proposals included uniform medical licensing, competitive examinations for public health positions, and a national ministry of health.

In the reaction following the revolutions of 1848, many of the more idealistic goals of the social hygienists were dropped, and the movement concentrated on sanitary engineering, improved working conditions, and more effective health administration. Lorenz von Stein formulated the more moderate position in 1867, arguing that the individual's health became a social issue when people, suffering the effects of noxious conditions over which they had no control, became a social burden. It was the government's duty to protect society against such influences, to assist those affected by them, and to reestablish a healthful environment. There was a powerful surge of opinion in favor of an active public health program, and following Germany's unification in 1871, a central public health office was planned and established (1873–1876). The Bismarckian program of national health insurance and workers' compensation followed.

Though France began earlier than other continental states, until the revolution of 1848 relatively little was done for public health administration. In 1848 and 1849, however, a trial of Louis Blanc's national workshops was undertaken, local health councils were set up, and a public health advisory commission was established. Neither the central nor the local boards possessed administrative powers, however, and they were, therefore, much less effective than their English counterparts. In Russia, on the other hand, where there was a long tradition of associating public health issues with the central government, administrative responsibility was divided among several government agencies, including the ministries for finance, public enlightenment (education), military affairs, and the interior. The *zemstvo* reforms of 1864 created local governing councils with health responsibilities and medical staffs. In some cases, these councils proved to be effective. A centralized health administration did not actually appear in Russia until after the 1917 revolution, but when it did, the People's Commissariat of Health proved to be the most complete and administratively integrated institution of its kind in the world. Though hampered by poverty, social disorders, and technological backwardness, Soviet public health established effective disease control and a comprehensive system of health institutions which vastly improved the Soviet standard of living.

American Public Health to 1900 Centralized public health administration was very slow to develop in the United States. The first public health institutions appeared during the colonial period in response to epidemics. In 1798, for example, as the result of a severe yellow fever outbreak, the city of New York won the right to pass health regulations, and six years later, a city inspector of health was appointed. The city inspector, who until 1838 was under the police department, was charged with responsibility for administering health laws, controlling environmental problems and sanitation, and collecting vital statistics. There was also a state officer responsible for port quarantine rules, and a municipal physician was to watch for communicable diseases.

New York's arrangements were inefficient and susceptible to political influence and corrupt practices. On the other hand, New York, like most American cities, had relatively few problems until the first waves of European immigrants swamped municipal facilities. The city's population rose from 75,770 in 1805 to 123,000 in 1820 and then mushroomed to 515,000 in 1850. Similar growth was recorded in Boston, Philadelphia, and New Orleans, while such inland cities as Buffalo, Cincinnati, St. Louis, and Chicago bulged with new arrivals.

At the midpoint of the nineteenth century, American surveys similar to and inspired by Chadwick's work in England revealed comparable urban problems, with the landmark work of John H. Griscom, *The Sanitary Condition of the Laboring Population of New York* (1845), leading the way. This study was influential in the American sanitary movement for the next 30 years. The evidence showed high rates of illness, disability, and premature mortality among the urban poor, and the argument was made that these findings all could be altered because the causes of the conditions could be removed. Similarly, in Boston, Lemuel Shattuck produced a census in 1845 which showed a high general mortality, an astounding infant and maternal mortality, and a host of communicable diseases deadly to the poor. Shattuck was put in charge of a commission to study health conditions in Massachusetts, and his report, which appeared in 1850, became famous. The politicians, however, ignored it. The state board of health which it proposed was not established until 1869, and the balance of its recommendations was simply pushed aside.

Investigative work revealing public health problems continued through the 1850s, and a variety of organizations joined the public health cause, but there were no important advances until after the Civil War. In 1866, however, the Council of Law of New York's Citizens' Association drafted legislation to establish a metropolitan board of health modeled after the English municipal boards. The result four years later was the nucleus of the New York City Health Department, which provided a stable municipal health administration with the capacity to act effectively. It was this structure which facilitated the rapid implementation of new biological discoveries in public health later in the century. Progress across the country, however, was slow. Louisiana had organized the first state board of health in 1855, but it was not effective. The Massachusetts board, founded in 1869, was the first workable state health board, but over the next eight years, only eight states and the District of Columbia followed Massachusetts' lead. Beyond this, a national quarantine act was passed in 1878, and a national board of health was set up in 1879. Administrative inefficiency and state opposition led to its abolition in 1883. As the nineteenth century closed, urban centers in the United States had developed active public health programs, but both the states and the national government were lagging. The impetus to change came with the twentieth century, though an integrated national system did not appear until after World War II.

Bacteriology and After: 1880 to 1980 The sanitary movement had begun to affect the incidence of epidemic diseases before knowledge of bacterial causes had been assimilated. More broadly, the growing emphasis on public health policies contributed to an improving standard of living reflected in a basic change in general mortality statistics. In the second half of the nineteenth century, mortality per 1000 in England and Wales turned down from 20.8 in 1850 to 18.2 in 1900 and fell below 16 by 1905. Sanitary engineering and the protection of water sources reduced cholera's effects in England, Germany, and France; slum clearance, housing controls, cotton garments, and improved standards of cleanliness promised to eliminate typhus even before its mechanics of transmission were understood. In England and Wales, deaths per 1 million of population from typhus remained around 900 until 1870. In the next decade, however, they dropped precipitously to 374, and by 1906, there were no typhus deaths at all reported. The typhoid death rate also declined, though more modestly, from 332 per 1 million to 198 between 1880 and 1890.

Though public health efforts improved conditions of life before the bacterial causes for disease were firmly established, the proof of the germ theory of disease, the identification of specific causal agents, and the definition of the transfer mechanisms involved allowed a substantial rationalization of public health functions while placing a premium on laboratory work. The most important development was the introduction of publicly supported bacteriological laboratories for disease diagnosis and control, and in this field, the United States, which contributed little or nothing to the pioneering work on bacteriology, led the way. In 1887, Joseph Kinyoun of the Marine Hospital Service organized a bacteriological laboratory in the Staten Island Marine Hospital. Five years later it was moved to Washington, D.C., where it became the Hygienic Laboratory, with a Biologics Control Division to test serums, vaccines, and other biological agents. In 1888, public health laboratories were founded in Providence, Rhode Island, and for the Michigan State Health Department, and in 1892, New York City established a division of bacteriology and disinfection in the city health department. This office originated as an anticholera device inspired by a severe outbreak of cholera in Hamburg. Under Hermann M. Biggs, who was succeeded by William H. Park, it developed into a diagnostic laboratory where Park established the concept of the diphtheria carrier (1893) and developed the first diphtheria antitoxin outside Europe (1894). The laboratory became an important research center working on tuberculosis, dysentery, typhoid fever, scarlet fever, and the role of milk in communicating disease. It also became the model for similar laboratories for the state of Massachusetts (1894) and the city of Philadelphia (1895). By 1900, diagnostic laboratories were found in every state and in most major cities. Public health laboratories virtually took over the diagnosis of communicable diseases while providing biological products to practicing physicians and public health officers. The later establishment of federal disease control centers carried on the laboratory tradition begun in the cities and states.

In Europe, where bacteriological research was concentrated, the public health laboratory was slow to develop. Analysis and diagnosis were performed at the research institutes and universities, which carried the weight of scientific investigation. This created an uneven pattern of service, especially in England, where many areas were far removed from university seats and lacked the extensive laboratory facilities of the major hospitals. Laboratories would accept samples by mail, but the system was inconvenient, and there were often delays when speed was essential. A few cities founded municipal laboratories, the first being Liverpool (1897), but until World War II, much of Britain was without regular laboratory service.

The bacteriological approach led to the control of communicable diseases in advanced societies, but powerful as the bacterial explanation for disease was, twentieth-century medical science soon found its limitations. Deficiency diseases arising from shortages in specific food elements or from the environment itself were identified early, and the importance of diet and behavioral patterns as well as environment became increasingly clear for circulatory problems, heart disease, and cancer. Control over food and drugs, inspection and regulation of health conditions in schools, factories, and public institutions, training in nutrition, hygiene, and child rearing, and, more recently, the study and control of dangerous pollutants in the atmosphere, food chain, and water system generated a vast mosaic of private associations, public laws, regulatory agencies, and international programs. The Soviet Union was the first to integrate the whole of its public health activities into a single administrative entity. The United States, where public health has become a major interest and issue, until 1953 relied essentially on local jurisdictions to perform public health functions. The creation of the Department of Health, Education and Welfare under the Eisenhower administration marked an effort to bring some order to the hodgepodge of federal agencies and offices which had been created over half a century to deal with specific problems. Here the gradual development from local to national and from individual to integrated programs recapitulates the patterns of public health evolution in the industrialized world.

Conclusion Twentieth-century public health may well have reached its zenith in the years from 1950 to 1975. A radical rise in Soviet mortality rates first noticed in the mid-1970s suggests a significant decline in Soviet public health effectiveness and raises the possibility that Russia may be the first industrialized nation to reverse the general progress toward declining mortalities, reverting to ratios met more commonly in the developing world. This decline, which is still suspected rather than proved, has not been explained, though it may find parallels as a result of inflation and budget cutting in Sweden, Denmark, West Germany, and France. Both Great Britain's Conservative government, elected in 1979, and the Reagan administration in the United States, elected in 1980, have announced and begun to implement reductions in social programs relevant to the public's health. Just as the problems created by industrialism and urbanization led to broad health and social welfare programs in the period from 1880 to 1980, the problems of fully modernized societies moving into a postindustrial age appear to demand retrenchment in welfare spending. Whether this is a momentary aberration or a true historical trend remains to be seen.

ADDITIONAL READINGS: Jeanne L. Brand, *Doctors and the State: The British Medical Profession and Government Action in Public Health, 1870–1912,* Baltimore, 1965; C. Fraser Brockington, *Public Health in the Nineteenth Century,* Edinburgh, 1965; William Frazer, *A History of English Public Health, 1834–1939,* London, 1950; Stuart Galishoff, *Safeguarding the Public Health: Newark, 1895–1918,* Westport, Conn., 1975; Arnold J. Heidenheimer and Nils Elvander, *The Shaping of the Swedish Health System,* New York, 1980; Roy M. Macleod, "The Anatomy of State Medicine," in F. L. N. Poynter (ed.), *Medicine and Science in the 1860s,* London, 1968; George Rosen, *From Medical Police to Social Medicine: Essays on the History of Health Care,* New York, 1974; George Rosen, *A History of Public Health,* New York, 1958; Andrew W. Russell (ed.), *The Town and State Physician in Europe from the Middle Ages to the Enlightenment,* Wölfenbüttel, German Federal Republic, 1982.

See also BACTERIOLOGY; CONTAGION; EPIDEMIOLOGY; HOSPITAL; specific disease articles.

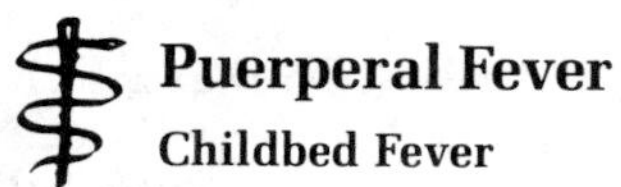

Puerperal Fever

Childbed Fever

Puerperal fever is a highly contagious hemolytic streptococcus infection which attacks the uterus after a woman has given birth. The disease can be identified in the Hippocratic *Epidemics,* but other classic authors including Celsus, Aretaeus, and Oribasius make no recognizable mention of it. Aetius, whose *Tetrabilion* gives 25 chapters to midwifery and 35 to women's diseases, has but a single reference to inflammation of the womb. Puerperal fever did not appear in an attested epidemic until the mid-seventeenth century, and it has been most prevalent in the eighteenth, nineteenth, and early twentieth centuries. Since puerperal fever was usually fatal, it was responsible for sharply elevating the maternal death rate, and its control has been statistically significant as a population factor.

Epidemic puerperal fever appeared with the expansion of hospital facilities and the shift toward doctors rather than midwives assisting at births. Hospitals were crowded with the sick, often filthy, and alive with infective bacteria of all kinds, including the ubiquitous streptococci. Doctors, especially surgeons, seldom cleaned themselves, their instruments, or their clothes, so when they worked with their maternity cases they literally bristled with infective potential. Traditional midwives were probably not much cleaner, but they were not exposed to the rich infective environment of the hospital wards, and even when they worked in hospitals, they were less likely to be directly exposed to infection. The largest part of their work was done in the home, and they were limited by knowledge, custom, and regulations in the kind of assistance they could offer. The doctors probed and manipulated freely, introducing whatever infections they carried directly into the parturient canal. Not surprisingly, women delivered at home by midwives were less likely to contract puerperal fever.

Although asepsis and the germ theory of disease belong to the second half of the nineteenth century, physicians had a general idea of how puerperal fever was communicated at least a century earlier, and successful control programs based on that understanding were implemented. Yet puerperal fever was still a serious threat to recently delivered mothers in advanced societies in the 1930s. In this case, the reason was neither medical nor scientific. The prerequisites for preventing puerperal fever were hygienic hospital conditions and a high standard of personal cleanliness on the part of doctors and attendants. The persistence of puerperal fever owed to intellectual complacency, insensitivity, arrogance, and ignorance.

Eighteenth-century English medical men were responsible for the best early work on puerperal fever. Among them, Charles White, the Manchester physician, surgeon, and male midwife, deserves special notice. White believed that puerperal fever resulted from the absorption of "infective matter" into the damaged tissues of the uterus which, like William Harvey, he thought of as "a vast internal ulcer." Therefore, he emphasized the drainage and self-cleansing of the uterus. He prescribed a special bed designed to permit the patient to rest at an angle which would enhance the flow of fluids. He also designed a special chair for this purpose. The natural flow could be aided by irrigations with antiseptic solutions to guarantee the removal of all "putrid matter." His strongest words, however, were reserved for arguing the necessity for cleanliness, for the isolation of infected patients, and for good ventilation. His book detailing his techniques appeared in 1773 and was published in French in 1774 and in German in 1775. An edition appeared in America in 1793.

White claimed never to have had a lying-in patient infected with puerperal fever, much less to have lost one. But successful as his record may have been, it lacked a theoretical dimension. This was provided by White's younger contemporary, Thomas Kirkland. Indeed, it was Kirkland rather than White, according to one modern authority, who was "the first man in this world to enunciate the true etiology, the import, and the prophylaxis of puerperal fever." Kirkland showed a more modern understanding of infective disease by shifting the focus of attention from the neohumoralist emphasis on flow toward consideration of an outside disease agent. He denied that puerperal fever was a disease in itself, considering it rather the product, or symptom, of a disease. He approached the notion that putrid fluids from one patient might produce disease in another, and he discussed fever as a symptom engendered by a particular and contagious cause contained in the infected matter.

Other writers, including Edward Foster, Philip Pitt Walsh, and Alexander Hamilton, accepted and expanded on Kirkland's views. Hamilton stressed the infectiousness of the condition, while Walsh believed that puerperal fever was not peculiar to lying-in women but was "no other than the common infectious fever, complicated with a more or less extensive inflammation of the peritoneum." Alexander Gordon, at the very end of the century, initiated the epidemiological study of puerperal fever and summarized the etiological view. Hew saw the similarities between puerperal fever and erysipelas (another streptococcal infection), and he pointed out that women who contracted puerperal fever were those who "were visited, or delivered by a practitioner, or taken care of by a nurse, who had previously attended patients affected with the disease." Moreover, he compared the infection which a surgeon might contract if he scratched his finger while dissecting a putrid body with the effect of "putrid matter" applied to the uterus.

A host of writers expanded on these ideas in the early nineteenth century. They identified the danger points for infection, the communicability of the agent causing puerperal fever, and the means to avoid it. Without a demonstrated germ theory, their explanations lacked specificity, but their practical programs were demonstrably effective. One notable example was the regimen which Robert Collins introduced at the Dublin Lying-in Hospital. Faced with an epidemic outbreak of puerperal fever in 1829, Collins introduced an intensive cleansing and purification plan. He filled each room with chlorine gas in condensed form, which he left for 48 hours. Chloride of lime with water was painted onto floors and woodwork to be left for another 48 hours. It was then washed off with fresh lime. Blankets and linens were scoured and cooked in a stove at 120 to 130°F. When patients used a room, it was repurified after departure, with blankets, quilts, and linens hung in the chlorine gas. The rooms when in use were kept thoroughly ventilated, straw ticks were changed regularly and always after two patients had used them, and any infected patients were isolated. Collins reported that during the time these measures were in effect, 10,785 patients were confined and delivered of whom only 58 died from all causes and none died from puerperal fever.

The conclusions to be drawn from the English work were well summarized by the American physician, essayist, and literateur Oliver Wendell Holmes in a paper prepared for the Boston Society for Medical Improvement in 1843. The society was deeply concerned over a series of fatal infections, some of which had claimed physicians' lives. Holmes's paper drove home the point that not only was puerperal fever contagious, but it was a pestilence that doctors carried. The paper was published in the *New England Quarterly Journal of Medicine and Surgery* in April 1843. The argument, though impressive, was flatly contradicted, and its effect was vitiated by two influential Philadelphia professors of midwifery, Charles D. Meigs, Jefferson Medical School, and Hugh L. Hodge, of the University of Pennsylvania. These men asserted the conventional wisdom that puerperal fever was not contagious and that most certainly it was not communicated by doctors.

Though puerperal fever was known and discussed in Britain and the United States for 75 years, the man most commonly associated with exposing its specific character was a Hungarian physician and surgeon, Ignaz Philipp Semmelweis, an assistant obstetrician in Vienna's General Hospital in 1847. In Semmelweis's time, there were two maternity wards. One was served by midwives, the other by students. The maternal death rate in the students' ward was 9.9 percent as compared with 3.4 percent in the midwives' ward. Semmelweis puzzled over this anomaly and discussed it with his colleagues to no effect until his associate and close friend Jakob Kolletschka died suddenly from an accidental infection contracted while dissecting a corpse. At the postmortem, Semmelweis was struck by the similarity of symptoms in Kolletschka's case to those exhibited by puerperal fever victims. This led him to consider the fact that the medical students often went directly from the dissecting rooms to the maternity wards where, in the course of examining their patients, they probed the genitals. He concluded that the infective principle which caused "cadaver fever" also caused puerperal fever, and he indicted "the examining finger" as the primary means for carrying it from dissecting room corpses to recently delivered mothers. He tested his insight by requiring those who examined patients to wash their hands first with liquid chloride, later chlorinated lime. The results were dramatic. A ward in which 1 out of every 6 or 7 women died saw its death rate drop to less than 2 of every 100.

Hand washing was Semmelweis's main prescription, and he concentrated on the link between the maternity ward and the dissecting rooms until further experience in the summer and fall of 1847 convinced him that a puerperal fever infection could be carried from another patient with an infected sore to the maternity ward. He considered communication other than by physical touch and concluded that puerperal fever could also be delivered "by foul air loaded with exhalations from putrifying animal matter, the putrid material finding its way through the air to the genitalia."

Although Semmelweis successfully reduced maternal mortality in his ward from 18 per 100 to less than 3, his ideas met general skepticism, and he was attacked sharply by leading members of the profession, most notably by Friedrich Wilhelm Scanzoni and Carl Braun. His supporters included Josef Skoda, who unsuccessfully urged Semmelweis to prove his case by animal experiments, and Ferdinand von Hebra, editor of the leading medical journal in Vienna. Hebra's report on Semmelweis's work only discussed cadaveric fever from the dissecting rooms, a condition peculiar to a general teaching hospital which would not occur elsewhere. Given the state of the medical art, there was no effective way to generalize the discovery. Consequently, even obstetricians willing to grant Semmelweis's conclusions could argue that the circumstances did not fit their practice and so could ignore the report. There was also considerable professional anger at the idea that the physician, the person responsible for healing, should be accused of carrying death.

Hebra published a second article in 1849, expanding on Semmelweis's conclusions and referring to his findings as equal in importance to Edward Jenner's discovery of smallpox vaccination. But the opposition was hardening. Semmelweis found professional advancement difficult, and when he finally gained the right to the title *privat-dozent* only to find he was cut off from clinical work and limited to theory, he resigned and left Vienna for Budapest, where he became head of the obstetrical division of St. Rochus Hospital in 1851. He introduced chlorine disinfection, and puerperal fever mortality fell below 1 percent. It was at St. Rochus that Semmelweis identified dirty bed linens and bandages as additional carriers for puerperal fever, thus bringing him around to the general sanitary views of earlier English writers. He also became convinced of the need for effective ventilation.

Semmelweis published a major book on puerperal fever in 1861. His mental health was weakened in the course of his controversies with unbelieving colleagues, however, and in 1865 he was admitted to a Viennese mental hospital. There he was found to have contracted an infection in his right hand, which spread and finally killed him. Semmelweis was the victim of the same type of infection which he had identified with puerperal fever.

Within the decade, Semmelweis's views were

entirely vindicated. Joseph Lister's use of antisepsis in surgery came in 1865, four years after Semmelweis published on the etiology of puerperal fever, and in the very year he died, J. L. Bischoff at Basel applied Lister's principles to midwifery, introducing carbolic hand washings, dressings, and bandages impregnated with carbolic acid. Midwifery clinics which employed these techniques were soon reporting the virtual disappearance of puerperal fever.

In 1874, Theodor Billroth, the famed Vienna surgeon, first saw the streptococcus in a sample of pus. The infective principle which Semmelweis and his predecessors had battled blindly was identified. Subsequently, it was found that several streptococcus strains produced puerperal fever, and since there was no effective treatment for the disease until the introduction of antibiotics, the rigid practice of asepsis remained the best defense against it. That, however, was not easily maintained. In Germany, Switzerland, and France, where midwifery was recognized and tightly regulated, puerperal fever was controlled. In the United States, on the other hand, where medical regulations were lax, and where midwifery was neither recognized nor regulated, puerperal fever remained a serious threat.

By 1921, strong rules governing the practice of midwifery had made a start on that aspect of the problem, while significant reforms in medical education combined with professional peer pressure forced even the most resistant of the old-guard physicians to accept cleanliness as a first principle in obstetrics and surgery. Maternal mortality and the incidence of puerperal fever fell significantly between 1930 and 1937, while the subsequent use of antibiotics substantially reduced the dangers of streptococcus infection in general and puerperal fever in particular.

ADDITIONAL READINGS: Irving S. Cutter and Henry R. Viets, *A Short History of Midwifery*, Philadelphia and London, 1964, chap. V; Harry F. Dowling, *Fighting Infection: Conquests of the Twentieth Century*, Cambridge, Mass., 1977; Sherwin B. Nuland, "The Enigma of Semmelweis—an Interpretation," *Journal of the History of Medicine and Allied Sciences* 34 (July 1979): 255–272.

See also ANTISEPTIC; BACTERIOLOGY; MIDWIFERY.

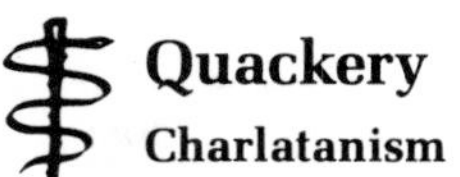

Quackery

Charlatanism

A quack, according to the *Oxford English Dictionary*, is "an ignorant pretender to medical or surgical skill; one who boasts to have a knowledge of wonderful remedies; an empiric or impostor in medicine." More generally, a quack is "one who professes a knowledge or skill concerning subjects of which he is ignorant." The first English reference to the word appeared in 1659, but it would appear to be descended from an earlier low Dutch term, "quacksalver," "one who quacks (boasts) about the virtue of his salves" and "an ignorant person who pretends to a knowledge of medicine or of wonderful remedies." Though the distinction is sometimes difficult to maintain, quackery should be separated from irregular, alternative, or sectarian forms of medical practice (see Irregular Medicine). The established medical profession has been quick to label deviating and competitive therapeutic systems "quackery," but when those systems are compared with their medical contemporaries in history, in terms of curative effects or explanatory power, there often is little to choose among. What distinguishes the quack is the determination to gull and mislead the unwary for personal gain.

The golden age of quackery came before science provided reliable criteria to guide health regulators; most governments lacked the means and the will to control medical frauds, and the population in general was disposed to credulity. Though a significant phenomenon from the sixteenth century on, quackery reached its zenith in the eighteenth-century Enlightenment, and it was most dramatically visible at court and in the service of the well-to-do. Though famous quacks were found throughout Europe, England nurtured the largest brood, while France probably stood in second place. Several factors contributed to this phenomenon. Quackery thrived in great cities with a concentration of wealth. London and Paris were Europe's leading urban centers. Moreover, there was little effective regulation over medical practices in England, and in the expansive Georgian era, there was no interest in promoting it. France had a longer regulatory tradition, but in the era before the revolution, there was little interest in invoking it. In the German states, Austria, and Russia, however, quacks met official hostility, and while the death penalty for quackery threatened in earlier days was almost never invoked, both Austria's empress Maria Theresa and Russia's Catherine II expelled known medical charlatans or forbade their entering the country.

While the great quacks sought the rich or used association with the powerful and great to enhance their effect among the poor, quackery spread outward into society to meet a social need. Formal medicine was generally for the well-to-do. Ordinary people—peasants, tenants and smallholders, artisans, shopkeepers, laborers of all sorts, and the vast class called indigents—turned to irregular practitioners for their medical services. Some of these, such as midwives, pharmacists, and apothecaries, had some formal standing, though often they served functions beyond their training. Others, as the smith or carpenter who also set bones, or the butcher or pig gelder who occasionally performed operations, had no standing beyond what experience conferred. The local pastor or priest was often medically helpful—John Wesley, the founder of methodism, was a noted "empiric" who published a treatise on treatments entitled *Primitive Physic* (1745)—and itinerants who made their way through villages and towns sold a wide variety of services.

This wandering population was particularly large in the strife-torn sixteenth and seventeenth centuries, but it was still a recognized factor in the eighteenth century. Among the itinerants who sold various health services were failed medical students, wandering herbalists and barber-surgeons, lithotomists, or stonecutters, and specialists in cataract couching, hernia repair, urine casting, face gazing, and worm extermination. In addition to the services they offered, many peddled elixers, salves, ointments, health amulets, restoratives, liniments, and cures for every known condition, acute or chronic.

Plague periods brought additional specialists who claimed powers that would assist people to avoid infection. Many itinerants were skilled in the operations they performed; others were not, and the fraud quotient was particularly high among the diagnostics, or prognosticators, and medicine men. In effect, quackery was an integral part of popular medicine, contributing to a medical culture in which regular systematic medicine was only indirectly involved. In comparison with formal medicine, very little is known about this broad phenomenon, though it is clearly one key to health in history.

Quackery specializes in simple answers to difficult problems, promising immediate relief for bothersome symptoms and a miraculous cure. The mysterious aspect is strong, since the fundamental premise is to activate hidden forces by arcane methods. The alchemist's promise to transform base metals into gold is the precedent for modern quackery. The leading quacks of the sixteenth century were alchemists first, and the tradition persisted through the eighteenth century. A growing recognition of nature's forces capped by Sir Isaac Newton's demonstration of the principle of gravity opened wider horizons, and eighteenth-century experiments with magnetism and electricity were worked into new forms of therapeutic magic. Elixirs, potions, and miraculous ointments remained the stock in trade for medical mountebanks, but elaborate equipment and rituals which allegedly awakened nature's fundamental forces added drama and scientific cachet.

The acknowledged prince of eighteenth-century charlatans was Count Alessandro Cagliostro, or Guiseppe Balsamo, who was born in Palermo in 1743. Cagliostro claimed to be an alchemist and magician whose special powers aided him in compounding restoratives, an elixir of life, and a mixture guaranteed to make ugly women beautiful. He sold these products successfully throughout Europe. He was also a forger, a confidence man, an exploiter of women, a false Freemason, and an intriguer. The darling of boudoir society, Cagliostro was imprisoned in the Bastille when he became implicated in the scandal over Marie Antoinette's diamond necklace. Released, he left France for England, where he was charged with fraud and imprisoned at Fleet Street. Again released, he was rearrested in Rome in 1789 by the Inquisition. The church tried and convicted him for heresy, sentencing him to death. The sentence was commuted to life imprisonment, and he died in 1795 in the fortress of San Leo. An out-and-out rascal whose whole career was dedicated to deceit, Cagliostro epitomized the exploitive spirit of quackery, while his victims showed the will to be fooled which makes chicanery so profitable.

Style was everything in quackery, as Cagliostro's career testified. Chevalier John Taylor made a point, no matter how poor he was, to appear grandly dressed, in a coach drawn by four white horses. A self-styled eye doctor, Taylor studied with William Cheselden in London, took a degree at Basel, and was received there and in Paris into the College of Physicians. He was also appointed oculist to King George II. Handsome, witty, and an effective speaker, Taylor toured Europe and traveled through Asia Minor to Persia. He carried testimonials from great men, including monarchs, displayed titles and degrees from distinguished institutions, and claimed expertise in eye surgery. Though reputed to have operated successfully to correct a squint, Taylor was more effective as a salesman than he was as a surgeon, and the patients he treated were frequently blinded. Despite numerous attempts to catch and punish him, Taylor remained free, finally to die in a monastery in Prague.

Michael Schüppach employed style in a different way. A heavy, jovial, good-humored man of peasant origin, Schüppach set up near Bern as a "mountain doctor" who understood the mysteries of "magnetic currents." His greatest success, however, was as a urine tester, and at the height of his career, he "read" from 80 to 100 patients a day. Seemingly a simple child of nature, Schüppach died a rich and respected man.

Joshua Ward, who died in 1761, was particularly effective in promoting his medications. Ward offered a pair of panaceas called the "drop" and the "pill." Both were compounds of antimony which, when ingested, acted as an expectorant, an antipyretic, and an emetic. The drop was a violent purgative which affected the bowel like calomel. These preparations were potentially very dangerous. Overdoses of the pill could produce fatty degeneration of the liver, while the drop in large doses could be responsible for gastroenteritis, colitis, and nephritis. It was also capable of killing by shock and circulatory collapse. Nevertheless, Ward's remedies were highly regarded, and Ward himself was well-respected. He became the minister of medicants for George II and ended his days a wealthy man.

Nature's curative powers were regularly invoked by quacks. Berlin became infatuated in 1780 with a former stocking weaver named Weisleder, a "moon doctor." Weisleder had his patients bare the sick portion of their anatomies to the moon's rays while the "doctor" put his hands on the exposed area and, looking to the moon, murmured incantations known only to himself. Weisleder began his work among the poor, and then the rich discovered him. At the height of his career, he treated hundreds of people at a time.

A contemporary of Weisleder, the Scot James Graham, invoked natural powers of another sort. Visiting America in 1772, Graham was introduced to Benjamin Franklin and electricity. Returning to London, Graham opened the Temple of Health, where he dispensed his "nervous aetherical balsam" as an elixir, used a huge air pump in certain of his treatments, and installed a "metallic conductor" to concentrate the electrical forces. Graham was strong on special effects. He dispensed his elixirs from a throne with a dumbwaiter at the side which delivered potions to his hand on signal. His patients were left in a darkened room listening to mysterious chants while stars twinkled on the ceiling and a "goddess of health" appeared in a niche, glimmering in a pearly light. He claimed to have invented earth baths and soil packs which allowed the patient to absorb elements from the ground itself; and he featured a "grand celestial bed" whose powers could overcome impotency and infertility in any who slept there. The use of the bed ranged from a stiff £50 per night to a princely £500. The room's decor was intended to promote sexual response, and the advance show for the Temple of Health included attractive young women displaying their bodies as a testimony to the value of Graham's treatments.

Elisha Perkins, an American, also called on nature's magnetic force. He claimed that drawing a metal "tractor" downward on the body would focus the natural magnetic flow and remove disease-producing blockages. Achieving some notoriety, he sent his son, Benjamin Douglas Perkins, to England, where he successfully presented his treatment to the Royal Society, and he opened the Perkins Institute and Dispensary, ostensibly for the poor. His claims were challenged and his credibility ruined when two physicians arranged for wooden rather than metal tractors to be used to attain the same results, and the younger Perkins fled London in disorder, though he carried away the equivalent of $50,000. The Perkins system had much in common with mesmerism, and there were parallels with Graham's methods as well.

Quackery in the grand tradition succumbed in the nineteenth century to medical systems and organized resistance. The career of John Long demonstrates the point. Born in County Limerick in 1798, Long was trained in painting and design in Dublin, but opportunities were slight and he removed to London, where he found work doing anatomical drawings. He also began to treat people. In 1826 one of his "patients" was so pleased with his cure that he mentioned Long in a letter, and a growing number of people sought him out. Long's specialty was an ointment which he rubbed on the skin as a first step in diagnosis. If the patient were well—that is, if no disease were present—there would be no reaction; but if there was illness in the system, the skin would develop a red rash and even ulcerate. The theory was that the ointment brought the illness to the surface, and further applications drew it out.

Long's methods attracted so many patients that the regular physicians became concerned. A group of 80 successful doctors organized to drive Long out of practice by impugning him and his ointment. Long counterattacked, criticizing the failures of regular medicine and pointing out that whatever else he did, he never weakened or undermined his patients' strength. He condemned bleeding and strong purges, pointing to the deadly consequences of weakening already wasted bodies. When two patients he was treating died, Long was charged with murder. Though he was acquitted, the second case dealt his reputation a blow from which it never recovered. Ostensibly specializing in consumption (tuberculosis), Long had some success in treating female hysterics, though he failed utterly with patients who were clinically insane. In the end it was consumption rather than his medical rivals that terminated his career, as he died from tuberculosis in 1834 at the age of 36.

In the second half of the nineteenth century, the character of quackery changed. Disciplinary specialization and professionalism reshaped the health services, while improved licensing and registry procedures guaranteed a minimum level of medical competence. By the twentieth century, the irregular, or sectarian, medical systems either had been recognized as special medical fields or had been absorbed into regular medicine. All these tendencies, when combined with expanding hospitals, dispensaries, and public health facilities, reduced quackery's natural market. In Europe, national health insurance was followed by national health programs to make regular medicine more readily available to the mass of the people. Medical quackery receded to the fringe occupied by touch doctors, food faddists, and, on a different level, religious sects such as Mary Baker Eddy's Church of Christ, Scientist, movement, which rejected regular medicine entirely.

The new era was by no means free of quackery. On the contrary, the products quacks traditionally sold—elixirs, restoratives, rejuvenators, panaceas, and the entire panoply of compounded cures—enjoyed an extraordinary expansion and enlarging popularity. Corporate organization, new techniques of production, and the development of mass advertising campaigns permitted unprecedented market expansion. And the therapeutic revolution which accompanied the establishment of the germ theory of disease initially reinforced and further enlarged the field for magical medical preparations. Claiming Pasteur as their scientific father, bactericides and germ killers which were asserted to be effective against all disease causes appeared on the market. The work of the Curies and Roentgen's x-ray were similarly exploited by manufacturers claiming their products were "irradiated" and therefore effective against cancer as well as a variety of lesser afflictions. Continental Europe, where pharmacy and the drug industry had a different history, was less affected by industrial quackery than were Britain and the United States, and the problem was particularly intractable in America.

Even before the twentieth century, nostrums and patent medicines were multi-million-dollar businesses, and there was fierce resistance to their regulation. Chemists could identify the active ingredients in many compounds and could thereby raise doubts about the claims which might be made. But publicizing such analyses had only a limited effect, and there was deep resistance in both legal and industrial circles to restricting advertising claims. The passage of the Pure Food and Drug Act (1906) gave some regulatory powers, but nostrum manufacturers were not intimidated. They believed that the existence of the act would help the public to think that whatever was sold had received some form of government approval and hence would be acceptable.

The creation of laws governing advertising

claims and the parallel problem of drug safety and effectiveness occupied the first half of the twentieth century in the United States. The tightening of the federal Food and Drug Act in 1938 and the reevaluation of effect of prescription drugs beginning in the early 1960s gave needed substance to controls over professional pharmacy (q.v.). Advertisements for nonprescription items, however, proved harder to control, and the introduction of new substances promising miraculous cures has generated profound controversies. The laetrile cancer cure is only one of the most recent. Because advertising's purpose is to stimulate people to buy, the problem of determining a reasonable congruity between claims and a product's actual effect is a difficult one.

There are thousands of products in the modern economy of health which fall outside the controls over prescription drugs. Such products are commonly tested for their safety, but the question of effectiveness remains. Beyond that, health and diet plans, gadgets to strip off weight, increase vitality, or otherwise improve life, and the mountains of literature which health-conscious people read daily attest to the persistence of quackery's spirit in the modern world. Regulation has shrunk the most dangerous aspects of the problem to a manageable minimum, but the claims for health aids of all sorts, from breath sweeteners to cold cures, from headache remedies to germicides to diet supplements, have never been louder or more insistent. Quackery in its classic individual form has been modernized and made respectable. Moreover, in today's world, the modern version of that ancient art plays a critical role in popular health culture, just as in an earlier time quackery was an integral part of medical service for all people.

ADDITIONAL READINGS: Oscar E. Anderson, Jr., *The Health of a Nation: Harvey W. Wiley and the Fight for Pure Food,* Chicago, 1958; M. N. G. Dukes, *Patent Medicines and Autotherapy in Society,* The Hague, 1963; Morris Fishbein, *Fads and Quackery in Healing,* New York, 1932; Grete de Francesco, *The Power of the Charlatan,* New Haven, 1939; Eric Jameson, *The Natural History of Quackery,* Springfield, Ill., 1961; Morton Mintz, *The Therapeutic Nightmare,* Boston, 1965; Otis Pease, *The Responsibilities of American Advertising: Private Control and Public Influence, 1920–1940,* New Haven, 1958; Richard H. Shryock, *The Development of Modern Medicine, an Interpretation of the Social and Scientific Factors Involved,* New York, 1947; Richard H. Shryock, *Medicine in America: Historical Essays,* Baltimore, 1966; James Harvey Young, "Device Quackery in America," *Bulletin of the History of Medicine* 39 (March–April 1965): 154–162; James Harvey Young, *Medical Messiahs: A Social History of Health Quackery in Twentieth Century America,* Princeton, 1967; James Harvey Young, *The Toadstool Millionaires: A Social History of Patent Medicines in America Before Federal Regulations,* Princeton, 1961.

See also BROWNIAN SYSTEM; IRREGULAR MEDICINE; MEDICAL PROFESSION; MESMERISM; PHARMACY.

Quinine

Quinine is the active alkaloid in the bark of the cinchona tree which suppresses the action of malaria parasites and also acts as a preventive. Quinine was the best and only remedy for malaria for 300 years. It was essential for Europeans who needed to live and work in tropical or subtropical areas where malaria was endemic, and it was of particular significance in the opening of Africa in the second half of the nineteenth century.

The circumstances under which quinine came to Europe are obscure. Jesuit missionaries in Peru apparently discovered the efficacy of cinchona bark in treating fevers. The first recorded instance of the bark's use was as a treatment of the viceroy of Peru in 1630. Although the Indians in Peru used Peruvian balsam for fever, they apparently did not know the curative powers of cinchona. The earliest reliable accounts of cinchona in Peru fall in the period between 1630 and 1635; the first clear description of the remedy in Europe was in a treatise by Herman van der Huyden published in Belgium in 1643.

In its pulverized form, quinine was known as "Jesuit powder." The association was unfortunate, for it added ideological heat to the medical controversy over the powder's efficacy. Oliver Cromwell, who died of a malarial fever in 1658, absolutely refused what he called a "Jesuit treatment" for the recurrent fever which had plagued him all his life. Gideon Harvey, author of *The Family Physician and the House Apothecary,* mentioned Jesuit powder in his 1667 edition but anathematized it in 1683. Harvey detested Jesuits, "with whom the less a man have to do either sick or well, it's the better," and he was convinced that if the Jesuits "had kept their *Indian Bark* to themselves ... hundreds would be on this side the Grave whose Bones are now turned into their first element." Thomas Sydenham, England's best-known seventeenth-century physician, was at first uncertain of the bark, but in 1666 he granted grudgingly that the Jesuit powder was effective against certain agues and fevers. Ten years later he gave it his unqualified endorsement. Other authorities wholeheartedly approved Peruvian bark, and when it was reported to have worked cures on King Charles II as well as the French dauphin, its reputation rose further.

By 1712, the curative powers of cinchona bark were specifically associated with intermittent fever, and in 1735, a French expedition to Peru found and identified the "quinaquina" tree. Linnaeus, the great Swedish naturalist, classified and named the tree "cinchona" in 1742. The name was derived from a story current in the seventeenth century which told of the miraculous recovery from fever of the countess Chinchon, wife of the Spanish viceroy to Peru. The countess, in gratitude for her recovery, is supposed to have distributed cinchona to the Peruvian poor and to have brought the remedy to Europe, where she gave it to the peasants on her estates. Historians have found no evidence to corroborate this story, though it is still repeated. When intermittent fevers were prevalent in England from 1765 to 1777, James Lind, author of the *Treatise on Scurvy* (1753) and a pioneer in naval hygiene, used Peruvian bark routinely in his treatments; and by the last decade of the eighteenth century, Britain alone imported 634,783 pounds of bark in just five years. Continental usage was on a comparable scale.

The controversy over fever bark was fed by the varied quality of powders on the market. This owed to the difference in quinine content in various cinchona barks and to systematic adulteration. As the demand for cinchona bark rose, the supply diminished, and Peruvian balsam, which had little effect on intermittent fevers, was added to cinchona, adulterating the product and producing a less effective remedy. This problem was finally solved in 1820 when two French chemists, Pierre Pelletier and Joseph Caventou, extracted quinine from cinchona bark. The quinine extract, or sulfate of quinine, became immediately available. It was far stronger and more effective than the bark powder, but it was also costly and produced severe side effects, including headache, rashes, vomiting, disturbed vision, and impaired hearing. Powders made from bark remained important, but it was now possible to test and grade them according to their quinine sulfate content.

The Peruvian cinchona supply was unreliable, and intensive harvesting without replacement threatened to end the trade entirely. But in the mid-nineteenth century, the Dutch began to experiment with cultivating cinchona trees on plantations in the East Indies. After considerable difficulty, they succeeded in establishing and maintaining varieties of cinchona trees that yielded high-quality bark, and the Dutch became the world's main quinine supplier until the Japanese seized the plantations early in World War II. Work had begun on synthetic quinine, however, long before the Japanese overran the Netherlands East Indies. Chloroquinine, a quinine derivative, appeared in 1934, and on the eve of World War II, mepacrine hydrochloride (Atebrin) became available. Originally compounded in 1930, Atebrin was used extensively and successfully in the Pacific theater of war, Burma, and New Guinea as a preventive against malaria infection and as a suppressant for malaria symptoms. Atebrin was especially effective in stopping blackwater fever, a particularly lethal form of malarial infection. Though an improvement on quinine sulfate, or chloroquinine, Atebrin also had side effects, which included overall yellow skin tint, vomiting, and sometimes emotional excitement. During the Vietnamese war it was replaced by pyrimethamine and sulfametozine given in single inoculations. Synthetics have now largely displaced natural quinine for both therapy and prevention.

ADDITIONAL READINGS: A. W. Haggis, "Fundamental Errors in the Early History of Cinchona," *Bulletin of the History of Medicine* 10 (October–November 1941): 417–459, 568–592; Dale C. Smith, "Quinine and Fever: The Development of the Effective Dosage," *Journal of the History of Medicine and Allied Sciences* 21 (July 1976): 343–367; J. W. W. Stephens, *Blackwater Fever*, Liverpool, 1937, 445–599; Leo Suppan, "Three Centuries of Cinchona," *Proceedings of the Celebration of the Three Hundredth Anniversary of the First Recognized Use of Cinchona, Missouri Botanical Garden Bulletin 18, no. 9 (November 1930): 29–138; Norman Taylor, Cinchona in Java: The Story of Quinine*, New York, 1945.

See also MALARIA.

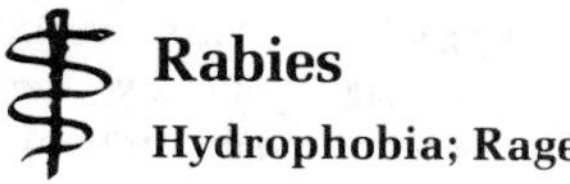

Rabies

Hydrophobia; Rage

The conquest of rabies was a major achievement for medicine and especially for immunization. Though hardly a mass disease like plague or smallpox, rabies is a particularly dreadful disorder which has terrified people for centuries. It is also a complicated disease which posed critical issues to investigators at the very outset of the bacteriological revolution. Rabies investigation was impossible following the methods established by Henle and Koch because the causal agent was too small to be seen, and it refused to be cultured in nonliving matter. Louis Pasteur's solution to these technical problems was the first major step on the road to successful research with viruses, and his work on antirabies vaccine opened new vistas on the mechanisms of immunization. These achievements were of greater long-term significance than finding the means to combat rabies, yet that achievement was important in itself and played a major part in winning public acceptance for immunization as well as veneration for Pasteur himself.

Disease Characteristics Rabies is an acute viral encephalitis which reaches humans most often through the saliva of infected animals, especially dogs. Usually the virus is introduced by biting. All rabid animal bites are dangerous, but the probability of rabies developing in any one case depends on the location and the depth of the bite. The virus introduced through the bite travels to nerve centers via the peripheral nerves. Incubation of the disease occurs in 3 to 8 weeks and no more than 90 days. Variations in the incubation period arise according to where the bite occurred: on the leg, 50 days; on the trunk of the body, 40 days; on the head, 30 days; and on the face, 20 days.

The disease which develops may be a furious rabies in which, after initial headache, general malaise, vomiting, eye watering, and nasal discharge, intense mental excitement develops, together with painful spasms of the jaw, pharynx, and larynx. It is in this phase that the sight or sound of water arouses a terrible dread. Swallowing becomes impossible, there is profuse sneezing and spitting, and the patient may try to bite anyone nearby. Normal behavior returns when the spasms go off, but the symptoms always recur and grow more intense until paralysis, exhaustion, or coma follows. The victims die from heart failure or asphyxia, most commonly in the midst of a convulsion.

Paralytic rabies is less common. It begins suddenly with a high fever and paralysis appearing first in the bitten zone, followed by paralysis of the muscles of the trunk, bladder, bowel, face, tongue, and eye. Death usually comes in three to seven days. Antirabies vaccine can arrest the progress of the disease if it is administered in time, but once symptoms begin, rabies infection in humans is virtually always fatal.

Early History Rabies is a disease which humanity has known and feared from very early times. In Greek myth, the hounds which savaged and killed Acteon the hunter when he surprised Diana bathing are considered rabid; Sirius, the Dog Star in the constellation Orion, was associated with mad dogs; the Greeks venerated Apollo's son Aristaeus for the protection he offered against rabies. Artemis played a comparable role in western Asia. When Greeks spoke of rabies, they called it "lyssa" or "lytta" ("madness"), while the word "rabies" itself is a Latin derivative from the ancient Sanskrit word *rabbas,* which meant "to do violence." The German word for rabies, *Tollwut,* has been traced back to an Indo-Germanic verb, *dhvar,* meaning "damage," combined with the Middle High German *wuot,* meaning "rage."

The earliest medical description of rabies has been ascribed to Democritus (ca. 500 B.C.). There are references to the disease in the Hippocratic writings of the fifth century B.C., and Aristotle's *Natural History of Animals,* refers to a madness which dogs suffer. Aristotle also reported, however, that the human being was exempt from the condition, a proposition which suggests that the disease was uncommon in the fourth century B.C. Plutarch was better-informed, mentioning not only that dog bite was dangerous but also that the condition could be spread by the bite of a rabid dog. Other classical writers from the Greek historian Xenophon through the Latin poets Vergil, Horace, and Ovid not only accepted the communicability of rabies by dog bite but thought that rabid persons could spread the disease by biting others.

Celsus, writing around A.D. 30, summarized contemporary knowledge and gave as accurate an appraisal of rabies as there was to be until the nineteenth century. He pointed out that the saliva of infected animals contained a virus or poison which was communicated through a bite to the victim to produce a disease which the Greeks called *hydrophion,* "a most wretched disease in which the sick person is tormented at the same time with thirst and the fear of water, and in which there is but little hope." Celsus gave many suggestions for treating those bitten. These included caustics, burning, cupping, cauterizing, and bloodletting. His recommendations included throwing patients without warning into a pond, and, if necessary, holding them under the water until they were forced to swallow water. This procedure was to alleviate thirst and overcome the dread of water.

Rabies retained an important place in the medical literature of the Mediterranean region, especially Greece, Sicily, and Crete, through the third century. It also was known farther east. Aetius, a sixth-century physician from Mesopotamia, described the dog disease in detail, and there are Syrian references to it from the ninth century which stress that is was incurable. Al Razi and Avicenna, the classic Arab authorities of the tenth and eleventh centuries, both described and prescribed against rabies, and we find a reference to the disease in eleventh-century Britain in the laws of Howel the Good of Wales, which were revived in 1026. St. Hubert, the patron saint of hunters, was believed to work miraculous cures on rabies victims. By the fifteenth century, however, appeals to St. Hubert were criticized by the humanist theologian John of Gerson; and in the seventeenth century, the learned doctors of the Sorbonne formally condemned "superstitious practices for the treatment of rabies." But the common people retained their faith in St. Hubert into the nineteenth century.

The first recorded epizootic of rabies occurred in Franconia in 1271, when rabid wolves attacked herds, flocks, and people. At least 30 people died. Spain had widespread canine rabies in 1500, and rabies became epizootic among dogs in Flanders, Austria, Hungary, and Turkey in the sixteenth century. The disease was especially widespread in the eighteenth century in both Europe and North America, and towns began to introduce dog control measures. When rabies appeared in London in 1752, all dogs were ordered shot on sight. In 1759 and 1760, a plague of rabies forced city officials to order all dogs confined for a month. Dogs on the streets were to be killed, and a two-shilling bounty was offered for each dead dog. Similar steps were taken on the Continent. In Madrid, 900 dogs were slaughtered in one day. Such measures proved unavailing, however, and the disease continued. By 1774, rabies had become general in England, people were discouraged from keeping dogs, paupers were forbidden to own dogs, and a five-shilling bounty was established for each mad dog killed.

Rabies was transferred to the North American colonies. Wild animal populations became infected, and between 1768 and 1771, the first major epizootic took place with dogs and foxes carrying the disease. Rabies was also common in the Caribbean islands. Throughout the new world, domestic animals and livestock suffered, and there were persistent reports of human deaths.

Rabies continued active into the nineteenth century, with severe outbreaks in France, Germany, and England. An epizootic in eastern France at the foot of the Jura Mountains lasted from 1803 to 1835. Hundreds of dead foxes littered the woodlands, and people as well as dogs, pigs, and other livestock were bitten. The disease was also active in Switzerland, the Black Forest, Thuringia, upper Austria, Hesse, and Hanover. Severe outbreaks occurred again in London and the English countryside throughout the first half of the nineteenth century, and rabies began to spread into South America, especially Peru and Argentina.

The plague of rabies continued unabated in the second half of the nineteenth century, with reports of the disease arriving in Europe from far-distant China. The first case in Hong Kong was in 1857, but throughout the next decade rabies reports were received from Guangzhou, Tianjin, and Shanghai. In most cases, infected European dogs were involved. By the third quarter of the nineteenth century, rabies was a worldwide problem which threatened both human and animal life and which had broad economic consequences. Moreover, it seemed that the disease was steadily increasing. The numbers were infinitesimal when compared with the numbers of victims claimed by such mass killers as plague or smallpox, but infection was a constant threat, death was inevitable, and the spread of rabies in the animal populations seemed literally endless. The *Lancet*, Britain's leading medical publication, reported with concern on the steady growth of rabies cases over the 15 years from 1860 to 1875, when the rabies death rate rose from 0.3 to 0.9, 1.8, and finally 2 per 1 million of population. The 1877 rate in London was rising as well. Political action followed. Local authorities were given the power to muzzle dogs in 1887, and when they failed to do so effectively, muzzling was brought under central control. Cases of canine rabies fell from 129 in 1890 to 38 in 1892. Public opinion forced relaxation of the muzzling regulations, and by 1895, canine rabies soared to 727 cases, and 463 were reported in 1896. In 1897, a new rabies order and a regulation controlling the importation of dogs went into effect. The control system worked, and by 1902, rabies had disappeared.

Dog controls were effective in England because there was no wild reservoir of disease, and once rabies was exterminated among the dog population, the problem was to prevent its importation. A rigid six-month quarantine was established for dogs and cats which worked until 1918 when returning soldiers smuggled pets into the country. Rabies reappeared at Plymouth, an epizootic began which spread to Devon and Dorset, where 129 cases were reported, and an additional 190 cases were recorded in other parts of the country. That outbreak was controlled by 1922, and since that time, Britain has been virtually free of rabies.

Such legal procedures as Great Britain used were of limited use in other nations where contiguous boundaries and sylvatic reservoirs made control extremely difficult. Rabies had been recognized among fox populations in the American colonies, and in the nineteenth century, the disease became established among skunks. The difficulty of enforcing muzzling and control regulations over so vast and diverse a country, when combined with natural reservoirs of disease, meant that rabies remained a serious problem in the United States until inoculation of pets reduced the danger in the twentieth century. Rabid skunks and squirrels are still dangerous in the rural United States. Among continental European countries, the coordination of different national policies on rabies control posed major problems, while, as in the United Statels, substantial reservoirs of rabies in wild animal populations have made the quest for control more difficult.

Immunization: Louis Pasteur Pasteur's discovery of an effective vaccine was the most important scientific achievement in the campaign against rabies, but it also marked a milestone in the history of immunization. Pasteur grew up in the Jura region of eastern France where rabies was a serious problem, and he may have been drawn to seek a solution for it by the childhood experience of seeing a rabid wolf running amok through the village. He began work on rabies in 1880, supported by Pierre Émile Roux and Charles Chamberland. Roux was trained for medicine, while Chamberland was a superior bacteriological technician. Both men had worked with Pasteur on his earlier anthrax studies.

In 1881, in his first report on rabies, Pasteur recorded his conviction that rabies attacked the central nervous system and "especially the bulb which joins the spinal cord to the brain." Saliva was not the sole seat of the virus. Efforts to identify or grow a rabies organism failed, but with the spinal cord and brain identified as the disease center, Pasteur began to experiment by injecting infective matter, usually nerve tissue from rabid animals, into the brains of rabbits. This produced a more virulent virus which, however, attained a stable incubation period. A virus so stabilized was called a "fixed virus," that is, a virus with fixed pathogenic power.

Pasteur also found that the virus became weakened, or attenuated, for dogs, guinea pigs, and rabbits when it was passed through a succession of monkey brains. This made a reliable vaccine possible. By 1884 he had developed a method by which a "fixed virus" was injected into rabbits. When they died, the spinal cords were removed and suspended at room temperature in sterile air over a drying agent. Oxygen penetrated the cords, attenuating the virus. The cords became almost nonvirulent in 2 weeks. A vaccine could be prepared by emulsifying bits of dried cord in a saltwater solution. The length of drying time produced the degree of nonvirulence in the cord. Thus, in 15 days, it was possible to protect a dog against the most virulent virus. On the first day, a vaccine made with rabbit cord which had dried for 14 days was injected. On the second day, a cord dried for 13 days was used, and so on until the end, when a fully virulent virus could be injected and tolerated.

Further tests showed that the attenuated cord could be used as a preventive for dogs already bitten. This was possible because the incubation period for the virus was so very long. In 1885, despite considerable resistance and opposition, Pasteur transferred his efforts from animals to a human case. The patient, a 9-year-old boy named Joseph Meister, had been bitten 14 times by a rabid dog. Rabies was considered a certainty. Pasteur began his injections 60 hours after the attack. The treatment was carried through 14 days when, for the last inoculation, Pasteur gave fully virulent material. The boy exhibited no rabies symptoms and returned to live a normal life. A 14-year-old boy, Jean Baptiste Jupille, was Pasteur's second patient, and he, too, recovered. The first failure was a girl, Louise Pelletier, who was bitten on the face and whom Pasteur did not see until 37 days after the event. He gave treatment on the pleading of the girl's parents, but there was little hope. The wound was in a critical area, and too much time had passed. Louise Pelletier developed rabies within 11 days of completing the treatment and died soon after.

During the next 15 months, Pasteur's vaccine was given to 2500 people, but as the requests for it multiplied, so also did the criticism. The vaccine was blamed for deaths, while successes were explained by arguing that the patients who recovered were not infected in the first place. One powerful argument which was difficult to answer was that natural rabies was a very rare disease, and Pasteur was actually infecting patients with laboratory rabies. This led to accusations of homicide by carelessness, the threat of lawsuits, and a violent conflict which spilled out of the Academy of Medicine into the chamber of deputies and the political journals. The medical fraternity divided between pro- and anti-Pasteur factions, and even Pasteur's laboratory colleagues were affected. Roux, for example, abandoned work on rabies, though he eventually returned to support Pasteur. Pasteur himself suffered from these attacks; his health began to fail, and in 1887, he had two serious strokes. An official English commission which investigated his work entirely confirmed the validity of his conclusions and the positive results of his treatments. The commission also pointed out, however, how difficult it was to make any absolute determination because the treatment had to be initiated before there was any way of predicting the likelihood of infection. The British government concentrated on quarantine and control, a point which Pasteur's critics were quick to exploit.

Though Pasteur's enemies chose to interpret British caution as a defeat for the rabies vaccine, subsequent experience showed that the critics were entirely wrong. Pasteur antirabies institutes were founded throughout Europe, South America, and Mexico, and in 1915, a 10-year study showed that in 6000 cases where rabies was confirmed, mortality among treated persons was just 0.6 percent as compared with 16 percent where no vaccine treatment was employed. Subsequently, the Pasteur method was refined with notable improvements in the methods for producing the vaccine itself, particularly a phenol treatment developed by David Semple which was recommended for the British armed forces. A 1927 world conference on rabies reaffirmed the Pasteur dried cord method but approved rabies virus killed or attenuated with phenol or ether as well. This conference also urged annual rabies vaccinations for dogs in areas where rabies was active. The live Flury vaccine, made from a strain isolated in 1940 and developed in hen and duck embryos between 1948 and 1954, was found to produce satisfactory immunities when injected in dogs and has been widely used to broaden protection. The introduction of antiserum to treatment and more recently to vaccination has made both more effective.

Rabies remains an active disease today everywhere except in Great Britain, Australia, and certain other islands. The way the disease functions is known and the means both to protect against it and to control it when contracted are available. These achievements owe primarily to the work of Louis Pasteur and his associates.

ADDITIONAL READINGS: P. B. Adamson, "The Spread of Rabies into Europe and the Probable Origin of This Disease in Antiquity," *Journal of the Royal Asiatic Society of Great Britain and Ireland* 2 (1977): 140–144; George M. Baer, *The Natural History of Rabies*, 2 vols., New York, San Francisco, and London, 1975; René Dubos, *Louis Pasteur: Free Lance of Science*, New York, 1950, 1976; J. H. Parish, *A History of Immunization*, London, 1965, chap. 4; René Vallery-Rodot, *The Life of Pasteur*, R. L. Devonshire (trans.), London, 1923.

See also IMMUNOLOGY.

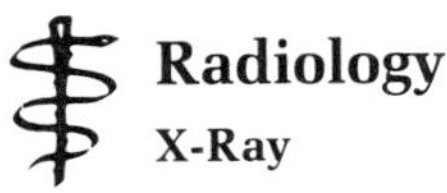

Radiology

X-Ray

Radiology is a specialized field of study which deals with the use of radio waves. Its medical application covers both diagnostic work and therapy. The requirements of these subspecialties are very different, and their separation occurred relatively early in the history of modern radiology. As an applied specialty, radiology dealt first with x-rays and then began to include the rays given off by radioactive substances in process of disintegration; it has come to include the products of atomic accelerators and nuclear reactors. Studies on the effects of radiation as separate from its diagnostic and therapeutic functions have formed a major and growing field in medicine and public health since 1945.

Modern radiology was born on November 8, 1895, when Karl Wilhelm Roentgen noticed an unexpected greenish fluorescence on his workbench while testing a Crookes tube. The light was produced by some unknown rays from the tube striking a screen treated with barium platinocyanide. Roentgen, a professor of physics at Würtsburg University, experimented with the tube, repeatedly sending electrical current through it and noting the behavior of the new rays that were given off. By December 28, he had found that his unknown, or "x," rays passed easily through wood, cloth, and paper but that they were resisted by denser materials. Photographs of the rays' effects showed bones clearly, but flesh did not appear. Roentgen set out his observations in a communication to the president of the Würtzburg Physical-Medical Society which was printed and distributed to the membership. His "Eine neue Art von Strahlen" ("A New Kind of Ray") reached the newspapers in Vienna and on January 6, 1896, was publicized in a special story in the London *Daily Chronicle*. The London *Standard* gave the story a worldwide release on the same date. The following day, the first x-ray photographs for clinical purposes were made by Alan Archibald Campbell Swinton.

Roentgen gave his first public lecture on x-rays at Würzburg on January 23, 1896, demonstrating how the rays permitted photographs to be made of the bones in a colleague's hand. Three scientific papers which he published the following year proved to be definitive. These papers were concerned with the effects of electrical currents, magnets, tube size, and distances on x-ray production; the rays' behavior in magnetic fields; and the linear character of x-ray movement. By that time, however, his discovery had also become a gigantic popular sensation, sparking music hall turns and several generations of x-ray jokes. Some people wondered if an x-ray "instrument" would make it possible for voyeurs to look at people's private parts, a fear which led one enterprising underwear manufacturer to advertise his garments as "x-ray proof." Roentgen himself was decorated by the imperial German government, and Bavaria granted him the right, which he never exercised, to use the aristocratic "von" in his name; but he gained nothing financially from his discovery.

The fact that certain substances released active radiation as they degenerated was less amenable to instant recognition and exploitation. At the end of the nineteenth century, the French physicist and engineer Antoine Henri Becquerel included the study of properties of rare earths among his interests; it was Becquerel who encouraged the penniless Polish expatriate Marie Sklodowska Curie to do her doctoral research on rays emanating from uranium. Marie Curie informed the Academy of Sciences in April 1898 that there was probably a new element to be found in pitchblende which was powerfully radioactive. Joined now by her husband, Pierre, Marie Curie embarked on a course of research which resulted in their identifying polonium in July and radium in December. During the next four years, with almost no support and under the most primitive conditions, the Curies worked to extract the more powerful of the two elements, radium, from the ton of pitchblende slag which the Austrian government gave them.

In 1901, Becquerel suffered an accidental burn from carrying a radium sample in his pocket, and Pierre Curie deliberately gave himself a burn to confirm the element's action. Treatments for lupus and malignancy followed. The Curies and Becquerel received the Nobel prize for physics in 1903, and by 1904, it had been proved that radium waves killed diseased cells preferentially. This aroused commercial interest in the element. Although Pierre Curie was killed in 1906 in a street accident, Marie carried on the work that she had begun in her doctoral research and won a then-unprecedented second Nobel prize, this time in chemistry, in 1911. At the time of her death in 1934 from the effects of radiation poisoning, she had won recognition as one of the leading figures in twentieth-century science and a pioneer in radiation research.

Radium's medical application was therapeutic

from the start, while the x-ray was more important initially as a diagnostic tool. It was not, however, a simple tool to use, and as the dangers of prolonged radiation exposure were not understood at first, the x-ray misled physicians often enough to strengthen resistance to its use. Broken bones, bullet wounds, and solid objects lodged inside the body posed only minor problems, but diagnoses involving soft tissue, including tumors, were very difficult. The first problem was to establish sufficient contrast for a readable picture to be taken; the second was to read the picture. Various bismuth compounds were used in the stomach and intestinal tract with some success; silver protein solutions, sodium bromide and thorium were among the materials which proved unsuccessful or dangerous. It was not until 1922 that lipidol was introduced to provide a bland and harmless substance that permitted effective photography. Lipidol remained in general use until the early 1950s when it was supplanted by a variety of aqueous-viscous agents which could be tailored to the particular x-ray function intended.

Reading x-rays accurately required a comparative approach in which normal and diseased conditions were studied and contrasted. It was this technique which America's first radiologist, Francis H. Williams, developed. Williams was both a physicist and physician who worked with the Massachusetts Institute of Technology and Boston City Hospital. His method was to study normal conditions in detail and then contrast the pathological against the normal. It was a difficult process to use effectively, however, and despite some notable successes during World War I, many physicians resisted it. As late as 1920, a noted cardiologist remarked that it was "doubtful if an x-ray examination of the heart has ever thrown the slightest light upon any cardiac condition."

Radiology showed a high degree of specialization and professionalism very early. Practicing physicians found that learning to use x-ray machines and applying them without help was time-consuming and inefficient. Thus a demand for specialists appeared by the turn of the century. Many students had worked with x-rays after their discovery, and those with specialties in physics or engineering or with experience as photographers or electricians returned to qualify as physicians with radiological skills. In 1910, a questionnaire circulated by the American Roentgen Ray Society showed that 27 percent of the society's membership were exclusively radiologists. Special curricula and licensing procedures followed.

Through the first half of the twentieth century, x-ray was used more and more frequently in treating neoplasms and skin conditions and in preparation for surgery. Chest x-rays and fluoroscopic examination became a standard method for identifying tubercular lesions and during World War I permitted rapid examinations of thousands of recruits. The x-ray also advanced the study of the central nervous system and, as techniques were refined, contributed to improved levels of success in neurosurgery. Radiation therapy also advanced rapidly, and for conditions which both reached, radiation had some natural advantages. X-ray equipment was clumsy and difficult to use. It was also imprecise. There was no standard unit of measurement for x-ray intensity, and therefore it was difficult to manage treatments rationally. Radium, on the other hand, was fully defined. Its atomic weight was established in 1907, an international standard specimen was prepared in 1911, and the unit of measurement (curie) was recognized. Even greater efficiency and accuracy were achieved by treatment with implants, a procedure introduced in 1905, as well as by the development of radiation "seeds," or raions. A unit of measurement for x-ray based on the rate of ionization, a process Roentgen had noted, was not defined until the Second International Congress of Radiologists in Stockholm in 1928, and the unit of ionization, or "r," was not made official until 1937. It was not until 1958 that the definition of a "rad" as 100 ergs per grain was agreed upon. After 1920, x-ray therapy gained again on radiation because of the relatively low power of radium implants and the capacity of x-ray to multiply its force. When plutonium, cobalt, and radioactive isotopes entered the therapeutic picture after World War II, however, the balance shifted back. In the end, both methods have special applications. Radiation therapy has been most useful on "close" treatments for carcinomas in the rectum, bladder, uterus, vagina, and esophagus, while x-ray is most effective for surface treatment, as in skin cancer.

The most recent development in radiology is the introduction of radioactive isotopes, which the cyclotron has made available in large quantities at relatively low cost. Recognized in 1910, isotopes were first generated in 1932, but they were not produced in quantity until after 1942, using uranium fission. They were first marketed in 1945, and by 1957, the U.S. Atomic Energy Commission had made 14,106 isotope shipments from Oak Ridge, Tennessee, alone. The isotopes were first used in 1936 to study metabolism and to treat leukemia. They have proved especially valuable for studying gland functions, tumor locations, and blood conditions. They have a variety of therapeutic uses, especially against cancers.

Though warnings on the use of radiation and x-rays were common enough in the early years of the twentieth century, the long-term consequences of heavy radiation, repeated exposure, and long exposure were not understood. Radium burns were considered temporary conditions, and dangers connected with handling x-ray machines, or fluoroscopes, were largely ignored. Fluoroscopes were not used only for medical purposes but were employed routinely in shoe stores and entertainment centers. X-rays were used freely in dental work and prenatal studies. The realization that radiation was dangerous grew during the 1920s and 1930s, but the reduction of unnecessary radiation exposure only became a major concern after World War II. This was largely a result of the atomic energy program. The dangers of radioactivity, so dramatically demonstrated in 1945, became the basis for elaborate research on the effects of different kinds and quantities of rays. Prewar work on tolerance for radiation was recognized to be inadequate, and in 1942, in response to potential dangers of research on atomic power and the eventual use of atomic weapons, tolerance estimates were dramatically reduced. The effects of radiation, however, were so complex that the only reasonable approach was to build safeguards into all radiation-producing equipment while reducing all radiation exposure to the lowest possible level. This conclusion started national policy debates over atmospheric testing of nuclear weapons as well as providing the background to current arguments over the safety of nuclear power stations. But it also meant a conscious effort to reduce radiation exposure in medicine. The earlier tendency to use x-ray or radium for all manner of conditions ended. Exposure was to be limited to what was necessary. Improved x-ray technology—higher voltage, filtered beams, faster film, and intensified field screens—substantially reduced radiation exposure. The amount of tissue irradiated was held to a minimum and the use of radiation therapy for benign conditions virtually disappeared. Though it is difficult to measure quantitatively, one recent study by the U.S. Public Health Service indicated that substantial progress in reducing unnecessary radiation exposure was being made, and a study by the Radiological Society shows marked improvement in the life expectancy of radiologists. Between 1934 and 1939, the average age of death for radiologists was 56; in the 1950s, this age was 64; and in the 1960s, 70. Improved equipment and recognition of the dangers involved account for much of the gain.

ADDITIONAL READINGS: A. R. Bleich, *The Story of X-rays: From Roentgen to Isotopes*, New York, 1960; Ruth and Edward Brecher, *The Rays: A History of Radiology in the United States and Canada*, Baltimore, 1969; Stephen B. Ewing, *Modern Radiology in Historical Perspective*, Springfield, Ill., 1962; Robert William Reich, *Marie Curie*, New York, 1974; David Sutton (ed.), *A Textbook of Radiology*, 2d ed., London, 1975.

Rheumatism

"Rheumatism" is a general term used popularly to designate painful conditions in muscles, joints, and bones. It has been replaced in medical terminology by particular names for specific diseases, such as "rheumatic fever" and "rheumatoid arthritis," which indicate both the condition and a specific cause. The activating agent for rheumatic fever is a group A hemolytic streptococcus, and the so-called "rheumatoid factor" in 75 percent of people with rheumatoid arthritis results from an immunological reaction to bacterial or viral infections.

Rheumatic fever was once widespread and dangerous. Twentieth-century medical statistics show that every spring, one-fourth of New York's hospital beds were occupied by rheumatic fever patients. Between 1930 and 1934, 3445 patients with rheumatic heart disease were treated in Philadelphia, and 20 percent died. Rheumatoid arthritis affects the lives of millions of people, but the effect is one of discomfort and inconvenience rather than mortal danger. This is serious enough for those who suffer it, and the annual losses in productivity which rheumatic conditions engender run to the millions of dollars.

Rheumatic conditions are believed to have existed for a long time, though the historical evidence is thin. Neither radiological assay nor macroscopic analysis has been able to demonstrate rheumatoid arthritis in prehistoric skeletons and though early medical writings on fevers hold clues, the descriptions are too general to identify rheumatic fever precisely. The closest we may come is in the Hippocratic writings of the late fifth century B.C., which describe an arthritis in which "fever comes on, acute pain affects the joints of the body, and the pains which vary from mild to severe flit from joint to joint." This condition appears to have been common, and it attacked "the young more frequently than the old" and was seldom mortal. This would appear to describe an acute rheumatic fever. After Hippocrates, the clinical detail receded in importance, and by Galen's time (ca. A.D. 150) the diagnostic image of rheumatism was firmly lodged in the humoral explanations for arthritis, where it remained until the sixteenth century.

The idea of a fever which produced pain and swelling in the joints was revived by the Italian physician Jerome Cardan and by Jean Fernel, the French humanist. Real de Colombo, the author of a major anatomical study published in 1559, recorded what may be the first evidence of a pathologic consequence to the heart from such a fever. The French physician and anatomist Guillaume de Baillou, a member of the medical faculty at the University of Paris, was the first to use the word "rheumatism" to describe an acute polyarthritis, separate from gout, in which "the joints are wracked with pains so that neither foot, hand, nor finger can be moved without pain and protest." This disease, which made the victim hot and which was worse at night than in the daytime, led to a chronic arthritic condition.

The best early modern clinical description for rheumatism came in the next century, when Thomas Sydenham described autumnal attacks, chiefly on the young, of a disease which began "with shivering and shaking," moved on to "heat, restlessness, and thirst," and broke into severe pain and swelling in the joints. Sydenham noted that this condition, when unattended by fever, was commonly mistaken for gout, though it "differs essentially" from gout. Hermann Boerhaave approved and followed Sydenham's description while adding the idea that rheumatism attacked "Brain, Lung, and Bowels" as well as joints. His students, Baron Antonius Störk and the Austrian court physician Gerard L. B. van Swieten confirmed these observations by postmortem examination and noted the danger when the disease attacked the brain or lungs.

By the opening of the nineteenth century, rheumatism had been separated from gout, and while its primary effect as an acute arthritis had been identified, the outline of a rheumatic disease which attacked the viscera was also taking shape. Work on the idea that an acute rheumatic attack damaged the heart began to be published in 1797. In the early nineteenth century, it was common to refer to rheumatism as a disease entity affecting both skeleton and viscera. Jean-Baptiste Bouillaud, a physician with the Sick Children's Hospital in Paris, published a major study which first presented rheumatic heart disease as a complete clinical and pathological entity. Bouillaud believed that rheumatic pericarditis and endocarditis were frequent occurrences, and he also believed they would always be a part of that disease's nature.

In 1900, Dr. F. J. Poynton and Dr. A. Paine discovered a diplococcus in the blood and joint fluid of eight living children with rheumatism. Their conviction that this "diplococcus rheumaticus" was the causal agent in acute rheumatism could not be confirmed. But their view of a mechanism involving a microorganism which set up immunological reactions was sound, although identification of the streptococcus involved and proofs for the immunological reaction were not established until the middle 1970s.

The first effective specific for rheumatism was found by accident in the eighteenth century, when the Reverend Edmund Stone, reporting to the Royal Society on April 25, 1763, ventured to draw the public's attention to willow bark. Stone had tasted the bark and found it bitter (like Peruvian bark). Moreover, because the willow grew in the damps where agues and fevers abounded, and because it was widely believed that God (or nature) grew herbs to cure diseases in the same place diseases originated, he thought there were grounds for trying it as a remedy. The Reverend Stone gave his willow bark to some 50 persons who had rheumatic fever symptoms, and he reported satisfactory results in nearly every case. The active ingredient in willow bark is salicin, which has an effect similar to that of the basic component in aspirin. Stone's discovery had no resonance, but just under a century later, Dr. Thomas MacLagan of Glasgow, following reasoning like Stone's (though aided by the extraction of glucoside of salicin in 1839), hit on the same remedy. It was very costly to extract, however, and it remained to chemistry to produce the salicylate group of drugs and sodium acetylsalicylate itself (1899) and put aspirin into the hands of millions of rheumatism sufferers. Other remedies for the effects of rheumatic fever and rheumatoid arthritis appeared with cardiac surgery after 1925 and with the steroid hormones in 1949. Modern preventive measures emphasize the use of sulfonamides and antibiotics to prevent reinfection from hemolytic streptococci. Though there is no cure, the means to alleviate symptoms and to manage the disease are well-developed, while successful prevention has substantially reduced the incidence of rheumatic heart conditions.

ADDITIONAL READINGS: W. S. C. Copeman, "Rheumatism," in Walter P. Bett (ed.), *The History and Conquest of Common Diseases*, Norman, Okla., 1954, 115–123; W. S. C. Copeman, *A Short History of Gout and the Rheumatic Diseases*, Berkeley and Los Angeles, 1964; G. E. Murphy, "The Evolution of Our Knowledge of Rheumatic Fever: An Historical Survey with Particular Emphasis on Rheumatic Heart Disease," *Bulletin of the History of Medicine* 14 (July 1943): 123–147.

See also ARTHRITIS; GOUT.

Rickets

Rickets is a bone disease which deforms and cripples children in the first two years of life. The cause for rickets is a vitamin D deficiency which can result from inadequate diet, insufficient exposure to ultraviolet rays, or a combination of the two. Rickets has been most common in temperate zone cities among the children of poor or working-class parents. Early diagnosis of the disease is difficult because the initial symptoms are unremarkable. Children developing rickets are often pale, irritable, and sleepless. They perspire profusely and are prone to diarrhea and, in severe cases, tetany and convulsions. Rickets seldom kills its victims, but it retards mental as well as physical growth and leaves permanent disabilities.

Though rickets was known for centuries, it is essentially a modern disease which peaked in the industrial age. Francis Glisson gave the first detailed description of the disease early in the seventeenth century, and in deference to his work, it was called "the English disease." Its high incidence in seventeenth- and eighteenth-century England gave the name an additional significance. Rickets was seen on the Continent during the early industrial revolution and in the course of the nineteenth century became epidemic throughout urban-industrial Europe and in the United States. In the last quarter of the nineteenth century and the first quarter of the twentieth, rickets was nearly universal among children in the Glasgow and London slums, and it was hardly less widespread in other urban manufacturing cities in the United Kingdom. On the Continent, a 1907 survey of hospitals in Paris revealed that every other child between the ages of six months and three years admitted to the hospitals suffered rickets to some degree. New York reported a similar incidence, and it was concluded in 1921 that fully 75 percent of all infants in New York and similar large American cities had rickets. The disease was particularly widespread in black and Italian neighborhoods, where children free from rickets were unusual.

Since rickets resulted from a combination of socioeconomic, environmental, and geographical factors, a successful campaign against it was only possible when the disease mechanism was understood and organizations capable of dealing with it on a mass basis were available. This conditions were not fulfilled until the early twentieth century when the etiology of rickets was firmly established by Edward Mellanby and Harriet Chick in England and E. V. McCollum in the United States. A variety of substances headed by different fish-liver oils was found to be effective against rickets, and public health and welfare administrations were available to distribute and administer these dietary supplements. The British effort was exemplary. A network of child care centers was established under government auspices, and a daily dose of cod-liver oil was given to every child attending. In 1911, there were just 100 centers, but in the next 20 years, the number grew to 1400 and their work was supplemented by health visitors. These efforts were intensified during World War II.

Though rickets has largely disappeared from the urban-industrial world, it is still found in developing nations, most notably in Africa and India. The incidence, however, does not approach that which occurred in the temperate regions, and other deficiency diseases are considered to be more serious. Nevertheless, especially as urbanization and industrialization expand in poverty-stricken areas, there is a potential for new outbreaks of rickets which needs to be watched.

ADDITIONAL READINGS: W. R. Aykroyd, *Conquest of Deficiency Diseases: Achievements and Prospects*, Geneva, 1970; Harriet Chick, *Studies of Rickets in Vienna, 1919–1922*, London, 1923; A. F. Hess, *Rickets, Including Osteomalacia and Tetany*, Philadelphia and London, 1929, 1930; G. F. McCleary, *The Early History of the Infant Welfare Movement*, London, 1933; George Rosen, *A History of Public Health*, New York, 1958.

See also DEFICIENCY DISEASES; VITAMINS.

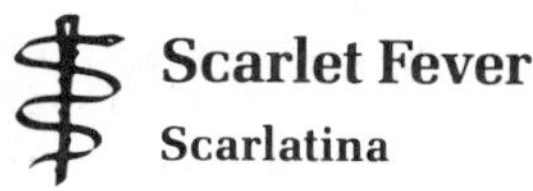

Scarlet Fever

Scarlatina

Scarlet fever is a common disease with an uncommon and highly complex etiological character. In the nineteenth century, as one of several diseases which were still widespread and dangerous, scarlet fever contributed to high mortality rates, especially among children. Its effects were restricted to Europe and North America, and its control in the twentieth century has followed from increased knowledge of streptococcal infections as well as the development of modern drug compounds, especially sulfonamides and penicillin.

Disease Characteristics Scarlet fever is an acute, highly infectious fever which is caused by a subcluster of hemolytic streptococcus bacteria called Lancefield group A. Scarlet fever rash results from reaction to an erythrogenic toxin; its symptoms, complications, and mortality are the direct effect of streptococcus germs which lodge in the throat. The symptoms include sore throat, a bright red rash spread evenly over the skin, fever, and a coated tongue with red papules (strawberry tongue). The most common complications are abscesses in the throat and tonsils, sinusitis, and inflammation of the lymph nodes and middle ear. Historical descriptions mention heavy discharges from the nose and ears, and death was not uncommon. The disease shows many faces. Sometimes scarlet fever is mild and relatively easy to manage; in other instances it develops a high rate of incidence and considerable mortality. Variations in the streptococci and in the resistance the host organism offers account for the varieties of intensity among scarlet fever outbreaks. Conditions of life—diet, housing, cleanliness, poverty or wealth—also have a bearing on the effects which scarlet fever may have.

Scarlet Fever History Whether scarlet fever was a factor earlier than the fourteenth century is simply not known, nor is there any hint of when, where, or how it made its appearance in Europe. According to J. F. C. Hecker, the leading nineteenth-century authority on medieval diseases, the earliest reference to scarlet fever was a fourteenth-century description by Gentile da Foligno of what he called a *malum rosatum*. There was also a report of a disease in 1527 among the children of Modena which a contemporary writer called *male di scarlatina* which may have been scarlet fever. August Hirsch, however, considered the 1543 account by Giovanni Filippo Ingrassia of an epidemic in Sicily to be the earliest verifiable historical record of a scarlet fever outbreak. Ingrassia, who was an early authority on public health and legal medicine, omitted the usual sore throat from his account, but in all other respects his description was consistent with scarlet fever.

The first unequivocal record of scarlet fever with all its distinctive symptoms appeared in 1627 in accounts of epidemics at Wittenberg and Breslau written by Daniel Sennert and his brother-in-law, Michael Düring. Sennert accurately recorded the sequence in which the rash appeared and then declined, being the first to note the "scaling," or "desquamation," which followed the rash. He was also the first to report the complications which scarlet fever was likely to produce, most notably a dropsy from kidney inflammation and polyarthritis from involvement in the joints.

The outbreak which Sennert and Düring witnessed was followed by a remission of the disease in northern Europe. During the middle and later years of the seventeenth century, however, scarlet fever became general across the Continent, and it appeared as well in England. In 1676, Thomas Sydenham added a short chapter titled "Febris Scarlatina" to the third edition of his *Medical Ob-*

servations (*Observationum medicarum*) which established the name "scarlet fever" for the disease and filled out the clinical description. Sydenham described a mild disease which was different from measles and which came on in late summer. His advice on treatment was simple and conservative: Keep the patient indoors and on a light diet. Bloodletting and heart remedies were unnecessary. Contemporaries, including the famous diarist Samuel Pepys, similarly used the phrase "a scarlett fevour," and it seems to have been a common designation.

Other English sources confirmed Sydenham's account of scarlet fever as a mild disease, and it seems certain that Sydenham never saw a severe case. Richard Morton, who also practiced in London in the second half of the seventeenth century, failed to distinguish between measles and scarlet fever, but some of the cases of fever he described in his *Pyretologia* (1694) were definitely severe scarlet fever. The difference between Sydenham's and Morton's descriptions may reflect the different classes of patients they saw. Sydenham worked among the well-to-do while Morton treated the poor. There is evidence that scarlet fever was more severe among the working classes, the poor, and the indigent than it was among the wealthy.

Epidemic outbreaks of scarlet fever were reported throughout Europe and the American colonies in the eighteenth century, and physicians developed a detailed clinical picture of the disease. Scarlet fever as they described it began with shivering and nausea, fever, a crimson rash, and a sore throat. Sometimes the rash and sore throat occurred separately. The rash scaled off by the sixth or seventh day, and the disease appeared to be over around the eighth or ninth day. Dropsy was frequent, and some patients died of it after about a month. In other cases, there was suppuration of the neck glands. In severe cases, the rash might appear on the first or second day, and the patient might then die. Those who lived recovered very slowly, while some lived through the disease only to die after a month or six weeks of debility.

Relatively little work was done on scarlet fever between 1800 and 1830, and the disease itself was quiet. Then new and more vigorous outbreaks began in Ireland (1831–1834) and England (1840; 1844; 1848), followed by a very active period from 1850 to 1890. Charles Creighton, the eminent nineteenth-century physician and epidemiologist, called scarlet fever in this period the most deadly of infectious childhood diseases. It was a significant factor in the high average mortalities in England and Wales, which reached 972 per 1 million of population between 1861 and 1870 and then, with the disease declining sharply, fell back to 338 for the decade 1881 to 1890.

The experience in the United States was similar. In New York City, for example, between 1805 and 1832, there were only 43 scarlet fever cases recorded, but between 1822 and 1847, the number reached 4074, and there were 579 in 1837 alone. A brief decline followed, and then came a new attack. In 1857, 1325 cases were registered in New York City, and in subsequent years the figures remained high there and throughout the United States. The severity of the disease abated by 1880, and in 1900, the scarlet fever death rate per 100,000 of population stood at 9.6. By 1935, it had dropped to 2.1, and in 1970 it was between 0 and 0.5.

Cyclical patterns of scarlet fever infection show high incidence in the early and middle nineteenth century and in the early twentieth century. Mortality, as in other infectious diseases including typhoid, tuberculosis, and diphtheria, steadily declined. Improved living standards account in part for the decline, but there also may be a cyclical pattern at work in the streptococci responsible and in their relationship with the host.

Understanding Scarlet Fever Knowledge about scarlet fever multiplied in the nineteenth and twentieth centuries. In 1861, Armand Trousseau established an accepted clinical basis for differentiating scarlet fever from other diseases, and the search for the casual agent began. Friedrich Loeffler, who discovered the diphtheria bacillus, identified streptococci in scarlet fever patients in 1884. In 1886, thanks to this lead, streptococci from an infected cow's udder were identified as the cause in a scarlet fever epidemic. But further progress was slow. Additional research failed to find streptococci in the skin sloughed off from scarlet fever rash or in the blood of any but the most severe scarlet fever cases. Nor was the presence of streptococci definitive proof of causation. In 1893, André Bergé, a Parisian physician, correctly identified scarlet fever as "a local infection" caused by a streptococcus which "grows in the crypts of the tonsils" where it secretes "an erythrogenic [rash-producing] toxin." Bacteriologists were unable to find the toxin, however, and there was uncertainty over how it worked. In 1905, a theory suggested that while the streptococcus was responsible for the complications which the disease developed, some still unknown factor caused the disease itself. This idea, rather than Bergé's approach, influenced research and was a prevailing misconception for two decades.

In 1924, George Dick and Gladys Dick, working at the University of Chicago, correctly identified hemolytic streptococcus as the causal agent in scarlet fever and were able to infect one of two volunteers after swabbing their throats with a culture obtained from the throats of scarlet fever patients. They also were able to establish a test for immunity to scarlet fever (the Dick test) by injecting the filtrate, or fluid, left after the streptococcus in a culture had been removed. If the patient was susceptible to infection, a red spot developed at the injection point. If he or she was immune, there was no reaction. This achievement was important for managing scarlet fever outbreaks, but the Dicks' conviction that the rash-producing toxin was also responsible for the disease symptoms and the complication was disproved in 1926. Their corollary view that one special variety of streptococcus was responsible was refuted in 1933 by Rebecca Lancefield at the Rockefeller Institute. She demonstrated that a group of streptococci provided the causal agents. Lancefield's work was confirmed the following year by Frederick Griffiths, an English bacteriologist who developed the method for classifying the different types in the group. There are more than 40 streptococcus types in what now is called Lancefield group A hemolytic streptococcus.

Over the last 40 years, research has established the complex causal patterns involved in a streptococcus-scarlet fever outbreak. A person infected with group A hemolytic streptococcus who is not immune to the rash-producing toxin will develop scarlet fever. If he or she is immune to the toxin or if there is no toxin, the person will develop a streptococcal sore throat. If the person is immune to the invading streptococcus as well, there will be no reaction at all. Attempts to develop serum treatment and vaccines, a process in which the Dicks were deeply involved, were only partially successful, and immunization was primarily used to protect physicians and nurses in hospitals and other institutions. Sulfonamides were used with some success against streptococcus carriers during World War II, but drug-resistant streptococci also appeared, leading to sanctions in attempting any further blood chemoprophylaxis. Sulfonamides also offered a partially effective treatment, but penicillin, which began to be used against streptococcal infections after World War II, proved to be much more effective, both in curing a particular infection and in preventing recurrence. Since penicillin was very expensive, it was at first used only in those cases where sulfonamides failed. Repeated demonstration of its effectiveness between 1947 and 1954 and a decline in its cost with mass production have made penicillin the preferred specific for streptococcal infection generally and scarlet fever in particular.

Scarlet fever is no longer the problem that it was, and medical science now understands its cause, dynamics, and how best to manage it. But one central problem is unresolved. The patterns of lesser and greater severity in historical outbreaks cannot be explained on the basis of present knowledge. Improved living conditions and an effective specific can account for some of the progress in controlling scarlet fever. The degree to which this favorable outcome was aided by cyclical decline in the malignant powers of the streptococci is not known. Therefore, it is possible that scarlet fever could again become a dangerous disease and that drug-resistant strains of the streptococcus could reduce the efficacy of the known penicillin treatment.

ADDITIONAL READINGS: Harry F. Dowling, *Fighting Infection*, Cambridge, 1977; H. J. Parish, *A History of Immunization*, London, 1965, 196–204; George Rosen, "Acute Communicable Diseases," in Walter R. Bett (ed.), *The History and Conquest of Common Diseases*, Norman, Okla. 1954, 26–38.

See also PENICILLIN.

Scurvy

Scurvy is a disease which results from diets deficient in vitamin C (ascorbic acid), an element present in large quantities in citrus fruits but occurring as well in potatoes, tomatoes, green peppers, and cabbages. This deficiency produces capillary weakness, which results in hemorrhaging into the tissues, bleeding gums, loose teeth, anemia, and a general debilitation. In infants and small children, there may be interference with bone development. Victims suffering from scurvy become dull and lethargic, body temperatures often fall below the normal range to 96 or 97° F, and there may be dropsical effects in the lower limbs as well as shortness of breath and painfully swollen joints. In severe cases, death is common.

Scurvy has been best known as a sailors' disease, but in fact, it has existed wherever people are forced to subsist without fresh fruits or vegetables. Disasters of all sorts which have interrupted normal provisioning have brought scurvy in their wake. Scurvy followed the potato blights in Ireland and Scotland of 1846 and 1847, attacked the French armies in the Crimea (1854–1856), was rampant on both sides of the line in the Civil War (1861–1865), interrupted explorations in the arctic and antarctic regions between 1875 and 1905, and generated major problems among Australian, Indian, and Turkish troops in the 1915 Gallipoli campaign of World War I.

Though obviously a serious problem, scurvy attracted little attention from major urban hospitals. It was not commonly met in cities, and since its diagnostic image was unclear and its pathology not really understood, it was likely that many individual cases went unrecognized. But scurvy was well-known at sea. When Vasco da Gama first rounded the Cape of Good Hope (1497–1499), more than half his complement succumbed to scurvy, and the disease remained a serious threat on long-distance voyages for the next 400 years. There were advances, most notably in the British navy. In the eighteenth century, James Lind, a Scottish naval surgeon, discovered that fresh fruit or lemon juice could prevent and cure scurvy. He published his findings, collected on a 10-week cruise in 1746, as *A Treatise on the Scurvy* (1753), and when Capt. James Cook made his famous voyages to the South Pacific (1772–1775), he modified Lind's rules, firmly enforced a strict hygienic discipline, and kept his company free from scurvy. The British navy's later success in blockading Napoleonic France owed in part to its ability to control scurvy. The disease continued to affect merchant crews on long voyages until 1844, when Parliament mandated a regular issue of lime juice on merchantmen. It was this practice which gave English seamen the nickname "limey," a term which by extension became a slang name for Englishmen in general.

The royal navy's success rested on Lind's careful observation, good discipline, and luck. There was, in fact, great confusion about scurvy, and a rigorous scientific definition of its symptoms and pathology was lacking until the late nineteenth century. Even so, improved maritime technology meant shorter voyages and better storage facilities, and both factors tended to improve shipboard diets; this, in combination with citrus juices, kept scurvy at bay. In 1860, however, the royal navy began to buy West Indian lime juice rather than the more costly lemon juice from Malta it had used previously, and in 1875 there was a severe outbreak of scurvy on two British ships engaged in arctic exploration. Subsequent expeditions also suffered unexpectedly and heavily, and it was not until 1919 that Alice Henderson Smith connected the reappearance of scurvy with the switch to West Indian limes. Smith's work was historical, but laboratory tests confirmed that the West Indian sour lime had a very low antiscorbutic factor which in preservation effectively disappeared. Such lime juice had no effect on scurvy.

It had been suspected for some time that many foods could prevent scurvy. The nineteenth-century pathologist and historian of disease August Hirsch identified potatoes as antiscorbutic, and doctors in London hospitals who suspected scurvy in children treated them with diets of meat, milk, potatoes, and citrus juices. Even with success, however, there was uncertainty over what produced it. It was found that while several foods seemed to ward off scurvy, some, such as apples, lemon juices, and cabbage, lost their antiscorbutic effects when they were heated. By 1907, however, Axel Holst and Theodore Froehlich were able to demonstrate that scurvy could be produced and cured by diet.

During World War I, a group of women scientists at the Lister Institute in London began a series of painstaking investigations into the antiscorbutic qualities of different foods. Harriet Chick, Margaret Hume, Ruth Skelton, and Margorie MacFarlane, backed by the historical researches of Alice Henderson Smith, classified which foods under what conditions were effective against scurvy. Ultimately, Arthur Harden, also of the Lister Institute, separated citric and other acids from lemon juice, leaving a residue with a high antiscorbutic effect which the acids in themselves lacked. It was also shown that antiscorbutics could not replace either the fat-soluble A factor or the water-soluble B factor in the diet of rats immune to scurvy. The rats' condition improved when the antiscorbutic was added to diets with A and B included. By 1919, the antiscorbutic factor had been recognized as an essential nutrient, and Jack Cecil Drummond named it "water-soluble C." Vitamin C was isolated in 1927, and it was synthesized in 1932. The picture was then complete. The cause and cure for scurvy were known, and its eradication became a political, social, and economic problem.

ADDITIONAL READINGS: James Lind, *A Treatise on the Scurvy*, 1753, reprint ed., Edinburgh, 1953; Alice Henderson Smith, "A Historical Inquiry into the Efficacy of Lime Juice for the Prevention and Cure of Scurvy," *Journal of the Royal Army Medical Corps* 32 (1919): 93–116, 188–208; Leonard G. Wilson, "The Clinical Definition of Scurvy and the Discovery of Vitamin C," *Journal of the History of Medicine and Allied Sciences* 30 (January 1975): 40–60.

See also DEFICIENCY DISEASES; VITAMINS.

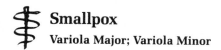

Smallpox

Variola Major; Variola Minor

Smallpox is a highly infectious disease of great antiquity which is communicated directly from person to person. The agent of infection is a filterable virus. Other diseases with a similar agent include measles, influenza, mumps, polio, encephalitis, yellow fever, and the common cold. There is no known treatment for smallpox, though penicillin may be used to counteract secondary effects. The disease can, however, be prevented through vaccination, and it is now considered to have been eradicated. Since there were still hundreds of thousands of cases as late as 1967, the antismallpox campaign is one of the triumphs of international public health and preventive medicine.

Smallpox was particularly dreaded for its high mortalities, especially among virgin populations or populations where its incidence had been low, and for its disfiguring, crippling, and blinding side effects. Untreated, and attacking a previously uninfected population, smallpox has recorded mortalities of up to 90 percent of those infected. It is more common, however, for death rates during an attack by variola major, the most virulent form, to hold between 20 and 40 percent of recognized cases. Mortalities in variola minor are of a different order of magnitude, running as low as 1 percent of the case incidence.

The smallpox virus spreads in droplets discharged from the nose or mouth. Indirect infection from clothing or bedding which infected persons have used is possible but infrequent. Most infection involves face-to-face exposure. An incubation period of 10 to 16 days usually precedes the first symptoms, which include high fever and aching limbs. This stage resembles influenza. In from 2 to 4 days a rash appears over the entire body but most densely on the face, arms, and legs. The rash papules enlarge and fill, first with a clear serum and then with pus. In severe cases, the pustules overlap, obliterating normal skin. Victims in this stage may become so swollen and disfigured as to be unrecognizable. Scabs form between the eighth and the tenth days, and by the third week they drop off, destroying pigmentation and leaving deep pits and scars. Blindness is one common consequence of severe smallpox, but eye damage can result from even mild attacks.

It is possible that the earliest identifiable case of smallpox was the Egyptian pharoah Ramses V, who died about 1160 B.C. In India, temples in which a deity of smallpox was worshiped hint at even more ancient beginnings. Diseases identifiable as smallpox do not appear in western sources, however, until after A.D. 500. Neither early Greek nor Hebrew writings record its presence, and while it is surmised that the Antonine plague which decimated Rome in the second century A.D. may have been smallpox, the evidence, including Galen's own descripton of it, is entirely uncertain. In the sixth century, Gregory of Tours refers to skin eruptions, rash, and fever in describing a pestilence which could have been smallpox, but it was not until the ninth century that the celebrated Persian physician Al Rhazi gave clearly identifiable diagnostic descriptions of smallpox and measles and distinguished between them. It appears from his account that these diseases were present in the Mediterranean and west Asian world for some time before he wrote. It is probable, therefore, that smallpox was established in western Asia and the Mediterranean early in the first millennium.

Smallpox is a disease of man which does not

depend on animal hosts or insect vectors. Moreover, humans who survive a smallpox attack are not infected again. Consequently, in areas where the disease has been active, adults seldom contract it, having developed immunities when they were children, while children are the most common victims. The infective chain, therefore, is easily broken in thinly settled areas, and high population density is a prerequisite for the disease to persist. This fact helps to explain the absence of smallpox until the Roman period from the thinly settled west and its presence in the densely settled areas of India and China in early times.

Chinese historical sources which accurately describe smallpox date from the fourth century A.D., though there is some question as to when the epidemic reported by the physician He Gong actually occurred. Japan appears to have received smallpox with its first recorded mainland contacts in the sixth century, and there were severe epidemics over the next 200 years. By the ninth century, the disease had established itself there, adults had developed immunities, and smallpox was considered to be a children's disease. The situation with India is rather different. There is abundant cultural evidence of smallpox from very ancient times, but written descriptions do not appear until the thirteenth century. It is uncertain, therefore, at what time the disease became established among Indian populations.

By the end of the fifteenth century, smallpox was firmly rooted throughout Europe, and Europeans had developed adult immunities to it. New world populations, however, had no such immunities. When the Spanish began the conquest of Mexico and Peru in the sixteenth century, viral diseases which the European invaders carried with them played a critical part, and smallpox was absolutely devastating. Both Aztecs and Incas were infected while fighting against the Spanish. The resulting outbreaks, working on peoples with no immunities whatsoever, were of such force as to destroy utterly the Indian cultures' capacity to resist. The psychological impact was as great as the mortality was high. Between 1518 and 1531, it is estimated that over one-third of the total Indian population died of smallpox, while the Spanish remained immune, a fact which was interpreted as proving that the gods favored the invaders. In a powerfully religious society, this conclusion undermined the will to resist and made it possible for relatively small bands of Europeans to conquer well-established and highly civilized cultures with combined populations of millions. But the initial smallpox outbreaks were only the beginning. The smallpox epidemics were followed by waves of measles, influenza, and finally typhus, all of which generated extraordinary mortalities. By the end of the sixteenth century, it is estimated that up to 90 percent of the indigenous populations had died in the successive waves of disease, and the Spanish began importing slaves to meet the labor demands created by catastrophic disease mortality.

Smallpox had a similar impact among North American Indians as European settlements were established along the Atlantic coast and began to spread inland. There are no mortality figures for the native Indian populations, but contemporary reports in the later seventeenth and throughout the eighteenth centuries speak of whole villages and even tribes succumbing to smallpox.

In North America, however, the European colonists also suffered, because their settlements were remote from one another, the infective chains broke down, and as generations of adults began to appear with reduced or low immunities, smallpox became a dangerous threat. This fact, when combined with the high mortality among Indian tribes, made English colonists especially responsive to control measures such as variolation. The Spanish, on the other hand, resisted controls, relying on their natural immunities. Spanish colonial policies which rotated personnel between the homeland and the colonies regularly brought immune adults into the infection zones. The Spanish did not introduce control procedures until early in the nineteenth century.

The significance of disease in the European colonization of the new world can hardly be exaggerated. Smallpox, measles, influenza, and typhus not only destroyed the indigenous peoples' capacity to resist but also effectively leveled cultural barriers to expansion. Disease was probably at least as important as technological superiority in the European penetration of North America, and it had profound effects on ethnic development in all the colonial territories.

Smallpox was considered a serious threat to European populations until the nineteenth century, though in the modern period nothing comparable to its ravages in the new world was recorded. Adult immunities developed over generations of exposure placed limits on the disease's extension, and the average mortality of 20 percent for those afflicted was markedly lower than that suffered during the bubonic plague outbreaks. English mortality records showed an estimated 5000 cases annually for London between 1680 and 1690, with an average of 1000 deaths per year. At the opening of the nineteenth century, it was believed that some 45,000 people died annually of smallpox in Great Britain, that possibly 40,000 died in Prussia, and that France's annual mortality may have reached 150,000.

Although these mortalities did not compare in magnitude with earlier plague outbreaks or with smallpox in the new world, the disease terrified Europeans, who feared its disfiguring and crippling effects as much as its death-dealing powers. This led to dramatizing the disease by extrapolating known mortality figures to broader and broader geographical areas to convey some sense of what smallpox meant to humanity. In the middle of the eighteenth century, for example, the noted mathematician Daniel Bernoulli set a figure of 15 million every 25 years as the toll which smallpox claimed. In light of what we now know about smallpox in the nonwestern world, this estimate, stunning as it was in the eighteenth century, was probably conservative; but it does dramatize what Europeans believed was a major and continuing threat to prosperity, progress, and social well-being. The realization, especially in England, that smallpox was a scourge for which there were effective control measures available undoubtedly added to the determination to emphasize as well as publicize smallpox's effects in order to generate public interest in specific actions to control it.

Long before the bacteriological age, folk wisdom in China, India, and western Asia encompassed preventive measures against smallpox. The basic fact was that an exposure which produced a minor infection conferred immunity. Ritual practices developed which involved breaking the skin, either between thumb and forefinger or in the nose, and implanting infected matter from a smallpox pustule. The resulting infection brought the desired immunity, though there was a real danger that the person infected might develop a full-scale case. There was the further danger that the person so infected, though developing an immunity, might in the "giving" stage which lasts about four weeks pass the disease to someone else who could develop an undiluted case and start a new chain of infection. Even so, variolation, as this procedure came to be called, was widely practiced outside Europe, and in the early eighteenth century it was introduced into Europe itself. Lady Mary Wortley Montague, wife of the British ambassador to the Ottoman empire and an inveterate traveler as well as author and grand hostess, popularized the practice when she returned from Istanbul in 1721. Deaths in the British ruling house, which complicated the succession in times of political uncertainty, had already aroused interest in smallpox control measures, and the Asian procedures received close attention and careful study from British scientists. It was discovered that variolation produced a death rate scarcely one-tenth that of a natural smallpox infection, and the procedure was used and improved until in the 1740s it was possible to offer it on what was very nearly a mass basis.

In rural England, where population clusters existed which had relatively low exposure to smallpox and therefore low adult immunity levels, variolation was welcomed and widely practiced. The same was true, and for much the same reason, in New England and the Middle Atlantic colonies. In London, however, where exposure levels were high and adult immunities well-developed, smallpox tended to attack small (and often, perhaps, unwanted) children, and the procedure, which did hold some danger for the adults treated, was less popular. On the European continent, attitudes were different, and resistance to variolation was stubborn and substantial. Wolfgang Amadeus Mozart's father was typical: He rejected inoculation for both his son and his daughter, declaring that it was sinful to interfere with God's will. Mozart contracted smallpox but lived. Empress Catherine II of Russia, however, accepted the English view and introduced inoculation into her territories, beginning with herself, her son, and the court. Her motive was to promote social welfare and population growth, and she financed a program which immunized some 2 million of her subjects before the end of her reign. Interest in inoculation rose in France after King Louis XV died of smallpox in 1775, but it was not until Napoleon's time that a concerted effort against the disease was made, and that particularly in the army. Prussia also began to immunize after 1775.

Resistance to immunizing procedures reflected fears about their safety, but in 1796, Edward Jenner, an English country physician, established a technique which proved to be both effective and safe. Observing that milkmaids who contracted cowpox, a benign eruptive disease passed between bovines and the people who cared for them, seemed immune to smallpox, he inoculated an eight-year-old boy named James Phipps with matter from a cowpox lesion and then repeated his procedure six weeks later using matter from a smallpox eruption. The cowpox inoculation produced a mild reaction; the smallpox, however, produced none at all. His paper describing this operation was refused by the Royal Society in 1797, so the following year he published a small book describing his original experiment and subsequent confirming cases. His argument was widely tested, and as additional experiments showed that the procedure was relatively safe, vaccination, as it came to be called, spread rapidly. In 1803, the Spanish sent vaccination teams into Mexico and then throughout their holdings; Napoleon ordered his armies vaccinated; and the procedure became general. Rapid population growth after the mid-eighteenth century throughout the European world but particularly in England and in North America owed in part to early and increasingly effective control measures against smallpox. The persistence of the disease in the nineteenth century, though substantially modified, showed insufficiencies in both military medical organization and public health delivery systems. Moreover, governments were not consistent in carrying out antismallpox programs. The French, for example, abandoned Napoleon's vaccination program after 1815 and as a consequence suffered heavy smallpox casualties as late as the Franco-Prussian War (1870–1871). Even so, actual techniques of inoculation in the nineteenth century left much to be desired, and the idea that smallpox could actually be eradicated was not considered practical until after World War II.

Regular vaccination had largely eliminated smallpox from Canada, the United States, and most European countries by the 1940s, and significant headway was being made in the Philippines and Central America. Between 1950 and 1959, with technical support from the Pan-American Sanitary Bureau, a concerted attack on smallpox eliminated the disease from all but five countries in the Americas. In 1959, the Soviet Union initiated a proposal in the World Health Assembly to open a global campaign to eradicate smallpox. It was not until 1966, however, that the World Health Assembly voted the program a special budget of $2.5 million. Vaccines of a quality acceptable to the World Health Organization were developed and distributed to the areas of smallpox infection; a bifurcated needle and simplified antiseptic methods meant a vaccination kit which fitted into a shirt pocket, thus increasing efficiency and mobility; finally, a systematic approach to reporting and investigation of cases made accurate definition of problem areas possible. It was discovered that the extent of infected zones and the number of existing cases were far greater than originally thought. But substantial progress was made between 1967 and 1971. Smallpox was eliminated from all of Africa except for Ethiopia, the southern Sudan, and Botswana. The last case in the Americas occured in April 1971, in Brazil, and Indonesia had its last case in January 1972. What remained were infection centers in Bangladesh, northern India, Nepal, Pakistan, and Afghanistan. Initial investigations uncovered unexpected foci of infection in presumably clean areas in India, but consistently improving investigative procedures, more efficient vaccination delivery systems, and, above all, an intensive public relations campaign brought success. On October 16, 1975, the world's last-known case of variola major was reported.

Since 1975, the discussion of smallpox has focused on whether the last-known natural smallpox viruses, which are kept under close security, should be kept alive. The accidental death of a laboratory worker has given emphasis to this argument. Though there are skeptics, it now appears that humanity's victory over smallpox is complete, and this promises well for other control programs carried out on a worldwide basis and aimed at diphtheria, whooping cough, tetanus, measles, poliomyelitis, and tuberculosis.

ADDITIONAL READINGS: Derek Baxby, *Jenner's Smallpox Vaccine: The Riddle of Vaccinia Virus and Its Origin*, London, 1981; John Z. Bowers, "The Odyssey of Smallpox Vaccination," *Bulletin of the History of Medicine* 55 (Spring 1981): 17–33; John Duffy, *Epidemics in Colonial America*, Baton Rouge, La., 1953; Donald A Henderson, "The Eradication of

Smallpox," *Scientific American* 235 (October 1976): 25–33; Donald R. Hopkins, *Princes and Peasants: Smallpox in History,* Chicago, 1983; William H. McNeill, *Plagues and Peoples,* New York, 1976; Peter Razzell, *Edward Jenner's Cowpox Vaccine: The History of a Medical Myth,* Firle, Sussex, 1980; K. B. Roberts, *Smallpox: An Historic Disease,* St. Johns, Newfoundland, 1978; Harry Wain, *A History of Preventive Medicine,* Springfield, Ill., 1970; Ola Elizabeth Winslow, *A Destroying Angel: The Conquest of Smallpox in Colonial Boston,* Boston, 1974.

See also IMMUNOLOGY; INOCULATION.

Sphygmomanometer

The sphygmomanometer is an instrument which measures blood pressure by applying sufficient force to make the pulse disappear. The pressure required to make the pulse disappear is the same as the pressure within the arterial system. The sphygmomanometer is a standard instrument today and performs a variety of diagnostic functions, especially in connection with heart disease and circulatory problems. Its general use for clinical purposes, however, only became practical in the late nineteenth century, though studies on blood pressure in both humans and animals began much earlier.

In 1628, the English anatomist William Harvey published his classic work on circulation of the blood (q.v.). Harvey observed that when arteries were severed, the blood spurted as if under pressure of some kind. The pressure persisted through the system because the blood flowed back to the heart. This phenomenon caught the attention of Stephen Hales, a clergyman and amateur scientist who became a fellow of the Royal Society in 1718 and whose interest in the phenomenon of sap rising in plants had been encouraged by Sir Isaac Newton. Stephen Hales wanted to measure the force which pushed arterial blood, and to this end, he prepared a glass tube at least 11 feet long which was then inserted into the artery of a horse. The height to which the blood rose in the tube provided a measure of the force behind it. Stephen Hales published these and other findings in a collection of "statistical" essays which appeared in 1733.

Nearly a century later, in 1828, a French physiologist, Jean Leonard Marie Poiseuille, eliminated the long glass tube by using a U-shaped tube containing mercury. The weight of the mercury counterbalanced the pressure of the blood, and the distance moved could be recorded in millimeters. Poiseuille was able to demonstrate that blood pressure was the same at the extremities as it was at the center of the body. Hales's apparatus had shown a huge disparity between measurements taken near the heart and those taken at a distance.

Other refinements followed, but so long as the measuring instrument had to be inserted into the artery, clinical use of the technique was limited. Even so, Frederick Akhbar Mahomed connected changes in blood pressure with different diseases. After joining the staff at Guy's Hospital, he regularly checked the blood pressure of scarlet fever patients and identified elevated blood pressure as a premonitory symptom of acute nephritis, a disease similar to rheumatic fever which sometimes complicates streptococcus infections. This work and other of Mahomed's observations were ignored until much later, and Mahomed himself died of typhoid fever in 1884 at age 35.

Samuel Siegfried von Basch developed the first sphygmomanometer that did not require breaking the skin, and he published a description of it in 1881. The machine was inaccurate and was soon abandoned. An Italian physician, Scipione Riva-Rocci, created the prototype of today's instrument in 1896. Riva-Rocci provided an inflatable band which was put around the upper arm, and air was then pumped in until the pulse disappeared. Air was then released from the band until the pulse reappeared, and the reading was taken. Riva-Rocci's instrument measured blood pressure in the artery when the ventricles were contracting (systolic pressure). It was recognized, however, that diastolic pressure, that is, pressure taken when the ventricles relaxed, was more important. Using a stethoscope, Nikolai Korotkoff, a Russian physician, devised a technique in 1905 for recording diastolic pressure. If one listened to the brachial artery at the elbow, when air was released from the sphygmomanometer band, a slight tapping could be heard. This was the systolic pressure. As more air was released, the sound became clearer and then disappeared. A reading at that point gave diastolic pressure. Since Riva-Rocci, there have been various modifications in design details, but the basic principle of his device has remained standard while the uses to which blood pressure readings were applied have multiplied.

ADDITIONAL READINGS: P. E. Baldry, *The Battle Against Heart Disease*, Cambridge, Mass. 1971; Stanley Jod Reiser, *Medicine and the Reign of Technology*, Cambridge, 1978; Charles Singer and E. Ashworth Underwood, *A Short History of Medicine*, 2d ed., Oxford, 1962.

Stethoscope

The stethoscope, an instrument for listening to sounds within the body as an aid to diagnosis, was invented in 1816 by René Théophile Hyacinthe Laënnec. Until the eighteenth century, clinical observation was restricted to externals. Only postmortem examination permitted judgments on conditions within the body. The first step toward observing internal conditions was taken when a Viennese physician, Leopold Auenbrugger, developed a technique called percussion, which involved thumping the chest and listening to the different tones to determine how organs were positioned, whether fluid was present, and where lesions might be located. Auenbrugger's technique, which he described in a pamphlet published in 1761, was sound and effective, but it gained no followers until Jean Nicolas Corvisart, a leading clinician of the period and Napoleon Bonaparte's personal physician, translated and annotated the work in 1808. Laënnec studied under Corvisart at La Charité Hospital and was an enthusiastic exponent of diagnostic auscultation. In 1816, confronted by a stout young woman with an apparent heart condition, Laënnec found that he was unable to use hand or ear to examine the patient without embarrassment, so he had recourse to a tightly rolled sheaf of papers, one end of which he placed against the precordial region and the other to his ear. As he wrote three years later, "I was both surprised and gratified at being able to hear the beating of the heart with much greater clearness and distinctness than I had ever done before." So valuable did this instrument seem that Laënnec described it and the results he obtained by using it at a session of the Academy of Sciences in February 1818; and in 1819, he published a two-volume study on what he called "mediate oscultation" by the instrument he called a stethoscope.

Though his first instrument was a rolled tube of paper, Laënnec later developed a wooden stethoscope which was a tube 9 inches long and 1½ inches in diameter. One version had a single-diameter hole the length of the body, while another had a bell-shaped opening which reduced to a small-diameter hole. The instrument was in two pieces which screwed together and had a detachable chest piece and earpiece. As the stethoscope became a standard diagnostic instrument, its design was refined and improved. In 1850, Pierre-Adolphe Piorry reduced the circumference, enlarged and changed the shape of the chest piece, and modified the earpiece. His version remained standard in France until about 1910. By 1850, pliable tubing was used to create a fully flexible monaural stethoscope, and George P. Cammann, an American physician, developed a binaural instrument with a tube for each of the physician's ears in 1852. In 1878, the microphone was invented, and a version which would amplify chest sounds was incorporated into the stethoscope. Physicians feared, however, that amplification would create distortion, and many resisted this improvement. Some went so far as to say that auscultation was the physician's art and that mediating instruments coarsened sound. To achieve auditory purity, these physicians returned to applying their ears directly to the patient's chest, though with a thin handkerchief to keep skin from touching skin. For most, however, the stethoscope remained a basic and valuable diagnostic tool, especially for chest conditions. It remains in use today, though its importance has diminished with improved x-ray examination and diagnostic tests. Its decline will continue because many younger physicians have not been trained in its use. In experienced hands, however, it is still acknowledged to be a useful, if limited, instrument.

ADDITIONAL READINGS: P. E. Baldry, *The Battle Against Heart Disease*, Cambridge, Mass. 1971; Sir William Hale-White, *Selected Passages from De l'auscultation mediate by R. Theophile Laënnec with a Biography*, London, 1923; Stanley Jod Reiser, "The Medical Influence of the Stethoscope," *Scientific American* 240 (February 1979): 114–122; Stanley Jod Reiser, *Medicine and the Reign of Technology*, Cambridge, 1978.

See also TUBERCULOSIS.

Sulfonamides

The sulfonamides are a group of antimicrobial drugs which are effective in varying degrees in preventing or treating bacterial infections. Their general chemical structure is a benzene ring to which an amino group ($-NH_2$) and a sulfonamide group ($-SO_2-NH_2$) are attached. The sulfonamides work by bacteriostatic action; that is, they prevent multiplication by replacing a necessary chemical group in the bacteria with a compound the bacteria cannot metabolize. Though less effective than antibiotics, the sulfonamides were the first "miracle drugs" and ushered in the era of chemotherapy.

Sulfonamides were first identified in 1908 by a Viennese student, Paul Gelmo, who recorded his discovery in his doctoral dissertation. Further indications of the group and its possible use against bacteria appeared in the United States just after World War I, but the group only came into prominence in 1935 when Gerhard Domagk, research director in experimental pathology and bacteriology for the I. G. Farben drug subsidiary of the Bayer Company, announced that Prontosil, an azo dye, cured laboratory mice of a lethal streptococcus infection. It also proved both effective and safe in human tests. The active ingredient in Prontosil was sulfanilamide, which was released, as the French chemists Dr. and Mme. Jacques Tréfouël of the Pasteur Institute in Paris showed, by chemical action within the body. Prontosil has only a weak antibacterial action when tested in test tubes. Sulfanilamide was isolated, synthesized, and prescribed without restraint because earlier publication had made the product and the process unpatentable. It was obviously superior to Prontosil, if only because it did not turn patients red.

Between 1935 and 1940, other members of the sulfonamide family came into existence. In 1938, a British research team under A. J. Ewins working for the pharmaceutical firm of May and Baker developed sulfapyridine; by 1940, American Cyanimid Company scientists and the Hoffman-La Roche Laboratories produced sulfadiazine and sulfasoxazole. Though sulfapyridine developed dangerous side effects, the other two seemed to be easier for the human system to tolerate while offering an effective treatment for puerperal sepsis, erysipelas, pneumonia, mastitis, and meningitis. The sulfonamides also proved effective against gonorrhea, providing the first demonstrably successful treatment for that perennial social problem. Experiments with the group as a pre-operation prophylactic in abdominal surgery, as an agent against sepsis in wounds, as an antiburn remedy, and as a general preventive against streptococcus infections indicated that a truly all-purpose therapeutic substance was at hand.

Controls over pharmaceuticals were minimal in this period, and time and experience were required to discover that the sulfonamides were dangerous drugs which could also become ineffective with overuse. Indeed, sulfanilamide was involved, though it was not the lethal agent, in a tragic case which showed the insufficiency of U.S. drug laws. At least 100 persons died before a deadly brew of diethylene glycol and sulfanilamide was withdrawn from sale. The death-dealing agent was the diethylene glycol, which was used to make administering sulfanilamide to children easier. The product, known as Elixir of Sulfanilamide, had not been tested for safety by the firm which produced it, but when the case was investigated, it was found that there had been no significant infringement of the law. This resulted in 1938 in the passage by the U.S. Congress of the Food, Drug and Cosmetic Act, which mandated a demonstration of safety as a prerequisite to marketing a drug product in the United States.

Public interest in the sulfonamides was intense, and this contributed to overuse. Newspapers and magazines extolled the miraculous powers of the sulfa drugs, especially sulfanilamide for pneumonia, and professional medical journals saturated their readers with an outpouring of some 5400 articles in the years between 1935 and 1950, with 596 in 1943 alone. It has been estimated that in the United States in 1941, 1700 tons of sulfonamides were administered to between 10 and 15 million people. Sober scientific appraisals of side effects and adverse reactions were difficult to make with such astronomical quantities involved. Nevertheless, it began to appear that sulfonamides were dangerous, especially in heavy dosages. New York City reported 28 deaths from adverse reactions to sulfonamides in 1941, and with that number proved, there were doubtless many more that went undetected. The frequency of adverse response was difficult to establish, though it was suggested in that same year that 1 of every 1600 pneumonia cases treated with sulfonamides died as a direct result of the treatment. Adverse reactions were much less common and were seldom mortal when low dosages for prophylactic purposes were administered, though resistant bacterial strains soon appeared.

Adversity can have positive side effects. Research set in train by the action of sulfonamides produced other substances to treat apparently unrelated conditions. During the early stages of the German occupation of France, typhoid fever outbreaks multiplied, and a physician in Montpellier, Marcel Janbon, tried to treat typhoid in his area with a sulfonamide. Several patients died from undetermined causes, while others suffered convulsions and went into coma. The reason was that the victims were undernourished, the glucose levels in their blood were low, and it appeared that the sulfonamides used actually further lowered the glucose level, inducing hypoglycemia. Experiments with dogs confirmed this explanation. When German scientific investigators learned of the result, they began to look for analogs to the sulfonamides that could be used to lower blood sugar levels in diabetics. They succeeded in developing tolbutamide and carbutamide, substances which proved effective against the high glucose concentrations produced by diabetes mellitus. In a similar instance, British and American investigators discovered that sulfonamides increased the secretion of urine by inhibiting the action of carbonic anhydrase, an enzyme. American Cyanimid and Merck, Sharpe and Dohme synthesized more effective inhibitors which were the prototypes for a variety of drugs to be used for different kidney diseases, high blood pressure, and conditions affecting the fluid system of the eyes.

Limitations on the effectiveness of the sulfonamides also became apparent. The substances had no effect on true fungi, viruses, yeasts, the rickettsias, *Treponema pallida* (the bacterial cause for syphilis), or tuberculosis. Tularemia, whooping cough, Weil's disease, and leprosy were similarly unaffected. Worse, those bacteria which the sulfonamides did affect soon showed resistant strains. Resistance appeared early when the sulfonamides were used to prevent streptococcus infections among recruits in World War II. In time, a high percentage of gonococci became resistant, and the same development occurred with meningococci. The shigellae responsible for bacterial dysentery, though originally susceptible to sulfonamides, had by 1953 become between 80 and 90 percent resistant. The death rate from shigella-caused dysentery had dropped significantly in the United States, from 8.2 per 1 million from 1935 to 1939 to 2.7 from 1945 to 1949. Antibiotics helped account for the lower more recent figure, but sulfonamides were the effective agent earlier. That considerable effect was lost by the 1950s.

The sulfonamides, though greeted as miracle-working drugs, failed to become the hoped-for panacea, but they represented a major step toward control of bacterial diseases. They have proved effective in shortening the course of diseases, in lowering fatality rates, in reducing the number of complications, and even in preventing individual cases of illness from becoming epidemic. Their development spurred research on other antibacterial agents and promoted analogous substances which added to the number of specifics available to the practicing physician. And in combination with antibiotics, the sulfonamides have been effective in treating a wide range of diseases. Rheumatic fever sufferers who cannot take penicillin can use sulfonamides, and they are still considered very useful for burn therapy. Resistant strains, dangerous side effects, and safer and more effective compounds have substantially reduced the number of bacterial infections in which sulfonamides will be the "drug of choice." The group remains useful, however, and its historic place as the first of the miracle drugs and a major component in the development of modern therapeutic techniques remain secure.

ADDITIONAL READINGS: Helmuth M. Boettcher, *Miracle Drugs: A History of Antibiotics*, Einhart Kawer (trans.), London, 1963; H. F. Dowling, *Fighting Infection: Conquests of the Twentieth Century*, Cambridge, Mass. 1977; Edward Kremers and George Urdang, *A History of Pharmacy*, 4th ed., Philadelphia and Oxford, 1976; David M. Wilson, *Penicillin in Perspective*, London, 1976.

See also CHEMOTHERAPY.

Surgery

Surgery is one of the oldest forms of medical treatment for which direct evidence exists. It is also the most practical of the medical disciplines. Since it deals with repairing damaged or malfunctioning body structures, surgery traditionally has been associated with anatomy. In recent years, as surgical procedures have been developed to repair or even replace vital organs, physiology has also become important to it.

From a historical perspective, surgery changed relatively little for more than 5000 years. Some societies at different periods proved more adept or more venturesome than others, but the catalog of possible operations before the end of the nineteenth century was short and dealt with the extremities while avoiding the body cavities, the central nervous system, and the brain. The discovery of anesthesias followed by the establishment of the germ theory of disease transformed surgical practice. Surgery became an elective procedure rather than a last resort, and surgical interventions were expanded until only a few body structures remain essentially inoperable. In this respect, surgery offers visible and dramatic evidence of the extraordinary changes which medical treatment has undergone in the last century.

Surgery in Ancient Times Trephining the skull is one of the oldest forms of surgery, and evidence concerning it dates at least from 10,000 B.C. Early operators used a polished stone cutting tool to remove circular segments of the cranium to relieve pressure created by a depressed skull fracture or to free a person from some tormenting "devil" believed to have lodged in the head. Primitive tribes have been found in modern times who not only trephine in the ancient manner but treat the wound as a mark of caste, giving it both ritual and cosmetic importance. There is similar evidence that bonesetting and amputations were performed very early, though amputations presented serious problems of infection, hemorrhage, and shock. Written sources show that most surgical operations were minor and that the common approach to surgery was conservative. The Egyptian medical papyri from the middle of the second millennium B.C. mention surgical treatments for abscesses and small tumors as well as malfunctions of the eye, ear, or teeth. Surgery in Hindu India was similarly conservative, though Indian healers developed great skill in cosmetic surgery, including remodeling and replacing noses, and they used a method of cutting for bladder stones (lithotomy) which Pierre Franco introduced into Europe in the sixteenth century A.D. The Hippocratic writings of the fifth and fourth centuries B.C. were very cautious in their approach to surgery, but where it had to be done, they emphasized cleanliness in wound management. The Hippocratic oath required physicians to leave cutting for the bladder stone to those who were expert at it, while in the writings as a whole, the surgical emphasis fell on fractures and dislocations, fistulas, hemorrhoids, and ulcers. Superficial cancers could be removed, but those "deep in the body" were to be left alone.

Subsequent writers dealing with surgery summarized the classic tradition and added little to it. Celsus, writing at the opening of the Christian era, gave the first detailed descriptions of lithotomy in the western literature. Paul of Aegina in the seventh century and the important Moslem authorities of the late tenth and early eleventh centuries, Albucasis and Avicenna, discussed cauteries with a white-hot iron to stop bleeding and for other therapeutic purposes. Both the Hippocratic writers and Celsus suggested cautery as a means for resisting putrefaction, though the Hippocratics held that when gangrene made amputation necessary, hemorrhage could best be avoided by cutting through "devitalized" rather than living flesh.

The Salerno school of medicine, which originated in the eighth century, introduced the idea of dry wound management, an idea that was repeated and expanded in thirteenth- and fourteenth-century treatises on surgery by Bruno di Longoburgo, Henri de Mondeville, and Guy de Chauliac. The last named, sometimes considered the most erudite surgeon of his time, published his *Grande Chirurgie* in 1363, which contained a discussion of open management for contaminated wounds that was not fully understood until the experience of World War I.

Early Modern Europe Surgery in Europe began to show signs of change in the sixteenth and early seventeenth centuries. In scientific terms, William Harvey's demonstration of the circulation of the blood (q.v.) established the basis for new physiological perceptions, while Andreas Vesalius's new anatomy (q.v.) provided the first accurate descriptions to guide surgical work. Ambroise Paré, probably the most influential figure in sixteenth-century surgery, had Vesalius's work translated into French to make it available to surgeons and barber-surgeons who were not university-trained and had no Latin. Finally, the introduction of gunpowder changed the nature of wounds in two ways. Rounded projectiles hurled by an explosive charge smashed and tore through flesh and bone, driving foreign matter deep into any wound. Infections, always serious, became a major problem, giving rise to the contemporary belief that a sort of "gunpowder poison" entered the wound. A second consequence was a significant increase in the number of amputations which had to be done, including amputations of the thigh, which previously were very rare and which were almost always fatal.

Ambroise Paré made notable contributions to solving some of the problems which the new wounds created. The most important of these were the Paré ligature and the substitute he developed for cauterizing open, uninfected wounds. Cauteries, both chemical and with hot irons, were normal procedures in the early modern period to stop bleeding and to cleanse wounds. In 1514, Giovanni de Vigo introduced boiling oil into wounds as a form of "thermal debridement" to counteract "gunshot poison" as well as to achieve hemostasis. Paré accepted this method despite the damage which it did, but in 1536, during the siege of Turin, the boiling oil ran out. Paré concocted an ointment, or "digestive," from egg yolk, rose oil, and turpentine which he applied directly to the wound. The mixture was successful. Wounds treated with it were less painful, were free of swelling, and were generally uninflamed. Paré abandoned the hot oil treatment, concluding in his classic *Method of Treating Wounds* (1545) that "gunpowder poison" was a myth and that gunshot wounds did not require cauteries—these should be reserved for gangrenous wounds, or to stop bleeding in diseased (infected) wounds. Where infection already existed, however, cautery was the favored method for treating it, a practice which continued into the twentieth century.

Paré's ligature was more important. Other writers from Celsus and Avicenna through Guy de Chauliac and Giovanni de Vigo recommended ligature, but Paré set about to show how it should be done and what results might be expected. Ligatures tied off the veins and arteries to establish hemostasis. Paré began using ligatures in 1552, and he published his conclusions on them in his *Ten Books* in 1564. In fact, Paré's ligature made successful thigh amputations possible. William Clowes reported doing one in 1588, and Fabricius apparently performed one in 1614. There was, however, one serious drawback. Fifty-three ligatures were necessary in a thigh amputation, and this required trained assistance. But helpers were scarce, and the people available at the time of an operation were needed to restrain the patient. Consequently, ligatures could only come into general use when a method had been found to control the flow of blood mechanically until the surgeon could tie the blood vessels. This was accomplished in the eighteenth century in France when J. L. Petit invented an effective tourniquet. Versions of the tourniquet had been proposed as early as the fourteenth century, but Petit's was the first that was practical. He published descriptions of his invention in 1718 and 1731. The Petit tourniquet was fixed to the abdomen for thigh amputations and put pressure directly on the main artery. This extremely valuable instrument permitted the elimination of cauteries to prevent hemorrhage and made Paré's ligatures practical.

Apart from amputations and wound management, lithotomy was the most widely performed operation in the early modern period. Bladder stones, or *vesicul calculi,* were widespread in Europe and America until the latter part of the nineteenth century. They are still common in southeast Asia, India, Pakistan, and the Middle East. The reasons for their prevalence and disappearance are equally obscure. There were essentially two forms of lithotomy: the suprapubic and the perineal. The suprapubic was the less common of the two since until the advent of anesthesia the more complicated perineal was actually less dangerous.

At least until the eighteenth century, most lithotomists (stonecutters) were itinerants, often barber-surgeons, who learned the technique from some more experienced practitioner. Some lithotomists were thieves, vagabonds, and charlatans; others were extraordinarily skilled practitioners and achieved dramatically good results. Lithotomists were public figures, and their operations were an open show. Style, publicity, and operative success meant wealth for a few, and the competition was brutal. The Colot family, for example, developed a successful technique which they kept a family secret for 200 years. Their entrepreneurial spirit and capacity for secretiveness rivaled that of the more famous Chamberlen family which similarly monopolized the obstetrical forceps (q.v.). Johann Jacob Rau, probably the most famous lithotomist of the early eighteenth century and evidently one of the best, ended his career in the chair of anatomy at Leyden. Not only was he secretive about his methods, but he taught his assistants and students a dangerously flawed technique. Rau was also accused of operating where no stone existed and palming one at the critical moment to fool his patient and the crowd. He claimed to have performed over 1500 lithotomies without a death, but in at least one place where his word could be checked, Amsterdam, records showed that 4 of his patients died in the course of 22 operations.

One of the most colorful of the lithotomists was a Franciscan lay brother named Jacques de Beaulieu, or Frère Jacques, who practiced in Louis XIV's Paris. Frère Jacques claimed to have learned his operation from an itinerant Italian. When he came to Paris, he became an overnight sensation for the violence and speed with which he worked. It was said that he "plunged his knife like a dagger into the perineum until it ground upon the stone, then with his fingers in the anus extruded it through the perineal wound." There were protests about Frère Jacques's technique which were possibly inspired by jealous rivals, and he was finally required to engage in further study before performing any more operations. It is said that when he slowed his style, he also lost his address and certainty, and with them his ability to operate effectively.

Before anesthesia, all surgery depended on operating speed to minimize the patients' pain. The lithotomists were no exception. In 1698, at the Hotel-Dieu in Paris, Frère Jacques did 10 lithotomies in less than an hour. The early-eighteenth-century English surgeon William Cheselden was even faster, performing the operation in less than 30 seconds. Speed was not all, however. Claude Pouteau, a French surgeon of considerable distinction, developed a "slow" technique which required up to 6 minutes. Pouteau believed that his patients suffered less if he took the time to be gentle. He was also unusual in stressing cleanliness. The results were impressive. Pouteau performed a series of 120 lithotomies in which he lost only 3 patients, an outstanding record for any surgical procedure before anesthesia and antisepsis.

Some very difficult and dangerous operations were performed in the premodern period. One of the most controverisal was the cesarean section performed on a living mother, which many authorities, Paré included, believed was inevitably fatal. Nevertheless, this operation, though uncommon, has been documented for the eighteenth and nineteenth centuries, and there are indications that it was done much earlier as well. Records from the city archives in Frankfurt-am-Main report 7 cesarean sections before 1411; François Rousset, personal physician to the duke of Savoy, published evidence in 1581 of 15 cesarean sections performed over a period of 80 years. In one case, the same woman was reported to have had 6 cesareans.

The first fully documented cesarean section was performed on April 26, 1610, by Jeremiah Trautman in Wittenberg. The mother lived 25 days and then died, probably of sepsis. The child lived to be nine years old. In 1689, Jean Ruleau performed a successful cesarean on a woman who suffered from rickets. The first documented cesarean in the British Isles was an emergency operation performed by an Irish midwife, Mary Donally, in 1738. By the end of the eighteenth century, the operation was no longer a curiosity, and despite a mortality rate estimated at 50 to 75 percent, it was defended strongly.

In the early seventeenth century, Florian Matthias, a barber-surgeon of Brandenburg, recovered a 9-inch knife which a Bohemian knife swallower had let slip handle first into his stomach. A similar emergency brought fame to Daniel Schwabe, a wound surgeon and lithotomist, who was called in by the Medical College of Königsberg in 1635 to recover an accidentally swallowed knife. By 1886, 26 such gastrotomies were known. They were for the most part successful. The first effort to correct a gastric problem as such, however, was not made until 1849, and it proved unsuccessful.

The Modern Period Though new operations were relatively rare in the years from 1550 to 1850, operating techniques did improve, new instruments were introduced, there was a steady accretion of knowledge concerning the body and disease, and the social character of the medical profession, surgery included, changed significantly. Surgery remained a practical art, but in France and England, it became bonded to the general field of medicine, and surgeons left the ranks of artisans to join physicians in the middle class. The evolution was slow and was probably not completed until the nineteenth century, when surgeons became indistinguishable from physicians in training and social status. The change followed a slightly different course in the German-speaking countries, where barber-surgeons were the rule until the end of the eighteenth century. One important difference which the change in status brought was a different set of educational requirements. Those who became surgeons in the first half of the nineteenth century had a much broader base in scientific knowledge than their predecessors, accepted science as a legitimating standard for the profession they pursued, and began to identify themselves with the academic, scientific, and medical elite. The surgeon was also better prepared to integrate current scientific knowledge into his work or to reject it. In either case, the surgeon acted within the framework of scientific medicine.

The development of surgery in England showed the characteristic pattern of movement toward higher levels of formal education as the definition for the surgeon's professional standing. In the middle of the eighteenth century, largely in response to a movement led by William Cheselden of St. Thomas' Hospital, London, surgeons and barber-surgeons separated, with the surgeons' company becoming a strong trade guild. At the end of the century the company was elevated into the Royal College of Surgeons, though surgical training remained on an apprentice basis. This situation held until the Apothecaries Act of 1815 gave apothecaries legal standing and strengthened their competitive position. The apothecaries' society had set up strong educational qualifications for their guild in England and Wales. Apprentices were to be articled for five years and were to have had two courses of lectures in anatomy and physiology and two in the theory and practice of medicine. They were also to have performed six months of ward duty. Apothecaries were permitted to practice surgery, and to compete with them, the Royal College of Surgeons established similar educational requirements, including ward work. In 1844, the Royal College of Surgeons legislated new and more stringent requirements for admission as a fellow. There was to be an examination which required a written account of six clinical cases together with set papers on anatomy, physiology, surgery, pathology, and therapeutics. Candidates could be subjected to a further oral examination as well as being required to perform dissections or operations on a cadaver. Qualifications to be admitted to the examination included a minimum age of 25 years, good character, six years of professional study, three of which had to have been in a recognized London hospital, and one year as house surgeon or surgical dresser in a recognized hospital in the United Kingdom. The first examinations were given in December 1844, and there were 24 successful candidates.

Similar patterns for defining professional status appeared on the European continent and in the United States, though the development, particularly in the latter, was markedly slower. But England led in more than training and licensing surgeons through the middle years of the nineteenth century. London became the world's leading surgical center between 1840 and 1870, supplanting Paris, whose leadership was tarnished in the upheavals after 1789, and Edinburgh. The latter owed its preeminence to such extraordinary teachers as the three Alexander Monros, the first two of whom dominated surgery at Edinburgh from 1720 to 1790. The third, though less influential than his father and grandfather, continued the tradition until 1846. Robert Knox, another superb teacher, drew over 500 students for his anatomy lectures in 1828 in a theater designed for only 200, but it was also Knox whose career at Edinburgh ended in the Burke-Hare scandal (see Anatomy).

Scots played an important part in London's rise to eminence. Among the most important was John Hunter, born near Glasgow in 1728, who studied with William Cheselden at St. Thomas' and Percivall Pott at St. Bartholomew's. Hunter served four years as a military surgeon before joining the surgical staff at St. George's Hospital and founding his famous school for anatomy and surgery in Leicester Square. His pupils included John Abernathy, who became a well-known surgeon at St. Bartholomew's Hospital, and the truly brilliant Astley P. Cooper, the first man to amputate a leg through the hip joint and the man who made the surgical reputation of Guy's Hospital. Another of Hunter's students was Philip Syng Physick, an American who carried Hunter's methods across the Atlantic and who has been called "the father of American surgery."

Part of the reason for London's leadership in the surgical field was the mounting number of hospitals (q.v.) founded in the eighteenth and nineteenth centuries, which provided training and the opportunity to practice. And as one of the two largest urban complexes in western Europe, with an aggregate population in greater London of more than 1 million by 1801 and twice that figure (2,235,344) by 1841, London offered the demographic and economic base to support an expanding profession. This vast urban system drew people who were looking for opportunity, and surgeons were notable among them. As John Hunter came to London in the eighteenth century, so other distinguished surgeons came from the north in the nineteenth. Charles Bell arrived in 1804, though he returned to Edinburgh in 1835, the year Robert Liston left Edinburgh for University College, London. Liston carries the reputation for being "the most famous operating surgeon of his time," and he was joined by another distinguished northern expatriate, William Ferguson, who was appointed to the King's College Hospital surgical staff. By 1840, such men as these had brought London the leadership in surgery which the city was to enjoy over the next three decades. Then the center of gravity shifted once more, this time to German Europe, and specifically to the new German empire. German surgeons dominated the field until the end of World War I, when surgery in the United States took the lead in the western world, a position it still holds today.

Though attaining recognition and status as a professional discipline, surgery at the midpoint of the nineteenth century was general rather than specialized, though elements of specialization were beginning to appear. Moreover, despite the hordes of students, it was a field in which a handful of practitioners dominated the scene. Hospital appointments were the key, for they conferred prestige and status which could be transformed into income. Hospital surgeons were able to charge high fees for their services, and as their students graduated from the status of fee payers to that of practitioners, their mentors could expect referrals. Astley Cooper, for example, earned the stupendous sum of £15,000 from indentures, fees from pupils, and consultations, and as one of London's leading surgeons, he could stand well up in the city's affluent commercial and professional establishment. This, however, was a social status for which most surgeons were not yet ready. Rough, uncultured, and ill-mannered, surgeons still tended to be men whose extraordinary physical strength, manual dexterity, and domineering personalities defined them. Robert Liston, in this respect, was typical: Crude, loud, abrasive, insensitive, and brutally rough on patients, he was also swift, dexterous, and the absolute master of what he did.

On operating day, a weekly event at London's hospitals, the famous surgeons peformed in order of seniority for an appreciative audience of colleagues, students, and the general public. Two hundred observers was not unusual, and crowds as large as 600 were reported. In the cockpit of the operating chamber, a wooden chair with heavy straps or a plain deal table was the center of the tableau, and it was there in an explosion of agony, gouts of blood, and rapid movement that the surgeon did his work. If the nineteenth century was an age of virtuosos, the operating surgeons were the virtuosos of the medical profession.

The number of operations performed was by twentieth-century standards very small. A large teaching hospital might have 200 operations in a year; a comparable institution today would have 10,000. And the types of operation were also comparatively few. Probably the most common form of surgery was amputation made necessary by tubercular infections which produced what was then called necrosis of the bone. Road accidents were another major cause for amputating limbs. The mortality in such procedures averaged 40 percent with infection as the most important though not the only cause of death. Excruciating pain attended all operations, and the surgeon's only weapon against it was speed. In 1824, Astley Cooper amputated a leg through the hip joint in 20 minutes; 10 years later, James Syme did the same operation in just over 1 minute. Even so, operations could take as long as 2 hours, and in a few cases the operating time reached 8 hours. Under these conditions, surgery was not an elective procedure. Even the most superficial operation was potentially mortal, and any decision to operate involved the question of whether the operation or the condition was the greater threat to life. Nevertheless, a catalog of new and difficult operations was performed, ranging from tying off an artery to bypass a weakening in the arterial wall to removing a tumor to making a bowel incision for a newborn child with an imperforate anus. The surgeons' only guides were extensive and precise anatomical knowledge, experience, and skill.

With relatively few operations to perform, only

a handful of surgeons were able to make their living from surgery alone, and most mid-nineteenth-century surgeons engaged in general medical practice. There was a sort of division of labor. Physicians tended to deal with underlying, or "profound," problems in the body's functions; surgeons, however, worked with what was on the surface: wounds and broken limbs, twisted frames, growths, skin and venereal diseases. The orthopedic (q.v.) content in surgery was very large, as was the gynecological, and the primary emphasis was on repair. Interestingly, when the Royal College of Surgeons first drew its regulations at the opening of the nineteenth century, it refused to accept as candidates practitioners who were only (or exclusively) dentists, aurists, oculists, chiropodists, or orthopedic surgeons. Such specialization was thought to be too close to the irregular practitioners—the bonesetters, lithotomists, or cataract couchers. In time, of course, education for general surgery proved to be the first step toward surgical specialization and the division of the field into areas defined by particular organs: ophthalmic surgery and ophthalmology (q.v.) were among the earliest; urology, the direct descendant of lithotomy, was another, and it joined orthopedic surgery and the surgical aspect of otolaryngology. Gastric surgery, cardiac surgery, and neurosurgery were further and more particular specialties developing out of general surgery. Before specialization could occur, however, surgery's operative potential had to expand, and this came in the second half of the nineteenth century.

The discovery of anesthesia (q.v.) in 1846 and Joseph Lister's work with antiseptics (q.v.) beginning in 1865 and 1866 radically changed surgery's potential. Both discoveries were important, but antiseptic surgery went to the heart of the problem of life or death. Anesthesias, however, had the more immediate effect. Even though ether and chloroform inhalants had unpleasant side effects and could produce unexpected fatal reactions, resistance to the use of anesthesias was never very serious. To banish pain from surgery was such an extraordinary benefit that people were not inclined to count the cost. For surgeons, a quiet patient meant far more effective operating technique, and even the most hardened was glad to be relieved from the tortured screams of the people they were trying to help. Antiseptics were quite another matter, because they involved accepting the germ theory of disease. That doctrine stood at odds with the conventional medical wisdom of the 1850s and 1860s. The resistance to antiseptic measures lasted into the twentieth century, though the main centers for surgical practice and leading surgeons themselves were using antiseptic surgery in the last quarter of the nineteenth century.

Asepsis was the key to antiseptic surgery, and by the early twentieth century, the primary emphasis in preventing infection fell on excluding bacteria from open wounds. Lister's carbolic spray was soon abandoned, but in its wake came face masks and rubber gloves, heat treatments to sterilize dressings and surgical tools, prohibitions on conversation during operations, surgical gowns, and the creation of special operating rooms designed for maximum cleanliness. Ambitious plans for washing or otherwise sterilizing the air proved ineffectual, but with heat sterilization it became possible to prevent infected materials from carrying bacteria into wounds. Antiseptic treatment for wounds themselves, however, was ineffective. Paul Ehrlich searched for a systemic chemotherapy against bacterial or viral infection, but it was not until the isolation of the sulfonamides in the 1930s and the introduction of penicillin and broad-spectrum antibiotics in the 1940s and 1950s that Ehrlich's idea was fulfilled. Until then, surgery used antiseptic measures to attain asepsis while fighting infection with traditional methods.

Anesthesia and antiseptics opened new fields to surgery and permitted more rapid development in established ones. Operating on the stomach was one of the first such new fields. Theodor Billroth, a brilliant surgeon and teacher who settled in Vienna, was the modern founder of gastric surgery. Billroth was trained in Berlin, was the professor of surgery in Zurich (1860–1867), and went to Vienna in 1867 to stay. His surgical school and clinic continued to 1938. Billroth resisted the germ theory of disease, but he accepted and practiced Lister's antiseptic techniques. He performed his first gastric cancer operation on January 29, 1881. The patient survived the operation but died of a renewed cancer attack 4 months later. Billroth used a chloroform anesthesia and spent an hour washing out the stomach. In the next 11 months, Billroth performed 21 operations for gastric cancer, and by 1890, he had done 41 gastric resections, of which 19 were operative successes. Even so, Billroth's operation remained extremely dangerous, and other methods for treating gastric cancer had to be explored.

By the end of the nineteenth century, a marked change was taking place in the number and kind of operations surgeons were performing. When compared with the period before Lister, the change was radical in the extreme, but Lister himself was a transitional figure, and the operations he performed in the last 16 years of his career (1877–1893) contrast markedly with the work of a comparably distinguished surgeon, William Watson Cheyne, through the years from 1890 to 1912. Cheyne was the beneficiary of a succession of medical advances which bore directly on surgical operations and which were too new to have a significant influence on Lister's work. Some of the most important stemmed from the new field of bacteriology (q.v.) and reflected growing sophistication in understanding disease causation, and particularly tuberculosis (q.v.). Such terms as "necrosis" and "caries," accurate enough for describing the state of a diseased bone or joint, were giving way to such words as "osteomyelitis" and, of course, "tuberculosis"; the rapid expansion of radiology (q.v.) greatly enlarged diagnostic and operative potential. The therapeutic revolution was in full swing, and its effects appeared dramatically in the changing character of surgical practice.

At the end of Lister's career and the beginning of Cheyne's there were few differences in their practices, and both practices were similar to the practices of surgeons before Lister in terms of the kind if not the quantity of cases. Fifty-nine percent of Lister's practice concerned accidents and orthopedic cases, with tubercular conditions prominent. In Cheyne's records, the comparable percentage was 48. There were, however, differences in the distribution. Virtually 33 percent of Lister's practice resulted from accidents. In Cheyne's practice, that percentage varied from 9 to 11. Sixteen percent of Lister's cases involved tuberculosis; Cheyne's records show a decline from 26 percent in 1890 to 11 percent in the decade from 1902 to 1912. Both Cheyne and Lister devoted between 13 and 14 percent of their time in 1890 to orthopedic repair, but Cheyne's practice in this field then dropped away to between 7.1 and 6.1 percent. More significantly, Lister's notebooks recorded no abdominal surgery to 1893, and Cheyne, in the comparable period, did just one bowel operation, and that was of sufficient interest to be described in the *Lancet*. But after 1890, Cheyne's abdominal surgery practice increased steadily from 4.3 to 16.5 percent in the period from 1902 to 1912; with elective hernia repair included, this portion of his practice reached 28.4 percent, thus becoming the most important single area in his practice. Improvement in operative techniques and the abilities to avoid infection and to control pain were turning surgery toward a truly general discipline in which the body cavities as well as the extremities were becoming regularly entered operative fields. Moreover, surgery itself, in place of being an emergency treatment or a last resort, had entered into the therapeutic armory and could be considered as an acceptable, even ordinary, method for dealing with diseases. To that extent, a surgical revolution had already been accomplished on the eve of World War I, and the new directions for surgical practice in the twentieth century were established.

The most dramatic advances in the new surgery concerned the brain and heart. Early efforts to perform brain surgery were almost always fatal, and as late as 1932 a textbook on surgery estimated that no more than 7 percent of brain tumors could be removed. Nevertheless, the field was established at the opening of the twentieth century through the work of Victor Horsley and Sir William Macewen. It was developed, however, by Harvey Williams Cushing, who learned his surgical technique from William Halsted at Johns Hopkins. Cushing established an early interest in neurosurgery, but when he went to England to work with Victor Horsley, the two men proved incompatible, and Cushing left London for Liverpool, where he worked with the great British neurologist Charles Scott Sherrington, on brain functions in the higher apes. He returned to Johns Hopkins in 1901, became associate professor of surgery in 1903, and, though he received little encouragement, worked intensively on neurosurgery with particular attention to trigeminal neuralgia (tic douloureux). In 1907 he performed an operation for this condition which has been termed the beginning of modern neurosurgery.

In 1905, Cushing became the first full-time neurosurgeon in the United States. His main contribution to the field was to develop techniques which steadily improved operative effectiveness. He promoted the gentle handling of tumors and brain material, used tiny silver clips at bleeding points in the brain to achieve bloodless operations, and reintroduced simple trephining, sometimes called palliative decompression, to relieve headache and other tumor-caused symptoms. Mortalities in brain surgery averaged about 40 percent, but Cushing continually improved the record. By 1915 he had removed 130 tumors with 8 percent mortality. Cushing's work established a new base for brain surgery and defined the techniques to pursue it.

Early work with heart surgery concerned nearby structures rather than the heart itself. There were attempts, for example, to treat pericardial effusion, a concentration of fluid, or frank pus, in the sac surrounding the heart. Jean Riolan had suggested a method for dealing with this problem in 1649 which was occasionally attempted until 1871. In 1866, however, Armand Trousseau proposed to approach the heart through an incision between the ribs. This method was tried in England at the urging of Clifford Allbutt, who studied with Trousseau. The tap was carried out and the patient recovered. Other procedures developed in the late nineteenth century, but none was particularly effective. In the early twentieth century, a rib resection method to reduce pressure on the heart from pericardial effusion was done, and some patients benefited. But this method, as well as most others, was considered of marginal utility.

A variety of operations on the heart was tried during the twentieth century with steadily improving effect. Efforts to suture stab wounds resulted in a mortality of 50 to 60 percent. Most deaths were due to infection. By 1914, the mortality had been reduced to 45 percent; during World War I, of 58 cases where suturing was required, only 14 died. In World War II, the record was even better. According to a report published in 1946, there were 134 cases of soldiers who had missiles lodged in or near the heart. All recovered, including 13 where foreign bodies were lodged in the heart itself. Using sulfa drugs and antibiotics, surgeons found that it was possible to open the heart without undue risk.

Another condition which surgeons learned to treat was mitral stenosis, which occurred when the mitral valve opening had been narrowed by vegetative growths caused by rheumatic fever. The procedure was to enlarge the mitral valve. This operation had been discussed as early as 1890, but it was first performed successfully in 1923 at the Peter Bent Brigham Hospital by E. C. Cutler and S. A. Levine. Henry C. Southar performed the same operation three years later at the London Hospital. In 1942 it was suggested that cyanotic congenital heart disease, the so-called blue baby disease, could be cured surgically. The operation for it was done successfully at Johns Hopkins in November 1944, by Alfred Blalock. This operation is often taken as the starting point for modern cardiac surgery.

Since 1944, there has been a series of dramatic advances in heart surgery. Between 1945 and 1952, the number of successful blind mitral valve operations increased substantially, while the use of low-temperature (hypothermic) techniques and a heart-lung machine permitted direct-vision open-heart surgery. This method, though having much to recommend it, produced severe brain damage in some cases. If the temperature were set at a relatively safe 28°C, the surgeon had just 6 to 10 minutes' working time. This led to entirely removing the heart from the body after an alternative system of circulation had been established. This idea had been raised in speculative form in 1812; in 1926, two Soviet scientists proved that it was possible to keep animals alive with a heart-lung machine. John Gibbon of Philadelphia began work on such a machine in 1935, but it was not perfected for animals until 1952, and it was first used on humans the following year. Three of the first four patients died. In that same year, Anthony Andreason and Frank Watson of the Buckston Brown Experimental Farm of the Royal College of Surgeons proposed the idea that a second person's heart could be used to circulate the patient's blood while the heart was out of the body. The method was used at the University of Minnesota in 1954. C. W. Lillihei and R. L. Varco repaired a congenital heart defect in a one-year-old boy with the child's father supplying the circulation. The method worked, as the child survived the operation, though he died of pneumonia 11 days later. Because there is some danger to the donor, who is then placed in a difficult moral position, Lillihei abandoned the idea in 1956. Finally, open-heart surgery was achieved by a combination of hypothermia and the heart-lung machine.

Surgery's achievements in the field of transplanting vital organs have been of major importance, though final success has remained elusive. Organ transplants began around 1875 when Jacques Reverdin, a Swiss surgeon, developed a technique for grafting human tissues. In 1912, the French surgeon Alexis Carrel found a way to connect blood vessels that permitted transplanted organs to function. The procedure was refined in the course of animal experiments dealing with various biological functions, and a successful human kidney transplant was done at Loyola University, Chicago, in 1950. In 1967, Christiaan Barnard of South Africa carried out the first human heart transplant, an operation which still attracts the public's attention.

The success of transplants varies according to the complexity of the organ or structure involved. Connective tissues and corneas, for example, transplant fairly successfully. Heart and kidney transplants have been more difficult, though in some cases they have lasted several years. The basic problem is an immune reaction in which the body rejects the transplanted organ. As a result, other methods of treatment are preferred, especially in heart cases, though transplanting remains an important therapeutic procedure and is invaluable for areas of experimental biology.

Heart surgery, which has provided the most dramatic of recent surgical breakthroughs, brought crowds back into the operating rooms, but of more significance are the thousands upon thousands of operations which surgeons perform daily with minimum discomfort for their patients and with minuscule loss of life. No operation could be taken less than seriously before 1850, and it has only been since 1935 that agents to fight infection with sufficient effectiveness have been available to make most operations routine. This is a major contribution to the health and welfare of modern society. The history of surgery is not so much a record of progressive steps toward an ultimate truth as it is one of the evolution of a socially useful trade whose potential was transformed in the second half of the nineteenth century and which has realized that new potential in the twentieth. The nineteenth century was surgery's heroic age—the twentieth has been its age of miracles.

ADDITIONAL READINGS: Frederick F. Cartwright, *The Development of Modern Surgery*, London, 1967; Guido Majno, *The Healing Hand*, Cambridge, Mass., 1975; J. F. Malgaigne, *Surgery and Ambroise Paré*, Wallace B. Hamby (trans. and ed.), Norman, Okla., 1965; Robert G. Robinson, *Surgery: Old and New Frontiers*, New York, 1968; Owen and S. D. Wagensteen, *The Rise of Surgery: From Empiric Craft to Scientific Discipline*, Minneapolis, Minn., and Folkstone, Kent, 1978.

See also ANATOMY; BARBER-SURGEONS.

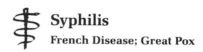

Syphilis

French Disease; Great Pox

Syphilis is a chronic venereal disease which reached epidemic proportions in Europe in the early sixteenth century. Its cause is the spirochete *Treponema pallidum*, an organism which is also responsible for nonvenereal endemic syphilis (bejel) and which is indistinguishable bacteriologically from the treponemata which cause yaws *(Treponema pertenue)* and pinta *(Treponema carateum)*. While these diseases show very different clinical characteristics, they are all related, and they appear to represent degrees on an evolutionary continuum from newest and most malignant (venereal syphilis) to oldest and least violent (pinta). Whether venereal syphilis is a new disease which first appeared at the end of the fifteenth century or whether it is a very old one which had a violent epidemic fling before reverting to a chronic condition is still uncertain. Modern chronic syphilis has a different profile than malignant epidemic syphilis, but it remains a serious danger to the public's health. Scientific medicine can diagnose and manage syphilis, but for social and cultural rather than medical reasons, syphilis incidence remains unacceptably high and may be increasing throughout the world.

Disease Characteristics Venereal syphilis is a disease whose only reservoir is human beings. It affects both men and women. The causal organism establishes itself in the genital system and is communicated by sexual contact. It is also possible for a fetus growing in a syphilitic mother to be infected and born with congenital syphilis. The disease first shows itself after an incubation period of 10 days to 10 weeks in the form of a small, hard, painless swelling at the point of infection. This is usually on the genital organs, near the anus, or on the mouth. This primary chancre (Hunter's chancre) enlarges slowly and sometimes breaks open to leave a shallow ulcer. Often, however, it will pass unnoticed, especially in women. Even without treatment, this first lesion will disappear in about 8 weeks. The infecting organisms move through the system, establishing themselves in the lymph nodes, and after 2 to 4 months skin lesions begin to appear. These vary greatly from an eruptive rash to ulcerating sores. They can appear before the primary lesion has healed. This marks a second stage in the disease. The second-stage lesions may heal in 2 to 6 weeks or last for a year or more. A latent period follows which may be interrupted by further external appearances. Although the disease may remain latent for years, it can be communicated to other persons, and it retains the capacity to produce severe damage at a later date anywhere in the system.

Syphilis has been called essentially a vascular disease, as the action of the treponema produces swelling and proliferation of endothelial cells together with reductions in vessel diameter. It also generates firm white lesions called gummas, which will measure up to 10 centimeters in diameter and which produce a considerable fibrosis on healing, especially in the liver. The gummas may appear in any internal organ. Modern chronic syphillis tends to develop its worst effects after a long period of latency. Those effects include a significant enlargement of the aorta and left side of the heart (cardiovascular syphilis) which often appears in middle age. There can also be severe damage to the nervous system (meningovascular syphilis; neurosyphilis). Any part of the nervous system can be invaded, and nerve damage usually appears only after a lapse of 15 to 25 years. The most common effect is a series of degenerative changes in the spinal cord (tabes dorsalis) or spinal nerves resulting in loss of sensory perception, progressive ataxia of limbs, and loss of reflex. This also can affect bladder, sexual, and rectal function. Syphilis attacking the brain produces what has been called a general paralysis of the insane (paresis; dementia paralytica) which is first marked by character changes, especially unstable emotions, grandiose visions, and loss of touch with reality. This condition, which affects men more often than women, can result in death within a year if untreated.

Modern treatments, especially the use of penicillin in early stages, have reduced the incidence of the most destructive late-appearing syphilitic conditions. Before antibiotics, however, dementia paralytica may have accounted for as much as 10 percent of admissions to insane asylums. While it is estimated that 66 percent of the people infected with syphilis who go untreated may live their lives with either no physical inconvenience or only minimal interference, a full 30 percent may expect to develop late destructive lesions. This proportion and the danger of further spread of the disease make early identification and treatment essential.

History It is difficult to establish precisely where the first outbreak of epidemic venereal syphilis occurred, though it appears to have been France, Spain, or Italy; the year was either 1493 or 1494. The Spanish scholar and physician Francesco López de Villalobos published a poem in Latin at Salamanca in 1498 concerning the disease named *las buvas*, or, as his editor and translator had it, "that which hath been known all along as the French pockes." The composition took place between 1493 and 1495, and while it described what its author observed, it also contained an immense erudition. Villalobos was certain that this disease was new, but to support his conviction, he believed it was necessary to review the medical classics. What he described was a pestilence which appeared "on the parts of shame" and which was a punishment for sexual excess, gluttony, drunkenness, and a dissolute life. Though he described a sore on the genitals, he did not connect it with the entry point of the infection, though others did. The previous year, another Spanish physician, Gaspar Torello, who served Pope Alexander VI, published a tract on the French disease, or *pudendagra*, as he called it, in which he described 17 cases he had attended. Torello recorded his conviction that the disease originated in France, probably in 1493, and spread from there to Spain and Italy.

In December 1494, Charles VIII of France, who had invaded Italy earlier that year with a cosmopolitan army, laid siege to Naples. Syphilis broke out among his troops, and when he withdrew the following year, his disintegrating army carried the infection throughout Europe. Though historians now point to the French invasion and retreat as critical events in syphilis's spread, the first reference to the event in any connected contemporary account of the epidemic was in a treatise by Giovanni di Vigo, a surgeon in the employ of Pope Julius II, who published in 1514.

There is substantial evidence that syphilis was active before he published on it. In August 1495, Emperor Maximilian I of the Holy Roman Empire published an edict on the *pösen Plättern* ("evil pocks") which warned that this unique disease was heaven's punishment on blasphemers. State and city governments recognized the existence of the disease and its venereal origin, and they began to expel prostitutes while establishing control measures based on the rules for isolating lepers. Medical inspection of prostitutes began in 1496.

The well-known Spanish physician Rodrigo Ruiz de Isla wrote his *Treatise on the Serpentine Malady* (i.e., syphilis) between 1510 and 1520, but he did not publish it until 1539. He claimed that he had treated victims of a syphilis epidemic in Barcelona in 1493. This would be the earliest dated experience with the disease, and it would place it in Spain before the French campaign in Italy. Rodrigo de Isla entered the further claim that it was Columbus's sailors who contracted the disease in the Caribbean and returned it to the old world after the initial voyage in 1492. There are serious errors in the text, however, which make this account questionable.

By the time Rodrigo de Isla published his book, the French disease had been epidemic in Europe for at least four decades, and in 1530 the Veronese physician and humanist Girolamo Fracastoro (Fracastorius) published his long poem, *Syphilis sive morbus Gallicus (Syphilis or the French Disease)*, which described the symptoms, course, and treatment of the great pox. It also told the story of a shepherd named Syphilis, who offended Apollo and was punished by a "pestilence unknown" which brought out "foul sores" upon his body which could only be washed away with quicksilver. Fracastoro thus gave the disease the name we know today, though the word "syphilis" was not actually used for it until the nineteenth century. Instead, it was called the pox, the great pox, or depending on who spoke, the French, Spanish, Portuguese, Italian, Neapolitan, Burgundian, German, or Polish disease. It was first and most commonly called the French disease. By 1546, when Fracastoro published his important treatise *On Contagion*, syphilis seemed to be losing its epidemic force, and by the opening of the seventeenth century, it had settled into the chronic pattern familiar to the modern world.

All accounts agree that the sixteenth-century syphilis epidemic was extremely malignant, swift-moving, and often fatal during its early stages. There was great physical suffering, and though death was less common than in plague or typhus, it was, by comparison with chronic syphyilis, very frequent, especially early in the disease. Moreover, the disease was almost universally considered new; that is, no epidemic of comparable character had occurred in the experience of those who wrote about it, nor could they find evidence of such an epidemic in the classic medical works.

The sixteenth-century diagnostic image of epidemic venereal syphilis was positive and very clear. Fracastoro, for example, reported a long, slow onset in which "the moon might circle the earth four times" before clear symptoms appeared after infection. The victim might be oppressed, slow, languorous, or heavy in spirit during this time. When the disease finally did appear it "arose in the generative organs" but would then race through the whole body or "eat away the groin." Severe pain came in the arms, shoulder blades, and calves of the legs; eruptions appeared on the skin's surface and at the extremities as "unsightly scabs break forth, and foully defile the face and breast." At this point, the malady often took a more serious turn when "a pustule resembling the top of an acorn, and rotting with thick phlegm, opens and soon splits apart flowing copiously with corrupted blood and matter," while the disease, now buried deep in the interior of the body, "feeds dreadfully upon it," leaving "joints stripped of their very flesh, bones rotting, and foully gaping mouths gnawed away, the lips and throat producing faint sounds." Fracastoro graphically described the destruction of a handsome young man as the "foul corruption fastened on his wretched limbs" and "the larger bones began to swell with loathsome abcesses," while ulcers destroyed his eyes and nostrils. This boy died, but many did not, living out their lives in hideous disfigurement.

The change from this malignant violence toward a more gentle onset, though with serious aftereffects, took place gradually. In 1736, Jean Astruc, the distinguished French venereologist, reviewed the contemporary literature to arrive at a progressive pattern of change in the disease symptoms. Between 1494 and 1516, syphilis was reported to begin with a small genital ulcer followed by a widespread rash and severe attacks which destroyed the palate, uvula, jaw, and tonsils. Gummy tumors (gummas) were common, there was agonizing pain, especially during the night in muscles and nerves, and an early death followed rapid physical deterioration. Between 1516 and 1526, two new symptoms appeared: bone inflammation with severe pain and eventual corruption of the bone and marrow, and hard genital pustules resembling warts or corns. Between 1526 and 1540, the malignancy abated, the number of pustules declined, there were more gummy tumors, and inflamed swelling of the lymph glands in the groin appeared. Astruc also mentioned the loss of teeth and hair, but this was probably owing to excessive doses of mercury rather than the disease alone. Between 1540 and 1560, the severe symptoms declined markedly, and something resembling gonorrhea became "the most common if not the perpetual symptom" of early syphilis. A further reduction in violence occurred between 1560 and 1610, with a noise in the ears the only new symptom.

Especially as the disease moderated, syphilis was regularly confused with gonorrhea. In 1767, the well-known physician and surgeon John Hunter attempted to settle the issue. He infected himself with pus from a patient who had a case of gonorrhea. Unknown to Hunter, the patient was also a latent syphilitic, and when Hunter developed both diseases, it appeared that there was a common cause. Despite Hunter's influence, Benjamin Bell argued for the separation of the two diseases in 1793, but while supporting evidence for his hypothesis accumulated through the nineteenth century, it was not until 1879 that the question was settled when Albert Neisser, a Breslau bacteriologist, isolated the gonococcus responsible for gonorrhea. In 1905, Fritz Schaudinn, a protozoologist at the Berlin Health Institute, discovered the spirochete *pallida (T. pallidum)*, the causal organism for syphilis. The next year, August von Wassermann and his associates developed the basic diagnostic test for syphilis. This development was the first step toward modern epidemic control.

Prevention campaigns against syphilis were organized in World War I which focused on identifying those who had the disease and treating them. Until 1939, these programs brought a sharp reduction in syphilis incidence. World War II reversed that trend, but after the war and into the late 1950s, syphilis resumed its steady pattern of decline. There has been a recrudescence of the disease, however, since 1958 which public health officials find alarming. The rise is especially notable in advanced societies and can be attributed to complacency about the disease, the rising cost of public health administration, the emergence of penicillin-resistant syphilis strains, new birth control devices which have made the condom outmoded, and a continuation of the twentieth-century revolution in sexual mores. Although it is unlikely that this rise in syphilis incidence prefigures another epidemic similar to the one in the early sixteenth century, the growing incidence of syphyilis in the advanced industrial societies must be accounted a major public health problem.

Theories on Origin Two essentially irreconcilable theories have emerged to explain the venereal syphilis outbreak at the end of the fifteenth century. The first argues that syphilis has been present under various names throughout human history, and that at the end of the fifteenth century, because of either social disorders which multiplied sexual contacts or a transformation in causal organisms, malignant epidemic syphilis swept Europe. The second thesis is simpler: Syphilis existed in the new world but not in the old. Columbus's voyages brought the disease to Europe, and a population without previous exposure suffered the explosive impact of a new disease.

The Columbian theory first appeared in 1539 in Rodrigo de Isla's *A Treatise on the Serpentine Malady* and received powerful backing from two contemporary historians of the Spanish empire, Bartolomé de las Casas and Gonzalo Fernández de Oviedo y Valdés. The strongest support for the Columbian theory, however, has come from modern anthropology. Detailed studies of old world bones yielded no unequivocal evidence of syphilitic lesions over the 5000 years before 1493. Comparative studies of new world Amerindian skeletons revealed apparent evidence of syphilitic lesions at least 500 years before 1493. The anthropological evidence lends force to the point that there is no positively identifiable description of a disease corresponding to syphilis in any medical work, classical, medieval, Arab, Indian, Egyptian, or Chinese, before 1493. Such descriptions are legion after 1493.

The anti-Columbian view argues the reverse on each issue. For anti-Columbians, the bone evidence is debatable, not definitive; the historical documentation on the outbreak of syphilis is not clear and is open to several interpretations; and there is abundant evidence from historical sources of the existence of venereal diseases. This appears to justify the hypothesis that syphilis was present and active long before 1493, though possibly in another form and under a different name. The most promising cover for syphilis is leprosy. Nineteenth-century authorities were certain that syphilis emerged from a *lepra* syndrome, a position which the distinguished historian of science and medicine Charles Singer repeated in his article on medical history in the 1937 edition of the *Encyclopedia Britannica*. More recently, the contention that something called a "venereal leprosy" in early documents was actually syphilis offers an additional argument to support the idea that not only was syphilis masked by other diseases, but the medical tradition contains direct evidence that this was so.

Neither the Columbian theory nor its opposite can be proved on the basis of available evidence, though a persuasive case can be made for either hypothesis. A third theory, which has been called unitary, or unitarian, has entered the field in the last four decades. This theory, though it could be made to fit the Columbian hypothesis, offers more support to the old world doctrine and is bacteriological rather than historical. While treponema-induced diseases differ greatly in their symptoms, the treponemata themselves are actually indistinguishable bacteriologically. This theory, therefore, postulates a common origin or ancestor for the treponema diseases and a version of Darwinian accommodation to explain how the spirochetes came to occupy different environments and different cultures and why there are such major clinical differences among them. The accommodation is reflected in the different disease syndromes which the treponemata engender. Pinta and yaws are surface infections communicated by skin-to-skin contact in climates sufficiently warm and moist for the spirochetes to exist outside the body. Endemic syphilis (bejel) appears in hot, dry areas where people are likely to be clothed, while the low humidity will destroy the spirochete immediately if it remains outside the body. The treponema accommodated by entering the more congenial environment of mucosal tissue. Transfer takes place by touch, with kissing being especially important. Infected implements can also carry the disease.

Venereal syphilis developed in temperate climates and urban cultures where temperature, humidity, and clothing forced the spirochetes into deeper penetration of the human system. Since sexual contact provided the most regular and reliable means of communication, while the genitalia provided a perfect interior environment, the adaptation to venereal disease took place. Variations on this thesis, most notably that it was yaws carried from a presumed African homeland which became the venereally transmitted syphilis in Europe, simply place different emphases on the evolutionary-historical process.

Like the leprosy approach, and even the Columbian doctrine, the unitary theory explains the outbreak of the sixteenth-century epidemic by reference to social violence, military conquests, and radically expanded sexual activity. The hypothesis is still unproved, though there is substantial evidence to support it, and it has yet to be fully synthesized with the historical data on epidemic syphilis. The unitary theory does, however, offer a significantly improved basis for interpreting the historical evidence, and it promises better answers than either the Columbian doctrine or its opposite has been able to produce.

Treatment Though epidemic syphilis called out quacks and curious remedies in great profusion, the basic treatment was relatively simple. In the early phases of the epidemic, bleeding was common, together with the application of *unguentum Saracenicum* to the sores. This specific, which contained mercury, had been used for years for skin eruptions. It proved effective against syphilis, and until arsenic compounds displaced it in the early twentieth century, mercury was the basic remedy. It was applied in huge quantities as an ointment, orally, and in vapor baths. Its first recorded use was in 1496 by a Veronese physician, Georgio Sommariva, while one of its many famous early adherents was Jacopo Berengario da Carpi, who treated Benvenuto Cellini, the famous Renaissance autobiographer and artisan.

The mercury treatment was sometimes referred to as "salivations," or "the salivary cure," because the point of the treatment was to start a heavy flow of saliva to wash out the poisonous phlegm. Since heavy salivation is also a symptom of mercury poisoning, the physicians were combating one serious evil with another hardly less damaging. Patients suffered the loss of their hair, "pains in the belly, foul ulceration of the mouth, loosening of the teeth," and it was no wonder that many victims, as the German humanist Ulrich von Hutton reported when describing his own case, preferred the agony of illness to the torture of the cure.

Among the gentler specifics, sarsaparilla was highly valued, though it was without therapeutic effect, and guaiacum tree bark was touted as a certain remedy. According to the doctrine that God placed the means to cure a disease in the place where the disease arose, guaiacum, which grew in the West Indies, both reinforced the Columbian theory of a new world origin for syphilis and held out hope for effective treatment. Shiploads of the substance were hauled to European ports, thousands were treated, and at least one banking house, the Augsburg Fuggers, made a fortune. In time, as syphilitic symptoms reappeared among those treated with guaiacum, the remedy fell into disfavor, thus supporting the critical attack which the outspoken medical gadfly Paracelsus leveled against the remedy in 1530.

Syphilis's tendency to disappear after the first phases had run their course gave comfort to quacks and a spurious validity to such remedies as guaiacum. In time, however, both stood revealed for the frauds they were. If, as the old saying had it, "a night with Venus meant a lifetime with Mercury," at least mercury had a record for good effect.

The use of mercury, though moderated from the heroic dosage of the epidemic era, continued to the opening of the twentieth century, when new syphilis treatments developed with advances in bacteriology. In 1889, Felix Balzer had proposed the use of bismuth, which killed spirochetes and was less dangerous than mercury. His proposal was not widely accepted. In 1904, Paul Ehrlich of Frankfurt developed the arsenic-based compound named 606 (for the number of experiments needed to produce it), or Salvarsan. Ehrlich was looking for a general antibacterial substance which could be injected without damage to the body to control a variety of dangerous germs. His compound was effective against *T. pallidum*, though not much else. Ehrlich's work, however, marked the beginning of chemotherapy (q.v.). Arsenic compounds supplanted mercury treatments for syphilis until the advent of antibiotics. In 1928, Sir Alexander Fleming of St. Mary's Hospital, London, isolated penicillin, but little was done with it until 1941, when a group at Oxford began testing it clinically. It became the major weapon against syphilis in 1943 when John F. Mahoney tested it in New York.

Penicillin is still the favored treatment for syphilis, but where there is sensitivity to penicillin, broad-spectrum antibiotics such as erythromycin or oxytetracycline may be substituted. Widespread penicillin dosage for other diseases may have had an unplanned effect on unrecognized syphilis cases, primarily in reducing latent syphilis infections, but there is also evidence that *T. pallidum* will develop penicillin-resistant strains. The most effective preventive is to identify and treat active syphilis cases and then to find all those who have had sexual contact with the patient within a three-year period and give them full antisyphilitic treatment. To establish and maintain such a campaign requires a highly developed public health system.

Conclusion It is virtually impossible to measure syphilis's effects. Though widespread and virulent in the sixteenth century, it soon lost its most destructive power, and it has had little or no effect on population development, economic growth, the formation of public health regulations, or even sexual attitudes. Dozens of famous people—artists, philosophers, politicians, royalty—have had syphilis in widely varying degrees of severity, and both modern incidence estimates and historical accounts indicate that millions of ordinary people also suffered from the disease. Syphilis's greatest potential for damage lies in its character as a long-term, insidious, degenerative disease which destroys individual lives. It is this rather than broad social consequences which makes syphilis control a pressing necessity and gives the rising incidence of syphilitic infections since the 1960s its most threatening aspect.

ADDITIONAL READINGS: A. W. Crosby, *The Columbian Exchange: Biological and Cultural Consequences of 1492*, Westport, Conn. 1972; H. F. Dowling, *Fighting Infection: Conquests of the Twentieth Century*, Cambridge, Mass. 1977; C. J. Hackett, "On the Origin of the Human Treponematoses," *Bulletin of the World Health Organization* 29 (January 1963): 7–41; R. C. Holcomb, "The Antiquity of Congenital Syphilis," *Bulletin of the History of Medicine* 10 (July 1941): 148–177; E. H. Hudson, "Treponematosis and Anthropology," *Annals of Internal Medicine* 58 (May 1963): 1037–1048; Theodore Rosebury, *Microbes and Morals: The Strange Story of Venereal Disease*, London, 1972; R. L. Williams, *Horror of Life*, Chicago, 1980.

See also GONORRHEA; LEPROSY.

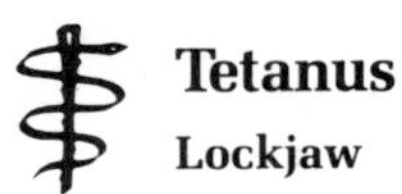

Tetanus

Lockjaw

Tetanus is an extremely dangerous disease caused by *tetanospasmin*, an element in the toxin secreted by the bacterium *Clostridium tetani*. The tetanus bacillus enters the body through wounds, and its toxin follows the nerve channels toward the spinal cord, where it becomes fixed in the anterior horn of the gray matter of the cord. Once it is established, the symptoms of tetanus begin, with headaches, toothache, sweating, and anxiety followed by increasingly severe muscular spasms in the head and neck (called "lockjaw") and throughout the system. If the case is mild, there may be a favorable prognosis; the death rate, however is above 40 percent, with death occurring most commonly from respiratory disorder or cardiac arrest.

C. tetani is found through the world. Its natural habitat is richly manured soil, and it is therefore common wherever sanitation is poor, or where there are numbers of domestic animals. It is particularly prevalent in tropical regions. Good sanitary facilities and routine immunization procedures can reduce tetanus incidence to negligible proportions, but where these elements are lacking, the disease is a scourge. Tetanus is the fourth most serious cause of death in India, claiming hundreds of thousands of victims every year. By comparison, Sweden records less than 10 tetanus deaths annually. The expanding drug culture in the United States accounts for an estimated 80 percent of recent tetanus cases, as users infect themselves by injection.

Tetanus has been recognized for centuries as an adjunct to injuries, and a particularly dangerous one. In the *Aphorisms*, the Hippocratic writer notes, in an obvious reference to tetanus, that "a spasm supervening on a wound is fatal." Until the second half of the nineteenth century, however, little else was known. Work on tetanus became possible with the onset of bacteriological studies in the second half of the nineteenth century, and tetanus shares with diphtheria a central place in the study of immunology as well. No cure for tetanus has been found, but the means to prevent its occurrence were available before World War I.

The tetanus bacillus was discovered by Arthur Nicolaier at the Hygienic Institute in Göttingen in 1884. Nicolaier observed the bacillus and generated tetanus in laboratory animals by injecting them with garden soil, but he was never able to grow the bacillus in a pure culture. Shibasaburo Kitasato, who worked in Robert Koch's laboratory in Berlin, accomplished that feat in 1889. Kitasato discovered that the tetanus bacillus was an organism which grew when deprived of oxygen, an early example of the relatively large anaerobic bacteria group. He was also able to produce tetanus in laboratory animals by serum injections. Kitasato noted that even in fatal cases the bacillus was only found in local lesions. This led him to suggest that the casual agent was actually a powerful toxin secreted by the bacillus. This toxin, when injected at sublethal levels into laboratory animals, produced a serum with an element in it which destroyed toxins. Injected into mice, it permitted 300 times the usual lethal toxin dose to be administered without damage to the mouse. Emil von Behring joined Kitasato in this work, which the two men summarized in an article published on December 4, 1890. To describe the substance which resisted toxin, they coined the word "antitoxin," and they are to be credited with discovering antitoxic immunity.

Though the antitoxin serum was of little use for therapy, it opened the door to protecting people against tetanus infection. Accidents were a common cause for tetanus cases, and in the United

States, fireworks accidents during Fourth of July celebrations were a familiar occurrence which often led to tetanus. In 1903, there were 3983 such accidents reported, with 406 deaths. The American Medical Association opened a campaign against the sale of fireworks and in favor of antitoxin injections either as a general protection against tetanus or at the time of injury. The campaign against fireworks was less successful initially than the antitoxin effort. Reported injuries from fireworks mounted steadily to 5460 in 1908, while deaths from tetanus dropped from 406 to 91, and then declined steadily until 1914, when there were no tetanus deaths at all. (Reported injuries dropped significantly after 1909, the only year when mortalities were significantly higher than the year before.) The use of antitoxin undoubtedly contributed to the rapid fall of the mortality figures.

Throughout the nineteenth century tetanus and war were indivisible, but during World War I medical science learned to control the disease on the battlefield. Brigadier Sir John Smith Knox Boyd estimated that the incidence of tetanus in various nineteenth-century wars ranged from 12.5 per 1000 during the Peninsular War to 2 per 1000 in the Civil War and the Crimean War. He estimated incidence at 3.5 per 1000 in the Franco-Prussian War. In World War I, British forces had an overall incidence per 1000 of 1.47, but at the outbreak of the war, and through its early months, the incidence ran at 8 per 1000 with an 80 percent mortality. Antitoxin was in short supply. Supplies were increased in November 1914, and wounded men could receive antitoxin injections almost immediately. Then the incidence of tetanus fell back to 1 per 1000, the death rate was cut in half, and by 1918, the British army had a tetanus incidence of just 0.6.

Between the two world wars, immunization procedures improved. In 1921, two English scientists, J. B. Buxton and A. T. Glenny, mixed toxin with antitoxin to confer immunity, while in France, Gaston Ramon and Christian Zoeller at the Pasteur Institute were developing toxoid (anatoxin). The latter pair treated toxin with formaldehyde, later alum, to destroy its toxicity without affecting its capacity to generate antibodies. This was essentially the method used to produce diphtheria toxoid. After they tested toxoid first on animals, in 1927 Ramon and Zoeller began to immunize humans. They also developed a serotherapy which combined antitoxin and toxoid. Though there was a brief flurry of fear when toxoid injections produced some anaphylactic reactions, the problem was isolated and dealt with.

In 1938, active immunization against tetanus was introduced into the British army. The French also immunized, and the U.S. armed forces had developed a program by the time war broke out in 1941. The British plan involved active immunization and, after November 1942, annual toxoid reinforcement doses. A single antitoxin dose was given when a soldier was wounded. The U.S. forces dropped the antitoxin component and relied entirely on toxoids. The Army used three injections three weeks apart, the Marines used two doses four to eight weeks apart, and all had a reinforcement one year later in addition to special reinforcing doses for those in particularly dangerous zones. The results throughout were excellent. The British evacuated 16,000 wounded men from Dunkirk with not a single tetanus case among those with active immunization. What tetanus there was (8 cases) occurred in the 10 percent who refused protective innoculation. In the U.S. Army there were just 12 tetanus cases, only 4 of which involved men who had had the tetanus shots.

Since World War II, active immunization against tetanus has become the rule. In the United States, children in their third month begin a series of three intramuscular toxoid injections. Nonimmunized adults get two or three injections, and immunized persons generally receive a booster on injury. This approach has largely eliminated tetanus as a serious disease problem in the United States and other advanced societies.

ADDITIONAL READINGS: Harry F. Dowling, *Fighting Infection: Conquests of the Twentieth Century,* Cambridge, Mass., 1977; J. H. Parish, *A History of Immunization,* London, 1965, chap. 13 and 14, 166–183; Charles Singer and A. Ashworth Underwood, *A Short History of Medicine,* 2d ed., Oxford, 1962.

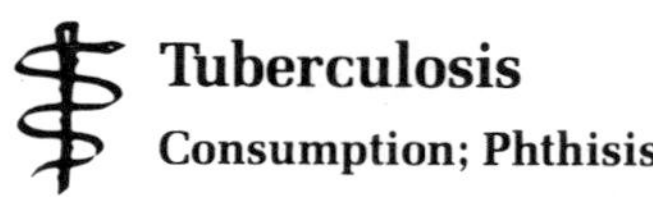

Tuberculosis is an infectious disease which exists worldwide, attacks humans and animals of all ages, varies greatly in its severity, and involves many different organs. Though currently controlled in advanced societies, tuberculosis remains a major cause of death elsewhere, and until the recent past it was the most important single cause of disease and death in Europe and North America.

Etiology The bacterial agent responsible for tuberculosis is the *Mycobacterium tuberculosis,* isolated in 1882 by Robert Koch. *M. tuberculosis* can affect nearly any part of the human system, but approximately 90 percent of modern tuberculosis is pulmonary. Tuberculosis also affects animals, and bovine tuberculosis *(Mycobacterium bovis)* can produce tuberculosis in humans who drink infected milk. In the United States, rigid regulations on identifying and destroying infected herds and mandatory pasteurization have virtually obliterated this source of tuberculosis; other nations have dealt with the problem by isolation of infected animals.

Tuberculosis is most commonly transferred by breathing infected droplets exhaled by an infected person. Since it is common for tubercular carriers to be unaware of their condition, public information campaigns aimed at unrestrained coughing or sneezing and indiscriminate spitting have been an important method for reducing tuberculosis incidence. Though it is less common, the disease can also be acquired through a break in the skin. Butchers, for example, who may handle tubercular carcasses, or surgeons who perform autopsies or operate where tuberculosis is present are especially vulnerable.

When ingested, *M. tuberculosis* is most likely to lodge in the lungs, where a primary infection will result. It can, however, pass into the system to produce tubercular infections in bones, joints, the intestines, the gastrourinary tract, the brain, the lymph nodes, the mouth, the throat, or nearly any place where infection is possible. Any point of infection can become the source of further infection. In general, the progress of the disease is slow, since the bacillus reproduces slowly. Galloping consumption, the swift wastage and death which so terrified the nineteenth century, was probably the culminating phase of an infective process begun months or even years earlier.

Wherever the tuberculosis germ may lodge, a number of processes take place, but there is no necessary pattern of development. This fact, combined with the long initial development stage, has made both diagnosis and prognosis extremely difficult. Before the bacillus was identified, tuberculosis was only diagnosed when its clinical symptoms appeared, that is, when the disease was far advanced. This helps to account for the belief that tuberculosis was virtually incurable.

Symptoms Much of early tuberculosis infection is symptomless, or the symptoms are such that they could signal a variety of chest conditions. Among the symptoms normally noted are lassitude, fatigue, irritability, and unrefreshing sleep. Fever, chills, and sweats may occur as well. Pulmonary tuberculosis will bring on coughing, production of sputum, shortness of breath, chest pains, wheezing, bloody sputum, and hemorrhage. Early descriptions of phthisis, or consumption, mention these characteristics, but they also stress physical wasting and febrile symptoms. One of the best and best-known early accounts of phthisis was written by Aretaeus of Cappadocia around the middle of the second century A.D. He described an acute case in which all excess flesh had disappeared, the fingers had become slender, and "of the bones alone the figure remains, for the fleshy parts are wasted." The appearance of this patient was greatly altered: "Nose, sharp, slender; cheeks prominent and red; eyes hollow, brilliant, and glittering; swollen, pale, or lined is the countenance; the slender parts of the jaw rest on the teeth, as if smiling . . . so also, in all other respects, slender, without flesh." Aretaeus also noted evening fever sweats and lassitude as accompaniments of the disease. There was little hope for any patient who reached so advanced a condition of decline.

Epidemiology The susceptibility of persons exposed to tuberculosis varies according to age, sex, race, occupation, and style of life. Sharp increases in tuberculosis mortality appeared in 1870 and 1871 when Paris was under siege and again on the outbreak of World War I in 1914. The increase appeared in neutral as well as belligerent countries. Blacks and American Indians have shown an extreme susceptibility, as have the inhabitants of New Caledonia and Hawaii. People with certain occupations, textile work or mining, for example, have proved to be more susceptible than other sectors of the population, and industrial workers generally have had higher tuberculosis rates than people in the professions. Correlations between tuberculosis and poverty, unsanitary living conditions, the absence of health care, and inadequate diet are very high, while the disease has generally been more active in urban than in rural areas.

People who have had no exposure to tuberculosis are assumed to be more susceptible than those who have had the chance to develop some natural immunities, but the mechanisms at work are poorly understood. Immunization has been successfully practiced in the twentieth century, and since 1947, increasingly effective methods of chemotherapy have sharply reduced mortality rates. On the other hand, the virulence of tuberculosis infection declined steadily after the middle of the nineteenth century, that is, before the bacillus had been identified and long before effective immunization and treatment were available. There is no present certainty that susceptibility will not rise again, or that currently successful immunization and therapy will not lose their efficacy.

The Ancient World Tuberculosis is a very old disease, but there is no reliable evidence on how widespread it may have been or whether it became epidemic before the seventeenth century. Skeletons from a Neolithic (ca. 4500 B.C.) site near Heidelberg show tuberculosis-type damage to the spine, and tubercular bone lesions have also been diagnosed in Egyptian remains from the Twenty-first Dynasty (ca. 1000 B.C.). A concentration of tubercular remains near Egyptian Thebes has suggested that a tuberculosis hospital may have been located there. Egyptian wall paintings which depict the dwarfs and hunchbacks favored at the pharaonic court add confirming evidence that tuberculosis infections were common. There are references in Sanskrit medical texts from the second and first millennia B.C. which are translated as "consumption" and which modern authorities believe refer to pulmonary tuberculosis. Finally, Chinese medical sources mention "lung fever" and "lung cough" with accompanying symptoms which indicate that they were tubercular.

The first extensive clinical material on tuberculosis is contained in the writings collected under the name of Hippocrates (ca. 460–375 B.C.). At first the Greeks had used the word "phthisis" to indicate any condition producing weight loss, but by Hippocrates's time, "phthisis" referred to a consumption with pulmonary symptoms. References to phthisis appear throughout the Hippocratic writings, and several of the Hippocratic aphorisms mention conditions which give rise to a phthisical reaction. The Hippocratics did not consider phthisis contagious. The clinical record in the Hippocratic writings is precise and clear, suggesting a familiarity based on many cases. This would indicate a substantial incidence of the disease. Since only cases reaching the stage where symptoms appeared are described, it is a fair assumption that there were many more cases in which the symptoms were not recognized.

Death was a common outcome for the disease, though again no precise estimate is possible for the number of deaths or even the number of advanced cases. Treatment in the Hippocratic tradition was gentle. Bleeding was used only in acute cases or to deal with some particular complication, while rest, baths, and a liquid diet were commonly prescribed. Chronic cases were fed richly. Milk, including human milk, was especially valued, and mild exercise was permitted. Some drugs were used, particularly to maintain bowel activity, and there was provision for a surgical incision and perforation at the level of the third rib "so as to give vent to a small portion of the fluid."

Subsequent Greek authorities added little to the Hippocratic tradition, which remained the main source for the study of phthisis until the work of Aretaeus of Cappadocia, quoted earlier, provided additional clinical detail. Galen, who was Aretaeus's contemporary and probably the greatest of the physicians of this period, actually contributed very little to the clinical description of consumption, but he did argue that the disease was contagious and that it was dangerous to live with a consumptive. Galen also stressed the importance of early recognition of the disease.

Medieval and Early Modern Europe Neither medieval Europe nor the Islamic world contributed any ideas of note on consumption, and because they left no clinical descriptions of the disease, there is no way to judge how rare or how extensive pulmonary phthisis may have been. There is, however, presumptive evidence of tubercular infections. Scrofula, a tuberculous infection of the lymph nodes of the neck, was apparently common in the Middle Ages because the king's touch (q.v.) was a popular ritual remedy in both England and France. There seems little doubt that medieval scrofula included the tubercular condition, though there is no way to tell what the incidence was because other diseases were also included under the term.

In the sixteenth century, postmortem studies performed by the Parisian physician Jean Fernel identified consumption (phthisis) with the chest cavity. His work suggested that the condition was a common one. In 1546, Paracelsus published a clinical study of phthisis among miners which underlined the prevalence of the disease and suggested why miners were susceptible to it. And in the seventeenth century, John Locke, the English political philosopher, asserted that consumption accounted for 20 percent of all deaths from disease to 1650.

Girolamo Fracastoro, the sixteenth-century physician whose germ theory of epidemic diseases laid the conceptual foundation for modern epidemiology (q.v.), considered phthisis highly contagious. His ideas became powerfully influential in southern Europe, where, as consumption became more common, elaborate programs for disease control were instituted. The Italian city of Lucca promulgated the first regulations governing anticonsumption prophylaxis in 1699; during the eighteenth century, such regulations became commonplace in southern Europe. In 1783, for example, Naples made reporting on consumptive patients mandatory. Violators incurred a huge 300-ducat fine with 10 years of imprisonment for subsequent offenses. Consumptives' personal belongings were inventoried. Those that could be were cleaned—the rest were destroyed. A consumptive's house had to be replastered "from cellar to garret" at the public expense; wooden door and window frames were removed, burned, and new ones installed; new houses were to stand empty for a year, or for six months after plastering. Heavy fines were levied for any interference with the administration of these rules or for noncompliance.

The Nineteenth and Twentieth Centuries It now appears that pulmonary consumption became epidemic in Europe in the seventeenth century, with the first peak occurring between 1650 and 1675. There was then a marked decline until 1730. By 1750, however, disease incidence again was rising, and by 1800 a contemporary could avow: "There is no more dangerous disease than pulmonary phthisis, and no other is so common . . . it destroys a very great part of the human race." In 1815, Thomas Young, a medical authority who had just completed a review of the writings available on tuberculosis, claimed that the disease had brought a "premature death" to at least a quarter of Europe's population and that this disease was "so fatal as to deter the practitioner even from attempting a cure."

Available statistics suggest that phthisis was an important element in the total mortality picture, though comprehensive modern studies with interpretations are lacking. Autopsy reports from the Charity Hospital in Paris (L'Hôpital de la Charité) in the early 1800s record tuberculosis as the cause of death in 250 out of 696 cases. Eastern seaboard cities in the United States between 1829 and 1845 had a tuberculosis mortality average around 400 per 100,000 of population. The low was 392 for Providence; the high was 618 in Philadelphia. Similar rates were common in nineteenth-century European cities. The peak was reached around 1850, when a steady decline in mortality began which continued into the twentieth century. By 1900, mortality in advanced societies was below 200 per 100,000 of population, and, with the exception of such anomalies as the sudden rise on the outbreak of World War I, it has continued to fall. The introduction of chemotherapy after World War II so substantially reduced mortality rates that they can no longer be used as an index for incidence. The answer to the question of whether preventive measures, including immunization, can contain another epidemic outbreak is part of the puzzle of the rate of epidemic decline in the early twentieth century.

Social and Cultural Characteristics Relatively little is known about the social impact of tuberculosis in ancient times, or even in the seventeenth century, and while the epidemic which bridged the eighteenth and nineteenth centuries was a highly visible social phenomenon, its consequences are unclear. That millions suffered the multiple physical, social, and economic effects of consumption is unquestionable; historians, however, have as yet to find a way to explain what that suffering meant. Tuberculosis produced neither mass hysteria nor public violence, and it was only at the end of the epidemic period, when antituberculosis campaigns elicited broad popular support, that there was any standard by which to measure the depth of social feeling which tuberculosis aroused. Because the period after 1750 was one of explosive growth in productivity and population, it is difficult to identify any chilling or inhibiting influence tuberculosis may have had on economic and social development. Yet in human terms, the debilitating character of the disease, its high mortality, and its broad prevalence among the indigent and working classes all argue for an enormous, if still unevaluated, impact.

The situation is different when we turn to the creative intelligentsia. Bubonic plague (q.v.) left identifying marks on late medieval and early modern art and literature, and the point has been argued, though not yet demonstrated, that plague coarsened and transformed the moral and spiritual fiber of European culture. Tuberculosis played a different role. As the disease carried off many brilliant, creative, and highly articulate people, it became a metphor for an era, shaping the romantic perception of genius, beauty, nature, fate, and death. Once the mystery of tuberculosis was revealed and it became a specific problem amenable to social and medical solutions, tuberculosis ceased to be aesthetically stimulating. Thus its impact on the tormented genius of the great modern Norwegian painter Edvard Munch remains an echo in the twentieth century of an outlook which was central in the nineteenth.

Only venereal disease could claim an incidence among the literati comparable to consumption, but the attitudes generated by syphilis and gonorrhea were very different from those which attended tuberculosis. Venereal disease was a matter for coarse joking, especially after the cruelly malignant sixteenth-century syphilis (q.v.) epidemic had passed; and while James Boswell might ruefully (or pridefully) repent the multiple infections his extraordinary sexuality exposed him to, it would be difficult to find anyone, ancient or modern, who regarded venereal disease as creative, or even interesting. On the contrary, fear of syphilitic infection and its association with physical corruption, even madness, contributed powerfully to what one recent writer calls "the horror of life" among late-nineteenth-century French literati.

The view of tuberculosis was quite different. George Gordon, Lord Byron, the very epitome of the romanitic poet, is supposed to have remarked that he wished he could die of consumption "because the ladies would all say, 'Look at that poor Byron, how interesting he looks in dying!' " Alexander Dumas sharpened the irony in Byron's wish when he reported that "in 1823 and 1824, it was the fashion to suffer from the lungs." Poets were especially prone to such a martyrdom, and for them it was considered good form "to spit blood after each emotion that was at all sensational, and to die before reaching the age of thirty." This, of course, is precisely what happened to John Keats, who died of tuberculosis in 1821 at the age of 26; Percy Bysshe Shelley was already advanced in tuberculosis at age 30 when he drowned.

Keat's biography, which is regularly reviewed in the literature on tuberculosis, reveals a young man who contracted the disease through prolonged exposure while nursing his consumptive brother and who suffered and finally died of the combined effects of consumption and the mismanagement which passed for treatment in his time. His suffering inevitably sapped his strength and weakened his creative power. But he, and to a considerable degree Shelley, symbolized a creative generation whose fate was written on its pallid face; and as they wrote despite their condition, and in the midst of a desperate search for relief from it, they came to be portrayed as the product of their disease, creators heated to the point of genius by consumption's inner flame. The American poet Sidney Lanier, who was consumptive, firmly believed that illness intensified his creative force; John Addington Symonds, a major historian and interpreter of the Renaissance, was convinced that tuberculosis gave him "a wonderful Indian summer of experience" by sharpening his perceptions of the world around him.

Consumptives had been thought for many centuries to have a life-enhancing, creative power. The Greeks referred to it as *spes phthisica*, apparently referring to the feverish, nervous energy which made consumptives' eyes glitter and drove them to exertions far beyond their waning strengths. Such vitality most often crested just before collapse. Even so, the belief in heightened sensibility which inhered in the feverishly ill became a cliché for the creative personality. This was only a short step from the idea that it was necessary to suffer in order to create, a conviction which led the Goncourt brothers to speculate that Victor Hugo would have been a far better poet if he had been less healthy.

The Goncourts belonged to the decadence of romanticism which found beauty in corruption and combined the most refined sensibility with an erotic fixation on crudity, ugliness, and filth. The nearly pornographic portrayal of social degradation and the linkage of death, disease, and sex in Munch and Aubrey Beardsley or in the pre-Raphaelites Dante Gabriel Rossetti and William Morris marked the fulfillment of the romantic association between disease and creative power. It was no accident that the ideal of feminine beauty was pale, languorous, consumptive; "elongated women with cadaverous bodies and sensual mouths." It might be added that the otherworldly, psychedelic quality which surrounded decadent romanticism was also related to the prevalence of opium abuse among the consumptive artistic community. Opium in its various forms was widely prescribed to relieve coughing, mental anguish, and diarrhea. Consumptives tended to become opium eaters, and the opium dream became an integral part of the late romantic style.

Diagnosing Tuberculosis Before Koch Until 1882, understanding and treating tuberculosis changed in various particulars but advanced relatively little. Diagnostic work on pulmonary tuberculosis improved when Jean Nicolas Corvisart, who had been professor of medicine at the Collège de France and who became Napolean Bonaparte's physician, rediscovered Auenbrugger's "technique of percussion," a method for tapping on the thorax to determine conditions in the chest and lungs. The data for diagnosis were greatly increased by Gaspard Laurent Bayle, who performed some 900 autopsies and combined his pathological observations with clinical work on tuberculosis patients. His friend René Laënnec connected tubercular manifestations in different parts of the body and in 1804 made the very important argument that these were the product of one single disease which showed itself in different ways. Laënnec's position was correct, but it was not yet susceptible to scientific proof.

Laënnec was also impressed by the diagnostic possibilities in listening to chest sounds, and it was he who invented the stethoscope (q.v.) and the technique of "mediate auscultation." Laënnec asserted in 1818 that the stethoscope made it possible to identify pathological conditions in the chest which then appeared in autopsies. Later in the century, the bronchoscope and the laryngoscope made direct inspection of the bronchial passages and the larynx possible. Like the stethoscope, these instruments were important for diagnosing pulmonary consumption.

Most research on consumption concentrated on the pathology of the tubercle, and in 1839, J. L. Schoenlein, professor of medicine at Zurich, named the whole complex of disorders "tuberculosis" since the tubercle seemed to be the anatomical base for it. The cause for tuberculosis, however, remained obscure. After the middle of the nineteenth century, Louis Pasteur's research on the bacteriological causes for fermentation and infection revived interest in the possibility that a germlike agent caused tuberculosis. This, of course, had been Fracastoro's conviction in the sixteenth century, and others, including a certain Benjamin Martin, who published in 1722, had argued the same position. However, there was no proof, though William Budd was converted to a contagion theory for consumption in the 1860s after observing the prevalence of tuberculosis among African blacks living in England, and Jean Antoine Villemine showed in 1865 that phthisis could be transferred by inoculation from a human or a cow to rabbits and guinea pigs. These were ignored because they contradicted the received wisdom that an "innate susceptibility" was the root cause for tuberculosis.

The Germ Theory The man who settled the matter was Robert Koch, a firm believer in the germ theory of disease who had already identified the bacterial cause for anthrax. Koch was a superb technician with a flair for finding the right method, and on March 24, 1882, he reported that he had identified a certain bacillus which was invariably present in tubercular lesions in animals and humans; that he had cultivated the bacillus in pure culture on blood serum; and that he had produced tuberculosis at will in healthy animals by inoculation. His discovery was "a technical achievement of such magnitude that many consider it the greatest single feat of bacteriological science, one of the most important in the whole history of medicine." Inevitably, Robert Koch was lionized. He became "the pope of medical science" for Europe and America, and in Japan he was nothing less than a demigod to whom a shrine was built. Koch's discovery was the critical first fact which during the next 75 years was qualified, modified, and extended to reveal the extraordinary complexities of tuberculosis infection. A new era had dawned.

Tuberculin and Diagnosis It was reasonable to assume that with the tuberculosis bacillus known, a means for immunizing against the disease would follow. Koch, possibly under pressure from the imperial German government, reported that he was on the brink of such a discovery, and his prestige was such that when he made partial disclosure of his vaccine, a glycerin extract of tubercle bacilli which he called tuberculin, his announcement was greeted with rejoicing. In this case, however, both the announcement and the joy were premature. Tuberculin proved to be both ineffective and dangerous. The medical profession soundly reprobated it, and Koch himself was severly criticized. Even if it was not successful as a vaccine, however, Koch's tuberculin proved to be a useful diagnostic tool because it generated an allergic reaction in persons who already had tuberculosis bacilli in their systems. The reaction would occur long after all clinical symptoms had disappeared, or even in cases where the original infection was too mild to have produced any symptoms at all. The importance of this kind of information for epidemiology can hardly be exaggerated.

Intensive research produced dozens of variations on the tuberculin compound and the method for administering the tests. The intradermal method, pioneered by C. Mantoux in 1908, has been favored for ease of administration and evaluation. Tuberculin was injected between skin layers. A reaction after five days measuring 10 millimeters was read as positive; if the reaction was between 5 and 9 millimeters retesting was ordered. Any reaction under 5 millimeters was considered negative. Before 1931, physicians usually did the testing, but a series of trials in New York and Minnesota showed that nurses could administer the tests. Before 1934, old tuberculin (essentially Koch's product) was employed. During the 1930s, however, Dr. Esmond Long, working under the auspices of the National Tuberculosis Association, produced a purified protein derivative which became standard. This form, PPD-S, has been supplemented with one using Baltey acid-fast bacilli (PPD-B). Since 1936, purified protein derivative tuberculin has been used on a worldwide scale. The tuberculin test is the master key to modern tuberculosis control programs. It is the only way to identify persons harboring the bacillus soon after infection; it is the only efficient way to locate sources of infection; it is the best method for determining the magnitude of a tuberculosis problem; and it provides a method for determining the effectiveness of any antituberculosis program by establishing a baseline for before and after comparisons.

Another technique of major epidemiological significance became available in 1895 when Wilhelm Konrad Roentgen stumbled on x-rays (see Radiology) while working on radiation. Professional acceptance was slow to come. In time, however, x-ray examination of the chest became routine, and Roentgenograms became a standard diagnostic device. The chest x-ray revealed evidence of infection before clinical symptoms could appear, though the very earliest stages of tubercular lesions remained invisible, and x-ray could not distinguish healing or healed scars from ones which were simply dormant. Bacteriological tests were necessary to confirm active tubercular infection. The chest x-ray was a simple and efficient way to determine whether further testing was necessary. It was used to good effect in military induction examinations during both world wars, and it became a critically important adjunct to clinical diagnosis.

The Sanitarium Movement Methods for treating tuberculosis developed slowly. In the nineteenth century, travel, especially to warm, sunny climates, was strongly recommended, but after Koch's discovery of *M. tuberculosis*, primary emphasis fell on isolation, rest, and gentle exercise. Rest centers, or sanitariums, for consumptives became the primary venue for treating tuberculosis and remained so until after World War I. Dr. George Bodington, a country physician in Sutton Coldfield, Warwickshire, who published a tract on consumption in 1840, may have originated sanitarium therapy for tuberculosis, but the first institution was established by Hermann Behrman in 1854. One of Behrman's patients, Peter Dettweiler, opened a reformed version in the Taunus Mountains in 1876. Two of the best-known sanitariums were founded by Otto Walther at Nordrach in the Black Forest and by Edward L. Trudeau at Saranac Lakes, New York. Walther's Nordrach sanitarium was noted for its highly structured therapy and firm discipline. It was particularly influential in England, where a large number of English sanitariums appeared around 1900 employing the Walther method and incorporating "Nordrach" into their names.

Edward L. Trudeau founded the sanitarium at Saranac Lakes in the Adirondacks as a personal retreat when he developed active tuberculosis in his left lung shortly after graduating from medical school at Columbia University. Certain that he would die. Trudeau instead found his health restored in the mountains, and in 1876 he planned a sanitarium on the site of his own recovery. He began to solicit funds, an undertaking for which he showed real talent, and he started building in 1884. The first patients were admitted in February 1885. The Saranac Laboratory was constructed soon after, and by 1900 the entire installation had become a major center for tuberculosis research. By 1925, alumni from the Trudeau Center included 261 physicians who either had been treated or had studied there and who were in sanitarium work throughout the United States and Canada.

The sanitarium movement reached its peak on the eve of World War I. Most followed the Walther system, though there was some support for the more active program constituted by Marcus Paterson at Brompton Hospital in 1905, which employed graduated and controlled physical labor. As treatments for tuberculosis moved toward surgical techniques and chemotherapy, sanitariums gave way to tuberculosis hospitals. Thomas Mann, the great twentieth-century German writer whose novel *The Magic Mountain* used the tuberculosis sanitarium as a powerful metaphor of mortality, remarked after World War II: "Such institutions as the Berghof [the sanitarium in *The Magic Mountain*] were a typical pre-war phenomenon. . . . The treatment of tuberculosis has entered on a different phase today; and most of the Swiss sanitaria have become sports hotels."

Surgical Therapy Surgical procedures for treating tuberculosis won a wide following. Pneumothorax, which a physician could perform, collapsed the lung by introducing sterile air into the pleural cavity. The theory was that by immobilizing the lung, the lesions would be encouraged to heal. In 1921, Sir James Kingston Fowler hailed artificial pneumothorax as one of "two real advances in the treatment of pulmonary tuberculosis" (sanitarium treatment was the other). This procedure, however, created a variety of problems for which other and more complex operations were needed. More effective methods for collapsing lungs were sought by performing extrapleural throacoplasty, an operation which involved removing segments of rib to allow the chest wall to collapse, or by interrupting the phrenic nerve in the neck to paralyze one side of the diaphragm. And in 1922, in place of air, oil was used in the pleural cavity when adhesions threatened the success of lung collapse. This procedure was abandoned because of complications.

Though surgery was extensively used in tuberculosis cases between 1920 and 1940, there was no conclusive evidence that it was valuable, and by 1949, pneumothorax had been very nearly abandoned. In that year, a distinguished Swedish physician, Gosta Birath, introduced a paper on pneumothorax at an international meeting by repeating the remark that "the pneumothorax needle [was] the most dangerous weapon ever placed in the hands of a physician." His paper was one of the last clinical studies of artificial pneumothorax.

Immunization After the failure of Koch's tuberculin, a number of scientists continued to look for a way to immunize against tuberculosis. The most advanced effort was that by Albert Calmette and Camille Guérin. Working in the Pasteur Institute in Lille, Calmette and Guérin produced a strain of *M. tuberculosis* in 1921 which was named Calmette-Guérin (BCG). In 1924, they declared that BCG was a fixed virus, that is, a virus which would always breed true to type. The vaccine was introduced and by 1928 had been given successfully to 116,000 infants in France and was widely used outside of the country as well. BCG came under attack, however, for statistical errors in the reports on its effectiveness, and more seriously, for not being a fixed virus. It was claimed that virulent strains were grown from three separate cultures of BCG, and the vaccine was very nearly withdrawn from use when 249 babies at Lübeck were given BCG and 67 of them died of acute tuberculosis. It was proved in this case, however, that the vaccine had been contaminated with a virulent virus from an outside source.

Though Germany and the United States refused to approve BCG, it was used successfully in Scandinavia, where it reduced the tubercular death rate significantly, and after World War II it was used in a Danish Red Cross program for vaccination in Hungary, Poland, and Germany. This program was placed under an international commission, and by September 1949, 8 million children and young adults had been inoculated. The following year vaccinations began in north Africa, the Middle East, south Asia, Pakistan, Ecuador, and Mexico. BCG was the vaccine employed. Tests in Britain over a 16-year-period confirmed that the vaccine was safe and that it produced a verifiable 79 percent reduction in case incidence.

Resistance to BCG persisted in the United States owing to conflicting reports on effectiveness, evidence that it produced positive results from tuberculin testing (thus confusing and vitiating a basic epidemiological tool), and a vehemently partisan campaign. U.S. opposition had no effect on European acceptance, however, and while there is still residual skepticism over the vaccine's use in underdeveloped and developing countries, largely for logistical reasons, BCG has been accepted as providing effective protection, and it probably represents the best hope for restraining tuberculosis in the underdeveloped world.

Chemotherapy and Cure During World War II, the final stage in the struggle to find an effective means for controlling tuberculosis began. In January 1944, Selman A. Waksman, a distinguished microbiologist at Rutgers University, isolated a new antibiotic, streptomycin, and reported his discovery. Streptomycin was tested by William H. Feldman and Horton G. Hinshaw of the Mayo Clinic and Institute, who found that it was well-tolerated by guinea pigs and that it had "a striking effect" on the human variety of *M. tuberculosis*. The tests were completed and the announcement made without undue publicity. Caution was the keynote, and it remained so in subsequent reports.

Streptomycin was subjected to mass testing organized by the American Thoracic Society, the clinical branch of the American Lung Association, with drugs provided by a consortium of commercial laboratories under the sponsorship of the U.S. Civilian Production Administration. Testing was also carried out by the Veterans Administration, the Navy, and the Army, acting together under a Joint Streptomycin Committee for Tuberculosis, "one of the most extensive research studies ever mounted," while work continued at the Mayo Clinic Foundation and at Cornell University Medical School. In 1947, encouraging reports appeared, especially for the use of the streptomycin in acute miliary tuberculosis and tuberculosis meningitis. It was also clear, however, that the tubercle bacilli had strains resistant to streptomycin which in long-term treatment rendered the antibiotic ineffectual. Nevertheless, in October 1948, the British Medical Research Council published its findings on streptomycin in a report which summarized a model clinical test for drug effect. Their results "offered the clearest possible proof" that "bilateral acute progressive tuberculosis could be halted by streptomycin."

Resistant strains posed a major problem, but parallel work on para-aminosalicylic acid (PAS) done by Jorgen Lehmann at the Stahlgrenska Hospital in Göteborg, Sweden, offered help. This work was began in 1946, and in December 1948 it was turned over to the Streptomycin Trials Committee of the British Medical Council, which tested PAS and issued an affirmative preliminary report at the end of 1949. A final report came the following year. It declared that PAS plus streptomycin "reduces considerably" the risk of the development of streptomycin-resistant tubercle bacilli. PAS had toxic side effects, however, and its use with streptomycin was still primarily for acute tuberculosis. It improved preparation for collapse therapy and lung resection, but it was not effective over the long term for pulmonary treatment.

In 1950 and 1951 testing began on a third antituberculous agent isolated simultaneously by Squibb and Hoffman-La Roche in the United States and I. G. Farben in Germany. This was isonicotinic acid hydrazide, or isoniazid, which produced the sought-after effects on pulmonary tuberculosis. The drug was potent, easy to administer, and cheap; as with streptomycin, however, there was evidence that it was prone to resistance. This drug was publicized prematurely in news reports published before the initial laboratory findings reached the public; and there was great disappointment and some resentment when it became clear that isoniazid was not the hoped-for miracle drug. While it improved the effect of PAS or streptomycin, it also left a large gap which had to be filled.

The deficiencies of isoniazid, PAS, and streptomycin were compensated for between 1953 and 1958, not by another new substance, but by the combination of the three basic drugs into a single long-term chemotherapy. The combination worked, and it is now considered to be "the sole treatment necessary for complete cure in uncomplicated . . . pulmonary or extrapulmonary disease." Professor John Crofton and a research team at Edinburgh played a critical role in working out the principle of the combination, and Crofton reported officially in 1959 that "the right use of modern methods of chemotherapy now makes it possible to aim at 100% success in the treatment of pulmonary tuberculosis." The only problem is that great care in prescription is essential. Individual cases must still be diagnosed and worked with individually, and successful treatment requires a "high degree of dedication and enthusiasm" from the physicians as well as maximum cooperation from the patients. Even so, chemotherapy in Britain brought a dramatic reduction in the national death rate and a clear reduction in the number of new cases. This result became general in industrial societies in the 1970s.

Society Against Tuberculosis: The Organizational Campaign Once the bacterial cause for tuberculosis was known, and with the successful campaigns against yellow fever and malaria to spur them on, people became convinced that tuberculosis, the most deadly fact of nineteenth-century life, could be controlled possibly even eliminated. But medicine could not accomplish this goal unaided. Society's resources needed to be mobilized to publicize what was known about the disease, to educate people to preventive techniques, to promote personal habits that would reduce the chance for infection, to fund the segregation and care of all tubercular patients, and to provide for further research. Between 1890 and 1900, in nearly every European country and throughout the United States, local, regional, and national associations sprang up to carry out the fight against tuberculosis. These societies were privately financed in most cases, and they had enormous social prestige. They were led by royalty in many European countries, and royalty found its allies among the elites of business, society, and the arts. Mass mobilization, as opposed to elite philanthropy, followed in the next decade.

The Pennsylvania Society for the Prevention of Tuberculosis, organized in 1892, created an action program which became a model for other groups. The core of the attack was to publicize the contagiousness of tuberculosis, to instruct the public on how to avoid it, and particularly to visit the poor who suffered from consumption, to supply them with medical assistance, and to inform them on hygienic principles. Hospital treatment for the consumptive poor was considered essential, but so was the legislative lobbying to strengthen preventive regulations and to support the existing boards of health.

Action programs raised significant policy problems. One of the most difficult concerned allocation of resources and the respective roles of government administrators, social workers, and physicians. When the American Lung Association (originally called the National Association for the Study and Prevention of Tuberculosis) was founded in 1904, the issue was faced squarely, and a policy statement was prepared in which scientific and medical work were given equal status with social aspects. The association accepted the principles set out three years earlier by A. S. Knopf of Philadelphia, whose pamphlet, "Tuberculosis as a Disease of the Masses and How to Combat It" became the Bible of the antituberculosis movement. "To combat consumption successfully," he wrote, "requires the combined action of a wise government, well-trained physicians, and an intelligent [informed] people." The association became the rallying ground for such an alliance.

Philanthropic organizations for various causes had appeared much earlier in the nineteenth century, but the tuberculosis societies marked a new departure. The creation of a corporate structure dedicated to a single purpose, in this case the eradication of a disease, while generating the income necessary to meet its goals was a peculiarly twentieth-century phenomenon which achieved its highest development in the United States. The American Lung Association was the model for the National Poliomyelitis Association established some three decades later, and it inspired other societies, including those for heart disease, meningitis, the problems of the blind, and cancer.

The central organizational problem was funding. Large gifts from individuals were inadequate to support long-term, broad-gauged programs, so the societies began to appeal for support to the general public. The key was small regular contributions made by millions of people. This type of fund-raising evolved slowly, and the Christmas Seal Campaign, which became the hallmark of the American Lung Association, occurred almost accidentally. The idea of selling a special tuberculosis stamp originated with Einar Holboell, a postal clerk in Denmark. It was brought to the United States in 1907 to be used for a local campaign in Delaware. The stamps raised about $3000, and the following year the American Red Cross sold Christmas Seals for the first time on a national basis. That effort yielded $135,000, and in 1910, an agreement was reached whereby the Red Cross continued to administer the sale of the seals but the funds went to the American Lung Association. After World War I, the association took over Christmas Seals, and in 1920, that source alone brought in nearly $4 million. Between 1935 and 1950, Christmas Seal sales climbed from $4.5 million to $20 million, and by 1972 the figure was $38 million.

While tuberculosis societies were dedicated to a variety of purposes, research included, their most important achievements were to publicize the nature of the disease and to convince the public of its contagiousness, its dangers, and the fact that individuals could take steps which would aid prevention. With broad public backing, governmental programs had a greater chance for success, and legislative support for tuberculosis campaigns was greatly strengthened. Ultimately, public funding for research, hospitals, epidemiological control, and treatment programs became necessary. When that happened, the basis in a favorable public opinion had already been laid. The public had been educated to cooperate.

The Current Scene Wherever a well-established public health system with adequate staff and hospital facilities exists, the standard chemotherapy against tuberculosis—streptomycin, PAS, isoniazid—works. Where such institutions are lacking, or where the level of national wealth is low, the approach to tuberculosis control through standard chemotherapy has been unsuccessful. A number of new drugs have been developed and used in an effort not only to provide a second line of defense for the standard attack but also to discover compounds which might provide more effective cures where public health apparatus is minimal. Thioacetazone with isoniazid proved effective in trials in east Africa, though not elsewhere, and a variety of other combinations and new substances has been tried. The most promising appear to be ethambutol hydrochloride, isolated by Lederle Laboratories in 1962, which can substitute for PAS without toxic side effects, and the family of rifamycins which was found in 1966. An oral form, rifamycin AMP (rifampicin in the United Kingdom, rifampin in the United States), shows bactericidal properties which are comparable to those of isoniazid. In 1969, after extensive testing, one authority referred to rifampin as appearing "to open a new era in anti-tuberculous chemotherapy." Further tests in the 1970s have supported this conclusion. Unfortunately, rifampin is extremely costly, and therefore it has not been accepted for general treatment.

Advances in chemotherapy raise the real possibility of treating tuberculosis on a short-term, nonsanitarium basis, something which is essential if the disease is to be controlled in poor societies. In 1956, an experiment was begun in Madras, India, in which tuberculosis cases were treated with PAS and isoniazid. The results were good so long as treatment and administration of the drugs were supervised. When self-administration was attempted, however, the results were mixed. This problem has led to experiments in Africa and Asia with short-course chemotherapy which would not require long-term oversight or reliance on self-administration. The results so far have been unsatisfactory. Furthermore, even as the search for a solution to the problem of long-term therapy in the underdeveloped world goes on, economic problems, especially inflation and the high cost of health care, are eroding the ability of advanced societies to identify and provide treatment for tuberculosis patients.

The medical answers to tuberculosis, including effective treatment, are now available. The problem for the present and the future is to implement controls and deliver the care required. This problem is most serious in underdeveloped and developing countries, but it is becoming a priority problem in advanced societies as well. Epidemiologists are uncertain whether the crests of tuberculosis activity in the seventeenth and mid-nineteenth centuries represent a pattern which will repeat itself. It would appear, however, that there is strong evidence for that possibility. The twentieth-century world possesses demonstrably effective means for interrupting that cycle; the question is whether it also possesses or will possess the requisite political, social, and economic power to implement those means.

ADDITIONAL READINGS: H. F. Dowling, *Fighting Infections*, Cambridge, 1977, chap. vi; René and Jean Dubos, *The White Plague: Tuberculosis, Man, and Society*, London, 1953; R. Y. Keers, *Pulmonary Tuberculosis: Journey Down the Centuries*, London, 1978; Anthony M. Lowell, *Tuberculosis Morbidity and Mortality and Its Control*, Cambridge, Mass. 1969; J. A. Myers, *Captain of All These Men of Death: Tuberculosis: Historical Highlights*, St. Louis, 1977; Selman A. Waksman, *The Conquest of Tuberculosis*, Berkeley and London, 1964.

Typhoid

Typhoid fever belongs to the enteric fever group; its causal agent is a member of the genus *salmonella*, and the disease can be either endemic or epidemic. Though typhoid fever is the most severe of the enteric fevers, it is often difficult to distinguish from the others, especially in less critical cases, and it is equally difficult to distinguish typhoid from several unrelated diseases. Though commonly confused with typhus, typhoid, when diagnosed clinically, can also be taken for septicemia, brucellosis, primary malarial attacks, infectious hepatitis, tuberculosis meningitis, tuberculosis peritonitis, miliary tuberculosis, Hodgkin's disease, or amebic liver abscess. Since modern physicians need laboratory tests and patient autopsy results to be certain of a typhoid diagnosis, it is virtually impossible to establish a definitive history for typhoid or to separate its effects from those of other epidemic-endemic diseases.

Etiology and Epidemiology *Salmonella typhi* lives in the human digestive system. It is transported from place to place by humans, and it is exposed in feces, vomit, and occasionally urine. Approximately 5 percent of the persons infected become long-term carriers; that is, though healthy themselves, they carry and transfer the salmonella bacillus. The best-known such carrier was Mary Mallon, called Typhoid Mary, a cook in the early twentieth century who is known to have infected some 53 people, 5 of whom died, and who is suspected of initiating an outbreak in Ithaca, New York, which developed 1300 cases.

People contract typhoid by eating food or drinking water which has been infected. Polluted water has been the most common source of typhoid, and water purification has been the most effective means for preventing the disease. Natural disasters such as floods which can infect water supplies are particularly dangerous. Houseflies can carry the typhoid bacillus on their bodies and deposit it directly on food. Fly control, therefore, is a second important method for preventing typhoid. Finally, carriers have to be identified and barred from work involving the preparation of food.

Typhoid has a worldwide distribution, but it is most common in tropical zones. India and Pakistan, including Bangladesh, have been major typhoid centers, contributing 66 percent of all known world cases in the period 1973–1977. Epidemiologically, culture is more important than climate, because prevention of typhoid requires close supervision and control of sewage, water supplies, garbage, and flies. Nevertheless, even in the underdeveloped world, the proved incidence of typhoid is less than that of cholera, another waterborne epidemic disease, or of malaria, which has recently been resurgent. According to figures published in 1978, there were just 206 verified typhoid cases throughout the world; the count over the period from 1973 to 1977 was 772. Since these figures come from areas where thousands of cholera cases are still reported, they suggest that typhoid was probably much less common in history than other mass infections. Individual epidemics, when a water supply is infected, can, however, be very severe. One outbreak at Worthing in England in 1893 produced 1411 cases with 186 deaths. Four years later Maidstone had 1847 cases with 132 deaths. Such outbreaks were common at the end of the nineteenth and the beginning of the twentieth centuries.

Symptoms Typhoid fever comes on gradually, with a developing fever, lassitude, loss of appetite, and muscular pains. Severe frontal headache, abdominal discomfort, cough, nosebleeds, and disturbing dreams accompany the early stages. When the onset is sudden, with high fever and delirium, death often follows by the second week. As the disease progresses, the mouth becomes dry, the tongue furred, and the bowels are constipated, though diarrhea is common in children. Temperature rises approximately 1°F per night. By the end of the first week, the patient's face is flushed, the mind is dull, and the expression heavy. A distended abdomen and loosening bowels develop, while the spleen enlarges and becomes tender. Jaundice appears in about 15 percent of the cases, respiration is rapid, and the primary physical complaints are thirst and headache. During the second week, a rash of pale pink papules appears on the abdomen and trunk. The rash may last for three or four days, and then it fades, leaving a brownish stain. The rash may reappear. During the second week, all symptoms may become more severe. The fever remains high, with marked distension of the abdomen and a violent, foul, liquid, yellow diarrhea, sometimes blood-colored. The pulse is slow, the heart sounds weak, and the patient is confused. Recovery usually begins in the fourth week. In extremely severe cases, all symptoms are exaggerated, and a "typhoid state" sets in characterized by delirium, severe dehydration, and cardiovascular collapse. There is severe distension of the abdomen with risk of internal hemorrhage and perforation. Convalescence is always prolonged after severe attacks.

Medical History The medical history of typhoid fever concerns the effort to identify and distinguish it from other continuous fevers. None of the medical classics, including the Hippocratic writings and Galen, offers a basis for definitive diagnosis because the clinical symptoms belong to several diseases and only autopsies show the intestinal lesions which are characteristic of the disease and make a definite identification possible. For the historian, it is not until the seventeenth century that evidence appears which seems to permit a historical diagnosis of typhoid. And this is questionable, because the separation of typhoid from typhus was not achieved until Sir William Jenner's successful work in the middle of the nineteenth century. Even then there was confusion—it was only at the opening of the twentieth century that both the etiology and epidemiology were set firmly in place.

When August Hirsch produced his classic handbook on historical and geographical pathology in the nineteenth century, though he identified references to typhoid in the medical literature of the sixteenth and seventeenth centuries, he had no evidence of any epidemic. Typhoid blended in with other distempers of the period. The first clinical description of typhoid was published in 1659 by Thomas Willis, a physician and scholar who observed the disease in King Charles I's army when it was encamped near Oxford in 1643. Fifty years later, Thomas Sydenham published as his last work the description of a fever resembling typhoid, and in 1680, he attended Lord Ossory, who appears to have had a severe attack of the disease.

It is possible that there was an outbreak of typhoid fever in the new world early in the seventeenth century. Scholars working on the early history of the colony at Jamestown, Virginia, note the very high death toll recorded between 1607 and 1624. In that period, 7549 colonists arrived at the James River, and 6454 died. It is suggested that the basic illness involved was a vitamin deficiency syndrome (beriberi) but that it was triggered by a typhoid outbreak. The colonists suffered swelling, or bloating, bloody fluxes, and burning fevers. If this was typhoid, it would be the first instance in which the disease achieved epidemic status in the seventeenth century.

A diagnostic image for typhoid began to take shape during the eighteenth and nineteenth centuries. Beginning with the Italian physicians Giorgio Baglivi and Giovanni Maria Lancisi, European doctors began to report a "new disease" whose symptoms, including intestinal lesions, correspond with those of typhoid. An epidemic at Lausanne in 1755 was studied by Simon-André Tissot, and the result was published in 1758. Tissot called the disease "putrid fever" and occasionally "bilious fever," but since he did no autopsies, a question remains whether the disease he described was in fact typhoid, though the presumption is that it was. An epidemic at Göttingen in 1762 was discussed by Johannes Georg Roederer, who was professor of medicine, and his assistant, Carl Gottlieb Wagler, who called the disease "morbus mucosus" but whose clinical descriptions, supported by autopsies, make a typhoid diagnosis virtually certain. There is evidence that typhus and malaria were also involved in this epidemic.

By the middle of the nineteenth century, the clinical and postmortem evidence demanded that typhus and typhoid be separated. Sir William Jenner, professor at University College, London, and physician to Queen Victoria, provided the definitive prebacteriological work on this project in 1847 through a rigid and highly disciplined clinical and pathological study of 36 cases. Ten years earlier, William Wood Gerhard of Philadelphia had made the first definite separation of typhoid from typhus. Karl J. Erberth isolated the causal organism for typhoid fever in 1880, thus providing the basis for definitive diagnosis.

In 1856 a Bristol physician, William Budd, who was a pioneer in connecting sanitation and sewage control with disease prevention, published the first of a series of articles arguing that the disease agent for what later was named typhoid fever was in the stools of typhoid patients. He connected epidemics with contact of well persons with the intestinal discharges of the sick and developed recommendations for disinfection of the discharges, boiling contaminated linens, and regular hand washing by attendants. He also pressed for disinfection of the cisterns into which discharges entered, for he believed the sewer was "a direct continuation of the diseased intestine," and he recommended boiling milk and water during epidemics. Budd was far in advance of his time, however, and his recommendations lacked the weight of well-established authority. Later research, of course, proved him correct.

Typhoid and Society Typhoid and typhus are both diseases which belong to periods of social breakdown and become active in times of war. Both respond to advances in public health, sanitation, and hygiene. In the Spanish-American War, typhoid fever attacked the new recruits in their U.S. encampments. Ninety percent of the volunteer regiments suffered typhoid outbreaks in the first eight weeks, and some 20 percent of the troops under arms contracted the disease during that year. Over 1500 typhoid deaths were recorded.

The incidence of typhoid in the Army reflected a generally high incidence of the disease in the country at large, and death rates in some American cities were as high as 144 per 100,000 (Pittsburgh) and 155 per 100,000 (Troy, New York). Sanitary regulations were reducing these figures, but in the Army camps, hygienic controls were still primitive. In this case, once the troops reached Cuba, yellow fever (q.v.) and malaria (q.v.) became more significant than typhoid. A special commission was appointed under Walter Reed to study tropical diseases and the U.S. Army in Cuba. This commission, whose work was the backdrop to subsequent work on yellow fever, finished its typhoid research in 1899 and published its report in 1904. The report enlarged existing knowledge on typhoid fever, particularly in relation to control through sanitation and military hygiene.

For British forces in South Africa, typhoid proved to be a terrible scourge. The British lost 13,000 men to typhoid, as against some 8000 battle deaths, and an additional 64,000 were invalided home. At the time of the Boer War, a vaccine against typhoid was available. In 1897, Almroth Wright, a bacteriologist, developed a preventive vaccine from killed typhoid bacilli. There was a great controversy over its efficacy, however, and only a fraction of the British army in South Africa (14,626 out of 328,244 men) received it. The controversy continued until a special antityphoid commission reported favorably on the vaccine in 1913, and the army then adopted a policy of vaccinating all men who were going abroad against typhoid. The results were dramatic. In the Boer War, typhoid incidence was 105 per 1000 men with mortality 14.6 per 1000. In World War I, incidence dropped to 2.35 per 1000, with a death rate of 0.139. Improved military hygiene was also a factor.

Earlier disease losses, as in the Napoleonic or Crimean wars, show that illness was more dangerous than enemy action, but it is unclear what proportion of the 270 men per 1000 who died from disease in the Napoleonic campaigns succumbed to any specific disease. Typhus (q.v.), however, was probably the most serious cause. The heavy typhoid losses in the Boer War, which can be validated, may have been an exceptional case. During World War I, neither typhus nor typhoid was significant on the western front, though both were scourges in eastern Europe. Advancing public health in western countries reduced the typhoid death rate significantly. In the years from 1871 to 1880, the typhoid death rate in England and Wales was 332 per 1 million of population. It dropped to 25 per 1 million in the period 1921–1925. A similar pattern appeared in the United States. In 1900, the typhoid death rate was 31.3 per 100,000. By 1935 it was down to 2.7, and in 1970, it was 0.

Typhoid remains a threat in underdeveloped countries or wherever circumstances breach public health defenses, particularly those guarding water supplies. But neither the world incidence of typhoid today nor the scattered historical data available suggest that typhoid has been one of the major diseases. It was always present with other diseases, and its particular impact was a reinforcing one, though the epidemic which broke out in Mexico in 1972 and generated thousands of cases is a reminder that typhoid cannot be considered a negligible threat.

ADDITIONAL READINGS: Harry F. Dowling, *Fighting Infection: Conquests of the Twentieth Century*, Cambridge, Mass., 1977; A. Glitzky, *Enteric Fevers: Causing Organisms and Hosts' Reactions*, Basel and New York, 1971; August Hirsch, *A Handbook of Geographical and Historical Pathology*, Charles Creighton (trans.), 3 eds., London, 1883, I, chap. XIII; W. Hobson, *World Health and History*, Bristol, 1963, chap. 8; J. H. Parish, *A History of Immunization*, London, 1965, chap. 5.

Typhus

Human, European, or classic, typhus is an epidemic disease which has regularly accompanied the worst of humanity's disasters and has always has been associated with filth, overcrowding, famine, and poverty. Typhus, as August Hirsch wrote in the nineteenth century, "is met with in association with the saddest misfortunes of the populace," and history is written "in those dark pages . . . which tell of the grievous visitations of mankind by war, famine, and misery of every kind." In 1935, when the cause for typhus was known, Hans Zinsser, in his classic book *Rats, Lice and History*, repeated Hirsch's point, stressing that typhus was the "inevitable and expected companion" of war and revolution and that the persistence of filth and unsanitary living conditions until nearly the end of the nineteenth century provided an optimum environment for typhus to flourish. The disease reached its widest distribution between the Thirty Years War (1618–1648) and the end of the Napoleonic era (1815), but it reappeared with devastating local effects during the world wars. Today, despite significant progress in epidemic control, sanitary engineering, and military hygiene, typhus remains a latent threat for advanced and backward societies alike which face civil disorder, political violence, and social disintegration.

Epidemiology Epidemic typhus is one of a group of diseases called rickettsias whose cause is a microorganism which stands midway between a virus and bacteria. The causal organism for the rickettsias lives in the blood of various animals, most notably rats, mice, and humans, and it is transferred by various insect vectors. The family may be classified according to host and vector. Tsutsugamushi disease or scrub typhus, is transferred by mites from rodents to humans, murine, or endemic, typhus (*Rickettsia typhi*) has the rat flea (*Xenopsylla cheopis*) for its vector; and Rocky Mountain spotted fever is vectored by a tick. Brill-Zinsser disease, or recrudescent typhus, depends on a previous infection and does not require a vector, though if lice are present, this form can become epidemic typhus. Epidemic typhus has the human louse (bodylouse, clothes louse) (*Pediculus humanus*) for its vector, and it is transferred from human to human.

P. humanus lives in clothes and hair, close to the warmth of the human body, and feeds on blood through the skin. The bites itch, and the victim scratches. When the louse feeds on a person infected with epidemic typhus, it draws the microorganisms into its stomach, where they multiply. *Rickettsia prowazekii* kills the body louse in from 10 to 12 days, but before the louse dies, it will defecate live typhus organisms while feeding, and the person bitten will rub or scratch them into the skin. The human is thus infected. An epidemic occurs as new human hosts carrying lice are infected and the lice carry the disease to other human hosts. Inevitably, people who live crowded together are most susceptible as the disease moves from body to body by way of the infected lice. Jails, ships, armies, and overcrowded dwellings all create the necessary environment. Even in an infected population, however, an epidemic will be of short duration if the linkage provided by lice can be broken.

In early medical works, typhus and typhoid (q.v.) were often confused, and it was not until 1837 that William Wood Gerhard first distinguished the two clinically. His conclusions were confirmed and reinforced by Sir William Jenner 10 years later. The cause for typhus was not established until the twentieth century, and the louse vector was actually identified before the causal agent itself. Charles Nicolle found the louse vector in 1909; the causal agent was identified by Stanislas J. M. von Prowazek in 1914 and described and named by the eminent Brazilian scientist Henrique da Rocha-Lima two years later. The agent was named after Howard T. Ricketts, an American scientist who first identified the rickettsia family in 1907, and Prowazek. Both men contracted and died of typhus in the course of their work.

In 1898, a New York physician, Nathan Brill, identified typhus cases among people who were louse-free but who came from eastern Europe where the disease had been epidemic. Hans Zinsser suggested in 1934 that these people carried *R. prowazekii* from previous exposures, and he hypothesized that if lice were present, the recurrent form could become epidemic. This suggestion helped to explain the carryover and transfer of the disease, and it was confirmed at Harvard medical school in 1951.

The further suggestion that rat colonies could carry epidemic typhus, passing it to humans through *X. cheopis,* the rat flea and primary vector for bubonic plague, was significantly modified when it was shown that *Rickettsia mooseri,* the rodent version, produced a different and milder disease than did *R. prowazekii.* Murine, or rat, typhus is natural to rodent populations, and where humans come into contact with them, as in Mexico or the southwest United States, there will be local outbreaks of murine typhus, a different disease from epidemic typhus.

Effective control of typhus requires breaking the infective chain by eliminating the louse vector. Modern insecticides, especially DDT, have proved extremely efficient for this purpose. During World War II, DDT was made up into a powder known as AL63, and this was used to spray soldiers' clothing at regular intervals. All underclothing was impregnated with the substance. This provided individual protection. DDT in powder form was also used on a mass basis for epidemic control. Immunization against typhus is also successful. Rudolph Weigle, a Polish physician, first cultured *R. prowazekii* in the intestines of lice in 1930. He was able to develop an effective vaccine, but the laborious method of culturing meant that the quantity of production was low and the cost was high. Harvey Cox, director of the U.S. Public Health Service, found in 1937 that the infectious material could be grown on fertilized hens' eggs, thus greatly simplifying production. Typhus vaccination could become a standard procedure. The combination of an effective vaccine and an efficient insecticide offers a high level of protection against typhus and the means to stop an epidemic if one starts. To control epidemic typhus, however, requires a high level of disciplined organization, and in areas where reservoirs of typhus infection may exist, the collapse of political authority threatens the ability to carry out disease control. It is also true that good personal hygiene, adequate diet, and a clean social environment form the first line of defense against typhus.

Symptoms The symptoms of true typhus are not so clearly marked as those of cholera or bubonic plague, and it is primarily in its epidemic form that historical identification of typhus has been most certain. During the onset of the disease, typhus resembles a severe influenza. The temperature rises to 103 or 104°F, there are chills and weakness in the limbs, the joints ache, and there is a severe headache. During the fourth or fifth day, skin eruptions begin on the shoulders and trunk, moving outward toward the extremities and sometimes appearing on the palms of the hands and the soles of the feet. The rash is pink in the beginning, but it turns toward a purplish brown-red and then to brown spots. The headache becomes excruciating, and patients often become disoriented and deranged with fever. By this stage, the disease is full-blown and readily identifiable.

In populations with no previous exposure to typhus or where other conditions have weakened the victims, the death rate can be very high, though typhus does not appear to have been so deadly as bubonic plague. Historians have recorded the decimation of whole armies by typhus, but the confirmed mortality for the disease ranges between 10 and 40 percent of the case incidence. In modern times, broad-spectrum antibiotics can reduce this mortality and shorten the period of convalescence, which in untreated cases lasts several weeks. In military situations, however, typhus's debilitating effects are as significant as the death toll. An army in the grip of typhus is unable to function. This gave the disease a dramatic role in wars, for on any given battlefield, typhus could turn victory into defeat.

Early Evidence of Typhus The early history of typhus is unclear. A case has been made that the plague Thucydides describes in his *History of the Peloponnesian War* is typhus, but despite the very detailed account that most modern of ancient Greek historians gave, the issue is not settled and probably cannot be. Whatever that outbreak may have been, it did not become epidemic, and this has made historians and epidemiologists skeptical that typhus was even present in Europe before the Middle Ages.

The early world distribution for the disease also remains mysterious. It was generally considered a disease of temperate zones, and it was thought that much of east and southeast Asia, India included, was free of typhus. North Africa, eastern Europe, the eastern Mediterranean, and western Asia have been accepted as historical centers of typhus infection. There are nineteenth-century accounts of typhus from Mongolia and northern China, however, including Beijing, which may indicate much older infection centers. This can only be speculation, since very little systematic work on Asian historical sources has been done to identify diseases. In the new world, it is generally agreed that typhus arrived with the European invaders, though it has been suggested that typhus may have preceded Columbus and Cortés in some regions. Once the European conquerors arrived, however, typhus played a major part in the epidemics which destroyed the indigenous Indian civilizations.

The first historical account of typhus comes from the Middle Ages and describes an outbreak at the La Cava monastery near Salerno, Sicily, in 1083. There are also passages in the Bohemian chronicle for 1096 which may refer to typhus. The chronicler recorded that the sick showed "no plague glands" but suffered from "soreness in the head." Apparently there were several outbreaks of what Germans came to call "head sickness" without plague swellings, and by the late fifteenth century this disease had attained a broad distribution in central and western Europe. If the identification of "head sickness" with typhus is correct, there would be nothing anomalous in such sporadic or intermittent outbreaks as the medieval sources suggest. But none of these outbreaks constituted an epidemic, and it appears that epidemic typhus did not occur in Europe until the end of the fifteenth century.

The Appearance of Epidemic Typhus The first true typhus epidemic began during the seige of Granada in 1489 and 1490. The disease was thought to have arrived with troops from Cyprus. In subsequent years, epidemic typhus spread rapidly across Europe, following the armies. Italy had become a battleground where France, the German emperor, the papacy, and various combinations of Italian principalities struggled for control. Germany was caught up in the first waves of religious warfare and peasant uprisings, while civil conflict exploded in France. In all cases, typhus stalked the land. Italy suffered heavy outbreaks at Bologna (1540), Padua (1549), and Ancona (1552). In the second half of the century there was typhus in Hungary which began in the midst of war and spread with an accompanying famine over Austria, Bohemia, Germany, the Netherlands, and back to Italy. Subsequently, war, crop failure, and typhus attacked the Netherlands, Germany, France, and Switzerland between 1572 and 1574. Sporadic typhus outbreaks occurred in England, most notably at what became known as the "Black Assizes," when jail fever among the prisoners infected judges, juries, and spectators at Cambridge (1522), Exeter (1568), and Oxford (1577). Similar outbreaks were recorded at Judge Jeffries's "Bloody Assizes" in 1685 and in the eighteenth century at Taunton and the Old Bailey in London.

Typhus activity expanded with the wars of the seventeenth century. The Thirty Years War

(1618–1648) brought it back to Germany to complete a devastation so thorough that it was said that wolves stalked the empty streets of German villages. The French campaigns against the Huguenots, the Baltic wars among Sweden, Norway, and Denmark, civil war in England, and a succession of famines in conjunction with war brought new typhus outbreaks. War casualties as such became a minor matter. It is estimated, for example, that in the first typhus outbreak at Granada, there were 17,000 disease deaths and 3000 deaths from military action. The French army at Rome in 1528 was almost totally destroyed by typhus, while casualties from enemy action were minimal. Disease losses in military forces in the sixteenth and seventeenth centuries were regularly in the tens of thousands, and it became quite literally true that victory belonged to the side best capable of preserving its health. Typhus was a particularly wicked participant in the wars, but its influence reinforced and was reinforced by syphilis, influenza, bubonic plague, and smallpox.

Typhus to 1815 Typhus accompanied the Spanish to Central and South America in the sixteenth century, but it did not reach North America until the eighteenth century, when it came as "shipboard fever" with trade and immigrants through the ports of Philadelphia, New York, Baltimore, Boston, and Portsmouth. This disease particularly concerned James Lind, who played a leading role in developing the field of naval hygiene, though he is now best known for his work on scurvy (q.v.). It was Lind's conviction that "ship fever" could be attributed to felons carrying "jail distemper" (jail fever), and to unclean impressed seamen, as well as to lower-class passengers. Lind was convinced that the disease traveled on human bodies, in clothing, on fabrics, and even on wooden surfaces. He recommended radical cleansing to prevent the disease from spreading, and he strongly advised systematic efforts to eradicate dirt. Under his influence, it became common practice when pressed seamen came aboard to strip them, shave their heads and beards, scrub them down, and issue them clean clothes before putting them into the ship's company. Such efforts helped, and the British navy had a better typhus record than either its own merchant fleet or the vessels of other countries. The French, if contemporary accounts may be believed, were especially bad. Their ships were filthy, typhus-ridden, and a danger to every place they landed. In 1746, for example, a French vessel landed near Halifax in Nova Scotia. It left behind a quantity of clothing and blankets which were infested with infected lice. The Miniak Indians, who acquired the bedding and clothes, took typhus as well, and they were virtually exterminated.

Palatinate German immigrants brought typhus to Philadelphia, creating such an outbreak that in 1754 the authorities began systematically to inspect arriving vessels and passengers for evidence of the disease. The danger from typhus grew worse when the Revolutionary War broke out. The colonists were seriously hampered during the Long Island campaign in 1776, for example, when their commander, Gen. Nathanael Greene, and more than one-third of his command sickened with typhus.

Sanitary engineering was not even in its infancy through much of the eighteenth century, personal hygiene was not a matter of great concern, and the louse was ubiquitous in society, high and low. Administrative techniques for dealing with natural disasters, epidemics included, were most advanced in the German states, where the political doctrine known as cameralism led to improved governing techniques, especially on the local level. The German states were marginally more effective in promoting cleanliness and inhibiting disease, but they were most notably effective once a disaster occurred. European society as a whole, however, lived with haphazard waste disposal, open sewers, crowded tenements, and minimal personal cleanliness. Typhus thrived.

Heavy typhus outbreaks accompanied the French Revolution and the round of major wars which began the nineteenth century. No army was free from infection, and while typhus was not the only disease, it was a very important one. Napoleon's experience in Russia was symptomatic. The French crossed the Nieman into Russian territory in June 1812. During July and August, they suffered from dysentery and diarrhea, the first consequences of inadequate and inappropriate foods—Bonaparte's army lived off the countryside, and the countryside was devastated—but there was no typhus until after the battle of Bŏrodino and the fall of Smolensk in mid-August. Napoleon's army reached Moscow a month later to find the city abandoned. During the next five weeks, the French army suffered a major typhus epidemic. The first cases were noted after Smolensk, but by the time the grand army was ready to evacuate Moscow, tens of thousands of men had fallen sick. When the army left Moscow, it abandoned those who were unfit to travel. The pursuing Russian forces carried typhus as well, and it is possible that 60,000 Russians succumbed to the disease in the course of the campaign. But the French situation was worse. Thirty thousand typhus cases were abandoned to die in Vilna alone, and only a handful of French troops finally reached Warsaw. Of the 600,000 men Napoleon led into Russia, almost none returned, and typhus was a major reason. Inevitably, the remainder of the French army and its Russian pursuers spread typhus among the civilian population of western Russia and Poland. And typhus accompanied the allied armies into central and western Europe, where the final campaign which defeated Napoleon was fought in 1814.

Typhus in 1812 was an adjunct of war. It weakened the French, and the losses it occasioned complicated Napoleon's problems of raising new forces. But it attacked the Russians as well. Typhus did not create the impossible situation which confronted the emperor in Moscow, but it contributed significantly to the misery and attrition which his forces suffered. This was not a negligible factor, though it was not a determining one.

Typhus in Peace and War: 1815 to 1945 After 1815, western Europe was relatively free from typhus with the exception of Ireland, where severe epidemics occurred during the famines of 1816 and 1817 and again, more seriously, in the famine years of 1846 and 1847. Beginning in 1830, cholera displaced typhus as the major epidemic infection of the nineteenth century, and when neither the Civil War (1861–1865) nor the Franco-Prussian War (1870–1871) occasioned epidemic typhus outbreaks, it appeared that the disease was retreating before social progress. Away from western Europe and the United States, however, the picture was somewhat different. There were typhus outbreaks in the cold weather during the Crimean War (1854–1856), and the disease appeared to be endemic in the eastern territories of the Hapsburg empire, in Russia, and in the Ottoman empire. There were also reports of typhus in north Africa—in Ethiopia, and at Cairo, Tunis, and Algiers—in west Asia, especially Persia, and in China. It appeared that those nations most successful in controlling dirt as well as disorder were least likely to suffer typhus, or, as August Hirsch put it: "It is always and everywhere the wretched conditions of living which spring from poverty and are fostered by ignorance, laziness, and helplessness, in which typhus takes root and finds nourishment."

World War I confirmed Hirsch's judgment that typhus was most dangerous for those nations which were least developed and least stable. Though over 1 million cases of trench fever, a rickettsial disease, were recorded on the western front, there was no outbreak of epidemic typhus. In the east, however, a savage typhus epidemic began in Serbia at the outset of the war. By November 1914, 2500 new cases a day were being admitted to the military hospitals, and the number of civilian cases was three times as high. In less than six months, there were 150,000 typhus deaths, a figure which included 30,000 Austrian war prisoners. But this was only the beginning. There were large reservoirs of infection in eastern Europe, and it was not surprising to find over 100,000 cases in Russia in 1914 and 1915. By 1916, that number had risen to 154,000, and with the collapse of the military front, the revolutions of 1917, and the onset of civil war, typhus simply ran riot. One commonly quoted figure for Russia between 1917 and 1921 is 25 million typhus cases with 2.5 to 3 million deaths. This was the most serious typhus outbreak in history; it is significant not only that it occurred in the less-developed east but also that it came in the midst of the most violent and destructive period Russian history had yet known. That Russia avoided a comparable outbreak in the wake of World War II attests to significant accomplishments by the Soviet regime in public health, hygiene, and social development. In 1917, however, the old formula worked once again: Relatively low cultural development, the breakdown of authority, and an era of intense warfare reinforced by famine unleashed a devastating typhus epidemic.

Similar patterns recurred in the course of World War II, though not in the Soviet Union. There were heavy outbreaks of typhus in Japan and Korea in 1945 and 1946 and again at the end of the Korean war, but the most notable action of the disease was in Europe. There was a severe typhus epidemic in Naples in 1943 when the Allies liberated the city, and the German extermination camps—Buchenwald, Bergen-Belsen, Dachau, Flassenberg, Mounthausen, Auschwitz, and others—were rotten with the disease.

Typhus apparently came to Naples from north Africa and Sicily with Italian soldiers, though the epidemic actually began among prisoners from Tunisia and Yugoslavia. The Allies arrived on October 1, 1943, as the epidemic was gaining force, and on December 15 opened a campaign against it. The critical procedure was dusting with DDT to destroy lice. Between December 15, 1943, and May 31, 1944, 3,265,786 persons were dusted. The epidemic peaked in January and was over by March, and for the first time in history, a typhus epidemic was stopped by direct action.

In Germany, there was no typhus west of the Rhine until the eastern front collapsed and refugees poured into the west in February and March 1945. Typhus first appeared in Munich, Gladbach, and Cologne. DDT dusting again proved effective. In the German concentration and extermination camps, however, the problem was more serious. At Dachau, there were some 40,000 inmates, with the dead and living crushed together in unspeakable conditions. By June 1, 1945, there had been 2336 typhus cases with 311 deaths. At Bergen-Belsen, typhus apparently arrived with a group of Hungarian Jews in January 1945. Conditions in the camp were indescribable. People were jammed into confined spaces with no sanitary facilities, so they lived steeped in their common excrement. There was no food or water. In desperation, the prisoners drank urine and ate excrement and even one another to stay alive. In such a chamber of horrors, typhus, which the Germans made no effective efforts to control, was very nearly welcome. When British forces liberated the camp on April 15, 1945, there were 55,000 inmates, of whom 10,000 were dead; 13,000 more died. There were at least 3500 typhus cases, though it is thought that at some time in the winter and spring nearly all the inmates had had typhus, and before the epidemic could be brought under control, there were an additional 13,000 cases. Once effective delousing began, however, the number of new cases dropped radically, and the epidemic was over by May 14.

Today, typhus holds no significant epidemiological secrets, and the measures for its prevention and control are well-known. Historically, however, there is much that is obscure. Typhus has not captured historians' interest the way bubonic plague, cholera, syphilis, or, more recently, tuberculosis and cancer have done. Almost nothing is known of typhus outside the west beyond the fact that it occurred, and though the disease was rampant during the early bubonic plague outbreaks and had a considerable extension throughout the modern period, scholars have ignored the problem of its effects on society and have done relatively little even to establish the actual magnitude of its incidence. Typhus offers opportunities for further historical research, but until that work is done, we will have to be content to identify it as the disease of poverty and disaster, an affliction which thrives in conditions of cultural backwardness and social disorder.

ADDITIONAL READINGS: Gaines M. Foster, "Typhus Disaster in the Wake of War: The American-Polish Relief Expedition, 1919–1920; *Bulletin of the History of Medicine* 55 (Summer 1981): 221–232; G. J. Harrington, "Epidemic Typhus and History," *Marquette Medical Review* 31 (1965): 147–190; August Hirsch, *Handbook of Geographical and Historical Pathology*, Charles Creighton (trans.), London, 1883, 3 vols., I, chap. XI; W. Hobson, *World Health and History*, Bristol, 1963; Frank L. Horsfall, Jr., and Igor Tamm (eds.), *Viral and Rickettsial Infections of Man*, 4th ed., Philadelphia, 1965; T. E. Woodward, "A Historical Account of the Rickettsia Diseases," *Journal of Infectious Diseases* 127 (May 1973): 583–594; Hans Zinsser, *Rats, Lice, and History*, Boston, 1935.

Vitamins

Vitamins are the "accessory food factors" which must be present in addition to requisite quantities of proteins, fats, and carbohydrates to maintain a healthy life, to promote growth, and to facilitate reproduction. Diseases resulting from vitamin deficiencies include scurvy (vitamin C), beriberi (vitamin B_1, or thiamine), rickets (vitamin D), and pernicious anemia (vitamin B_{12}). Other more complex deficiency diseases are brought about by protein-energy malnutrition, which reinforces the effects of specific vitamin deficiencies.

Though nutritional science in the eighteenth and nineteenth centuries established the quantities of proteins, fats, carbohydrates, mineral salts, and water necessary for life, the absence of certain elements came to be connected with specific diseases. In 1753, the Scottish physician and naval surgeon James Lind linked the prevention of scurvy (q.v.) with lemon juice. At the end of the nineteenth century, a Dutch colonial researcher on Java, Christiaan Eijkman, noted the similarities between polyneuritis in chickens and pigeons feeding on polished rice and beriberi (q.v.). His observations and those of his associate, Gerrit Griijn, formed the backdrop to the work done by Sir Frederick G. Hopkins in 1906. Hopkins observed that rats fed on artificial milk failed to grow but that when natural cow's milk was added to their diet, growth resumed. The following year, Axel Holst and Theodore Froehlich demonstrated that a dietary deficiency caused scurvy and that the disease could be cured by replacing the missing element. The word "vitamin," used to describe the accessory food factor, was coined in 1912 by Casimir Funk, a Polish-American biochemist. Funk believed that the secret element was an amine, or derivative from ammonia, and he called it "vitaamine," or "vitamine." When it was found in 1920 that the amine connection was incorrect, the final "e" was dropped.

The first vitamin identified was B_1 (thiamine). This was the element Funk named in 1912, though it was not isolated in pure form until 1926 and it was not synthesized for 10 more years. Vitamin A (retinol) was suspected in 1913, but its chemical character was not established until 1933, and it was finally synthesized in 1947. This vitamin is especially important for vision. Its absence causes night blindness, and a prolonged deficiency produces lesions and finally blindness. Vitamin C (ascorbic acid) was the hidden factor in citrus juices which counteracted scurvy. It was chemically isolated in 1927, and its antiscorbutic action was defined in 1932. In that same year, vitamin C became the first vitamin to be synthesized in the laboratory. The Hungarian biochemist Albert Szent-Gyorgyi received the Nobel prize for this work. Other vitamins, including the members of the B vitamin group, vitamin D, and vitamins E, G, H, and K, were discovered in the 1930s and 1940s. Vitamin B_{12}, the anti–pernicious anemia vitamin, was isolated in 1948 and 1949 and reported by Karl Folkers (United States) and Alexander R. Todd (Great Britain). The discovery and synthesis of vitamins completed a stage in the development of scientific nutrition while providing the means to combat and even eliminate a number of specific diseases arising from deficient diets.

ADDITIONAL READINGS: R. J. Kutsky, *Handbook of Vitamins and Hormones*, New York, 1973; E. V. McCollum, *A History of Nutrition*, Boston, 1957; Leonard G. Wilson, "The Clinical Definition of Scurvy and the Discovery of Vitamin C," *Journal of the History of Medicine and Allied Sciences* 30 (1975): 40–60.

See also DEFICIENCY DISEASES; NUTRITION.

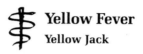

Yellow Fever

Yellow Jack

Yellow fever is a dangerous endemic-epidemic disease which played a significant role in the early history of American coastal cities and which was a continuing barrier to colonizing and developing the Caribbean islands, tropical Central and South America, and west Africa. Though the disease is largely controlled in twentieth-century urban areas, vast reservoirs of infection continue to exist in tropical rain forests which endanger more settled regions. Nevertheless, successful epidemic control measures have improved living and working conditions in affected areas, and the early successes against yellow fever inspired further and more intensive efforts against such diseases as dengue fever, malaria, dysentery, and typhoid.

Etiology and Epidemiology There are now two recognized varieties of yellow fever: urban and jungle. Urban yellow fever is the historic disease which flourished from the seventeenth to the twentieth centuries. Jungle yellow fever was not identified until the 1930s. The infective agent in yellow fever is a group B virus which is communicated by insect vectors. The sole vector in urban yellow fever is the female of the *Aëdes aegypti* mosquito (formerly *Stegomyia fasciata*). The mosquito draws infected blood into its stomach; incubation requires about three days, after which the mosquito is fully infective until it dies in from two to four months. The main reservoir of infection is the human being. Monkeys are the main infective reservoirs for jungle yellow fever, though other mammals may also be involved. A variety of forest mosquitoes act as vectors, with the most important being *Haemogogus capricorni*, *Haemogogus spegazzini*, and *Haemogogus spegazzini* *falco*. Human beings contract jungle fever from mosquito bites when they enter the forests or when an infected monkey enters the human zone and is bitten by a domestic mosquito and that mosquito in turn bites a human.

The historic yellow fever outbreaks occurred in developed human environments and were the work of *A. aegypti*. This specialized, house-haunting mosquito breeds in small ponds or pools, water jugs, barrels, pitchers, or any other holder with a hard, smooth bottom in which water can accumulate and stand. Its flight range is not over 100 yards. Ships' water supplies were natural breeding grounds for *A. aegypti* and made long-distance transmission of yellow fever possible. An established population of *A. aegypti* mosquitoes is prerequisite for an urban yellow fever epidemic. The presence of the yellow fever virus is not sufficient in itself. This helps to explain the absence of yellow fever from settled regions before the mid-seventeenth century and the close association between the disease and port cities. After the role of *A. aegypti* in yellow fever transmission was established in 1902, mosquito control became the focal point for yellow fever campaigns. This remains the first and most important measure in settled regions. Because insect control is impractical in jungle environments, immunization is the only effective measure against jungle yellow fever. The World Health Organization's communicable disease watch provides a warning system should enzootic yellow fever threaten to become epidemic.

Clinical Characteristics The incubation period for yellow fever is relatively short, with the first symptoms appearing four or five days after infection. These symptoms include a rising temperature, flushed face, and reddened lips and tongue. Soon, however, the temperature falls to subnormal levels, the skin turns a lemon yellow, and the victim begins to vomit a colorless liquid which soon changes to dark brown or black. This "black vomit" gave yellow fever one of its many names, and it is one of the most important evidences for historical identification. Black vomit results from blood partially digested in the stomach, and the amount of blood indicates how severe the attack is. The virus attacks internal organs and often severely damages the kidneys and liver. It is this action of the virus which most commonly causes death. When yellow fever is endemic, the incidence and mortality of the disease are greatest among children. Adults develop immunities, and the overall effect of the disease will often be limited. Where no natural immunities exist, however, both incidence and mortality may be very high, and the disease affects all members of the population without regard for class, age, race, or sex. As a whole, death rates vary grossly, ranging from 10 or 12 percent to 80 percent of known cases, and in one particularly awful outbreak in Rio de Janeiro, the mortality reached 94.5 percent of the reported cases. Yellow fever is especially dangerous for such small, self-contained populations as a ship's company or the inmates of a prison, and its effects within a city can be devastating. Because yellow fever tends to remain localized and because its geographical distribution has been on the fringe of the world's great population centers, it does not count among history's worst killers. Nevertheless, yellow fever's local effects were often very severe, and an outbreak was a terrible experience which frequently had significant immediate effects on society and the local economy.

Early History There is an unresolved argument concerning whether yellow fever existed in Central America and tropical South America before Columbus landed. Mayan historical records suggest that this might be true, but the evidence is slight. Beginning in 1495, there are reports of what appears to be yellow fever on Santo Domingo. This could support the hypothesis that yellow fever antedated Columbus's arrival and that his men caught it in the new world, but it also could mean that the Spanish adventurers brought the disease with them. Since the first firm evidence that yellow fever existed in the Caribbean comes 140 years later, the reports from the late fifteenth century or earlier seem doubtful.

By 1635, yellow fever was definitely present in the Caribbean, and in 1647 there was a severe epidemic on Barbados. Slavers from the west African coast probably brought the virus in their human cargoes and the mosquitoes with their water. Black African slaves showed immunities to the disease, but Europeans and Amerindians alike proved highly susceptible. In 1648 and 1649, yellow fever spread to the Yucatán, St. Kitts, Guadeloupe, and Cuba. Although the earliest written evidence for yellow fever in west Africa is from

Sierra Leone in 1764 and Senegal in 1778, the relative immunity of African slaves transported to the Caribbean argues strongly for yellow fever's presence long before the historical record identifies it.

Yellow fever probably reached colonial North America at the end of the seventeenth century. Boston port authorities were concerned about the pestilence reported from the Caribbean in the 1640s and contemplated action to prevent the infection from entering the colony, but there is no indication that the disease arrived. Noah Webster, the nineteenth-century American lexicographer who was an early historian of medicine as well, referred to an "autumnal bilious fever" in New York in 1668, a designation which has been interpreted to indicate yellow fever. However, the description of the disease included neither the anticipated high mortalities common in a virgin population nor any reference to black vomit, Webster's account may well refer to some other illness which reached epidemic proportions. The first detailed account of an authentic yellow fever epidemic in North America comes from Cotton Mather, who in 1693 described a disease brought to Boston on a British man-of-war. He spoke of "a most pestilential Feaver" which carried off his neighbors "with very direful symptoms of turning *Yellow*, vomiting, and bleeding every way." There seems little doubt that this was yellow fever, and it was part of the American landscape until 1906.

The Eighteenth and Nineteenth Centuries

Yellow fever attained its widest extension in the eighteenth and nineteenth centuries. Extremely active in the Caribbean, it became general in South America midway through the nineteenth century. In west Africa, yellow fever was active throughout the entire period, and together with other tropical diseases it gave this area its reputation as "the white man's graveyard." Farther north, yellow fever began to appear on the Iberian peninsula. Cádiz suffered five separate epidemics between 1700 and 1780, and Lisbon (1723) and Málaga (1741) were also visited. None of the eighteenth-century occurrences spread out from their beginning points, but in the nineteenth century, the Iberian peninsula was more generally invaded. There were also occasional cases of yellow fever at west European ports, but there were no serious outbreaks. The most active areas for the disease included west Africa, the Caribbean, Central America, and the North American port cities.

In view of a rapidly expanding trade with the Caribbean islands and the African coast, the appearance of yellow fever in North American ports is not surprising. Charleston, South Carolina, New York, and Philadelphia were the cities most regularly visited in the eighteenth century; in the nineteenth century, New Orleans became the yellow fever capital of the United States. Charleston and Philadelphia had their first epidemic in 1699, and the first New York outbreak came in 1702. In each case, both incidence and mortality were high. In the New York epidemic, for example, at least 570 people died, an estimated 10 percent of the city's entire population, and life was severely disrupted.

Charleston had a series of yellow fever outbreaks in the first half of the eighteenth century, building to a peak in 1758. In the second half of the century, there was a 40-year intermission, followed by six severe epidemics between 1790 and 1799. The 1740s were particularly hard for New York and Philadelphia. After nearly 35 years without a yellow fever epidemic, the disease returned to New York in 1741 and 1747 and to Philadelphia from 1743 to 1745 and again in 1748. As in Charleston, there was a remission in the second half of the eighteenth century, but in the last decade of the century yellow fever returned, more virulent than ever. In 1793, Philadelphia suffered one of the worst yellow fever epidemics on record when over 4000 deaths were recorded between August and October. This was not surpassed until the New Orleans outbreak of 1853.

In 1802, Napoleon Bonaparte sent an army to Haiti to suppress a native uprising led by Pierre Toussaint-Louverture. The uprising failed, but the French army was almost totally destroyed by yellow fever. This event helped Napoleon to decide to rid himself of his new world holdings and played a part in his offer to sell the Louisiana Territory to the United States. In 1820, Savannah, Georgia, lost nearly 2500 citizens out of a population of 7500 to yellow fever; Norfolk, Virginia, was devastated in 1855 when a fever-ridden vessel was permitted past the quarantine, and New Orleans lived through a succession of yellow fever epidemics which culminated in the outbreak of 1853 when 10,000 people, about one-tenth of New

Orlean's population, died. New Orleans continued to suffer yellow fever outbreaks in the second half of the nineteenth century and in fact had the last major yellow fever epidemic in the United States in 1906. By that time, the mosquito vector was known, and effective control measures were available. After 1906, yellow fever ceased to be a serious problem in the United States.

Yellow Fever and Society Yellow fever struck American cities during the summer months, with the disease peak generally occurring in late August or September and the epidemic lapsing in October as mosquito activity dropped off with cooler weather. The attacks were sporadic and their focus limited. Despite high losses in particular epidemics, there was little reinforcement of mortality, and incidence tended to be spread across the whole spectrum of society. Nevertheless, the poorer classes suffered higher mortalities because they were the first affected by shortages in food or facilities and were the least resistant to disease. However, with a high birthrate and substantial immigration, yellow fever had at most a passing effect on urban population patterns. This does not mean that yellow fever was without effect. Any number of personal tragedies were recorded as families were decimated and promising young people carried off. Daily life was seriously disrupted, the entire energy of whole communities being necessary simply to care for the sick and bury the dead. Labor was impossible to find, commerce slowed to a mere trickle, and merchants, especially those whose goods were perishable, suffered heavy losses. Such a combination of factors, for example, accelerated Philadelphia's decline and loss of place to New York as America's first port city during the yellow fever of 1793.

Contemporary accounts from the last decade of the seventeenth century through the middle of the nineteenth century make it clear that while people feared yellow fever, it hardly generated the hysterical terrors or mass responses that attended the first wave of cholera (q.v.) or the medieval black death (see Bubonic Plague). The most common reaction was for people to take steps to avoid any contact with the fever or its victims. It was normal for the urban middle classes to leave the cities during the hot summer months, and in such a place as New Orleans, this annual migration might carry as many as 50,000 people away from a city which at its peak winter population in 1850 would have numbered some 150,000. The same was true of the Atlantic seaboard cities. The threat of yellow fever increased the exodus. Philadelphia in 1793 was described by contemporaries as very nearly a ghost town, with only the wheels of the hearses to break the unnatural silence. In that case, the college of physicians had recommended that people should avoid public gatherings, that the dead should be transported in closed vehicles, that the church bells should not toll, and that citizens going abroad should cover their noses with a cloth or handkerchief soaked with vinegar or camphor. The real fear was of contact with the contagion or miasma, and while the physicians plainly hoped to avoid scenes of riot and disorder, they contributed as well to the citizens' practice of personal isolation. People avoided meeting one another on the street, a proffered handshake was considered to be a threat, and while some physicians told their clients that flight was the best policy, the fugitives were not welcome outside the city. New Jersey, Maryland, and Delaware all closed their borders to travelers from Philadelphia, though other traffic was permitted to pass freely, and strangers coming into rural communities were not allowed to stay. The yellow fever epidemics produced relatively little violence. There were bitter complaints about price gouging, callousness, incompetence, exploitation, and the cowardice of public officials, but over nearly two centuries, a whole group of towns becoming cities accepted the disease with a surprisingly philosophical spirit.

Eighteenth- and nineteenth-century physicians could do relatively little for yellow fever sufferers. Fever treatment traditionally involved purges and bleeding, and to that end, Dr. Benjamin Rush, one of Philadelphia's most noted physicians, promoted a radically heroic version of this therapy which he carried out despite mounting criticism on the more than 100 patients he saw daily. Others who emphasized nursing and a more gentle approach claimed better results, and the profession divided on the issue. New influences were beginning to make themselves felt, but it would be an exaggeration to say that the yellow fever was especially significant in promoting them. By the middle of the nineteenth century, medical procedures had improved, but southern doctors remained wedded to the heroic therapies inherited from the eighteenth century. The resounding failure of southern medicine in the New Orleans yellow fever outbreak led directly, as John Duffy has shown, to reforms in licensing procedures and medical education in the south. In this respect, the 1853 New Orleans epidemic was significant medically, for it gave impetus to the modernization of the southern medical profession.

Yellow fever played a role in the development of sanitary policies, public health institutions, and the growth of municipal responsibility for public welfare. In 1794, and in response to the yellow fever outbreak, the state of Pennsylvania instituted boards of health to provide the continuity of leadership and administration on health affairs which the epidemics showed were profoundly needed. Baltimore also created a health commission in 1794, and it began to legislate on conditions affecting public health in 1797. Two years later, Philadelphia initiated a public water supply system, an example followed by other east coast cities in the next two decades. The decline and finally the disappearance of yellow fever from the coastal cities of the north during the first decades of the nineteenth century owe something to these changes. Improved quarantine policies more effectively administered were one factor. Enclosed water supplies, better waste disposal, and improved drainage reduced mosquito breeding areas. But there is the further possibility that the decline was only marginally affected by improved public services and that it owed to changes in sugar refining centers and trade patterns which affected the introduction of active yellow fever into American ports.

The ideology of private charity and self-help was a persistent control on the development of public institutions in America, and nowhere was this attitude stronger than in rich and vital antebellum New Orleans. Here yellow fever had a considerable effect. During the 1853 epidemic, when the disease first appeared in the city, the common reaction was to ignore reports about it or to deny them. It was only when the death toll rose above 250 per day that New Orleans reacted to the danger. It was clear that charitable organizations could not handle the problems of caring for epidemic victims, though heroic efforts were made. Ultimately, it was the municipal government which proved effective. Under the strong leadership of Mayor A. D. Crossman, city officials remained on duty and, with the full cooperation of the business community, maintained firm order throughout the epidemic period. New Orleans absorbed over 10,000 deaths without disorder or disruption, and by fall, though new cases were still being reported, the people of the city seemed already to have forgotten it. The yellow fever tested and strengthened municipal organization, leading toward a consolidation of public services and the centralization of their administration. This did not mean, however, that New Orleans became forward-looking on matters pertaining to yellow fever prevention. On the contrary, the 1853 epidemic was considered an incident to be forgotten, a crisis that had passed and that simply proved that the city could deal with any comparable crisis in the future. It was only after the 1906 epidemic that New Orleans took up a serious anti–yellow fever program, and by that time the technology of control was sufficiently advanced to guarantee success.

Endemic yellow fever in the Caribbean or in Africa had a different kind of significance for Americans and Europeans. While local populations developed immunities, aliens entering the einvironment were extremely vulnerable. The first tentative efforts in the early nineteenth century to explore the heart of Africa failed because of the disease barrier, and the introduction of large numbers of nonimmune European or American soldiers or workers in Latin America and the Caribbean was an invitation to disaster. Yet in the nineteenth century, these areas were becoming increasingly important. Expanding industrialization and world trade provided a powerful impetus to enter and develop new territories and to cut transportation costs by shortening sailing routes as well as by exploiting the new maritime steam technology. During the 1860s, the Suez Canal radically reduced the time and the cost of shipping to and from south Asia and the far east, and this success revived the idea of driving a canal across the Isthmus of Panama to connect the Atlantic and Pacific oceans. Ferdinand de Lesseps, the French engineer responsible for the Suez success, attempted the Panama project but failed. Though other factors were involved, disease, particularly yellow fever but also malaria, proved an insurmountable barrier. Between 1881 and 1888, thousands of European workers sickened and died in the jungles, eventually forcing abandonment of the project. When the United States went to war with Spain over Cuba and subsequently declared its interest in developing a canal through Panama, the control of yellow fever became a matter of national priority. Yellow fever epidemics may have played only a marginal role in the urban history of the United States, but political interests and military needs gave yellow fever control new significance at the opening of the twentieth century.

The Defeat of Urban Yellow Fever Early control measures against yellow fever were limited to enforcing quarantines. Vessels found to have the disease on board flew a yellow flag (the yellow jack, which became a nickname for the disease itself), while health boards concentrated on maintaining cleanliness and good order. Quarantines assumed that yellow fever was contagious, but there was a growing body of opinion during the nineteenth century that filth was the source of disease. Anticontagionists believed that putrefaction generated noxious and dangerous airs and that "heat acting on moist animal and vegetable matter, produced putrid exhalations." Benjamin Rush accepted and propagated the idea that the Philadelphia yellow fever began with a cargo of rotting coffee which had been dumped on the dockside; and even at the opening of the twentieth century, after the germ theory of disease had been established, public officials in the United States and abroad remained convinced that sanitation was the key to disease control. They argued that bacteria bred in filth, an argument appropriate to many epidemic diseases but not, as it happened, to yellow fever. Anticontagionists fought quarantines in the early nineteenth century, and their successors in the sanitary movement remained unconvinced that the way to control yellow fever was by destroying mosquitoes. The truth was, however, that until the mosquito vector was discovered, there was no effective method of control.

The discoveries which led to successful yellow fever control belong to the first period of the bacteriological age and owe heavily to American medical development. Various theories had accounted for yellow fever before 1900, including miasma, spontaneous generation, and contagion. One of the first men to challenge this approach was an Irish-born, Dutch-educated former surgeon for the East India Company named John Crawford (1746–1813) who settled in Baltimore in 1796. He argued that decay and disease both were the products of minute organisms, and that plague, yellow fever, and all other fevers "must be occasioned by eggs inserted without our knowledge into our bodies." Crawford's curious idea was only one of many precursors of a germ theory for disease. In 1848, Dr. Josiah Nott of Mobile, Alabama, suggested an infective agent for yellow fever which had to have an intermediary to communicate it. Six years later, Dr. Louis Daniel Beauperthuy, a native of Guadeloupe who was educated in Paris, made precisely the same point. Both men thought the mosquito was a possible vector, but neither was prepared to offer the needed experimental evidence. Dr. Carlos Finlay, a Havana physician educated in Cuba and Europe, followed the same reasoning. In 1818, he presented a paper in which he not only suggested the mosquito as the yellow fever vector but called attention specifically to *A. aegypti.* But Finlay's problem was the same as that of those who preceded him: He lacked experimental evidence. Ironically, though his positions were in general correct, he was never able to communicate yellow fever using a mosquito vector under laboratory conditions. He remained active in the field despite his disappointments, and in fact he proposed a program aimed specifically at mosquito control (as opposed to general sanitary reforms) which was similar to that later successful program Maj. William Gorgas instituted. Dr. Finlay became a member of Dr. Walter Reed's Yellow Fever Commission in 1900.

In 1897, an Italian bacteriologist, Dr. Guiseppi Sanarelli, who was working on the island of Flores off Montevideo, Uruguay, announced that he had identified a bacillus (*Bacillus icteroides*) in a substantial number of yellow fever patients which could be the causal agent for yellow fever. The U.S. Medical Corps appointed doctors Walter Reed and James Carroll to investigate Sanarelli's discovery. They were joined by an assistant army surgeon, Dr. Aristedes Agramonte, and Dr. Jesse W. Lazear, a bacteriologist.

The commission's first results were negative. They could find no evidence that the Sanarelli bacillus caused yellow fever, and they concluded that when it was present, it was a secondary invader irrelevant to yellow fever causation. This left the commission with no starting point for further work. Statistical studies on yellow fever in Mississippi by Henry R. Carter, however, provided the clue that was needed. The Carter studies showed a differential of from two to three weeks in the causal chain from the first infected case to the first group of cases. This once more indicated the possibility of a vector. Sir Ronald Ross's recent identification of the mosquito vector in malaria and the growing evidence on insect roles in other diseases including African sleeping sickness (q.v.) led the commission to turn back to test Finlay's hypothesis.

With Finlay's full cooperation, and even using some of his mosquitoes, the commission began to work on an outbreak of yellow fever among American troops some 200 miles from Havana. Despite the undoubted presence of the disease, however, they failed to transmit it under laboratory conditions until, in part from carelessness, an infected mosquito bit Dr. Carroll, who developed a full case of yellow fever. He recovered, but a similar accident took Jesse Lazear's life. The problem had arisen from the failure to allow for extrinsic incubation of the infective material in the mosquito. Once the mechanism was understood, the commission moved ahead rapidly to prove that yellow fever could not be communicated by direct exposure, on goods, or by personal belongings.The commission's conclusion was that there was incontrovertible evidence that yellow fever followed the bite of an infected mosquito and that there was no evidence to support any other method of transfer.

The Reed commission's work led directly to the plan to control yellow fever by destroying mosquitoes. William C. Gorgas devised and initiated the program in February 1901. The Gorgas campaign built on the knowledge that the yellow fever mosquito was found around houses and used clean water standing in smooth, hard receptacles in which *A. aegypti* would breed. Every household in Havana inventoried such jars, pitchers, basins, or catchments where water might collect. Everything that could be emptied was emptied, kerosene was spread on the surface of larger collections, wells and cisterns were screened, and the most minute attention was given to every potential breeding place, regardless of its remoteness or difficulty of access. Gorgas also carried out a plan for identifying and isolating yellow fever patients, though this was less important than the antimosquito campaign. The campaign was a success. The infective chain was disrupted, and within three months the yellow fever had vanished. Shortly thereafter, Oswaldo Cruz carried out a similarly successful campaign in Rio de Janeiro.

In 1904 Gorgas tackled yellow fever and malaria mosquitoes in Panama. By 1905, he had again proved that mosquito control was an effective way to control disease, and in this case, his efforts were extended to include a significant malaria problem. However, Gorgas had to overcome heavy resistance from military and administrative leaders who refused to accept the need to eradicate mosquitoes but remained convinced that the disease bred in filth. Since Gorgas's campaign paid little attention to normal cleanup techniques, they found much about which to complain, though it soon was clear that the Canal Zone had become an area where Americans or Europeans could live and work. Gorgas's success was the principal factor in the completion and successful operation of the Panama Canal.

Walter Reed died following an operation for appendicitis in 1902. Before his death, however, he also contributed, with James Carroll, to the discovery of the causal agent for yellow fever. Reed was aware that the agent which caused hoof-and-mouth disease was small enough to pass the finest filter. In October 1901, he and Carroll subcutaneously injected three volunteers with 3 cubic centimeters of a diluted, filtered serum taken from an experimentally infected yellow fever patient. The three recipients were nonimmune. Two of the three developed yellow fever. Reed and Carroll presented a joint report concluding that yellow fever was caused by an ultramicroscopic agent which could pass a filter which would retain the smallest known bacteria. Though the agent was not identified, this was the first time that a filterable virus was proved to be the cause of a specific human disease. The identification and classification of yellow fever types, the development of an effective vaccine, and further contributions to the methods of modern virology all took place after World War I.

Worldwide Eradication and Control: 1913 to 1939 The opening of the Panama Canal raised the very serious question of how to prevent the spread of yellow fever to Asia. The Japanese government protested the canal's opening, and the Indian Medical Service carried out an investigation which led to recommendations for yellow fever quarantine stations in Panama, Hong Kong, and Singapore. The commission also originated a mosquito control campaign in India. The danger of yellow fever establishing itself as an epidemic disease in densely settled Asian countries raised justifiable fears, and American medical and sanitation experts, including William Gorgas, Dr. H. R. Carter, and Dr. J. H. White, testified before the commission that eradication was the best and most effective answer to the danger.

With successful programs already carried out in Cuba, Panama, and Brazil, a worldwide eradication program seemed feasible. In 1913, the foundations were laid with the newly created Rockefeller Yellow Fever Commission. The assumption was that yellow fever was vectored only by *A. aegypti* and that there were a very few places where the disease was endemic. If these centers could be destroyed, it followed that yellow fever would disappear. Monitoring stations were planned for east and central Brazil, the southern Caribbean, Mexico, and west Africa, though it was thought that the only endemic center of yellow fever in South America was at Guayaquil, Ecuador.

World War I halted the campaign, but once the war was over, the program was carried out vigorously. By July 1919, it seemed that it had been entirely successful, and the quarantines were lifted at Guayaquil in 1920. Other successful programs were carried out in Guatemala, Peru, Brazil, Honduras, El Salvador, Nicaragua, and Mexico. Findings in Africa, however, forced a change in approach. In 1925, the Rockefeller Foundation West African Yellow Fever Commission picked up the work which had been recommended earlier and which had barely been begun in 1920. It was this commission which found the previously unsuspected jungle variety of yellow fever and began to study the complexities of its epidemiology. By 1927, the African study team was able to prove that monkeys as well as humans were susceptible to yellow fever, and while they clung to *A. aegypti* as the only vector, they accepted the view that yellow fever could pass from humans to monkeys and vice versa. Subsequent studies showed that a variety of mosquitoes vectored yellow fever infection, and by the 1930s it had become quite clear that there was no practical way to carry out eradication against arboreal mosquitoes. The only protection for humans venturing into the jungles was immunization. By 1932, a method for cultivating yellow fever virus had been found, and five years later an effective vaccine using the 17D strain of yellow fever virus was available. A mass vaccination program begun in French West Africa in 1939 introduced what became the approved method of prevention in areas where mosquito eradication was not practical.

Yellow Fever Today Yellow fever outbreaks have continued to be major health problems since World War II. Unlike the historic variety, which ended in 1906, these epidemics affect underdeveloped, rural areas near jungle centers of infection. The association among yellow fever, trade, and cities no longer holds, thanks to mosquito control, a worldwide disease intelligence network, and vaccination. But in the nonurban areas, the problem has continued. For nine years, from 1948 to 1957, Central America, and especially Panama, suffered from jungle yellow fever. The disease has been most persistent in Africa, however, with localized outbreaks in 1958 and 1959 in the Congo region (Zaire) and in the Sudan. There were 5000 yellow fever deaths in Ethiopia between 1960 and 1962, and outbreaks were recorded in Senegal (1965), Mali, Nigeria, and Upper Volta in 1969 and in Angola and Nigeria in 1972. The World Health Organization reported an increase of cases for Africa and South America for 1974 and 1975, though the incidence declined in 1976.

In 1953, the World Health Organization approved a standardized vaccine based on the 17D strain, and it has since sponsored vaccination programs in endemic areas. The relatively low numbers of cases reported in localized outbreaks during the 1960s and 1970s suggest an improving situation, though the massive Ethiopian epidemic underlines the persistent danger which unattended yellow fever poses. A vaccination program for Trinidad in 1979 exemplifies the current direction for yellow fever control and emphasizes that only close international cooperation and effective public health administration can provide continuing protection in the modern world. Yellow fever cannot be eradicated, but it can be controlled.

ADDITIONAL READINGS: Sir Robert Boyce, *Mosquito or Man? The Conquest of the Tropical World*, 3d ed., London, 1910; Macfarlane Burnet and David O. White, *The Natural History of Infectious Diseases*, 4th ed., Cambridge, Mass., 1972; H. R. Carter, *Yellow Fever: An Epidemiological and Historical Study of Its Place of Origin*, Baltimore, 1921; John Duffy, *Epidemics in Colonial America*, Baton Rouge, 1953; John Duffy, *Sword of Pestilence*, Baton Rouge, 1965; Richard Fiennes, *Zoonoses of Primates*, Ithaca, New York, 1967; John M. Gibson, *Physician to the World: The Life of General William Gorgas*, Durham, N. C., 1950; August Hirsch, *Handbook of Geographical and Historical Pathology*, Charles Creighton (trans.), 3 vols., London, 1883; H. A. Kelly, *Walter Reed and Yellow Fever*, 3d ed., New York, 1923; William L. Poud, "This Is Yellow Fever," in D. H. Clarke and J. Casals, *Viral and Rickettsial Infections of Man*, 4th ed., Philadelphia, 1965; J. H. Powell, *Bring Out Your Dead: The Great Plague of Yellow Fever in Philadelphia in 1792*, Philadelphia 1949; George K. Strode (ed.), *Yellow Fever*, New York, 1951; Max Theiler, "Yellow Fever," in T. M. Rivers and Frank M. Horsefall, *Viral and Rickettsial Infections of Man*, 3d ed., Philadelphia, 1959; World Health Organization, *Yellow Fever Vaccination*, Geneva, 1956.

Index

Index